BASIC PHARMACOKINETICS

SECOND EDITION

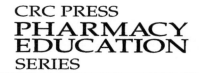

CRC PRESS
PHARMACY EDUCATION
SERIES

BASIC PHARMACOKINETICS

SECOND EDITION

MOHSEN A. HEDAYA
Kuwait University, Kuwait

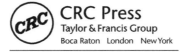

CRC Press
Taylor & Francis Group
Boca Raton   London   New York

CRC Press is an imprint of the
Taylor & Francis Group, an **informa** business

CRC Press
Taylor & Francis Group
6000 Broken Sound Parkway NW, Suite 300
Boca Raton, FL 33487-2742

© 2012 by Taylor & Francis Group, LLC
CRC Press is an imprint of Taylor & Francis Group, an Informa business

Printed by CPI on sustainably sourced paper
Version Date: 2011928

International Standard Book Number: 978-1-4398-5073-2 (Hardback)

Library of Congress Cataloging-in-Publication Data

Hedaya, Mohsen A.
  Basic pharmacokinetics / Mohsen A. Hedaya. -- 2nd ed.
    p. ; cm. -- (Pharmacy education series)
  Includes index.
  ISBN 978-1-4398-5073-2 (alk. paper)
  I. Title. II. Series: CRC Press pharmacy education series.
  [DNLM: 1. Pharmacokinetics. QV 38]

615'.7--dc23   2011037484

Visit the Taylor & Francis Web site at
http://www.taylorandfrancis.com

and the CRC Press Web site at
http://www.crcpress.com

To the memory of my parents, may God have mercy on their souls

Contents

Preface

Pharmacokinetics involves a quantitative description of the absorption, distribution, metabolism, and excretion of drugs, the processes that govern the drug concentration–time profile in the systemic circulation and different organs and tissues. This discipline has been of great interest to scientists involved in the discovery, development, and preclinical and clinical evaluation of drugs, and to practitioners involved in the clinical use of drugs. Because pharmacokinetics is a quantitative discipline, the different processes affecting drug pharmacokinetic behavior can be described mathematically, and the different pharmacokinetic parameters can be related by mathematical equations. Although mathematical relationships are important for understanding different pharmacokinetic concepts, those with limited mathematical background usually have difficulty in grasping these concepts when they are described solely utilizing mathematical relationships. This book utilizes different approaches for presenting pharmacokinetic principles to suit readers from different scientific backgrounds. The mathematical equations that describe the concepts are presented in addition to exploring the underlying concepts and how they are related to the physiological processes in the body. This is in addition to the graphical presentations and computer simulations that allow visualization of the interplay between the different pharmacokinetic parameters by observing how the change in the pharmacokinetic parameters of the drug is reflected on the drug concentration–time profile in the body. This book consists of two different parts: the textual printed materials and the highly interactive computer-based presentations and simulations included in the companion CD. This combination should provide a useful learning environment for readers to understand basic pharmacokinetic principles.

The contents of this book have been expanded and updated to provide an in-depth coverage of the different basic pharmacokinetic concepts that will satisfy the needs of pharmacokinetic learners in various biomedical fields. The book starts with a basic introduction to pharmacokinetics and its related fields and reviews the mathematical operations commonly used in pharmacokinetics in Chapters 1 and 2. Chapters 3 through 5 cover the basic pharmacokinetic concepts and discuss drug distribution and drug clearance and how these two processes affect the rate of drug elimination that is reflected on the drug profile in the body after a single intravenous dose. Chapters 6 through 11 cover the factors affecting drug absorption following extravascular drug administration, the rate and extent of drug absorption, and drug bioequivalence. The steady-state concept during constant rate intravenous infusion and during multiple drug administration is then introduced in Chapters 12 and 13. Chapters 14 through 18 cover additional basic concepts such as renal drug elimination, drug metabolism, multicompartment models, nonlinear pharmacokinetics, and drug administration by intermittent intravenous infusion. This is followed, in Chapters 19 through 22, by a discussion on additional specialized concepts that cover pharmacokinetic–pharmacodynamic modeling, noncompartment pharmacokinetic data analysis, clearance concept from the physiological point of view, and physiological modeling. Chapters 23 through 27 introduce the reader to the clinical applications of pharmacokinetics, including therapeutic drug monitoring, drug pharmacokinetics in special populations, pharmacokinetic drug–drug interactions, pharmacogenomics, and applications of computers in pharmacokinetics. The contents of the companion CD, which have been expanded, are described in Chapter 28. In addition to self-instructional tutorials, two sections that allow pharmacokinetic simulations and pharmacokinetic–pharmacodynamic simulations have been included in the CD. Suggested pharmacokinetic simulation exercises have also been included throughout this book to link the contents of the textual materials and the contents of the CD and to reinforce the different pharmacokinetic concepts. I have tried to include the basic pharmacokinetic information that can be useful for those interested in pharmacokinetics in all biomedical fields. I hope readers find this book beneficial.

For MATLAB® and Simulink® product information, please contact:
The MathWorks, Inc.
3 Apple Hill Drive
Natick, MA, 01760-2098 USA
Tel: 508-647-7000
Fax: 508-647-7001
E-mail: info@mathworks.com
Web: www.mathworks.com

Author

Mohsen A. Hedaya, PharmD, PhD, is a professor at the Faculty of Pharmacy, Tanta University, Tanta, Egypt, and is currently on leave to work at the Faculty of Pharmacy, Kuwait University, Kuwait City, Kuwait. He received his BSc in pharmacy (1980) from Tanta University, and his PharmD (1984) and PhD (1989) from the University of Minnesota, United States. After completing his graduate studies under the supervision of Professor Roland Sawchuk, Dr. Hedaya continued to work with him as a postdoctoral research fellow at the University of Minnesota. Dr. Hedaya was appointed in 1990 as a lecturer of clinical pharmacy, Faculty of Pharmacy, Tanta University. In 1993, he joined the College of Pharmacy, Washington State University, United States, as an assistant professor of pharmaceutical sciences. After returning to Egypt in 1999, he was promoted to the rank of associate professor and then to professor of clinical pharmacy. He served as the chair of the clinical pharmacy department and vice dean for academic affairs at the Faculty of Pharmacy, Tanta University.

Dr. Hedaya's interest is in pharmacokinetics. He has taught basic and advanced pharmacokinetic classes to professional pharmacy students and graduate students in Egypt, the United States, and Kuwait. His research interests include pharmacokinetic drug interactions, drug delivery to the brain, pharmacokinetic computer simulations, and bioequivalent study design and data analysis. This is in addition to his interest in the development and assessment of computer-aided instructional materials in the area of pharmacokinetics.

Dr. Hedaya is a member of numerous international scientific associations and has received several prestigious teaching and research achievement awards. He has to his credit extensive scientific publications in national and international journals and frequently gives presentations at national and international scientific meetings. The computer-based educational materials developed by Dr. Hedaya in the area of pharmacokinetics are currently being used by more than 300 educational, research, and industrial institutions around the world.

1 Introduction to Pharmacokinetics

OBJECTIVES

After completing this chapter you should be able to

- Define biopharmaceutics, pharmacokinetics, pharmacodynamics, clinical pharmacokinetics, population pharmacokinetics, and toxicokinetics
- Discuss the different applications of pharmacokinetics and its related disciplines in the biomedical fields
- State the major differences between linear and nonlinear pharmacokinetics
- Describe the general approaches utilized in pharmacokinetic modeling
- Describe the rationale for pharmacokinetic–pharmacodynamic modeling
- Discuss how pharmacokinetic simulations can be used to demonstrate the basic pharmacokinetic principles

1.1 INTRODUCTION

Pharmacokinetics and its related fields have numerous applications in all stages of the drug development process. This includes studying of the drug pharmacokinetic behavior in different animal species, which can be utilized to predict the absorption, distribution, metabolism, and elimination of the drug in humans. Also, designing and preparing a suitable dosage forms of the drug for use in the preclinical and clinical phases of drug development. Moreover, identification of the range of blood drug concentration, which is associated with the optimal therapeutic effect and minimum toxicity. In addition to determination of the factors that affect the drug pharmacokinetic behavior in the different patient populations, which is important for individualization of drug therapy to achieve the optimal therapeutic outcome in all patients. The following discussion covers a brief introduction to the general principles of the field of pharmacokinetics and its related fields.

1.2 GENERAL DEFINITIONS

1.2.1 BIOPHARMACEUTICS

It is the field of science that involves using the drug physicochemical properties and the biological and physiological characteristics of the human body to design and prepare dosage forms that provide the maximum drug availability at the site of drug action.

Scientists in this field usually investigate the chemical, physical, physiological, pathological, and formulation factors that can affect the drug absorption, distribution, and elimination processes. All these factors are important in determining the in vivo performance of drug products.

The physicochemical properties usually determine the drug stability, solubility, membrane permeability, and affinity to different tissue components. Knowledge of drug stability is important in determining the proper storage, transportation, and manufacturing conditions as well as the appropriate routes of drug administration. For example, heat-sensitive drugs should be stored and transported at low temperature, while moisture-sensitive drugs have to be formulated using dry procedures. Also, acid-labile drugs have to be administered orally in the form of enteric-coated dosage forms to avoid drug hydrolysis in the acidic gastric environment. Furthermore, the drug solubility is important in selecting the solvents used in liquid formulation and also in determining the rate and extent of drug absorption since the drug has to be in solution before crossing the biological membrane. Hydrophilic compounds are highly soluble in biological fluids but have poor membrane permeability, while lipophilic compounds have low solubility in biological fluids but have good membrane permeability. So a balance has to exist between the lipophilicity and the hydrophilicity of the compound for adequate diffusion across biological membranes.

The dosage form can be designed to control the rate of drug release, which influences the rate of drug availability at the site of absorption, and hence the rate of drug absorption. The rate of drug absorption and elimination are the major determinants of the time course of drug concentration in all parts of the body, including the site of action. This is an important factor in determining the time course of the drug effect. The physiological characteristics of the different systems of the body and the drug properties have been utilized to formulate specialized dosage forms such as inhalers and transdermal batches, which are more effective than conventional dosage forms under some specialized conditions.

1.2.2 PHARMACOKINETICS

It is the field of science that is aimed at studying the fate of any substance after administration to living organisms. Pharmacokinetics involves studying of the kinetics of drug absorption, distribution, metabolism, and excretion, including the rate and extent of each of these processes. These processes are the main determinants of the time course of the drug profile in all parts of the body, which determines the time course of the drug effect after drug administration. The pharmacokinetic principles are usually applied to drugs; however, the same principles can be applied to any compound such as nutrients, hormones, toxins, pollutants, pesticides, and others.

Studying the rate of drug absorption is important because faster drug absorption leads to faster onset of drug effect, an essential requirement for the treatment of acute conditions and in emergency situations. However, rapid drug absorption is not always desirable. During multiple drug administration for the management of chronic diseases such as hypertension or diabetes, the use of drug products with slow rate drug absorption may be more appropriate. This is because when the drug is absorbed slowly, small fluctuation in blood-drug concentrations is produced leading to steady therapeutic effect. Also, studying the extent of drug absorption is important because the amount of drug responsible for producing the drug effect is the amount of drug absorbed and reaches the systemic circulation.

Drug distribution to the site of action is necessary for the drug to produce its desired effect. The rate of drug distribution to its site of action affects the onset of effect and the extent of distribution determines the intensity of the effect. For example, an antibiotic that is very effective in the eradication of the bacteria causing meningitis in vitro can be useful in the treatment of meningitis only if it is distributed to the central nervous system in enough quantities to achieve concentrations above the minimum inhibitory concentration. Also, an anticancer drug is effective only when it is distributed in sufficient quantities into the cancerous tissues.

The rate of drug elimination is important in determining the required frequency of drug administration during multiple drug administration to compensate for the eliminated drug. Drugs that are eliminated faster require frequent drug adminis-tration to maintain effective drug concentrations all the time during multiple drug administration. Also, the function of the organs responsible for drug elimination determines the required dose adjustment in patients with eliminating organ dys-function. For example, patients with reduced kidney function require lower doses of drugs that are mainly eliminated by the kidney, while patients with liver dis-eases usually require lower doses of drugs that are mainly eliminated by hepatic metabolism.

The pharmacokinetic behavior of the drug is determined from the rate and extent of the drug absorption, distribution, metabolism, and excretion. Each of these pro-cesses is associated with one or more parameters that are dependent on the drug, the drug product, and the patient. These are the pharmacokinetic parameters that determine the rate and the extent of the different processes. The study of pharmaco-kinetics usually involves the determination of drug pharmacokinetic parameters and the factors that can affect these parameters to predict the pharmacokinetic behavior of drugs under different conditions.

1.2.3 CLINICAL PHARMACOKINETICS

It is the field of science that applies the basic pharmacokinetic principles in the clini-cal use of drugs. The goal is to select the optimal dosing regimen for each individual patient based on the patient's specific information and the drug pharmacokinetic characteristics. The optimal dosing regimen should produce the maximum thera-peutic effect and the minimum adverse effects. The patient's specific characteristics such as age, weight, gender, kidney function, liver function, diseases, hydration state, concomitant drug use, and any other factors that can affect the pharmacokinetics of the drug are used to predict the drug pharmacokinetics behavior in that particular patient. Also, the drug concentration-effect relationship, including the therapeutic and adverse drug effects, is used to determine the range of blood drug concentra-tions associated with the maximum therapeutic effect and minimum toxicity. The basic pharmacokinetic principles are used to predict an initial dosage regimen for the patient based on the patient's specific information and the drug pharmacokinetic behavior. When the patient starts receiving the drug, the blood drug concentrations measured at specific time points after drug administration can be utilized to determine the patient's specific pharmacokinetic parameters. A more accurate dosing regimen for the patient can be calculated based on the patient's specific pharmacokinetic parameters. If the patient continues taking the drug, the drug blood concentration together with the clinical monitoring parameters are used to modify the dosing regimen whenever it is necessary.

1.2.4 PHARMACODYNAMICS

It is the field of science that deals with the relationship between drug concentration at the site of action and the intensity of the drug effect. The existence of a relationship between drug concentration in the body and the resulting drug effect is obvious; however, this relationship can be different for different drugs. This is because different drugs produce their therapeutic effect by different mechanisms. The therapeutic effects of some drugs result from the direct effect of the drug on a receptor, an enzyme, or a specific tissue in the body. Drug concentration at the site of action of these directly acting drugs may or may not be at equilibrium with the drug in the systemic circulation. Also, some drugs produce their therapeutic effect by initiation of a sequence of events that leads to the therapeutic effect. In this case, the drug effect may appear after the drug is completely eliminated from the body such as in the case of oral anticoagulants and some anticancer drugs. Different techniques are used to describe the drug concentration-effect relationship in each of these conditions. Studying the drug concentration-effect relationship in the range of concentrations observed during the clinical use of drugs can be useful in determining the expected changes in the drug effect due to the change of the time course of the drug in the body. Also, characterization of the concentration-effect relationship is useful for designing more effective drug formulations and dosing regimens. Drug products can be formulated and dosing regimens can be designed to achieve drug blood concentration–time profiles that produce the optimal therapeutic effect.

1.2.5 POPULATION PHARMACOKINETICS

Population pharmacokinetics is the study of the sources of variability in the drug pharmacokinetic behavior among individuals who are the target patient population. The patients' specific characteristics that can alter the pharmacokinetic behavior of drugs are studied to identify measurable factors that can cause changes in the drug pharmacokinetic behavior. The effect of each factor on the drug pharmacokinetic behavior can be quantified and used in recommendations for the proper use of the drug in the different patient subpopulations. Also, the variability in the pharmacokinetic behavior of the drug that cannot be explained by specific patient characteristics and usually results from random variability is determined. The increase in the unexplained pharmacokinetic variability usually compromises the safety and efficacy profile of the drug. This is because in the presence of high variability in the drug pharmacokinetics, the same dose of the drug can produce a wide range of concentrations in different patients. These concentrations can be high (toxic), average (therapeutic), or low (subtherapeutic).

Pharmacokinetic studies are usually performed in a homogenous group of patients or volunteers with little variability. Intensive sampling is usually needed to determine the average pharmacokinetic behavior of the drug in the study population. However, population pharmacokinetic studies require the use of data obtained from a large number of patients with different characteristics and receiving the drug of interest under different conditions. The information used can be sparse or dense data obtained from patients taking the drug under different protocols. This is because the large number of patients allows the identifications of factors that can affect the drug pharmacokinetic variability.

1.2.6 TOXICOKINETICS

It is the field of science that applies the pharmacokinetic principles to determine the relationship between the systemic exposure of a compound and its toxicity. Toxicokinetic studies are pharmacokinetic studies performed to determine the absorption, distribution, metabolism, and elimination of the drug or chemicals during the toxicity studies. The information obtained from these toxicokinetic studies in laboratory animals is extrapolated to establish the drug concentration-toxic effect relationship in humans.

1.3 APPLICATION OF THE PHARMACOKINETIC PRINCIPLES IN THE BIOMEDICAL FIELDS

1.3.1 DESIGN AND EVALUATION OF DOSAGE FORMS

Drugs are usually administered as dosage forms by different routes of administration including intravenous, intramuscular, subcutaneous, oral, rectal, transdermal, inhalational, etc. The choice of the route of administration usually depends on the drug pharmacokinetic behavior after administration including the mechanism of drug absorption from the site of administration, the distribution of the drug to the site of action, and the elimination of the drug from the body. Performing pharmacokinetic studies is necessary to determine the appropriate route(s) of administrations and the suitable dosage form(s) that can achieve the optimum therapeutic outcome. Pharmacokinetic studies are also used to evaluate targeted drug delivery systems, which are prepared to preferentially deliver the drug to a specific target in the body such as a tumor.

1.3.2 EVALUATION OF DRUG FORMULATION

The pharmaceutical dosage forms usually contain the active pharmaceutical ingredient in addition to inactive additives that are used to give the dosage form its specific characteristics. The most important of these characteristics are the rate and the site of release of the active ingredient after administration, which usually influence the drug profile in the body. Pharmacokinetic studies are usually performed to evaluate the effect of different additives on the in vivo performance of the drug formulations for the same active drug from different manufacturers.

1.3.3 Pharmacological Testing

The drug concentration-effect relationship can be determined either in vitro using an appropriate experimental model or by performing the pharmacokinetic study and monitoring the pharmacologic effect of the drug simultaneously. Characterization of the drug concentration-effect relationship can help in predicting the therapeutic effect of the drug that should result from different drug concentration–time profiles. This is useful in determining the drug concentration–time profile that should achieve the desired drug effect.

1.3.4 Toxicological Testing

The pharmacokinetic studies are performed to determine the tissue exposure to the drug after a single-dose administration and also to determine tissue accumulation during multiple administration. The drug tissue exposure and accumulation are usually correlated with the observed toxicity of the drug. This information can be useful in determining the range of safe drug doses.

1.3.5 Evaluation of Organ Function

Determination of the pharmacokinetic parameters for specific markers can be used to evaluate the function of specific organs. For example, creatinine is an endogenous compound that is excreted completely by the kidney. Creatinine clearance, one of the pharmacokinetic parameters for creatinine, is used as a measure of the kidney function. Reduction of the kidney function leads to reduction in the creatinine clearance. Similarly, the clearance of markers that are completely eliminated by the liver can be used to evaluate the liver function.

1.3.6 Dosing Regimen Design

The relationships between drug concentration and the therapeutic and toxic effects are used to determine the range of drug concentrations required to achieve the maximum therapeutic effect with minimal toxicity. The pharmacokinetic principles are used to determine the drug pharmacokinetic parameters for specific patients. The patient's specific pharmacokinetic parameters are used to determine the appropriate dosage regimen (dose and dosing interval of a specific drug product) that should achieve drug concentrations in the desired range for each patient. This is known as individualization of drug therapy.

1.4 BLOOD DRUG CONCENTRATION–TIME PROFILE

The drug pharmacokinetic behavior in the body is characterized by obtaining serial blood samples after drug administration and measuring the drug concentrations in these samples to determine the blood drug concentration–time profile. This is because blood is the most readily accessible sampling site to monitor the change in drug concentration in the body with time. The blood drug concentration–time profile is dependent on the rate and extent of drug absorption, distribution, and elimination processes that occur simultaneously after drug administration. Drug absorption increases the amount and concentration of the drug in the body, drug elimination decreases the amount and concentration of the drug in the body, and drug distribution involves transfer of the drug between different parts of the body. The blood drug concentration–time profile can be described by mathematical equations that include the pharmacokinetic parameters for the drug absorption, distribution, and elimination processes.

The blood drug concentration–time profile is usually correlated with the drug effect-time profile with higher concentrations producing more intense effect. So modification of the blood concentration–time profile leads to modification of the therapeutic effect of the drug. The blood concentration–time profile can be affected by factors such as the dosing regimen, the dosage form, the patient characteristics, and the concomitant drugs used by the patient. All these factors can affect the drug absorption, distribution, and elimination, which in turn affect the drug therapeutic outcome.

Administration of the same dose of different drugs to the same patient usually produces different blood drug concentration–time profiles. This is because different drugs have different absorption, distribution, and elimination characteristics. Also, administration of the same dose of a drug to different patients usually produces different blood drug concentration–time profiles. This is because the same drug is usually absorbed, distributed, and eliminated differently in different patients. Figure 1.1 is an example of the blood concentration–time profile after administration of a single oral dose of a drug. The profile shows an initial increase in drug concentration representing the absorption phase followed by a decline in drug concentration representating the elimination phase. So it is important to investigate the factors that can affect the absorption, distribution, and elimination of drugs

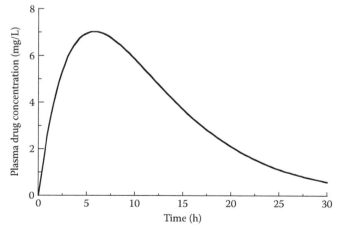

FIGURE 1.1 Representative example of the drug concentration–time profile after a single oral dose of a drug.

because these factors affect the blood drug concentration–time profile and hence the drug therapeutic outcomes.

1.5 LINEAR AND NONLINEAR PHARMACOKINETICS

1.5.1 LINEAR PHARMACOKINETICS

Linear pharmacokinetics is also known as dose-independent and concentration-independent pharmacokinetics because the pharmacokinetic parameters such as the half-life, total body clearance, and volume of distribution are constant and do not change with the change in drug concentration or the drug amount in the body. When a drug follows linear pharmacokinetics, the drug absorption, distribution, and elimination processes that affect the blood drug concentration–time profile follow first-order kinetics. Also, administration of increasing doses of the drug results in blood drug concentration–time profiles, which are proportional to the administered doses after single and multiple drug administration.

1.5.2 NONLINEAR PHARMACOKINETICS

Nonlinear pharmacokinetics is also known as dose-dependent and concentration-dependent pharmacokinetics because the pharmacokinetic parameters are dependent on the drug concentration or the drug amount in the body. At least one of the absorption, distribution, and elimination processes, which affect the blood drug concentration–time profile, is saturable and does not follow first-order kinetics. The change in drug dose results in disproportional change in the blood drug concentration–time profile after single- and multiple-dose administrations. Table 1.1 summarizes the differences between linear and nonlinear pharmacokinetics.

TABLE 1.1
Differences between Linear and Nonlinear Pharmacokinetics

Linear Pharmacokinetics	Nonlinear Pharmacokinetics
Also known as dose-independent or concentration-independent pharmacokinetics	Also known as dose-dependent or concentration-dependent pharmacokinetics
The absorption, distribution, and elimination of the drug follow first-order kinetics	At least one of the pharmacokinetic processes (absorption, distribution, or elimination) is saturable
All the pharmacokinetic parameters such as the half-life, total body clearance, and volume of distribution are constant and do not depend on the drug concentration	One or more of the pharmacokinetic parameters such as the half-life, total body clearance, or volume of distribution are concentration dependent
The change in drug dose results in proportional change in the drug concentration	The change in drug dose results in more than proportional or less than proportional change in the drug concentration

1.6 PHARMACOKINETIC MODELING

Pharmacokinetic modeling involves the development of a model that can describe the pharmacokinetic behavior of the drug in the body with an acceptable degree of accuracy. The different components of the model are related by mathematical expressions, which collectively can describe the pharmacokinetic behavior of the drug. These mathematical expressions include the pharmacokinetic parameters that govern the drug absorption, distribution, and elimination processes, in addition to constants such as the dose and the frequency of drug administration. Some pharmacokinetic models include physiological and biochemical parameters. The choice of the modeling strategy is usually based on the objective of the modeling process. Pharmacokinetic modeling can be performed to estimate the pharmacokinetic parameters that can be used to predict the drug pharmacokinetic behavior under certain conditions, to evaluate the factors affecting the drug pharmacokinetic behavior, to assess the variability in the drug pharmacokinetic behavior, to determine specific organ exposure to the drug, or to utilize the pharmacokinetic information to improve the drug therapeutic outcome, etc. When selecting the pharmacokinetic model, one has to make sure that all the model assumptions are fulfilled, and the information required to determine the model parameters can be obtained. Pharmacokinetic studies are usually designed to obtain the necessary information including drug concentration in blood, tissues, or other body fluids at different time points. The obtained data are fitted to the model equations to estimate the pharmacokinetic model parameters that can be used to fulfill the objective of the modeling process. The common modeling strategies used in pharmacokinetics are described below.

1.6.1 COMPARTMENTAL MODELING

In compartmental modeling, the body is presented by one or more compartments depending on the rate of drug distribution to the different parts of the body. When the drug is rapidly distributed to all parts of the body, the body is considered behaving as one compartment, and the drug follows the one-compartment model, while when the drug distribution to some organs is faster than its distribution to other organs, the body behaves as two different compartments, and the drug follows the two-compartment model. The model usually includes parameters that describe drug absorption, distribution between the compartments, and elimination from one or more of the compartments. These models differ in the number of compartments and the arrangement of the compartments relative to each other as shown in Figure 1.2. Compartmental modeling is data-based modeling, because the obtained blood drug concentration–time data after drug administration are used to choose the best pharmacokinetic model that can describe the drug pharmacokinetic behavior.

1.6.2 PHYSIOLOGICAL MODELING

In physiological modeling, the body is divided into a series of organs or tissue spaces and the model describes the uptake and disposition of the drug in each of these organs. The model is usually constructed to include organs and tissues for drug site of action, drug toxicity, drug elimination, and any other organ of interest. Information about

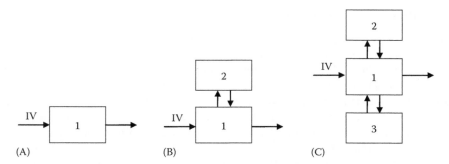

FIGURE 1.2 Representative examples of compartmental pharmacokinetic models: (A) one-compartment model, (B) two-compartment model, and (C) three-compartment model.

the organ size, organ blood flow, drug uptake to different organs, and drug elimination from different organs is used to build the model. An example of a physiological model is presented in Figure 1.3. The model parameters are modified until the model-predicted drug concentration in the blood and tissues is in agreement with the obtained experimental information. Then the model can be used to predict the drug pharmacokinetic behavior after administration of different doses by different routes of administration. The physiological models can be used in toxicological testing to determine specific organ exposure to the drug. This modeling technique is useful in predicting the differences in the drug pharmacokinetic behavior in different species including humans by using the size, the blood flow, and the elimination parameters for the organs of the different species. Also, these models can be used to predict the change in drug pharmacokinetic behavior due to physiological and pathological changes.

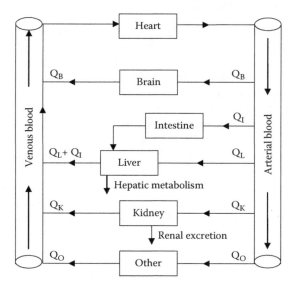

FIGURE 1.3 Representing example of a physiologically based pharmacokinetic model that includes the heart, brain, intestine, liver, kidney, and other tissues. The term Q represents the blood flow and the subscript indicates the organ.

1.6.3 Noncompartmental Approach

Pharmacokinetic models are usually associated with specific assumptions that cannot be confirmed sometimes. When the objective of the pharmacokinetic study can be achieved without making any model assumption, the noncompartmental (model independent) approach can be used. This approach uses some pharmacokinetic parameters that can be determined without making any assumption of a model to describe the drug disposition. For example, the maximum blood drug concentration, the time of the maximum blood drug concentration, and the area under the plasma concentration–time curve can be determined without making any assumption of a specific model. These three parameters are used to compare the rate and extent of drug absorption after administration of two different drug products for the same active drug in bioequivalence studies.

1.7 PHARMACOKINETIC–PHARMACODYNAMIC MODELING

The main emphasis of pharmacokinetics is to study the absorption, distribution, and elimination of drugs, the processes that affect the drug concentration–time profile in the body. However, the interest usually is to relate the drug concentration–time profile of the drug to the drug effect-time profile. The drug in the systemic circulation is distributed to all parts of the body, including the site of action, and equilibrium is established between the drug in blood and the drug at the site of action. The drug at the site of action usually produces the drug effect as presented in Figure 1.4.

The intensity of the drug therapeutic effect is dependent on the drug concentration at the site of action. Several pharmacodynamic models have been developed to describe the relationship between the drug concentration at the site of action and the resulting effect. The pharmacokinetic principles are used to describe the relationship between the dosing regimen and the drug concentration–time profile at the site of action, while the pharmacodynamic principles are used to describe the relationship between the drug concentration at the site of action and the resulting drug effect. Combining both principles, the relationship between the drug dosing regimens and the resulting drug effect can be described. This allows the selection of the dosing regimen that should achieve the desired therapeutic effect with minimum adverse effects. More complicated relationships can be developed to relate the drug concentration–time profile to the drug effect for indirectly acting drugs, or when the drug effect results from a long sequence of events.

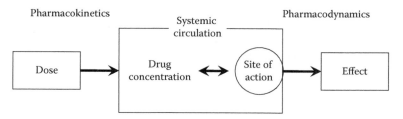

FIGURE 1.4 Schematic presentation of the relationship between pharmacokinetics and pharmacodynamics.

1.8   PHARMACOKINETIC SIMULATIONS

Simulation of the pharmacokinetic behavior of the drug under different conditions can be used in teaching, training, and research. The idea of the pharmacokinetic simulation is to change one or more of the pharmacokinetic parameters and examine how the change in this particular parameter affects the drug pharmacokinetic behavior. This can be very useful in visualizing the effect of different pharmacokinetic parameters on the drug concentration–time profile and understanding the interplay between the different pharmacokinetic parameters.

For example, the drug plasma concentration–time profile after a single oral dose of the drug can be described by the following equation:

$$Cp = \frac{FDk_a}{Vd(k_a - k)}(e^{-kt} - e^{-k_a t}) \qquad (1.1)$$

where
   Cp is the drug plasma concentration at any time t
   D is the dose of the drug
   F is the drug bioavailability that is a measure of the extent of drug absorption
   k_a is the absorption rate constant
   k is the elimination rate constant
   Vd is the volume of distribution

The plasma drug concentration can be calculated at different time points by substituting the value for each of the pharmacokinetic parameters and using different values for time. The calculated plasma concentrations at the different time points are plotted to simulate the drug concentration–time profile. The values of the parameters included in Equation 1.1 can be changed one parameter at a time, and the simulation is repeated to visualize the effect of changing that particular parameter on the drug concentration–time profile. For example, the dose can be changed to simulate the effect of changing the dose on the drug concentration–time profile. Also, the bioavailability can be changed to simulate the effect of using different drug products with a different extent of absorption on the drug concentration–time profile. Furthermore, the absorption rate constant can be changed to simulate the effect of using different drug products with different rates of absorption on the drug concentration–time profile. Moreover, the elimination rate constant can be changed to simulate the drug concentration–time profile after administration of the drug to patients who eliminate the drug at different rates. Additionally, the volume of distribution can be changed to simulate the drug concentration–time profile after administration of the drug to patients with different body weight.

2 Review of Ma... Fundamentals

OBJECTIVES

After completing this chapter you should be able to

- State the basic mathematical operations commonly used in pharmacokinetics
- Discuss the basic rules for mathematical operations for exponents and logarithms
- Explain the rationale for curve fitting and its application in pharmacokinetics
- Plot the experimental data on the Cartesian and the semilog scales and estimation of the slope and y-intercept graphically
- Discuss the basic applications of calculus in pharmacokinetics

2.1 INTRODUCTION

Pharmacokinetics is the discipline of science that is concerned with the study of the rate and extent of drug absorption, distribution, metabolism, and excretion. Understanding the characteristics and the mechanisms of these processes allows writing mathematical expressions that describe the drug profile in the body. Characterization of the drug concentration–time profile is important because it is usually related to the time course of the therapeutic effect of the drugs. Understanding the basic mathematic principles that are used frequently in pharmacokinetics can be very useful in grasping the basic pharmacokinetic concepts. This can help in understanding how the mathematical expressions that describe the different pharmacokinetic processes are derived. Also, comprehending the basic mathematical principles can assist in understanding the interplay between the different pharmacokinetic parameters. Furthermore, knowing the basic mathematical principles allows the correct utilization of the pharmacokinetic equations to predict the drug pharmacokinetic behavior in the body. This is in addition to application of the proper pharmacokinetic data analysis techniques in research and clinical practice. This chapter reviews the basic mathematical principles that are commonly used in pharmacokinetics such as exponents, logarithms, graphs, and curve fitting.

NTS

on is a mathematical operation that involves two numbers, the base "a" ,ponent "n", and it is usually written as a^n. It is usually read as "a" raised power.

he rules of exponents:

- When the exponent is a positive whole integer: Exponentiation is the repeated multiplication of the base, n times.
  Example: $a^4 = a \times a \times a \times a$
  e.g., $2^4 = 2 \times 2 \times 2 \times 2 = 16$
- When the exponent is one: Any number raised to the power 1 is the same number.
  Example: $a^1 = a$
  e.g., $5^1 = 5$
- When the exponent is zero: Any number raised to the power 0 is equal to 1.
  Example: $a^0 = 1$
  e.g., $4^0 = 1$
- When the exponent is a negative number: Exponentiation is the repeated division of 1 by the base, n times.
  Example: $a^{-3} = 1/a^3$
  e.g., $3^{-3} = 1/3^3 = 1/27$
- One raised to any power: It is equal to 1.
  Example: $1^n = 1$
  e.g., $1^{12} = 1$
- Zero raised to any power: It is equal to 0.
  Example: $0^n = 0$
  e.g., $0^7 = 0$
- Minus one raised to any power: It is equal to −1 if n is an odd number and is equal to 1 if n is an even number.
  Example: $-1^n = 1$ if n is even number
  $\qquad -1^n = -1$ if n is odd number
  e.g., $-1^8 = 1$
  $\qquad -1^5 = -1$
- Multiplication of two numbers both having the same base but raised to different exponents: It is equal to the base raised to the sum of both exponents.
  Example: $a^n \times a^m = a^{n+m}$
  e.g., $2^3 \times 2^4 = 2^7$
- Division of two numbers both having the same base raised to different exponents: It is equal to the base raised to the difference between the two exponents.
  Example: $a^n/a^m = a^{n-m}$
  e.g., $2^5/2^3 = 2^{5-3} = 2^2$
- A number consists of a base and an exponent raised to an exponent: It is equal to the base raised to the product of both exponents.
  Example: $(a^n)^m = a^{n \times m}$
  e.g., $(3^2)^3 = 3^6$

- The nth root of a number is equal to the number raised to a power equal to $1/n$.
  Example: $\sqrt[y]{a} = a^{1/y}$
  e.g., $\sqrt[3]{a} = a^{1/3}$

2.3 LOGARITHMS

The logarithm of a positive real number (N) to a given base is the power to which the logarithm base should be raised in order to get the number N. There are two bases that are commonly used. The first base is for the common logarithm function (log) and it is equal to 10, and the second is for the natural logarithmic (ln) function and it is equal to e (e = 2.718282).

If $A = b^x$, then $\log_b A = x$

For example: $1000 = 10^3$ then $\log_{10} 1000 = 3$
                $1 = 10^0$ then $\log_{10} 1 = 0$
                $0.01 = 10^{-2}$ then $\log_{10} 0.01 = -2$

Taking the antilogarithm of a number is equal to 10 raised to a power equal to this number. So, in the aforementioned example, the anti-logarithm of 3 is equal to 10^3 which is equal to 1000. It is common to convert mathematical expressions that have the natural logarithm (base = e) to the common logarithmic function (base = 10). In this case

$$2.303 \log N = \ln N$$

The logarithm has no units. So, if the plasma drug concentration after drug administration is 100 mg/L, the logarithm of the drug plasma concentration after drug administration is equal to 2.

Rules of Logarithm:

- The logarithm of two multiplied numbers is the sum of the logarithm of each number.
  Example: $\log N \times M = \log N + \log M$
- The logarithm of two divided numbers is the difference of the logarithm of each number.
  Example: $\log N/M = \log N - \log M$
- The logarithm of a number raised to a power is equal to the power multiplied by the logarithm of the number.
  Example: $\log N^m = m \log N$
- The logarithm of a number is equal to the negative value of the logarithm of the reciprocal of this number.
  Example: $\log N = -\log 1/N$
  $\log N/M = -\log M/N$

- The logarithm of 10 raised to any power is equal to this power.
  Example: $\log 10^m = m$
- The natural logarithm of e raised to any power is equal to this power.
  Example: $\ln e^m = m$

2.4 GRAPHS

Graphs are usually used to present the relationship between two or more variables. In pharmacokinetics, graphs are commonly utilized to represent the drug concentration in the systemic circulation or drug pharmacological effect as a function of time after drug administration. In the two-dimensional graphs that are commonly used in pharmacokinetics, the drug concentration or drug effect (the dependent variable) is plotted on the y-axis, while time (the independent variable) is plotted on the x-axis. There are two types of scales that are commonly utilized in pharmacokinetics, the Cartesian scale and the semilog scale.

2.4.1 CARTESIAN SCALE

In the Cartesian scale, both the y-axis and the x-axis are linear. Each point can be plotted on the Cartesian scale by a pair of numerical coordinates that determine the perpendicular distance of the point from the x-axis and the y-axis. Although negative or positive values can be used for the coordinates in the Cartesian scale, only positive coordinate values are used to present plasma concentration versus time profile. Figure 2.1A is an example of the Cartesian scale. The scale used on the x- and y-axes is determined from the range of values to be plotted for the independent and dependent variables, respectively. Plotting the available data on the largest possible portion of the graph paper

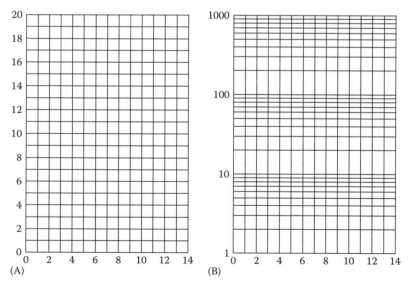

FIGURE 2.1   Example of (A) the Cartesian scale and (B) the semilog scale.

improves the data presentation and makes it easier to describe the graph characteristics. While squeezing the data on a small portion of the graph paper may result in missing important information from the graph and decreases the plotting accuracy.

2.4.2   Semilog Scale

The semilog scale has a logarithmic scale on the y-axis and a linear scale on the x-axis, as in Figure 2.1B. This type of graph is useful in plotting values that are changing exponentially. On the semilog graph the spacing of the scale on the y-axis is proportional to the logarithm of the number, not the number itself. Plotting data on the semilog scale is equivalent of converting the dependent variable values to their log values, and plotting the data on the linear scale. The semilog graph paper consists of repeated units called cycles. Each of these cycles covers a single $\log_{10}$ unit, or 10-fold increase in number. The semilog graph paper is available in one, two, three, or more cycles per sheet. Figure 2.1B represents a three-cycle semilog scale. The choice of the number of cycles depends on the range of the values to be plotted.

To plot data on the semilog scale, the first step is to determine the range of values for both the dependent and independent variables. The values for the dependent variable are arranging in the ascending or descending order and the range of values is used to determine the number of cycles needed to plot the data. Using the graph paper with the correct number of cycles is important for good data presentation. Plotting data that covers three $\log_{10}$ units (three orders of magnitudes) on a two-cycle graph paper leads to missing some of the data points, and plotting data that covers one $\log_{10}$ unit (one order of magnitudes) on a five-cycle graph paper squeezes the plot on small part of the graph paper and decreases plotting accuracy.

Example

Plot the following drug concentration–time data on the semilog scale:

Time (h)	Drug Concentration (ng/mL)
1	500
3	303
6	143
10	53
14	19
18	7.1
24	1.6

Answer

- The scale on the x-axis is chosen to make the time points cover the largest portion of the x-axis.
- The drug concentration values are used to determine the number of cycles needed.

500	303	143	53	19	7.1	1.6

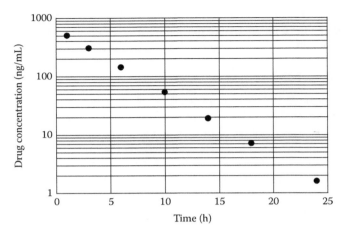

FIGURE 2.2   Data plotted on the semilog scale.

Three cycles are needed to plot these values.

First cycle covers	1–10
Second cycle covers	10–100
Third cycle covers	100–1000

Figure 2.2 represents the drug concentration–time data plotted on a three-cycle graph paper.

2.5   CURVE FITTING

Curve fitting is a mathematical procedure that involves finding the specific equation that describes the relationship between a set of variables. The first step in the curve fitting procedures is to find the general form of the equation that can describe the relationship between the variables of interest, based on some theoretical, biological, or physiological background information. For example, if the theoretical background information suggests the existence of linear relationship between the two variables such as in case of zero-order processes, the data are fitted to the straight-line equation. While if the evidences suggest that exponential relationship exists between the two variables such as in first-order processes, the data are fitted to the equation that describes this exponential relationship, or the log-transformed dependent variable values and time are fitted to the straight-line equation. While when the relationship between the variables is expected to be related by hyperbolic function such as in case of the relationship between the enzymatic reaction rate and substrate concentration, the data are fitted to the equation that describes this hyperbolic relationship. Characterization of the model that describes the relationship between variables can be achieved by fitting the data to the different equations for different models. The equation that provides the best fit for the data is for the best model that can describe the relationship between the variables.

Once the general form of the equation is determined and the experimental data are generated, the next step is to determine the specific mathematical equation that quantitatively relates the variables together. This is usually achieved by estimation of the equation parameters using the curve fitting procedures. For example, determination of the specific equation that describes the linear relationship between two variables is achieved by calculation of the slope and the y-intercept for this linear relationship. Determination of the specific equation that can relate the variables is important because this equation can be used to predict the behavior of the variables under different conditions. Curve fitting can be as simple as finding the straight-line equation that describes the linear relationship between two variables which can be performed using a simple scientific calculator. However, curve fitting can be a complex procedure such as in case of fitting experimental data to a multi-exponential equation that describes the pharmacokinetic behavior of drugs, a procedure which usually requires powerful computers and specialized data analysis software.

2.5.1 LINEAR REGRESSION ANALYSIS

When a dependent variable is related to an independent variable by a linear relationship, this means that this relationship can be described by a straight-line equation (i.e., $y = a + bx$).

The slope and y-intercept are usually estimated experimentally by taking several measures for the dependent variable at different values of the independent variable and then performing the simple linear regression. Each experimental data point has some error with varying magnitude associated with it. So the data points do not have to fall exactly on the straight line. So it is important to evaluate the appropriateness of the estimated line in describing the data.

2.5.1.1 Graphical Determination of the Best Line

The line of best fit can be determined graphically by drawing the line that makes all the experimentally obtained data points as close as possible to the line, and all points fall randomly around the line. Graphical determination of the best line is not accurate because it is subjective since different individuals may draw different lines for the same set of data. When the line is determined graphically, the y-intercept is determined by back extrapolating the line to the y-axis. The slope of the line is $\Delta y / \Delta x$, which can be determined by taking two different points on the line and these two points are used to calculate the slope as in Figure 2.3. The slope of the line can be determined as in Equation 2.1 for the Cartesian scale, and as in Equation 2.2 for the semilog scale.

$$\text{Slope} = \frac{y_2 - y_1}{x_2 - x_1} \tag{2.1}$$

$$\text{Slope} = \frac{\log y_2 - \log y_1}{x_2 - x_1} \tag{2.2}$$

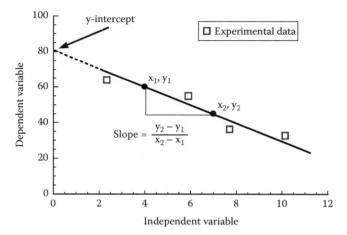

FIGURE 2.3 Estimation of the y-intercept and the slope of a straight line graphically.

The slope of the best line should not be calculated by substituting the values of two of the experimental data points in Equation 2.1 or 2.2. This is because when calculating the slope from two data points only, it is assumed that these two data points do not have any error associated with them, and all the other data points are ignored. In this case, the calculated slope can be different depending on which two points were used in the calculation.

2.5.1.2 Least Squares Method

The least squares method is a statistical approach used to calculate the best slope and y-intercept values for the best line that can describe the experimental data. The idea of the linear regression is to choose the line which can minimize the sum

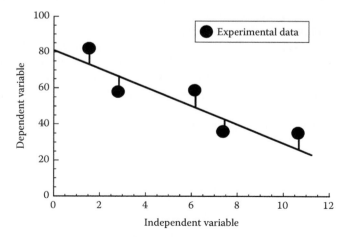

FIGURE 2.4 Least squares method determines the line that can minimize the sum of the squared distance between the experimental data and the line.

of the squared perpendicular distances between each experimental data point and the line as in Figure 2.4. This approach is known as the least squares approach. The calculated slope and y-intercept using the linear regression analysis will be the same for a given set of data. The linear relationship between the two variables can be evaluated by calculating some parameters as the correlation coefficient, r, and the coefficient of determination, R^2, which determine how much of the variability in the dependent variable results from the change in the independent variable. Values for r and R^2 that are close to unity indicate strong linear relationship between the two variables. Most of the scientific calculators can perform the linear regression analysis.

2.6 CALCULUS

Calculus is a branch in mathematics that focuses on limits, functions, derivatives, integrals, and finite series. If geometry is the study of shapes, and algebra is the study of operations, calculus is considered the study of change. It has two major branches, which are differential calculus and integral calculus.

2.6.1 DIFFERENTIAL CALCULUS

Differential calculus is the study of the derivative of a function. Loosely speaking, a derivative can be thought of as how much one quantity is changing in response to changes in some other quantity. For example, the derivative of the amount of the drug in the body after an IV dose with respect to time is the instantaneous rate at which the drug is eliminated over a very short period of time.

2.6.2 INTEGRAL CALCULUS

Generally speaking, integral calculus is the reverse of differential calculus. It is used to sum all the small infinitesimally small units of changes into the whole value of the variable over the integration limits. For example, summation of all the changes in the plasma drug concentration after drug administration gives the area under the plasma concentration–time curve.

2.6.3 PHARMACOKINETIC APPLICATIONS

The drug absorption, distributions, metabolism, and excretion processes cause changes in the drug concentration and drug amount in the different parts of the body. The main objective of most of the pharmacokinetic studies is to describe how the plasma drug concentrations change with time after drug administration. The basic calculus principles are very useful in driving mathematical expressions that can describe the plasma drug concentration as a function of time. This is usually achieved first by writing the differential equation that describes the rate of change in the plasma drug concentration at an infinitesimal period of time, which should include all the variables that can affect the plasma drug concentration. This differential equation describes the rate of change in the plasma drug concentration at any time after drug concentration. However, the differential equation cannot be used to determine the drug concentration at a specific time. Integrating (solving) this differential equation gives an equation that describes the drug concentration as a function of time. Substituting for a specific value for time in the integrated equation gives the drug plasma concentration at that particular time.

PRACTICE PROBLEMS

2.1 Calculate the values of each of the following:
   a. $7^3 \times 7^{-1}$
   b. $12^5/12^3$
   c. -1^9
   d. $\log 1000 - \log 10$
   e. $\log (10{,}000/100)$
   f. $\log 100^3$

2.2 The linear relationship that describes the change in the drug amount (A) in mg, as a function of time (t) in h, can be described by the following equation: $A = 120\,\text{mg} - 2\,(\text{mg/h})\,t$.
   a. Calculate the amount of the drug remaining after 10 h.
   b. What is the time required for the drug amount to decrease to zero?

2.3 In an experiment to study the chemical decomposition, a drug solution was prepared and an aliquot of the drug solution was obtained at different time points. The drug concentrations in the samples and the results were as follows:

Time (h)	Drug Concentration (mg/L)
2	274
6	260
12	246
24	202
36	180
48	140

   a. Draw the drug concentration against time on the Cartesian scale and graphically estimate the slope and y-intercept.
   b. Write the equation that describes the change in drug concentration with time.

3 Drug Pharmacokinetics Following a Single IV Bolus Administration
Drug Distribution

OBJECTIVES

After completing this chapter, you should be able to

- Describe the difference between the perfusion rate-limited and permeability-limited distribution
- Discuss the influence of the rate of drug distribution on the drug pharmacokinetic behavior
- Describe the principles of the commonly used methods for the determination of the plasma protein binding
- Define the volume of distribution and describe the relationship between the amount of drug in the body, plasma drug concentration, and volume of distribution
- Analyze the effect of changing plasma protein binding and tissue binding on the drug distribution characteristics and Vd
- Estimate the Vd after a single IV bolus dose
- Calculate the appropriate IV dose required to achieve a specific drug concentration

3.1 INTRODUCTION

Intravenous (IV) bolus administration of the drug involves direct introduction of the drug into the systemic circulation over a very short period of time. In the systemic circulation, drugs can bind to blood constituents mainly plasma proteins and cellular components leaving a fraction of the drug unbound. The drug is distributed with the blood circulation to all parts of the body including the site(s) of action and the eliminating and noneliminating organs. The free, unbound drug can diffuse across the capillary membrane to reach the tissue interstitial space. Drug passage across the capillary membrane can be transcellular by passive diffusion, paracellular through the junction between the capillary endothelial cells, or through a specialized transport protein. Once in the tissue interstitial space, the drug can cross the cellular membrane and distribute inside the cell.

3.2 DRUG DISTRIBUTION PROCESS

Different drugs have different distribution characteristics in the body. This includes differences in the rate of distribution and the extent of distribution to different parts of the body. The drug distribution process is affected by factors related to the tissues such as tissue blood perfusion, the presence or absence of anatomical barriers, the tissue composition, and the physiological function of the tissue. Drug-related factors that can affect the drug distribution include the physicochemical properties of the drug, drug binding to plasma proteins, and drug binding to tissue components. The following discussion will consider the distribution of the drug to noneliminating organs or tissues.

3.2.1 RATE OF DRUG DISTRIBUTION

Drugs are distributed to all parts of the body with the blood circulation. If the capillary membrane and the cellular membrane do not act as anatomical barriers to the drug tissue distribution, the tissue blood perfusion becomes the important factor in determining the rate of drug distribution to that tissue. In this case, the rate determining step in the drug distribution process is the rate of drug delivery to the tissue via the blood circulation. This is called perfusion rate-limited distribution. Consequently, the rate of drug distribution will be faster in highly perfused tissues such as the lung, liver, and kidney compared to the poorly perfused tissues such as fat. Therefore, the equilibrium between the drug in blood and the drug in highly perfused tissues is achieved faster than the equilibrium between the drug in blood and the poorly perfused tissues.

The biological membranes in some organs have special characteristics that make the membrane act as a barrier to protect the organ from the distribution of many substances in the blood. An example of these barriers is the blood brain barrier (BBB) that is characterized by the presence of tight junctions between the endothelial cells of the blood capillaries supplying the blood to the brain. The BBB prevents the distribution of many polar compounds in the blood to the brain tissues. Only lipophilic compounds can distribute across the BBB by passive diffusion. In this case, the distribution of polar compounds across these biological barriers is slow and the rate determining step for the distribution process is the rate of drug diffusion across the barrier. This is called permeability-limited distribution. Consequently, nonpolar drugs usually distribute to the tissues faster than polar drugs. Hence, the equilibrium between the drug in the blood and the drug in tissues is achieved faster for nonpolar drugs compared to the more polar drugs.

3.2.2 EXTENT OF DRUG DISTRIBUTION

The physicochemical properties of the drug and the tissue characteristics are important in determining the extent of drug distribution to different tissues and organs. The extent of drug distribution to a particular tissue can be expressed as the tissue distribution coefficient (Kp_T), which is the ratio of the total (free + bound) drug concentration in the tissue (C_T) to the total (free + bound) blood drug concentration (C_B) when the drug in tissues and in blood is at equilibrium, as in Equation 3.1:

$$Kp_T = \frac{C_T}{C_B} \tag{3.1}$$

Drugs with high Kp_T in a certain tissue are extensively distributed to that tissue and C_T is higher than C_B, that is, high tissue to blood total drug concentration ratio. Since a drug can have different distribution characteristics in various tissues, a drug can have different Kp_T for various tissues. The drug Kp_T reflects the total drug concentration ratio at equilibrium, but does not indicate how much drug is distributed into a particular tissue. To determine the amount of the drug distributed to a particular tissue (Amount$_T$), one has to consider the volume of the tissue (V_T) in addition to C_T, C_B, and Kp_T as in Equation 3.2:

$$Amount_T = C_T V_T = Kp_T C_B V_T \tag{3.2}$$

The drug molecular weight, lipid solubility, and ionization in physiological pH are key factors in determining the extent of drug tissue distribution. Drugs with low molecular weight can diffuse across biological membranes and distribute to the tissues better than high molecular weight drugs. The lipophilicity of drugs measured as the octanol/water partition coefficient is also important, with lipophilic drugs diffusing across the lipoidal biological membranes and tissue anatomical barriers better than hydrophilic drugs. The degree of drug ionization in the physiological pH also affects the drug tissue distribution since the unionized drug molecules are more lipophilic than the ionized drug molecules.

The tissue characteristics and the whole body composition affect the extent of drug distribution to different tissues and also the fraction of the drug amount in the body that is distributed to the different tissues. Lipophilic drugs, for example, can distribute to fat-rich tissues much more than hydrophilic drugs. Consider administration of the same dose of a lipophilic drug to two different patients who have the same body weight but one of them is obese and the other is slim. These two individuals have different body composition with the body mass of obese patient having larger percentage of fat compared to the slim patient. A larger fraction of the administered dose of the lipophilic drug is distributed to the fat tissues in the obese individual leaving a smaller fraction of the dose for the other nonfat tissues, while in the slim individual, a larger fraction of the administered dose is distributed to the nonfat tissues. Also, alkaline drugs that are predominantly unionized in physiological pH can cross the biological membranes better than ionized drugs and can be distributed to the breast tissues. Once distributed into the breast tissues, alkaline drugs are ionized in the relatively acidic pH of the breast tissues and entrapped until they are excreted in the breast milk. This is because the ionized molecules cannot cross the membrane back to the blood. The drug binding in blood and tissues can also affect the drug distribution characteristics between the blood and tissues. Drugs that are highly bound to blood constituents such as plasma proteins and cellular components with little binding to tissue constituents usually have low Kp_T, while drugs that have high binding affinity to some specific cellular components in tissues and little binding in blood will be distributed to higher extent in tissues and usually have high Kp_T.

3.2.3 EQUILIBRIUM BETWEEN THE DRUG IN BLOOD AND TISSUES

Drug distribution to different parts of the body leads to the establishment of equilibrium between the drug in blood and in tissues with the concentration ratio depending on the drug properties and the tissue characteristics. The distribution of the drug to organs that can eliminate the drug such as the liver and kidney results in excretion of part of the drug in the blood. The decrease in the drug amount and hence drug concentration in blood due to drug elimination leads to disruption of the drug equilibrium between the tissues and blood. A fraction of the drug in tissues will have to redistribute to the blood to maintain the distribution equilibrium between the tissues and blood. So the reduction of the drug concentration in blood is accompanied by a proportional reduction in the drug concentration in the different tissues to maintain the tissue to blood distribution equilibrium. This condition can be described as a pseudo-equilibrium state since the rate of drug transfer from the tissues to blood is slightly more than the rate of drug transfer from the blood to tissues due to the eliminated drug.

3.3 DRUG PROTEIN BINDING

The drug in the systemic circulation can bind to plasma proteins such as albumin, alpha-1-acid glycoprotein, globulins, and lipoprotein. This is in addition to drug partitioning inside the blood cells by diffusion across the blood cell membrane and binding to blood cell constituents. The extent of protein binding in plasma can be expressed as the fraction bound, which is the ratio of the bound drug concentration to the total drug concentration in plasma, or the free fraction, which is the ratio of the free drug concentration to the total drug concentration in plasma. The extent of protein binding can also be expressed as percentage bound or percentage free. The percent of drug bound in plasma ranges from 0% (free fraction = 1.0), when the drug is not bound to plasma proteins, to >99% (free fraction <0.01), when the majority of the drug is bound to plasma proteins. This is dependent on the affinity of the drug to the plasma proteins. The binding of the drug molecules to plasma proteins is reversible and the percent bound and the free fraction are relatively constant for a given drug in a given individual. In some instances, the percent bound decreases and the free fraction increases at high drug concentration when the protein binding sites are saturated.

A simple model that describes the distribution of drugs between plasma and tissues is presented in Figure 3.1. The free and bound drug molecules in plasma are present at equilibrium as expressed by Equation 3.3:

$$D + P \leftrightarrow PD \tag{3.3}$$

where
   D is the free drug molecule
   P is the plasma protein
   PD is the drug bound to plasma protein

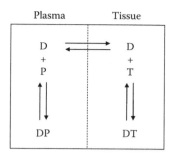

FIGURE 3.1 Diagram representing the distribution of the drug between the plasma and the tissues. D is the free (unbound) drug molecule in plasma and tissue, P is the plasma protein, DP is the drug bound to plasma protein, T is the tissue components to which the drug can bind, and DT is a drug bound to tissue components.

If the physicochemical properties of the drug allow its diffusion across the biological membranes to enter the tissues, only the free drug molecules in plasma can cross the membrane. Once free drug molecules are distributed to tissues, a new equilibrium is established in plasma and drug molecules are liberated from their plasma protein binding sites to maintain constant drug-free fraction in plasma. The drug molecules distributed to the tissues can bind to different tissue constituents depending on the drug affinity to these tissue constituents. The binding of the drug molecules to tissue constituents is also reversible and the ratio of the free to total drug concentration is relatively constant for a given drug in a given tissue. The binding of drug to tissue constituents can be expressed as shown in Equation 3.4:

$$D + T \leftrightarrow DT \qquad (3.4)$$

where
  D is the free drug
  T is the tissue protein to which the drug can bind
  DT is the drug bound to tissue protein

When the drug is distributed to tissues and equilibrium is established between the drug in plasma and the drug in the tissues, the free drug concentration in plasma should be equal to the free drug concentration in the tissues. However, the total (free and bound) drug concentration in tissues and plasma is different and their ratio is the tissue to plasma distribution coefficient (Kp_{TP}) similar to the tissue to blood distribution described in Equation 3.1. Dividing the total tissue concentration and the total plasma concentration by the free drug concentration (similar in plasma and tissues), the tissue to plasma partition coefficient can be expressed by the ratio of the free fraction of the drug in plasma (f_{uP}) to the free fraction in tissues (f_{uT}), as in Equation 3.5:

$$Kp_{TP} = \frac{C_T}{C_P} = \frac{f_{uP}}{f_{uT}} \qquad (3.5)$$

Drugs that are bound to tissue components more than their binding to plasma proteins, that is, have smaller free fraction in tissues, have higher tissue to plasma total drug concentration ratio, and are extensively distributed to the tissues, while drugs that are bound to plasma protein more than their binding in tissues will have low tissue distribution.

3.3.1 EFFECT OF CHANGING THE PLASMA PROTEIN BINDING

The binding of drugs to plasma proteins and to tissue proteins is an important factor in determining the drug distribution in the body. The extent of drug protein binding depends on the concentration of the drug and protein in addition to the affinity of the drug molecule to the protein. Any physiological or pathological conditions that can alter the concentration of the protein or affect the affinity of the drug to the protein can change the drug protein binding resulting in modification of the drug distribution characteristics.

3.3.2 DETERMINATION OF PLASMA PROTEIN BINDING

All analytical techniques used for the determination of drug concentration in plasma measure the total (free + bound) drug concentration. These procedures usually require sample preparation procedures that involve protein precipitation, liquid-liquid extraction, or solid-phase extraction, which usually denatures the plasma protein and causes liberation of the drug molecules from their protein binding sites. So the measured concentration represents the total drug concentration. Studying the drug protein binding or determination of the free drug concentration in plasma usually requires special procedures. The most common techniques used in these studies are ultrafiltration and equilibrium dialysis.

3.3.2.1 Ultrafiltration

In this technique, the plasma sample that contains the drug is filtered through special membrane filter that allows passage of the plasma water but not the large molecular weight plasma constituents including proteins. The free drug in plasma can pass through this membrane filter with the plasma water as presented in Figure 3.2. Since the membrane filter has very small pore size, the filtration process has to be aided by centrifugation at 37°C, since the plasma protein binding is dependent on the temperature. The drug concentration in plasma samples before filtration is the total drug concentration, while the concentration in the filtrate is the free drug concentration.

3.3.2.2 Equilibrium Dialysis

This technique utilizes a special dialysis chamber that is separated into two halves by a semipermeable membrane that allows the transfer of the free drug molecules but not the drug bound to proteins. The plasma sample that contains the drug is placed on one side of the chamber and the drug-free protein-free buffer solution is placed on the other side of the chamber. The dialysis chamber is maintained at 37°C since the drug protein binding depends on the temperature. The free drug in the plasma side can transfer across the semipermeable membrane until equilibrium is established between the free drug in both sides of the dialysis chamber as presented in Figure 3.3. At equilibrium, the free drug concentration in the plasma side is at

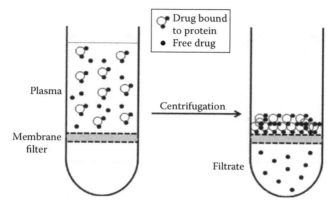

FIGURE 3.2 Schematic presentation of the ultrafiltration process. After filtration of the plasma sample, the filtrate drug concentration is equal to the free drug concentration in the plasma sample.

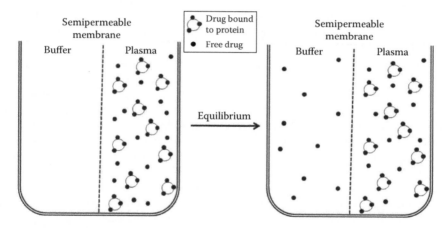

FIGURE 3.3 Schematic presentation of the dialysis chamber that is divided in halves by a semi-permeable membrane. After equilibration, the drug concentration in the plasma side is the total drug concentration, and the drug concentration in the buffer side is the free drug concentration.

equilibrium and is equal to the drug concentration in the buffer side of the chamber. So the drug concentration in the buffer side is equal to the free drug concentration, and the drug concentration in the plasma side is the total drug concentration.

In both techniques, the free fraction of the drug in plasma and the percent of drug bound in plasma can be determined as in Equations 3.6 and 3.7:

$$\text{Free fraction} = \frac{\text{Free drug concentration}}{\text{Total drug concentration}} \quad (3.6)$$

$$\% \text{ Bound} = \frac{\text{(Total-free) drug concentration}}{\text{Total drug concentration}} \times 100 \quad (3.7)$$

3.4   DRUG PARTITIONING TO BLOOD CELLS

In addition to binding to plasma proteins, the drug in the systemic circulation can distribute across the blood cell membrane and bind to the blood cell components. The approach used to describe the drug tissue distribution that is presented in Figure 3.1 can be used to describe the drug distribution to the blood cells. The drug blood to plasma ratio is the ratio of the drug concentration in whole blood (blood cells + plasma) to the concentration of drug in plasma, while the drug blood cell partition coefficient is the ratio of the drug concentration in the blood cells (without plasma) to the drug concentration in plasma. When equilibrium is established between the drug in plasma and the drug inside the blood cells, the free drug concentration in plasma is equal to the free drug concentration inside the blood cells. The drug blood to plasma concentration ratio depends on the drug binding to the blood cell components and the drug binding to plasma proteins. Drugs that can bind to blood cell components much more than their binding to plasma proteins usually have blood to plasma concentration ratio larger than one, while drugs that can bind more to plasma proteins usually have blood to plasma concentration ratio smaller than one. Drugs with equal binding to plasma proteins and blood cell components have blood to plasma concentration ratio equal to one.

The importance of the blood to plasma drug concentration ratio is that the pharmacokinetic parameters of drugs are usually calculated based on the analysis of drug concentrations in plasma rather than in whole blood. If the drug blood to plasma concentration ratio is equal to one, there will be no difference in the pharmacokinetic parameters calculated from plasma or whole blood concentrations. However, when the blood to plasma concentration ratio is different from one, differences in the calculated parameters using plasma and whole blood concentrations are observed. So when reporting pharmacokinetic parameters it is important to state whether the parameters were calculated based on plasma or whole blood drug concentrations. This issue becomes more complicated when the drug partitioning into the blood cells is concentration dependent, that is, the distribution ratio between blood and plasma is different at different drug concentrations.

The blood to plasma distribution ratio is also important when the drug is not equally distributed between the blood and plasma and there is a range of drug concentrations in the blood that is associated with the maximum therapeutic effect and minimum toxicity. This range of drug concentrations will be different depending on whether the drug is measured in whole blood or in plasma. The dose of cyclosporin A, an immunosuppressant drug used in organ transplant patients, is selected to maintain its concentration in blood or plasma within a certain range to ensure optimal therapeutic effect and to avoid toxicity. The range of the desired cyclosporine A concentration is 100–400 ng/mL for whole blood, and 50–150 ng/mL for plasma, depending on the samples used in the analysis. This is because cyclosporine A concentration in plasma is about 20%–50% that in whole blood. The therapeutic range for tacrolimus, which is another immunosuppressant drug, is also different depending on whether the sample used for drug determination is plasma or blood.

Similar to the drug tissue distribution, the blood to plasma concentration ratio depends on physicochemical properties of the drug. Large molecular weight drugs that cannot cross the blood cell membrane are distributed mainly in plasma with little or no partitioning into the blood cells such as in case of heparin and insulin. Many lipophilic drugs can cross the blood cell membrane and bind to the cell components to the same extent as their binding to plasma proteins producing blood to plasma concentration ratio around one. Few drugs can bind to the blood cell components to higher extent producing high blood to plasma concentration ratio such as the antimalarial drug chloroquine, which has high blood to plasma concentration ratio.

3.5 VOLUME OF DISTRIBUTION

After IV administration, the drug is distributed via the systemic circulation to all parts of the body, leaving only a fraction of the administered dose in the blood. Drugs are not distributed equally to all tissues since different drugs have different affinities for different tissues. This means that the drug amount, and hence the drug concentration, in the blood will be different for different drugs depending on the administered dose and the drug distribution characteristics. IV administration of drugs with high tissue distribution coefficient (i.e., have high affinity to tissues) results in the distribution of the majority of the administered dose to the tissues leaving only a small amount of the drug in the blood. When the distribution equilibrium is achieved, the blood drug concentration will be low, while for drugs with low tissue partition coefficient, only a small fraction of the administered dose is distributed to the tissues leaving the majority of the dose in the blood and producing high blood drug concentration. Also, IV administration of increasing doses of the same drug to the same individual results in proportional increase in the drug amount and the drug concentration in tissues and blood.

3.5.1 RELATIONSHIP BETWEEN THE DRUG AMOUNT IN THE BODY AND THE PLASMA DRUG CONCENTRATION

Addition of a known amount of a drug to a beaker that contains certain volume of a solvent will produce drug concentration that is dependent on the volume of the solvent. The relationship between the drug amount, drug concentration, and the volume of the solvent can be expressed as

$$\text{Drug concentration} = \frac{\text{Amount of the drug}}{\text{Volume of the solvent}} \qquad (3.8)$$

The volume of distribution (Vd) of the drug is the pharmacokinetic parameter that relates the amount of the drug in the body and the drug concentration in the plasma (the most common sampling site). It can be defined as the volume where the drug is distributed inside the body. Since the drug is not distributed equally to all parts of the body, Vd does not represent a real volume and is often known as the apparent volume of distribution. In other words, we can say that the body behaves as if it has a volume equal to Vd. The Vd is affected by the physicochemical properties of the drug, tissue characteristics, protein binding, and any factor that can affect the extent of drug tissue distribution. The relationship that relates the amount of the drug in the body, the plasma drug concentration, and Vd can be expressed as

$$\text{Plasma concentration} = \frac{\text{Drug amount in the body}}{\text{Vd}} \qquad (3.9)$$

Rearrangement of Equations 3.8 and 3.9 will give Equation 3.10:

$$\text{Vd} = \frac{\text{Drug amount in the body}}{\text{Plasma concentration}} \qquad (3.10)$$

Drugs with high Kp_T are extensively distributed to the tissues after IV administration leaving small amount of the drug in blood. The resulting plasma drug concentration will be low and the calculated Vd will be large. On the other hand, drugs with low Kp_T usually have a small amount of the drug distributed in tissues after IV administration leaving most of the drug in blood. The resulting plasma drug concentration will be high and the calculated Vd will be small. For example, highly polar drugs with high molecular weight like heparin and insulin have limited ability to cross the capillary membrane, which makes them distribute mainly in the vascular volume. These drugs usually have Vd approximately similar to the plasma volume. Small molecular weight highly polar drugs can cross the capillary membrane to the extracellular space; however, these drugs cannot distribute intracellularly because of their high polarity. The aminoglycoside antibiotics are hydrophilic drugs that distribute mainly in the extracellular space with small amounts distributed specifically to other tissues. These drugs have Vd roughly about the volume of the extracellular fluids. Other less polar drugs can distribute across the cell membrane and stay in the intracellular water without binding to any cellular components. Aminopyrine is a compound that is distributed mainly into the total body water, that is, the extracellular and intracellular fluids. This drug has Vd nearly similar to the total body water. Nonpolar drugs can distribute intracellularly and bind to specific cell components of different tissues. Drugs such as the cardiac glycoside digoxin and the tricyclic antidepressant drugs are extensively distributed to different tissues and can have very large Vd. The average Vd for the antiepileptic drug phenytoin is about 50L, for the antibiotic ciprofloxacin is nearly 120L, for cardiac glycoside digoxin is about 500L, and for the tricyclic antidepressant imipramine is around 1600L in a 70kg individual. Remember, Vd does not represent a real volume.

3.5.2 DRUG PROTEIN BINDING AND THE VOLUME OF DISTRIBUTION

When the drug is distributed to tissues and equilibrium is established between the drug in plasma and in tissues, the free drug concentration in plasma and in tissues is equal. Drugs that are highly bound to tissue components and have small free fraction in tissues compared to plasma usually have large Vd, while drugs that are highly bound to plasma proteins with small free fraction compared to tissues usually have small Vd. Based on this, the Vd of the drugs is dependent on the vascular volume, the volume of the tissues where the drug is distributed, and the tissue to plasma distribution coefficient. Since the drug tissue to plasma distribution coefficient can be expressed as the ratio of the free fraction of the drug in plasma and tissues as in Equation 3.5, Vd can be expressed as

$$Vd = V_p + V_t \left(\frac{f_{uP}}{f_{uT}} \right) \tag{3.11}$$

where
   Vd is the volume of distribution
   V_p is the volume of the plasma
   V_t is the volume of the tissues
   f_{uP} is the free fraction of the drug in plasma
   f_{uT} is the free fraction of the drug in tissues

This relationship indicates that changes in plasma protein binding or tissue binding can lead to changes in the drug Vd.

3.5.3 Effect of Changing the Plasma Protein Binding on the Volume of Distribution

Drug binding to plasma proteins can be reduced either by reduction in the concentration of the plasma proteins or a decrease in the affinity of the drug to plasma proteins. Conditions that cause reduction in plasma proteins concentration include liver diseases, nephritic syndrome, pregnancy, cystic fibrosis, burn, malnourishment, and old age. Accumulation of endogenous compounds that can compete with drugs for their binding sites results in reduction of the percent drug bound and increase in the drug free fraction. This can occur in conditions such as hyperbilirubinemia, jaundice, renal failure, and liver diseases. Moreover, exogenous compounds such as drugs with high protein binding affinity (e.g., warfarin, valproic acid, and nonsteroidal anti-inflammatory drugs) can compete and displace other drugs from their protein binding sites. All these conditions can lead to reduction of the percent drug bound to plasma protein and increase in the free fraction of drugs in plasma.

   Conditions that can reduce the drug protein binding in plasma without affecting the drug binding in tissues produce higher free drug concentration in plasma. Since the free drug in plasma and in tissues is at equilibrium, higher free drug concentration in plasma will lead to diffusion of free drug from plasma to tissues until new equilibrium is established. This means that reduction in plasma protein binding without change in tissue binding will result in shifting of drug from plasma to tissues. In other words, the drug will be distributed more to the tissues, and Vd will be larger. Conversely, if the binding of drug to tissue protein is reduced without affecting drug binding to plasma protein, this leads to shifting of the drug from the tissues to plasma. This means less tissue distribution and smaller Vd.

3.6 DRUG DISTRIBUTION AFTER A SINGLE IV BOLUS DRUG ADMINISTRATION

3.6.1 WHEN FAST EQUILIBRIUM IS ESTABLISHED BETWEEN THE DRUG IN BLOOD AND TISSUES

After a single IV bolus administration, the drug is distributed to all parts of the body, with the systemic circulation. If the rate of drug distribution to all tissues is fast, rapid equilibrium is established between the drug in blood and the drug in all tissues. The decrease in the drug concentration in blood due to drug elimination results in immediate and proportional decrease in the drug concentration in all tissues. For these drugs, the drug concentration–time profiles in blood and all tissues after single IV drug administration, although not equal, will decline at the same rate as in Figure 3.4. The rapid equilibrium between the drug in blood and tissues makes the body behave as one homogenous compartment. The Vd of the drug relates the amount of the drug in the body and the drug concentration in plasma at any time after IV drug administration. The drug in this case is said to follow one-compartment pharmacokinetic model. The one-compartment pharmacokinetic model can be presented by the diagram in Figure 3.5A.

3.6.2 WHEN SLOW EQUILIBRIUM IS ESTABLISHED BETWEEN THE DRUG IN BLOOD AND TISSUES

After IV bolus administration of some drugs, the rate of drug distribution is fast to some organs and tissues and slow to other organs and tissues. Rapid equilibrium is established between the drug in blood and some tissues, while the equilibrium takes longer time for other tissues. During the initial phase after IV drug administration and before establishing the equilibrium between the drug in blood and all tissues, the concentration of the drug in blood and all tissues is not proportional. However, once the distribution

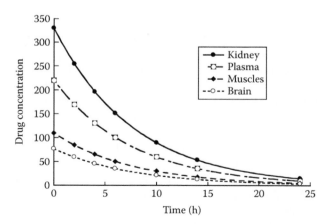

FIGURE 3.4 Hypothetical example of the drug concentration–time profiles in different organs on the linear scale for a drug that follows the one-compartment pharmacokinetic model and eliminated by first-order process. Rapid equilibrium is established between the drug in plasma and in all tissues after administration, so the drug concentration declines at the same rate in all tissues.

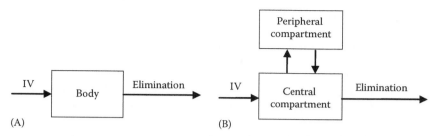

FIGURE 3.5 Diagrams representing the (A) one-compartment pharmacokinetic model where the drug distributes rapidly to all parts of the body and (B) two-compartment pharmacokinetic model where the drug distributes rapidly to the organs comprising the central compartment and slowly to the organs comprising the peripheral compartment.

equilibrium is established, the reduction of drug concentration in blood due to drug elimination is accompanied by a proportional reduction in the drug concentration in all tissues to maintain the tissue to blood distribution equilibrium. For these drugs, the drug concentration (and also amount) time profile in blood after single IV administration is parallel to the profiles in some tissues but not parallel to the profiles in other tissues as in Figure 3.6. The body in this case behaves as two different compartments, and the drug is said to follow two-compartment pharmacokinetic model. The first compartment includes the blood and the highly perfused tissues where rapid equilibrium is established between the drug in blood and tissues and is known as the central compartment, while the second compartment includes the slowly equilibrating tissues and is known as the peripheral compartment. Again, the drug concentrations in the different tissues comprising the central compartment and the peripheral compartment are not equal.

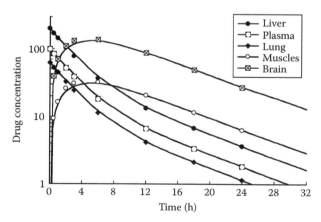

FIGURE 3.6 Hypothetical example of the drug concentration–time profiles in different organs on the semilog scale for a drug that follows the two-compartment pharmacokinetic model and eliminated by first-order process. The drug profiles in the organs comprising the central compartment (liver, plasma, and lung) are not parallel to the profiles in the organs comprising the peripheral compartment (muscles and brain) initially after drug administration; however, after establishing the distribution equilibrium between all organs, the drug profiles in all organs decline at the same rate.

The two-compartment pharmacokinetic model can be presented by the diagram in Figure 3.5B. In this model, the volume of distribution of the central compartment relates the amount of the drug in the body and the plasma concentration right after drug administration when the drug is distributed only in the central compartment. Other volume parameters can relate the amount of the drug in the body and the plasma drug concentration when the drug is distributed in the central and peripheral compartments. The multicompartment pharmacokinetic models will be discussed in detail in Chapter 17.

3.7 DETERMINATION OF THE VOLUME OF DISTRIBUTION

The Vd can be determined from the relationship between the amount of the drug in the body and the resulting plasma drug concentration. However, it is impossible to measure the amount of the drug in the body without using invasive procedures. The only time the amount of drug in the body is known is immediately after IV administration (at time zero), when the amount of drug in the body is equal to the dose. Immediately after IV administration, the relationship between the dose, the initial drug concentration at time zero (Cp_o), and Vd can be written as follows:

$$Cp_o = \frac{Dose}{Vd} \tag{3.12}$$

Since it is practically impossible to measure the plasma concentration at time zero, the initial drug concentration can be estimated. The plasma concentrations obtained at different time points after administration of a single IV dose are plotted and the plasma concentration–time profile that describes the obtained concentrations is determined. The plasma drug concentration–time profile is back extrapolated to the y-axis to estimate the initial plasma drug concentration as in Figure 3.7. The Vd is calculated from a rearrangement of Equation 3.12 as follows:

$$Vd = \frac{Dose}{Cp_o} \tag{3.13}$$

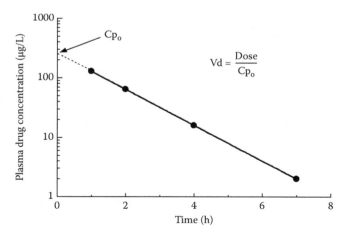

FIGURE 3.7 Initial plasma drug concentration after a single IV bolus dose is determined by back extrapolation of the drug concentration–time profile to the y-axis.

Vd has units of volume (e.g., liters). Since Vd depends on the weight of the patient, it can be expressed in terms of volume/weight (e.g., liters/kg).

Example

After a single IV bolus dose of 1000 mg of an antibiotic, the initial drug concentration was estimated as 20 mg/L. Estimate the volume of distribution of this drug and calculate the IV dose required to achieve an initial plasma drug concentration of 30 mg/L.

Answer

$$Vd = \frac{Dose}{Cp_o} = \frac{1000\,mg}{20\,mg/L} = 50L$$

$$Dose = Cp_o \times Vd = 30\ mg/L \times 50\ L = 1500\ mg$$

3.8 CLINICAL SIGNIFICANCE OF THE VOLUME OF DISTRIBUTION

Most drugs have specific therapeutic range where the drug is most likely to produce the optimal therapeutic effect with the minimum adverse effects. Often, it is necessary to select the dose of the drug that should achieve plasma drug concentration within this range. The Vd allows calculation of the IV bolus dose required to achieve a certain plasma concentration of the drug as in Equation 3.14:

$$Dose_{IV} = Cp_{Desired} \times Vd \qquad (3.14)$$

The Vd also allows calculation of the plasma drug concentration that should be achieved after administration of a certain dose. Increasing the dose in a given patient results in proportional increase in the initial drug concentration since Vd is constant. Drugs that are extensively distributed to the tissues will have large Vd and usually require larger doses to achieve a certain plasma drug concentration.

3.9 SUMMARY

- The Vd is the apparent volume in which the drug is distributed in.
- The Vd is the pharmacokinetic parameter that relates the amount of drug in the body to the concentration of the drug in the sampling site. It is not an actual volume, but it is a hypothetical volume determined by the drug distribution behavior.
- The size of the Vd is different for different drugs and ranges from 3 to 5 L to more than 25 L/kg. Drugs with high affinity for tissues have higher Vd.
- The Vd has units of volume or volume/weight.

PRACTICE PROBLEMS

3.1 Explain why some drugs may have Vd more than 1000 L in 70 kg patients.

3.2 What is the difference between the drugs that follow one-compartment pharmacokinetic model and those that follow the two-compartment model?

3.3 Explain why the plasma protein binding has to be performed at 37°C.

3.4 After IV bolus administration of 450 mg of a drug, the initial drug concentration was found to be 15 mg/L.

a. Calculate the Vd of this drug in this patient.

b. What is the IV bolus dose required to achieve an initial drug concentration of 20 mg/L?

c. If the patient receives a single IV bolus dose of 2 g of the drug, calculate the expected initial dug concentration after this large dose.

3.5 The plasma concentration–time profile after a single IV dose of 300 mg of a drug was back extrapolated and the y-intercept was 7.5 mg/L.

a. Calculate the Vd of this drug.

b. Calculate the dose that should achieve an initial drug concentration of 12 mg/L.

4 Drug Pharmacokinetics Following a Single IV Bolus Administration
Drug Clearance

OBJECTIVES

After completing this chapter you should be able to

- Define the total body clearance and the organ clearance
- Discuss the physiological meaning of the total body clearance
- Calculate the total body clearance using different methods
- Explain why the clearance and volume of distribution are considered independent parameters
- Describe the relationship between the clearance, volume of distribution, and elimination rate constant
- Discuss the clinical significance of the total body clearance

4.1 INTRODUCTION

After intravenous (IV) bolus administration, the drug is distributed to all parts of the body including eliminating and noneliminating organs. In noneliminating organs, the drug can distribute back and forth between the blood and the tissues to maintain the distribution equilibrium, while in eliminating organs, in addition to drug distribution, the drugs can be eliminated leading to reduction in the drug amount in the body. The drug elimination process can be defined as the process by which the drug becomes no longer available to exert its effects in the body. This can happen by excretion of the unchanged drug from the body without any modification of the drug molecule. Examples of unchanged drug excretion include the renal drug excretion in urine, excretion of drugs with bile into the gastrointestinal tract (GIT), lung excretion of volatile drugs during expiration, and excretion of drugs with body secretions such as saliva, sweat, or milk. The other major route of drug elimination is drug metabolism, which involves enzymatic modification of the chemical structure of the drug molecule to form a new chemical entity known as the metabolite. Since the metabolites are inactive molecules in most cases, drug metabolism is considered one of the elimination pathways. However, for few drugs, the metabolites possess therapeutic and/or adverse effects. Drug metabolism usually occurs in organs that contain the metabolizing enzymes such as the liver, small intestine, kidney, and lungs.

4.2 ELIMINATING ORGANS

The physicochemical properties of drugs usually determine the route by which the drug is eliminated from the body. Lipophilic drugs can easily cross the biological membranes and distribute to tissues, so they have higher probability to come in contact with the metabolizing enzymes. On the other hand, hydrophilic drugs cannot easily cross biological membranes and have lower tissue distribution. This makes hydrophilic drugs stay mainly in the systemic circulation until they are delivered to organs like the kidney where they can be excreted unchanged. Many organs are involved in the drug elimination from the body, and some organs can have both metabolic and excretory functions. The following discussion will focus on the two major eliminating organs, the liver and the kidney. The liver is the major organ involved in drug metabolism in addition to excretion of many drugs in the biliary system. The kidney is the major organ for drug excretion besides its ability to metabolize many drugs. The renal excretion of drugs and the hepatic clearance will be discussed in detail in Chapters 14 and 21, respectively.

4.2.1 LIVER

The liver is located in the upper right part of the abdomen just below the diaphragm, weighing approximately 1.6 kg in a 70 kg individual. The blood supply to the liver is around 1.5 L/min, with the portal vein that collects blood from the GIT providing 75% of that blood supply and the rest is provided by the hepatic artery. The basic functional unit of the liver is the liver lobule. Blood enters the lobules through small branches of the portal triad, which includes branches of the hepatic artery, portal vein, bile duct, and lymph vessel, then flows through the sinusoids until it is collected in a central vein. A liver sinusoid is a blood vessel with discontinuous endothelium, so it allows passage of blood components across its membrane. The hepatocytes are separated from the sinusoids by the space of Disse or the perisinusoidal space that allows protein and other plasma components from the sinusoid to be taken up by the hepatocytes. The network of central veins that collect the blood from the hepatic lobules is joined together to form the hepatic vein, which carries the blood from the liver to the vena cava. In the liver, the drug is transferred from the blood in the sinusoids to the hepatocytes where it can be metabolized or excreted unchanged in the bile. Figure 4.1 represents a simplified diagram for the hepatic lobule to demonstrate its basic components.

The liver has several functions including synthesis, and storage, in addition to the metabolism and excretion functions. The pharmacokinetic behavior of drugs is usually affected by the efficiency of the liver in metabolizing and excreting drugs. The metabolic and excretory functions of the liver are affected by several factors including drug properties in addition to other physiological and pathological factors. The drug lipophilicity and plasma protein binding are important factors since the drug has to cross the hepatocyte membrane to get in contact with the metabolizing enzymes,

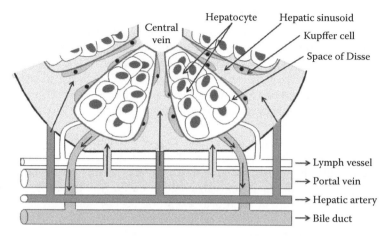

FIGURE 4.1   Simplified diagram showing the basic components of the liver lobule.

and only free drug molecules in plasma can cross the biological membrane. Also, diseases like hepatitis or chronic alcoholisms can significantly reduce the hepatic enzymatic activity. Furthermore, neonates and elderly patients usually have enzymatic activity lower than that of adults, and genetic factors can play an important role in the variability in the hepatic enzymatic activity. Moreover, concomitant administration of drugs that can induce or inhibit the enzymatic activity can affect the metabolic function of the liver. Since the distribution of the metabolizing enzymes in the liver is not homogenous, the change in blood flow to the liver can affect the amount of the drug delivered to the liver and also affect the distribution of the drug to different parts of the liver, which can in turn affect the drug metabolic rate.

4.2.2   KIDNEY

The kidneys are located behind the abdominal cavity in the retroperitoneum space one in each side of the body and weighing approximately 150 g each in a 70 kg individual. The blood flow to both kidneys is around 1.2 L/min supplied by the renal arteries and the renal veins returning the blood from the kidneys. The basic functional unit of the kidney is the nephron, with both kidneys containing about two to three million nephrons. The nephron consists of the glomerulus, followed by the proximal tubule, next is the loop of Henle, then the distal tubules, and finally the collecting tubules that transfer the formed urine to the urinary bladder where it is stored and then excreted. In addition to the endocrine, synthetic, and metabolic functions, the kidney plays an important role in the excretion of many drugs. Three processes are involved in the renal handling of drugs that leads to renal drug elimination. These are glomerular filtration, renal tubular secretion, and renal tubular reabsorption.

The blood reaching the glomeruli is filtered through the glomerular membrane. The filtration occurs depending on the molecular size of the compound. All the free drug molecules are filtered through the glomerular membrane, while proteins and protein-bound drugs stay in the blood. Drug molecules can be secreted in the renal tubules by active transport systems that are specialized for compounds with specific structure features. The drug in the renal tubules can undergo active or passive reabsorption. Passive reabsorption of drugs in the renal tubules involves passage of drugs across the tubular membrane so it is influenced by the drug lipophilicity. Lipophilic and unionized drugs can cross the renal tubular membrane so they can be reabsorbed back to the blood, while hydrophilic and ionized drugs stay in the lumen of the renal tubules and are excreted with the urine. Figure 4.2 shows the different components of the nephron and the different processes involved in the renal drug excretion.

The rate of drug excretion in urine is the sum of the rate of filtration and secretion minus the rate of drug reabsorption. The filtered and secreted drug can be reabsorbed completely in the renal tubules, so the drug in this case is not excreted in urine, while when the drug is not reabsorbed or partially reabsorbed, the drug is excreted in urine. The rate of renal drug excretion depends on many factors such as the drug properties, blood flow to the kidney, the renal function, plasma protein binding, and concomitantly administered drugs. Hydrophilic drugs have limited tissue distribution, so they stay mainly in the systemic circulation where they can be eliminated by the kidney. Also, drugs with limited plasma protein binding are filtered at higher rate in the glomeruli, and if not reabsorbed in the renal tubules, they are excreted in urine. Furthermore, the ability of the kidney to excrete drugs depends on the number of functioning nephrons. Patients with normal kidney function have more functioning nephrons compared to patients with renal failure. So the reduction in kidney function reduces the kidney's efficiency in excreting drugs. Moreover, concomitant drug administration may affect the renal excretion of drugs if they can compete for the same active secretion system or if one drug can affect the urinary pH, which can affect the ionization and tubular reabsorption of other drugs.

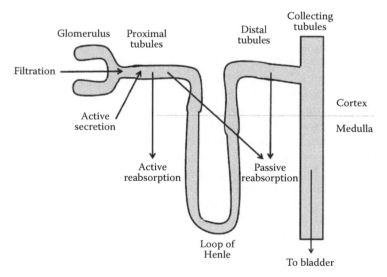

FIGURE 4.2 Simplified diagram showing the different components of the nephron and the processes involved in the renal drug elimination.

4.3 TOTAL BODY CLEARANCE

The total body clearance (CL_T) is defined as the volume of plasma or blood completely cleared of the drug per unit time. It is a measure of the efficiency of all eliminating organs in the body in metabolizing/excreting the drug from the body. The CL_T has units of volume/time (e.g., L/h or mL/min). It can be normalized for body weight and expressed in units of volume/time/weight (e.g., L/h kg, or mL/min kg). The CL_T of a drug in a particular patient is constant and is independent of drug concentration as long as the drug elimination process follows first-order kinetics. However, when the drug elimination process follows zero-order kinetics, CL_T will be different at different drug concentrations.

The CL_T represents the overall clearance of the drug from the body by all eliminating organs, while organ clearance represents the clearance of the drug by a specific organ. For example, the renal clearance can be defined as the volume of plasma or blood completely cleared of the drug per unit time by the kidney. So the CL_T is the sum of the clearances of all eliminating organs as expressed in Equation 4.1:

$$CL_T = \text{Renal clearance} + \text{Hepatic clearance} + \text{Lung clearance} + \cdots \quad (4.1)$$

Most drugs are eliminated by more than one elimination pathway. For example, the cardiac glycoside digoxin is eliminated partially by renal excretion and partially by hepatic metabolism. In this case, the CL_T is equal to the sum of renal clearance and hepatic clearance. In some special cases, the drugs are eliminated from the body by a single elimination pathway. The aminoglycoside antibiotics are eliminated only by renal excretion. For these drugs, the CL_T is equal to the renal clearance.

4.3.1 PHYSIOLOGICAL APPROACH TO DRUG CLEARANCE

The drug delivered to the eliminating organs is subjected to metabolism and/or excretion, resulting in the decrease in drug amount in the body. The fraction of the drug eliminated during a single passage through the eliminating organ depends on the efficiency of the organ in eliminating the drug. If the eliminating organ has high efficiency for drug elimination (high drug clearance), a large fraction of the amount of the drug delivered to the organ is eliminated during a single pass through the organ.

On the contrary, if the organ clearance is low, only a small fraction of the drug delivered to the organ is eliminated during a single pass. This fraction can be zero if the drug is not eliminated by the organ. The efficiency of the organ in eliminating the drug is reflected in the difference between the drug concentration in the blood reaching the organ and the drug concentration in the blood leaving the organ. Using the fraction of the drug excreted during a single pass through the organ and the blood flow to the organ, one can calculate the volume of blood that can be considered completely cleared of the drug per unit time. This is the clearance of the drug by that particular organ.

The fraction of the amount of drug presented to the eliminating organ which is eliminated during a single pass through the organ is a parameter known as the extraction ratio (E). The extraction ratio is a function of the intrinsic ability of the eliminating organ to eliminate the drug and the blood flow to the organ. It can be calculated from the ratio of the difference in the drug concentration in the arterial and venous blood to the drug concentration in the arterial blood in that organ, as presented in Equation 4.2:

$$E = \frac{Cp_a - Cp_v}{Cp_a} \tag{4.2}$$

where

    E is the extraction ratio for the drug in the eliminating organ

    Cp_a and Cp_v are the drug concentration in the arterial and venous blood of the organ, respectively

Multiplying the extraction ratio by the total blood flow to the organ (Q), the volume of the blood that is completely cleared of the drug per unit time can be calculated as presented in Equations 4.3 and 4.4:

$$CL_{organ} = Q \left[\frac{Cp_a - Cp_v}{Cp_a} \right] \tag{4.3}$$

$$CL_{organ} = QE \tag{4.4}$$

The organ clearance of a drug that is completely eliminated during single pass through the organ, that is, $E = 1$, is equal to the organ blood flow. This indicates that the maximum organ clearance for a drug is the blood flow to that particular organ. The product of drug concentration in the arterial side of the organ and the organ blood flow is the rate of drug delivery to the organ, while the product of drug concentration in the venous side and the organ blood flow is the rate of drug exiting the organ, as in Equations 4.5 and 4.6:

$$CL_{organ} = \frac{QCp_a - QCp_v}{Cp_a} \tag{4.5}$$

$$CL_{organ} = \frac{\text{Rate of drug delivery to the organ} - \text{Rate of drug exiting the organ}}{\text{Concentration of drug entering the organ}}$$

$$\tag{4.6}$$

The difference in the rate of the drug delivery to the organ and the rate of drug exiting the organ is the rate of drug elimination by the organ. So the organ clearance can be expressed using the rate of drug elimination and the blood drug concentration as in Equation 4.7:

$$CL_{organ} = \frac{\text{Rate of organ drug elimination}}{Cp_a} \qquad (4.7)$$

The same principle can be applied to any eliminating organ and also to CL_T, since it is the sum of all organ clearances. The CL_T can be determined from the overall rate of drug elimination from the body and the drug blood concentration.

4.3.2 TOTAL BODY CLEARANCE AND THE RATE OF DECLINE IN THE AMOUNT OF THE DRUG FROM THE BODY

The organ clearance is a measure of the organ efficiency in eliminating the drug, and CL_T is a measure of the efficiency of the whole body in eliminating the drug. The CL_T is the volume of blood completely cleared of the drug per unit time; however, it does not indicate how rapid the drug is eliminated from the body. When the drug is eliminated from the blood, the drug has to redistribute back from the tissues to the blood to maintain the tissue to blood distribution equilibrium. So the rate of drug disappearance from the body or the rate of decline in the drug concentration–time profile can be viewed as the fraction of the amount of the drug in the body eliminated per unit time. The rate of decline in the drug amount in the body is dependant on CL_T and also on the volume where the drug is distributed in, Vd. For example, if two drugs have the same CL_T and different Vd, the drug with the smaller Vd will disappear from the body faster than the drug with the larger Vd. This is because when the clearance is similar, it should take shorter time to eliminate a certain fraction of the drug with smaller Vd, and longer time to eliminate the same fraction of the drug with large Vd.

For example:

Gentamicin: $CL_T = 0.50\,L/h$ Vd = 14 L
Rifampin: $CL_T = 1.4\,L/h$ Vd = 70 L

The CL_T of rifampin is higher than that of gentamicin. However, because rifampin Vd is larger, the rate of decline of the plasma rifampin concentration is slower than that of gentamicin. So based on this, the CL_T of the drug by itself does not indicate the rate of decline of the drug amount or drug concentration in the body. Also, the Vd of the drug by itself does not indicate the rate of decline in the drug amount or drug concentration. However, both CL_T and Vd determine the rate of decline in the drug amount and drug concentration in the body.

4.3.3 TOTAL BODY CLEARANCE AND VOLUME OF DISTRIBUTION ARE INDEPENDENT PHARMACOKINETIC PARAMETERS

The CL_T of a drug is dependent on the intrinsic ability of the eliminating organ(s) to excrete or metabolize the drug. For example, when the drug is metabolized by the liver, the metabolic clearance is dependent on the activity of the metabolizing enzymes and the factors that can help the drug to get in contact with the enzymes. Also, the renal clearance of a drug is dependent on the ability of the kidney to excrete the drug in urine. On the other hand, the Vd of the drug is dependent on the physicochemical properties of the drug and the tissue characteristics that influence the affinity of the drug for the different tissues. For example, drugs with high affinity for distribution to different tissues have large Vd, while drugs that are poorly distributed to tissues have small Vd.

This indicates that changes in the ability of eliminating organs to eliminate the drug affect the CL_T of the drug, without affecting its Vd. Also, changes that can affect the distribution of the drug to different tissues can affect the Vd of the drug without affecting its clearance. For this reason, CL_T and Vd are considered independent pharmacokinetic parameters. The change in one of these two parameters does not lead to change in the other parameter. However, modifications in some biochemical or physiological factors can lead to changes in both CL_T and Vd. This does not contradict the notion that CL_T and Vd are two independent parameters. The independent parameters CL_T and Vd together determine the dependent pharmacokinetic parameters that describe the rate of decline in the drug amount and drug concentration in the body, which are the elimination rate constant and the half-life of the drug.

4.3.4 DETERMINATION OF THE TOTAL BODY CLEARANCE

Calculation of CL_T based on Equation 4.7 requires determination of the total drug elimination rate and the blood drug concentration. However, it is practically impossible to determine the total drug elimination rate from the body. So CL_T is usually determined using indirect methods by measuring other pharmacokinetic parameters that can be related to CL_T. The most common method used to calculate CL_T depends on Equation 4.8 that describes how the elimination rate constant (k), which is a dependent pharmacokinetic parameter, is related to the independent pharmacokinetic parameters, CL_T and Vd. Usually k and Vd can be estimated experimentally and then CL_T can be calculated:

$$\frac{CL_T}{Vd} = k \tag{4.8}$$

It is possible to calculate the rate of drug elimination by a specific organ such as the kidney since it is possible to determine the rate of drug elimination in urine over a certain time interval. So Equation 4.9 can be used to determine the renal clearance of drugs by collecting a urine sample over a certain time interval and calculating the rate of renal drug excretion over this collection interval. The renal clearance can be calculated from the renal excretion rate and the average plasma drug concentration. This will be discussed in detail in Chapter 14.

$$CL_{Renal} = \frac{\text{Renal excretion rate}}{\text{Drug blood concentration}} \tag{4.9}$$

4.4 CLINICAL IMPORTANCE OF THE TOTAL BODY CLEARANCE

The clearance of some markers that are eliminated by a specific eliminating organ can be used to determine the function of that eliminating organ. For example, creatinine is an endogenous byproduct of muscle metabolism, which is excreted only by the kidney. Creatinine is freely filtered in the renal glomeruli and does not undergo significant secretion or reabsorption in the renal tubules. The CL_T of creatinine is the same as its renal clearance since it is completely eliminated by the kidney. The creatinine clearance is used as a measure of the glomerular filtration rate that is the major determinant of the renal function. The decrease in creatinine clearance from its average normal value of 120 mL/min indicates a decrease in kidney function. Similarly, a special compound such as indocyanine green that is eliminated extensively by hepatic metabolism can be used to determine the liver function. Since this compound is extensively eliminated by the liver, its CL_T is very close to the hepatic blood flow. Determination of the CL_T of this compound after IV administration can be used to monitor the hepatic function. When the CL_T of this compound is much lower than the average hepatic blood flow in the patient population, this indicates reduction in the hepatic function.

Patients with eliminating organ dysfunction usually have lower ability to eliminate the drugs. If the eliminating organ dysfunction does not affect the drug distribution characteristics significantly, the lower elimination efficiency usually leads to slower rate of elimination. Patients with renal failure usually eliminate the drugs that are eliminated mainly by the kidney at a much slower rate and usually require smaller than average doses to produce the therapeutic effect. For example, the dosage requirement of the aminoglycoside antibiotics, which is mainly eliminated by the kidney, in a renal failure patient is much lower than the dosage requirements in patients with normal kidney function. Also, patients with hepatic cirrhosis eliminate the drugs that are mainly eliminated by hepatic metabolism at a slower rate and usually require smaller than average doses to produce the therapeutic effect. For example, the dosage requirement of the antiasthmatic drug theophylline, which is mainly eliminated by hepatic metabolism, in liver cirrhosis patients is much lower than the dosage requirements in patients with normal liver function. Moreover, patients with different degrees of eliminating organ dysfunction may require different degrees of dosage reduction, so doses should be individualized.

4.5 SUMMARY

- The total body clearance is the volume of the plasma or blood that is completely cleared of the drug per unit time. It has units of volume/time or volume/time-weight.
- The total body clearance for a drug is constant within a patient (dose and concentration independent) when the elimination processes follow first-order kinetics.
- The total body clearance is a measure of the efficiency of all eliminating organs in eliminating the drug, and it is the sum of all organ clearances (i.e., CL_T is the sum of the renal clearance, hepatic clearance, and all other organ clearances).

- The total body clearance by itself does not indicate the rate of decline in the drug amount or drug concentration in the body.
- The total body clearance and the volume of distribution are two independent pharmacokinetic parameters that together determine the rate of decline of the drug amount and drug concentration in the body.

PRACTICE PROBLEMS

4.1   The following are the pharmacokinetic parameters for a group of drugs:

Drug	Vd (L/kg)	Elimination Rate Constant (h⁻¹)
Theophylline	0.45	0.11
Ampicillin	0.3	0.6
Quinidine	3	0.08

a. Which drug has the highest CL_T?
b. Which drug has the lowest CL_T?

4.2   A drug is eliminated by the hepatic metabolism and renal excretion. Its hepatic extraction ratio is 0.2 and renal extraction ratio is 0.3. If the hepatic blood flow is 1.5 L/min and the renal blood flow is 1.2 L/min, calculate the following:

a. Renal clearance
b. Hepatic clearance
c. Total body clearance

4.3   A patient received an IV bolus dose of a drug that is eliminated mainly by the kidney by a first-order process. The calculated Vd was 20 L and the elimination rate constant was $0.3465\,h^{-1}$. The patient received the same dose of the same drug after developing renal disease, and the calculated Vd was 20 L and the elimination rate constant was $0.1733\,h^{-1}$. Explain the differences in the pharmacokinetic parameters before and after developing the renal disease.

5 Drug Pharmacokinetics Following a Single IV Bolus Administration
The Rate of Drug Elimination

OBJECTIVES

After completing this chapter you should be able to

- Define the order, the rate, and the rate constant for a process
- Describe the difference between zero-order and first-order drug elimination
- Define and calculate the half-life and area under the curve after a single IV bolus administration
- Estimate the pharmacokinetic parameters after a single IV drug administration when drug elimination follows zero-order and first-order elimination
- Describe the relationship between the clearance, volume of distribution, and elimination rate constant
- Utilize the mathematical expressions to calculate the plasma concentration at any time after a single IV drug administration
- Evaluate the effect of changing each of the pharmacokinetic parameters on the drug concentration–time profile after a single IV bolus dose, using the pharmacokinetic simulations

5.1 INTRODUCTION

The amount of the drug in the body decreases due to drug elimination leading to reduction in the plasma drug concentration. The rate of drug elimination affects the rate of decline in the plasma drug concentration, which has significant clinical consequences after single- and multiple-drug administration. Assuming the existence of direct relationship between the plasma drug concentration and drug effect, the duration of drug effect depends on the rate of decline in the plasma drug concentration. For example, the duration of effect of a general anesthetic that is eliminated rapidly from the body is shorter than the duration of effect of general anesthetics that are eliminated from the body at slower rate. During multiple drug administrations, drugs that are eliminated rapidly from the body have to be administered more frequently compared to drugs that are eliminated at slower rate. For example, the antibiotics that are eliminated rapidly from the body are usually administered every 4, 6, or 8 h, while those with slower rate of elimination are administered less frequently.

The drug CL_T is a measure of the efficiency of the body in eliminating the drug, but it does not indicate the rate of decline in drug concentration. This is because the CL_T is the volume of plasma cleared from the drug per unit time. Without knowing the volume in which the drug is distributed, that is, Vd, we cannot determine how fast the drug amount and concentration decreases. So after a single IV bolus administration, the rate of decline in the plasma drug concentration is dependent on both CL_T and Vd, the two independent pharmacokinetic parameters.

5.2   KINETICS OF THE DRUG ELIMINATION PROCESS

The rate of drug elimination from the body is not the same as the rate of decline in the plasma drug concentration or the rate of disappearance of the drug from the body. This is because the rate of drug elimination is the amount of the drug eliminated per unit time, while the change in plasma drug concentration or drug amount in the body as a result of drug elimination determines the rate of decline in the plasma drug concentration and the rate of disappearance of the drug from the body. When certain amount of the drug is eliminated over a period of time, the decline in the plasma drug concentration during the same time period depends on the total amount of the drug in the body. For example, if the elimination rate of a drug is 100 mg/h, this corresponds to 10% reduction in the plasma drug concentration per hour if the total amount of the drug in the body is 1000 mg at that time and 50% reduction in plasma drug concentration per hour if the amount of the drug in the body is 200 mg. So the rate of decline in the plasma drug concentration can be viewed as the rate of drug elimination from the body relative to the total amount of the drug in the body. In other words, it reflects the fraction of the drug amount in the body eliminated over a period of time. Different drugs can be compared by determining the time required for the elimination of a certain fraction of the drug amount in the body or the time required for the plasma drug concentration to decrease by a certain fraction. In fact, the half-life ($t_{1/2}$) is a pharmacokinetic parameter defined as the time required to eliminate 50% of the amount of the drug in the body or to decrease the plasma drug concentration by 50%. Drugs with shorter half-lives are eliminated from the body faster than the drugs with longer half-lives.

5.2.1   ORDER OF THE DRUG ELIMINATION PROCESS

The way the rate of a process is related to the drug amount or drug concentration available for the process is determined by the order of the process. The order of a process is the power to which the drug amount or concentration available for the process is raised to in the equation that describes the rate of the process. In other words, the rate of any process is dependent on the drug amount or concentration raised to a power. The value of this power is equal to the order of the process. In a process that follows zero-order kinetics, the drug amount (or concentration) in the equation that describes the rate of the process is raised to power zero. This means that the rate of a process that follows zero-order kinetics is independent on the drug amount and concentration, that is, the rate of zero-order process is constant and does not depend on the drug amount and concentration, while for a process that follows first-order kinetics, the drug amount (or concentration) is raised to a power equal to one in the equation that describes the rate of the process. This means that the rate of a process that follows first-order kinetics is dependent on the drug amount available for this process.

5.2.2 Rate of Drug Elimination

The rate of a process is the velocity at which it occurs. After IV drug administration, drug elimination is the only process that affects the change in the amount of the drug in the body. The rate of drug elimination is equal to the rate of change in the amount of the drug in the body. If A is the amount of the drug in the body, the rate of change in the amount of the drug in the body can be expressed as $-dA/dt$. The negative sign is used because the amount of the drug in the body is decreasing due to drug elimination. The rate of drug elimination is determined experimentally by measuring the decrease in the amount of the drug in the body over predetermined time intervals. Then the rate of drug elimination during each time interval is determined by dividing the amount of the drug eliminated by the length of the time interval. The units of the rate of elimination are units of mass per time (e.g., mg/h, g/day, or mg/min) or concentration per time (e.g., mg/L h, or μg/mL h). Based on the order of the elimination process, the rate of the drug may or may not depend on the drug amount in the body. The rate of elimination for processes that follow zero-order kinetics is independent of the drug amount in the body. So the rate of drug elimination is constant regardless of the amount of the drug in the body, while the rate of elimination for processes that follow first-order kinetics is dependent on the drug amount in the body. So the rate of drug elimination through first-order process is directly proportional to the amount of the drug in the body. After IV bolus drug administration, the rate of drug elimination initially is high because the amount of the drug in the body is high. As time proceeds, the rate of drug elimination decreases because the amount of the drug in the body decreases.

5.2.3 Rate Constant for the Drug Elimination Process

The rate constant for the elimination process is a constant that influences the rate of the elimination process. The way the rate constant influences the rate of elimination is dependent on the order of the elimination process. The rate of the drug elimination process that follows zero-order kinetics is constant and is equal to the rate constant for the zero-order elimination process. So the rate of elimination and the rate constant for the elimination process for the zero-order process are equal. The rate constant for the zero-order process has units of amount/time (e.g., mg/min, mg/h, or mg/day) or concentration/time (e.g., mg/L h, μg/mL h, or mg/L h). The rate of drug elimination for processes that follow first-order kinetics is proportional to the amount of the drug in the body and it is equal to the product of the first-order elimination rate constant and the drug amount. So the rate constant for the first-order elimination processes is constant and it has units of time^{-1} (e.g., day^{-1}, h^{-1}, or min^{-1}).

5.3   DRUG ELIMINATION BY ZERO-ORDER PROCESS

Zero-order elimination occurs when the elimination process of the drug occurs via a pathway that can be saturated during the clinical use of drugs. For example, if the drug is eliminated through drug metabolism by a low-capacity enzyme system and the amount of the drug in the body is much larger than the amount of enzymes, this leads to saturation of the metabolizing enzymes and the rate of drug metabolism becomes constant. The rate of drug metabolism does not change with the change in drug concentration as long as the metabolizing enzymes are saturated, since all the enzymes available are involved in drug metabolism. Also, when the elimination of drug occurs by the saturable active transport system in the renal tubule, drug elimination can follow zero-order kinetics. In this case, when the drug concentration in the body is high enough to saturate this transport system, the rate of drug elimination becomes constant and concentration independent. Only few examples of drugs are eliminated by zero-order processes after using therapeutic doses of the drug.

5.3.1   DETERMINATION OF THE ZERO-ORDER ELIMINATION RATE CONSTANT

The rate of a zero-order elimination process is constant and is equal to the zero-order elimination rate constant (K_o). The zero-order elimination rate constant has units of mass/time. If the amount of drug (A) is decreasing at a constant rate, then the rate of change of the amount of drug in the body (dA/dt) can be expressed by the following differential equation:

$$\frac{dA}{dt} = -K_o \tag{5.1}$$

where K_o is the zero-order elimination rate constant and the negative sign is used because the amount of the drug in the body decreases with time due to drug elimination. The integration of Equation 5.1 yields Equation 5.2, which describes the change of the amount of drug with time:

$$A = A_o - K_o t \tag{5.2}$$

where
   A is the amount of the drug in the body at any time t
   A_o is the amount of drug in the body at time zero that is equal to the dose after a
      single IV bolus administration
   K_o is the zero-order elimination rate constant

If the dose, the zero-order elimination rate constant, and the two constants in Equation 5.2 are known, this equation can be used to calculate the amount of the drug in the body at any time by substituting the value of time. Equation 5.2 describes a linear relationship between the amount of the drug and time. This is because it is in the same form of the equation of a straight line (y = a + bx), where y is the dependent variable,

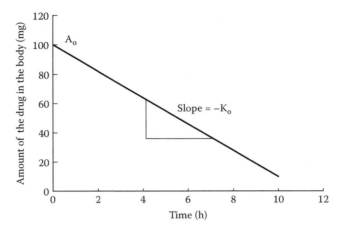

FIGURE 5.1 Plot of the amount of the drug versus time on the Cartesian scale when the elimination of the drug follows zero-order kinetics.

x is the independent variable, a is the y-intercept, and b is the slope of the line. A plot of the amount of the drug versus time on the Cartesian scale yields a straight line as in Figure 5.1. The y-intercept is equal to A_o, and the slope is equal to $-K_o$.

Example

A drug is known to decompose in acidic medium by a zero-order process. After addition of 500 mg of the drug in a beaker that has 0.01 N HCl, the following data were obtained:

Time (h)	Amount of Drug Remaining (mg)
2	432
4	356
8	221

a. Calculate the zero-order decomposition rate constant of this drug.
b. What will be the amount of the drug remaining after 12 h?

Answer

a. Calculation of the zero-order decomposition rate constant:
  - Plot the amount of the drug versus time on a Cartesian graph paper as in Figure 5.2.
  - Draw the best line that goes through the three data points.
  - Calculate the slope of the line by taking two points on the line (do not calculate the slope from two of the given data points).

$$\text{Slope} = \frac{(y_2 - y_1)}{(x_2 - x_1)}$$

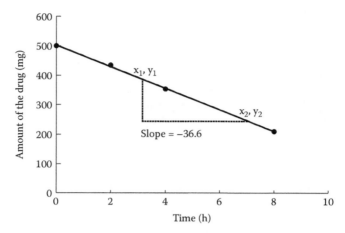

FIGURE 5.2   Plot of the amount of the drug remaining (undecomposed) versus time on the Cartesian scale.

From Figure 5.2:
The slope = $-K_o$ = -36.6 mg/h
So the zero-order decomposition rate constant = 36.6 mg/h
b. To calculate the amount of the drug remaining after 12 h, substitute in Equation 5.2 the value of A_o, K_o, and time.

Amount remaining after 12 h = 500 mg – 36.6 mg/h × 12 h = 60.8 mg.

5.3.2   DETERMINATION OF THE HALF-LIFE FOR ZERO-ORDER DRUG ELIMINATION

The half-life is defined as the time required for the drug amount in the body or the blood drug concentration to decrease by one half (50%). It indicates how fast the drug is eliminated from the body. When drug elimination follows zero-order kinetics, the rate of drug elimination is constant, that is, constant amount of the drug is eliminated per unit time. After administration of 100 mg of the drug as a single IV bolus dose, the time required for the 100 mg to decrease to 50 mg ($t_{1/2}$) is different from the time required for the 50 mg to decrease to 25 mg ($t_{1/2}$) and both are different from the time required for the 25 mg to decrease to 12.5 mg ($t_{1/2}$). This means that the $t_{1/2}$ for drugs that are eliminated by zero-order processes depends on the amount (and the concentration) of the drug, as presented in Figure 5.3.

The $t_{1/2}$ is the time required for the amount of the drug in the body (A) to decrease to 50% of its value. Substituting this information in the general form of Equation 5.2,

$$0.5A = A - K_o t_{1/2} \tag{5.3}$$

Solving Equation 5.3 for the half-life yields,

$$t_{1/2} = \frac{0.5A}{K_o} \tag{5.4}$$

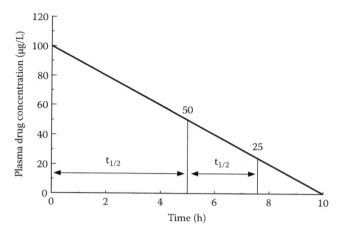

FIGURE 5.3 Half-life of the drugs eliminated by zero-order processes is dependent on the drug concentration.

This indicates that the $t_{1/2}$, when the elimination process follows zero-order kinetics, is proportional to the drug amount (A) or drug concentration and is inversely proportional to the zero-order elimination rate constant K_o. So the $t_{1/2}$ for the drug is longer when the amount of the drug in the body is large. This is important during the clinical use of drugs that are eliminated by zero-order process since an overdose of these drugs will produce high drug concentrations that will lead to long half-life and very slow rate of decline in the amount of the drug in the body.

Example

In the example presented in Figure 5.2, the zero-order rate constant for drug decomposition was calculated to be 36.6 mg/h. Calculate the $t_{1/2}$ for the decomposition process when the amount of the drug is 500 mg and when the amount of the drug is 300 mg.

Answer

Substitute in Equation 5.4 to calculate $t_{1/2}$.
    When the amount is 500 mg,

$$t_{1/2} = \frac{0.5A}{K_o} = \frac{0.5 \times 500\,mg}{36.6\,mg/h} = 6.8h$$

When the amount is 300 mg,

$$t_{1/2} = \frac{0.5A}{K_o} = \frac{0.5 \times 300\,mg}{36.6\,mg/h} = 4.1h$$

The half-life is longer when the amount of the drug is larger.

5.4   DRUG ELIMINATION BY FIRST-ORDER PROCESS

In first-order elimination, the metabolic and excretory systems have high capacity compared to the amount or the concentration of the drug in the body. Based on the probability theorem, the amount of the drug that can come in contact with the elimination mechanisms is proportional to the total amount of the drug available for elimination, that is, the rate of elimination is proportional to the amount of the drug in the body. There are factors that can help some drugs to get in contact with the elimination systems and possibly hinder other drugs from getting in contact with the elimination systems such as drug lipophilicity, protein binding, and the affinity of drug to the elimination mechanism. So the rate of drug elimination is usually different for different drugs. However, for a given drug in a specific patient, the rate of elimination of the drug is proportional to the amount of the drug in the body, when the elimination follows first-order kinetics. The elimination of the majority of the drugs used clinically follows first-order kinetics.

5.4.1   DETERMINATION OF THE FIRST-ORDER ELIMINATION RATE CONSTANT

In first-order elimination, the rate of drug elimination at any time is the product of the elimination rate constant (k) and the amount of the drug in the body (A). When the drug elimination process follows first-order kinetics, the rate of change of the amount of drug in the body (dA/dt) can be expressed as

$$\frac{dA}{dt} = -kA \tag{5.5}$$

where k is the first-order elimination rate constant and the negative sign is because the amount of the drug in the body decreases with time due to drug elimination. The rate of drug elimination decreases with time because of the decrease in drug amount in the body. Plotting the amount of drug in the body versus time on the Cartesian scale gives a curve with decreasing slope as shown in Figure 5.4.

Equation 5.5 is a differential equation that describes the rate of change of the amount of the drug in the body with time. The integration of Equation 5.5 with respect to time from time = 0 to ∞ yields Equation 5.6:

$$\ln A = \ln A_0 - kt \tag{5.6}$$

where
   $\ln A$ is the natural logarithm of the amount of the drug at any time t
   $\ln A_0$ is the natural logarithm of the initial drug amount in the body that is equal
      to the dose after an IV bolus administration
   k is the first-order elimination rate constant

The first-order elimination rate constant, k, is the overall rate constant for the elimination process that may occur by more than one first-order elimination pathways.

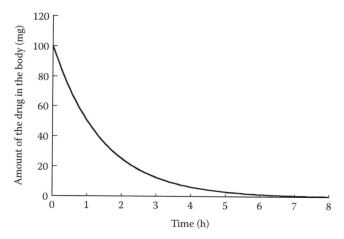

FIGURE 5.4 Plot of the amount of the drug versus time on the Cartesian scale when the elimination of the drug follows first-order kinetics.

Equation 5.6 is an equation in the form of the straight-line equation and describes a linear relationship between ln A and time. A plot of ln A versus time on the Cartesian scale yields a straight line. The y-intercept is equal to ln A_o and the slope is $-k$ as shown in Figure 5.5. Since ln A = 2.303 log A, Equation 5.6 can be expressed as

$$\log A = \log A_o - \frac{kt}{2.303} \tag{5.7}$$

Equation 5.7 describes a linear relationship between log A and time. A plot of log A versus time on the Cartesian scale yields a straight line. The y-intercept is

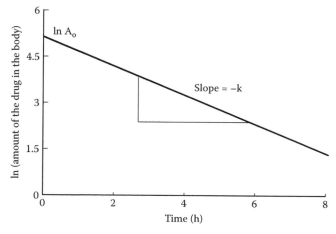

FIGURE 5.5 Plot of the natural logarithm of the amount of the drug versus time on the Cartesian scale when the elimination of the drug follows first-order kinetics.

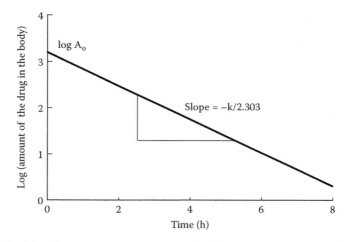

FIGURE 5.6 Plot of the logarithm of the amount of the drug versus time on the Cartesian scale when the elimination of the drug follows first-order kinetics.

equal to log A_0 and the slope is $-k/2.303$ as in Figure 5.6. Taking the anti ln of Equation 5.6 yields the following equation:

$$A = A_0 e^{-kt} \tag{5.8}$$

This is an exponential expression (nonlinear) that describes the change in the amount of the drug in the body with time. Plotting the amount of drug in the body versus time on the Cartesian scale gives an exponentially decreasing profile as in Figure 5.4, while a plot on the semilog scale gives a straight line. For A versus time plot on the semilog scale, the y-intercept is equal to A_0 and the slope is $-k/2.303$ as in Figure 5.7.

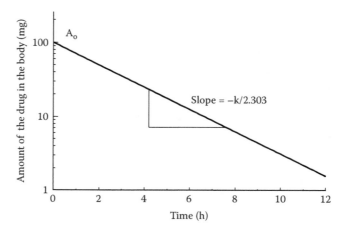

FIGURE 5.7 Plot of the amount of the drug versus time on the semilog scale when the elimination of the drug follows first-order kinetics.

In practice, determination of the plasma drug concentration is much easier than determination of the amount of the drug in the body. So dividing Equations 5.6 through 5.8 by Vd gives three similar equations that describe the change in drug concentration with time as follows:

$$\ln Cp = \ln Cp_o - kt \tag{5.9}$$

$$\log Cp = \log Cp_o - \frac{kt}{2.303} \tag{5.10}$$

$$Cp = Cp_o e^{-kt} \tag{5.11}$$

The equations that describe the change in the amount of the drug in the body with time or the change in the plasma drug concentration with time have two different parameters, the first-order elimination rate constant and the initial drug amount or concentration. The first-order elimination rate constant, k, influences the rate of decline in the drug amount-time profile and the drug concentration–time profile. Larger values of k indicate steeper decline in the plasma drug concentration, which indicates faster rate of drug elimination as in Figure 5.8. The other parameter in the equations is the initial amount of the drug in the body that is equal to the dose after IV bolus administration or the initial plasma drug concentration that is equal to dose/Vd.

After IV bolus administration, k can be determined by obtaining serial plasma samples and determination of the drug concentration in these samples. A plot of ln Cp versus time on the Cartesian scale is a straight line with slope equal to −k. Also, a plot of log Cp versus time on the Cartesian scale is a straight line with slope equal to −k/2.303. Moreover, a plot of Cp versus time on the semilog scale is a straight line with slope equal to −k/2.303. Since the drug concentration–time profile after a single IV bolus dose is decreasing, it always has a negative slope. This negative slope is equal

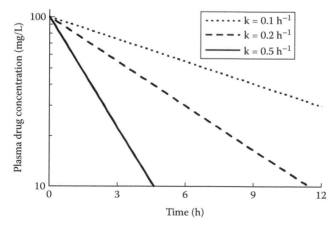

FIGURE 5.8 Drugs with larger first-order elimination rate constants are eliminated at faster rate.

to $-k$ or $-k/2.303$, depending on the plot used, and so the first-order elimination rate constant will always have a positive value and has units of time^{-1}.

Example

After a single IV bolus drug administration of a drug that is eliminated by first-order process, serial plasma samples were obtained and the concentrations are as follows:

Time (h)	Drug Concentration (mg/L)
1	310
3	200
6	125
8	80
12	40

Using a graphical method, calculate the elimination rate constant of this drug.

Answer

Plot the plasma drug concentrations on the semilog scale as in Figure 5.9 and calculate the slope.

$$\text{The slope on the semilog scale} \ = \frac{\log y_2 - \log y_1}{X_2 - X_1} = -0.08\,h^{-1}$$

$$\text{Slope} = -0.08 = \frac{-k}{2.303}$$

So $k = 0.184\,h^{-1}$.

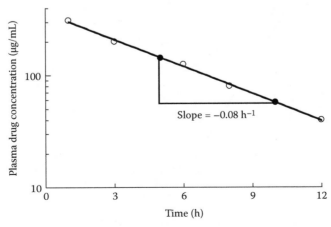

FIGURE 5.9   Plot of the plasma drug concentration versus time on the semilog scale.

5.4.2 DETERMINATION OF THE HALF-LIFE IN FIRST-ORDER DRUG ELIMINATION

The half-life is the time required for the drug amount or plasma drug concentration to decrease by 50%. Substituting this information in Equation 5.11 that describes the concentrations of the drug at any time gives the following equation:

$$0.5Cp_o = Cp_o e^{-kt_{1/2}} \tag{5.12}$$

Taking the natural logarithm of both sides of the Equation 5.12,

$$\ln 0.5 = -kt_{1/2} \tag{5.13}$$

By rearrangement,

$$t_{1/2} = \frac{0.693}{k} \tag{5.14}$$

When the drug elimination process follows first-order kinetics, the $t_{1/2}$ of the drug is constant and is related to k. In other words, the time required for the drug plasma concentration to decrease from 100 to 50 µg/L is the same as the time required for the plasma drug concentration to decrease from 15 to 7.5 µg/L as illustrated in Figure 5.10.

The $t_{1/2}$ can be determined graphically from the plasma drug concentrations after a single IV bolus dose of the drug. Serial plasma samples are obtained at several time points after IV bolus drug administration and samples are analyzed for the drug

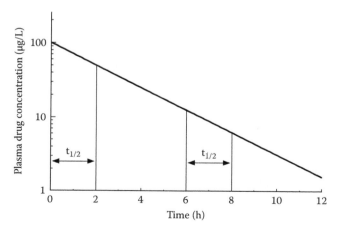

FIGURE 5.10 Half-life of the drug is independent on the drug concentration when the drug elimination process follows first-order kinetics.

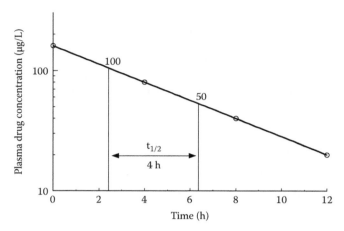

FIGURE 5.11   Graphical determination of the half-life.

concentration. The plasma drug concentrations are plotted versus time on a semilog graph paper and the best line that goes through the samples is drawn. Starting at any point on the line, the time required for the y-coordinate of this point to decrease by 50% is determined and it is equal to the $t_{1/2}$, as in Figure 5.11.

5.4.3   Mathematical Expressions That Describe the Plasma Drug Concentrations after a Single IV Bolus Dose When the Elimination Process Follows First-Order Kinetics

Equations 5.9 through 5.11 describe the time course for the plasma drug concentration after a single IV bolus dose when the elimination process follows first-order kinetics. These equations can be written in a more general form:

$$\ln Cp_2 = \ln Cp_1 - kt \tag{5.15}$$

$$\log Cp_2 = \log Cp_1 - \frac{kt}{2.303} \tag{5.16}$$

$$Cp_2 = Cp_1 e^{-kt} \tag{5.17}$$

where
   Cp_1 and Cp_2 are the plasma drug concentrations at two different time points, with
      time difference equal to t
   k is the first-order elimination rate constant

These three equations can be used in calculating useful pharmacokinetic information. Similar equations can be written in this general form to describe the time course of the drug amount in the body after administration of a single IV dose of the drug.

Example

Ampicillin is an antibiotic that is eliminated from the body by first-order process. The aforementioned mathematical expressions can be used to solve the following four questions:

a. Calculate the amount of ampicillin remaining in the body 6 h after IV administration of a single dose of 500 mg if the first-order elimination rate constant for ampicillin is 0.53 h^{-1}.

Answer

$$A_2 = A_1 e^{-kt}$$

$$\text{Amount remaining} = 500\,\text{mg}\ e^{-0.53h^{-1} 6h} = 20.8\,\text{mg}$$

b. Calculate ampicillin first-order elimination rate constant if the amount of ampicillin remaining in the body 6 h after administration of a single IV dose of 500 mg is 20.8 mg.

Answer

$$A_2 = A_1 e^{-kt}$$

$$20.8\,\text{mg} = 500\,\text{mg}\ e^{-k6h}$$

$$\frac{20.8\,\text{mg}}{500\,\text{mg}} = e^{-k6h}$$

$$\ln\frac{20.8}{500} = \ln e^{-k6h}$$

$$-3.179 = -k6h$$

$$k = 0.53h^{-1}$$

c. Calculate the time required for the amount of ampicillin in the body to decrease to 20.8 mg after IV administration of a single dose of 500 mg if the first-order elimination rate constant is 0.53 h^{-1}.

Answer

$$A_2 = A_1 e^{-kt}$$

$$20.8\,\text{mg} = 500\,\text{mg}\ e^{-0.53h^{-1}t}$$

You can solve for t, which will be 6 h.

d. Calculate the IV bolus dose of ampicillin administered if the amount of ampicillin remaining in the body after 6 h is 20.8 mg, and the first-order elimination rate constant of ampicillin is 0.53 h^{-1}.

Answer

$$A_2 = A_1 e^{-kt}$$

$$20.8 \text{ mg} = A_1 e^{-0.53 h^{-1} 6h}$$

You can solve for A_1, which will be 500 mg.

In this example, an equation in the general form of Equation 5.8 was used to solve these questions, however equations in the general form of Equations 5.6 and 5.7 can also be used to solve the questions.

5.4.4 RELATIONSHIP BETWEEN THE FIRST-ORDER ELIMINATION RATE CONSTANT, TOTAL BODY CLEARANCE, AND VOLUME OF DISTRIBUTION

The rate of drug elimination if the elimination process follows first-order kinetics is the product of the first-order elimination rate constant, k, and the amount of the drug in the body, A, as presented in Equation 5.18:

$$\text{Drug elimination rate} = kA \tag{5.18}$$

Since the amount of the drug in the body is the product of the plasma drug concentration and Vd,

$$\text{Drug elimination rate} = kCpVd \tag{5.19}$$

Rearrangement of Equation 5.19:

$$\frac{\text{Drug elimination rate}}{Cp} = kVd \tag{5.20}$$

$$\frac{CL_T}{Vd} = k \tag{5.21}$$

Equation 5.21 describes the relationship between the CL_T, Vd, and k. The first-order elimination rate constant is dependent on both CL_T and Vd. As discussed previously, the CL_T and the Vd are independent pharmacokinetic parameters, and k is the dependent pharmacokinetic parameter. This is despite the fact that the CL_T is usually calculated from the product of k and Vd.

5.5   AREA UNDER THE DRUG CONCENTRATION–TIME CURVE

The area under the drug concentration–time curve (AUC) is obtained by integrating the equation that describes the plasma drug concentration with respect to time from time zero to time infinity. It has units of mass-time/volume:

$$\int_{t=0}^{t=\infty} Cp\,dt = AUC \tag{5.22}$$

Integrating Equation 5.11 that describes the plasma drug concentration–time profile after administration of a single IV bolus dose when the drug is eliminated by first-order process yields the value of the AUC after a single IV bolus dose:

$$AUC\Big|_{t=0}^{t=\infty} = \int_{t=0}^{t=\infty} Cp_0 e^{-kt}\, dt \tag{5.23}$$

$$AUC\Big|_{t=0}^{t=\infty} = \frac{Cp_0}{k} \tag{5.24}$$

So the AUC can be calculated after a single IV bolus dose from the initial plasma drug concentration and the first-order elimination rate constant. Since Cp_0 is equal to the dose/Vd, the AUC after administration of a single IV dose can be expressed as

$$AUC\Big|_{t=0}^{t=\infty} = \frac{Dose}{kVd} = \frac{Dose}{CL_T} \tag{5.25}$$

Based on Equation 5.25 the AUC after administration of a single IV bolus dose is directly proportional to the administered dose as in Figure 5.12 and is inversely proportional to the CL_T as in Figure 5.13. Patients with different degrees of eliminating organ dysfunction have different clearance values for the same drug. Patients with

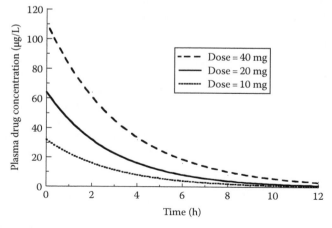

FIGURE 5.12   Area under the plasma concentration–time curve is proportional to the administered IV dose.

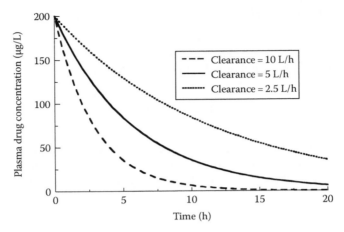

FIGURE 5.13   Area under the plasma concentration–time curve is inversely proportional to the total body clearance if the same IV dose is administered.

severe dysfunction usually have lower clearance while those with normal function have higher clearance. So after administration of the same IV dose, higher AUC is observed in the patients with lower clearance and lower AUC in patients with higher clearance as illustrated in Figure 5.13. So the AUC can be used to determine and compare the clearance of the same drug in different patients. Also, the AUC can be used to compare the clearances of different drugs in the same patients. Drugs with smaller clearance produce higher AUC while those with higher clearance produce smaller AUC if the same dose is administered. Furthermore, the calculated AUC after different routes of drug administration can be used to compare the amount of the drug that reaches the systemic circulation to calculate the drug bioavailability, a concept that will be discussed in detail in Chapter 10.

5.6   CALCULATION OF PHARMACOKINETIC PARAMETERS AFTER A SINGLE IV BOLUS DOSE

Serial plasma samples after IV drug administration are required to calculate the drug pharmacokinetic parameters. Samples are analyzed and the measured concentrations are plotted versus the corresponding time for each sample on the semilog scale. The best fitted line is drawn and is back extrapolated to the y-axis. The slope of the line is calculated and the y-intercept that represents the initial drug concentration (Cp_o) is determined.

- The elimination rate constant is calculated from the slope of the best fitted line. The slope of the drug concentration–time plot on the semilog scale is equal to $-k/2.303$.
- The $t_{1/2}$ of the drug is determined from k ($t_{1/2} = 0.693/k$). Also, the $t_{1/2}$ can be determined from the graph by finding the time required for any plasma drug concentration to decrease by 50%.
- The Vd is calculated from the dose and the initial drug concentration ($Vd = Dose/Cp_o$).

- The CL_T is calculated from k and Vd ($CL_T = k \times Vd$).
- The AUC is calculated from Cp_o/k. This method can be used only for the calculation of the AUC after a single IV bolus dose. The trapezoidal rule that is a more general method for calculation of the AUC after all routes of administration will be discussed in Chapter 10.

Example

After IV bolus administration of 1000 mg amoxicillin, the following plasma concentrations were obtained:

Time (h)	Concentration (mg/L)
0	72
1	45
3	18
5	7.1
7	2.8

a. Using a graphical method, calculate Vd, $t_{1/2}$, k, CL_T, and AUC of amoxicillin.

Answer

- Plot the plasma concentrations of amoxicillin versus time on a semilog graph paper.
- Draw the best line that goes through the plasma concentrations and back extrapolate the line to the y-axis.

a. From Figure 5.14, the Cpo = 72 mg/L

$$Vd = \frac{Dose}{Cp_o} = \frac{1000\,mg}{72\,mg/L} = 13.89\,L$$

The half-life is determined by taking any drug concentration (e.g., 38 mg/L) and calculating the time required for this concentration to decrease by 50%. From Figure 5.14, the half-life is 1.5 h.

$$k = \frac{0.693}{t_{1/2}} = \frac{0.693}{1.5\,h} = 0.462\,h^{-1}$$

Note that it is possible to calculate the elimination rate constant k from the slope of the line (slope = $-k/2.303$). Then the half-life is calculated from k:

$$CL_T = kVd = 0.462\,h^{-1} \times 13.89\,L = 6.417\,L/h$$

$$AUC = \frac{Cp_0}{k} = \frac{72\,mg/L}{0.462\,h^{-1}} = 155.8\,mg\,h/L$$

or

$$AUC = \frac{Dose}{CL_T} = \frac{1000\,mg}{6.417\,L/h} = 155.8\,mg\,h/L$$

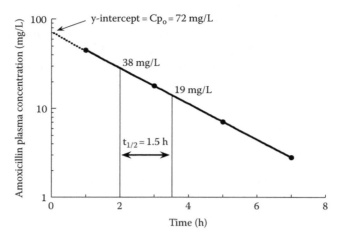

FIGURE 5.14 Plot of the plasma concentration–time curve.

5.7 CLINICAL IMPORTANCE OF THE ELIMINATION RATE CONSTANT AND HALF-LIFE

Drugs that have larger k have shorter $t_{1/2}$ based on the relationship between these two parameters as described by Equation 5.14. These drugs are eliminated from the body much faster than the drugs with smaller k and longer $t_{1/2}$. Drugs that are eliminated rapidly from the body have shorter duration of effect after a single-dose administration, because the drug concentration in the body falls below the effective concentration very quickly. During multiple administrations, drugs that are eliminated rapidly from the body will need to be given more frequently to maintain effective drug level in the body, while slowly eliminated drugs should be given less frequently. For example, penicillin G is eliminated from the body very fast, so it is usually administered every 4–6 h, while a drug like digoxin that is eliminated slowly from the body is usually administered once every day.

Patients with eliminating organ dysfunction usually eliminate the drug at slower rate compared to patients with normal eliminating organ function as illustrated in Figure 5.15. The $t_{1/2}$ is longer and k is smaller in patients with eliminating organ dysfunction. So the dosage requirement for patients with eliminating organ dysfunction is smaller than patients with normal function. Patients with eliminating organ dysfunction can also receive the doses of the drug less frequently compared to the patients with normal function. For example, the half-life of the aminoglycoside antibiotics is much longer in patients with kidney failure compared to patients with normal kidney function. So the dosage requirement from these antibiotics is much smaller in renal failure patients compared with patients with normal kidney function. Also, renal failure patients usually receive the aminoglycoside doses at longer dosing intervals. This is because the aminoglycoside antibiotics are eliminated mainly by the kidney, and the decrease in kidney function slows the rate of their elimination.

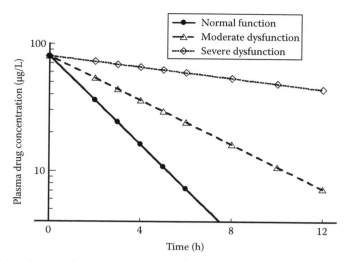

FIGURE 5.15 Plasma drug concentration–time profile in patients with different degree of eliminating organ dysfunction. Patients with eliminating organ dysfunction eliminate the drug at slower rate compared to patients with normal organ function.

5.8 FACTORS AFFECTING THE PLASMA DRUG CONCENTRATION– TIME PROFILE AFTER A SINGLE IV BOLUS DOSE

After a single IV bolus drug administration, the initial drug concentration depends on the dose and Vd of the drug. If the elimination process follows first-order kinetics, the plasma drug concentration–time profile declines at a rate dependent on k. The time course of the therapeutic effect of the drug including the intensity and duration of effect is related to the plasma drug concentration–time profile. For most drugs, there is a range of plasma drug concentrations that is associated with the optimal drug effect. Above this range there is a higher chance of developing toxicity and below this range the drug may not be effective. Changes in the drug concentration–time profile are usually reflected in the therapeutic effect of the drug. So it is important to examine how the change in each of the pharmacokinetic parameters affects the drug concentration–time profile. The plotting excercise of the IV bolus administration module in the basic pharmacokinetic concept section and the pharmacokinetic simulations section of the companion CD to this textbook can be used to run these simulations. Pharmacokinetic simulations can be very useful for this purpose, and the companion CD that comes with this textbook can be used to run these simulations.

5.8.1 Pharmacokinetic Simulation Exercise

Pharmacokinetic simulations can be used to examine how each of the parameters included in the equation that describes the drug concentration–time profile after a single IV bolus dose affects the drug profile. The parameters are changed one at a time while keeping all the other parameters constant, and the drug concentration–time profile is simulated. The resulting drug plasma concentration–time profile is examined to see how the change in the pharmacokinetic parameter affects the drug profile.

5.8.1.1 Dose

Administration of increasing doses of the drug in the same individual produces higher Cp_0 and higher AUC; however, changing the dose does not affect k, Vd, or CL_T if the elimination follows first-order kinetics. Higher doses may achieve high plasma drug concentration and increase the chance of developing toxicity, while lower doses achieve low initial drug concentrations that may not be adequate to produce therapeutic effect. Also, after administration of larger doses of the drug, the drug concentrations stay above the minimum concentration required for producing the effect for a longer period of time, resulting in longer duration of drug effect.

5.8.1.2 Volume of Distribution

Administration of the same dose of the same drug to a group of patients who have different Vd, for example, patients with different body weight, results in lower Cp_0 in the patients with larger Vd and higher Cp_0 in patients with smaller Vd. The rate of decline in the drug concentration–time profile depends on k. If the CL_T is similar in a group of patients who have different Vd, patients with smaller Vd have faster rate of drug elimination (larger k and shorter $t_{1/2}$), while patients with larger Vd have slower rate of drug elimination (smaller k and longer $t_{1/2}$). This is because k and $t_{1/2}$ depend on both CL_T and Vd. The AUC will not be affected by the change in Vd only. This is because AUC is dependent on the dose and CL_T. The change in Vd does not affect CL_T since Vd and CL_T are the independent pharmacokinetic parameters.

5.8.1.3 Total Body Clearance

Administration of the same dose of a drug to a group of patients who have different CL_T, for example, patients with different eliminating organ function, results in different rates of decline in the drug concentration–time profile if their Vd is similar. Assuming similar Vd, patients with higher CL_T have faster rate of drug elimination (larger k and shorter $t_{1/2}$), while patients with lower CL_T have slower rate of drug elimination (smaller k and longer $t_{1/2}$). This is because k and $t_{1/2}$ are dependent on both CL_T and Vd. The AUC will be smaller in patients with higher CL_T and larger in patients with lower CL_T. This is because the AUC is dependent on the dose and CL_T. Administration of the same dose of the same drug to a group of patients who have different CL_T will produce the same Cp_0 since the initial drug concentration is dependent on the dose and Vd. The change in CL_T does not affect Vd since the Vd and CL_T are independent pharmacokinetic parameters.

5.9 SUMMARY

- The first-order elimination rate constant is the rate constant for the elimination of the drug from the body, and $t_{1/2}$ is the time required to eliminate 50% of the drug in the body. Both parameters reflect the rate of drug elimination through all routes of drug elimination and determine how fast the drug is eliminated from the body.
- The first-order elimination rate constant and $t_{1/2}$ are dependent on the CL_T and Vd of the drug, the two independent pharmacokinetic parameters.

- The elimination rate constant and $t_{1/2}$ of the drug are constant within a patient (dose and concentration independent) when the drug elimination process follows first-order kinetics. However, different patients may have different k and $t_{1/2}$ for the same drug.

PRACTICE PROBLEMS

5.1 Two different drugs were administered to the same individual in different doses on different occasions, and the half-lives were calculated after each drug administration.

	Drug A	Drug B
Dose (mg)	Half-Life (h)	Half-Life (h)
40	6	4
60	6	6
80	6	8

a. Which of the two drugs is eliminated by first-order process? Why?
b. Calculate the elimination rate constant for the drug that is eliminated by first-order process.
c. Describe how the rate of elimination, the elimination rate constant, and the half-life change with the change in dose for both drugs.

5.2 A single 400 mg IV bolus dose of an antibiotic was administered to a patient. The amount of the drug determined at different times after drug administration is as follows:

Time (h)	Amount (mg)
0	400
2	378
4	356
8	312
12	268
18	202
24	136

a. Does the elimination process follow zero-order or first-order kinetics?
b. What is the rate constant for the elimination process?
c. What is the half-life of the drug immediately after drug administration?
d. What is the rate constant for the elimination process if the dose was 600 mg?
e. What is the amount of the drug in the body 20 h after drug administration?
f. What is the amount of the drug in the body 40 h after drug administration?

5.3 A single IV bolus dose of a drug was administered to a patient and the amount of the drug in the body was determined at different time points after drug administration.

Time (h)	Amount (mg)
0.5	396
1	315
2	198
4	79
8	12.4
12	1.96

a. What is the order of the elimination process of this drug?
b. What is the rate constant for the elimination process?
c. What is the dose of the drug administered to this patient?
d. What is the equation that describes the amount of the drug-time profile in the body?
e. Calculate the amount of drug in the body 10h after administration.
f. What is the half-life of the drug immediately after drug administration?

5.4 A single 1000 mg IV bolus dose of an antibiotic that is eliminated by first-order process was administered to a patient and the following blood concentrations were obtained:

Time (h)	Blood Concentration (mg/L)
0	33.3
1	26.5
2	21.0
4	13.2
6	8.33
8	5.25
12	2.08

a. Graphically estimate $t_{1/2}$, k, Vd, and CL_T.
b. Calculate the AUC after administration of the 1000 mg.
c. What is the initial drug concentration Cp_0, $t_{1/2}$, k, Vd, CL_T, and AUC if the administered dose was only 500 mg?
d. What is the dose required to achieve Cp_0 of 50 mg/L?

5.5 The following blood concentrations were measured after administration of a single 200 mg IV bolus dose of a drug that is eliminated by first-order process:

Time (h)	Blood Concentration (mg/L)
1	1.85
2	0.858
3	0.397
4	0.184
6	0.039

    a. Graphically estimate $t_{1/2}$, k, Vd, CL_T, and AUC.

    b. Calculate mathematically and graphically the time when the blood drug concentration is exactly 0.5 mg/L.

    c. What is the initial drug concentration Cp_0, $t_{1/2}$, k, Vd, CL_T, and AUC if the administered dose was only 400 mg?

    d. Calculate mathematically the drug blood concentration after 10 h of drug administration.

5.6 Draw the line that represents the following plasma concentration–time relationship on the semilog scale.

$$Cp = 25e^{-0.099t}$$

5.7 After administration of a single 400 mg IV bolus dose of a drug a plot of the blood concentration–time profile on semilog graph paper is linear with slope of $-0.1\,h^{-1}$ and y-intercept of 1 mg/L.

    a. Calculate $t_{1/2}$, k, Vd, CL_T, and AUC for this drug.

    b. What is the slope and y-intercept if the dose was 1000 mg?

    c. What is the length of time required for the initial drug concentration to decrease to 0.25 mg/L after administration of the 400 mg dose?

    d. What is the smallest dose required to achieve blood drug concentration above 1 mg/L for 6 h after drug administration?

5.8 A single IV bolus dose of 5 mg/kg was administered to a patient. A semilog plot of the plasma concentration–time profile was linear with y-intercept of 10 mg/L and a slope of $-0.06\,h^{-1}$.

    a. Calculate $t_{1/2}$, k, Vd, CL_T, and AUC for this drug.

    b. What is the slope and y-intercept if the dose was 20 mg/kg?

    c. What is the length of time required for the initial drug concentration to decrease to 1 mg/L after administration of 5 mg/kg?

    d. What is the dose required to achieve blood drug concentration above 1 mg/L for 12 h after drug administration?

5.9 The following are the pharmacokinetic parameters for a group of drugs:

Drug	Vd (L/kg)	Elimination Rate Constant (h)
Theophylline	0.45	0.11
Ampicillin	0.3	0.6
Quinidine	3	0.08
Propranolol	5	0.15
Procainamide	2	0.23
Lidocaine	1.3	0.4

    a. Which drug has the fastest elimination rate after IV administration of the same dose? Why?

    b. Which drug will produce the highest initial drug concentration if the same doses of the drugs are administered by IV bolus dose? Why?

    c. Which drug has the highest CL_T? Why?

    d. Which drug will require the highest dose to achieve Cp_0 of $15\,\mu g/L$? Why?

    e. Which drug will require frequent administration (larger number of doses every day) to maintain the drug concentration in the therapeutic range all the time? Why?

5.10 A patient received a single 600 mg IV bolus dose of a drug that is eliminated mainly by first-order excretion through the kidney. Two weeks later the patient developed acute kidney disease, he received another 600 mg IV bolus dose of the same drug. The following drug concentrations were obtained after administration of the drug before and after developing the renal disease:

	Drug Concentration (mg/L)	
Time (h)	Before Renal Disease	After Renal Disease
1	21.2	25.5
2	15.0	21.2
4	7.5	15.0
6	3.75	10.6
8	1.88	7.5
12	0.469	3.75

    a. Calculate the $t_{1/2}$, k, Vd, CL_T, and AUC for this drug before and after developing the renal disease.

    b. Explain the differences in the pharmacokinetic parameters in the two occasions.

5.11 A single 800 mg dose of a drug was given by IV bolus administration and the plasma concentrations were determined. A plot of the plasma concentration–time profile was linear on a semilog graph paper. The y-intercept of the plot was 20 mg/L and the slope of the line was $-0.043\,h^{-1}$.

    a. Calculate the $t_{1/2}$, k, Vd, CL_T, and AUC for this drug.

    b. Calculate the blood drug concentration 14 h after drug administration.

    c. What is the slope of the plasma concentration–time profile on semilog scale if a dose of 400 mg was given by IV bolus?

    d. Calculate the initial plasma concentration if the dose of this drug was 400 mg IV bolus.

5.12 A general anesthetic has a volume of distribution of 15 L and a minimum effective concentration of $2\,\mu g/mL$ (the drug is effective as long as the drug concentration is above $2\,\mu g/mL$). After administration of 120 mg of the drug as an IV bolus dose to a patient the drug produced anesthetic effect for 6 h.

    a. Calculate the half-life of this drug.

    b. Calculate the minimum effective concentration for the drug if the dose was 400 mg.

    c. Calculate the expected duration of effect if an IV bolus dose of 240 mg was administered.

    d. Calculate the lowest dose that will produce an effect for 3 h.

    e. Calculate the expected duration of effect if 20 mg was given as an IV bolus dose.

6 Drug Absorption Following Extravascular Administration

Biological, Physiological, and Pathological Considerations

OBJECTIVES

After completing this chapter you should be able to

- Describe the basic structure features of the cell membrane
- Discuss and differentiate between the general mechanisms of drug absorption
- Describe the different physiological and anatomical futures of the different components of the gastrointestinal tract that can affect the drug absorption
- Discuss the general anatomical and physiological characteristics that can affect drug absorption from the nasal cavity, the pulmonary system, and the skin
- Describe the advantages and disadvantages of the buccal, oral, colonic, rectal, nasal, pulmonary, and transdermal drug delivery system

6.1 INTRODUCTION

Drugs are usually administered for their local effect at the site of administration or for their systemic effects at one or more sites remote from their site of administration. Locally acting drugs are applied directly at their intended site of effect, so they exert their effect without the need for transfer to different parts of the body. However, drugs used for their systemic effects have to be absorbed from their site of administration to the systemic circulation where they are distributed to all parts of the body including their site of action. Studying the kinetics of drug absorption from the site of administration is important since the rate and extent of drug absorption have direct effect on the drug concentration–time profile in the body and, hence, the drug effect-time profile. Drug absorption is also important for locally acting drugs since the drug may be absorbed from its site of application producing undesirable systemic effects.

Drugs are usually administered by parenteral, enteral, topical application to a tissue or body space, in addition to specialized routes of administration such as inhalation, intranasal, and transdermal. Except for intravenous (IV) and intra-arterial administration where the drugs are directly introduced into the vascular space, drugs administered for their systemic effects have to be absorbed to the systemic circulation to produce their effects. Absorbed drugs are distributed via the systemic circulation to all parts of the body including their site of effect. The choice of the route of administration usually depends on many factors including the drug characteristics, drug product properties, the physiological characteristics of each site of administration, and the condition being treated. For example, many drugs are administered by the parenteral route because they cannot be absorbed after oral administration due to their inability to cross the biological membrane, or instability in the gastrointestinal (GIT) secretions. Also, drugs used to treat emergency cases are usually administered via the parenteral route to produce rapid effect. Furthermore, orally administered drugs that are extensively metabolized during their first-pass through the liver can be administered rectally or sublingually to bypass this first-pass metabolism.

There are many factors that can affect the rate and extent of drug absorption which include the anatomical, biological, physiological, and pathological characteristics of the different sites of drug administration. Also, drug properties including its physicochemical nature, solid sate characteristics, and chemical stability can affect the drug ability to overcome the biological barrier for drug absorption from the site of administration. Furthermore, drug products are usually designed to control the rate of drug release from the dosage form after administration, which can affect the rate and extent of drug absorption. This chapter will focus on the physiological factors which can affect the drug absorption process, while the following two chapters will cover the drug properties and drug product characteristics that affect the drug absorption process.

6.2   CELL MEMBRANE

The cells of an organ are individually functioning units surrounded by the cell membrane which physically separates the intracellular components from the extracellular environment. The cell membrane is selectively permeable to control the transport of substances to and from the cell. It contains a wide variety of molecules mainly lipids and proteins that are involved in different cellular processes such as cell adhesion, ion channel conductance, and cell signaling. Tissues and organs are made of groups of cells surrounded by a specialized cell structures called epithelia, which can be viewed as the organ's "outer membrane." In addition to holding the organ together, the epithelia have a wide variety of functions including transport, barrier, and secretory processes depending on the organ. The most important challenges in the drug delivery process are to overcome the absorption barriers, represented by the biological membranes, and to allow drug transport from the site of administration until it reaches its site of action. While doing so, the drug has to pass through a number of membranes, epithelia, and tissues. Understanding the structure and function of the cell membranes and epithelial tissues is very important in determining the factors affecting the drug absorption process and in developing strategies to overcome these absorption barriers.

6.2.1 STRUCTURE OF THE CELL MEMBRANE

The main structure feature of the cell membrane is a lipid bilayer consisting of amphipathic lipids, mainly phospholipids and other molecules such as glycolipids and steroids. Phospholipids are compounds in which two of the hydroxyl groups of glycerol are esterified with fatty acids and the third to phosphoric acid. The phosphate groups are joined with small hydrophilic organic groups such as choline, ethanolamine, inositol, and serine. The phospholipids have two very lipophilic tails and a hydrophilic region around the phosphate ester. The lipid bilayer components are arranged as a bilayer sheet in which the lipophilic tails are in the center of the membrane and hydrophilic groups are in the outer sides of the membrane. The membrane is held together by interaction of the lipophilic tails. This special arrangement prevents passage of hydrophilic molecules and allows passage of lipophilic molecules.

The bilayer components undergo continuous dynamic changes as the lipid molecules can move in the plane of the bilayer by lateral diffusion, or move from one side of the membrane to the other by transverse diffusion with the help of specialized membrane proteins. In animal cells, cholesterol is normally dispersed in varying degrees throughout cell membranes between the hydrophobic tails of the membrane lipids, where it influences the strength and rigidity of the membrane. The cell membrane contains different types of proteins and carbohydrates in addition to the lipid bilayer [1]. This includes integral proteins which contain a sequence of lipophilic groups that are embedded in the lipid bilayer, and the peripheral proteins which are surface proteins attached to the integral proteins. The integral membrane protein includes the transport proteins which are responsible for moving molecules in and out of the cell. It also includes the cell surface receptor which is the site of recognition of many hormones and mediators. Furthermore, glycoproteins are integral proteins attached to carbohydrate chain which is responsible for cell recognition and some immunological functions. Figure 6.1 represents a diagram that shows the basic structure features of the cell membrane.

6.2.2 EPITHELIA

The majority of the internal and external body surfaces are covered with epithelium. The epithelium consists of a layer of protein, normally collagen, which has one or more layers of epithelial cells on top of it. The difference in the characters of the epithelial cells depends on the tissue or the organ, and can vary from thin and permeable as in the blood vessels, thick as in the esophagus, to keratinized as in the skin. The epithelial cells have asymmetric distribution of transport proteins on the apical (outer) and the basolateral (inner) sides of the cell membrane. The cell membranes of adjacent cells in any tissue or organ are not in complete contact with each other, but have intermembrane space which is filled with the extracellular fluid. Small molecules can easily move from one site to another through this space. The cells of the

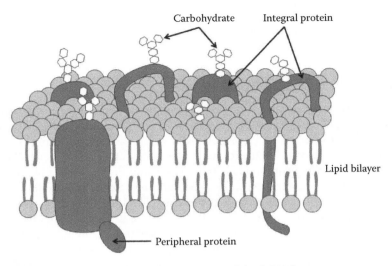

FIGURE 6.1   Diagram showing the basic structure of the lipid bilayer.

epithelial layer are bound together to form different types of junctions which act as barrier to prevent diffusion of solutes in between these cells. The cells in the epithelial layer can be bound together by special protein strands that attach the cells very closely to each other forming tight junctions that protect the interior of the tissue or organ such as in case of the blood brain barrier. Also, the gap junction is a common type of cell junction in which adjacent cells become very close and form a connection between adjacent cells allowing transfer of cytoplasm and solutes between the cells. Furthermore, desmosomes are small structures which bind adjacent cells together to enable a group of cells to function as a unit such as in cardiac muscles and skin epithelium [2].

6.3   MECHANISM OF DRUG ABSORPTION

The main function of the absorption barriers is to protect the tissues and organs from harmful compounds. In the mean time, these barriers are selectively permeable to many compounds with different properties including nutrients, vitamins, minerals, and other compounds which are useful for the normal functions of the body. These essential compounds can be absorbed by different mechanisms which can be utilized for the absorption of drugs [3,4]. Figure 6.2 includes a diagram showing the common mechanisms for drug transport across the biological membranes.

6.3.1   PASSIVE DIFFUSION

Passive diffusion is a process by which the molecules are transported from higher concentration to lower concentration with the concentration gradient. The diffusion process is called passive because it does not require energy and the driving force for the diffusion process is the concentration gradient. The rate of drug

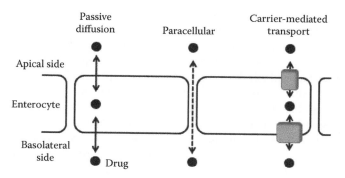

FIGURE 6.2 Common mechanisms for drug transport across biological membranes.

transport across the biological membranes can be described by Fick's law of diffusion as described in Equation 6.1:

$$\text{Rate of diffusion} = \frac{dA}{dt} = \frac{DKS}{h}(C_{abs} - C_p) \qquad (6.1)$$

where
   dA/dt is the rate of drug diffusion across the membrane
   D is the diffusion coefficient which is constant for a specific drug in a specific environment
   K is the drug partition coefficient
   S is the membrane surface area
   h is the thickness of the membrane
   $(C_{abs} - C_p)$ is the difference in the drug concentration between the absorption site and plasma, or more generally the difference in drug concentration on both sides of the membrane

After drug absorption from the site of administration it reaches the systemic circulation where it is distributed to all parts of the body. Distribution of the absorbed drug dilutes the drug concentration in the systemic circulation and makes the drug concentration in plasma very low relative to the drug concentration at the site of absorption. This will always make the drug concentration at the site of absorption much higher than the drug concentration in the plasma side, which is known as the sink condition. In this case, Fick's law can be simplified to

$$\text{Rate of diffusion} = \frac{dA}{dt} \cong \frac{DKS}{h}C_{abs} \qquad (6.2)$$

Since the parameters D, K, S, and h are constant for a specific drug when transported across a specific membrane, this equation describes first-order diffusion with the rate of diffusion proportional to the drug concentration at the site of absorption. This can also explain why the absorption of most drugs administered in the form of solution by different routes of administration follows first-order kinetics.

Examining Fick's law of diffusion allows determination of the factors affecting the rate of diffusion of a drug across the biological membrane by passive diffusion, and hence drug absorption by passive diffusion. The rate of drug absorption by passive diffusion is proportional to the increase in the drug lipid solubility, the increase in the surface area available for drug absorption, the increase in concentration gradient between the site of absorption and the plasma, and decreases with the increase in the thickness of the biological membrane. So lipophilic drugs can be absorbed by passive diffusion more than hydrophilic drugs. Also, the small intestine is the main site of absorption for orally administered drugs that are passively absorbed because of its large surface area. Furthermore, the absorption of topically administered drugs from the foot or palm is much less that the absorption from the chest or the abdomen because of the difference in the thickness of the skin.

6.3.2 CARRIER-MEDIATED TRANSPORT

Carrier molecules can be involved in the transport of drugs across the biological membrane. These carrier molecules are very specific for the transport of a particular drug or a group of drugs from one side of the membrane to the other side. The epithelial membrane is usually described as highly polarized since the distribution of the carrier molecules on the apical and lateral sides of the membrane is not the same. Since there is an infinite number of carrier molecules, the process of carrier-mediated transport is saturable. This means that the rate of drug transport increases as the drug concentration increases until it becomes constant at very high drug concentration. The rate of drug transport by a carrier-mediated system can be described by the following equation:

$$\text{Rate of transport} = \frac{J_{max}C_{abs}}{K_m + C_{abs}} \qquad (6.3)$$

where

J_{max} is the maximum rate of drug transport which is dependent on the amount of carrier molecules available

C_{abs} is the drug concentration at the absorption site

K_m is a constant that depends on the affinity of the drug to the transport carrier

At low drug concentration, when $C_{abs} \ll K_m$, Equation 6.3 is reduced to Equation 6.4 and the rate of transport becomes proportional to the drug concentration since both J_{max} and K_m are constants, which means that the drug transport follows first-order kinetics:

$$\text{Rate of transport} = \frac{J_{max}}{K_m} C \qquad (6.4)$$

While at high drug concentration, when $C_{abs} \gg K_m$, Equation 6.3 is reduced to Equation 6.5 and the rate of transport becomes constant due to saturation of the carrier, which means that the drug transport follows zero-order kinetics:

$$\text{Rate of transport} = J_{max} \qquad (6.5)$$

Carrier-mediated transport can be active transport where the drug is transported against the concentration gradient, that is, from lower to higher concentration. The active transport process requires energy. Carrier-mediated transport can also be facilitated diffusion where the drug transport is with the concentration gradient, that is, from higher concentration to lower concentration. The facilitated diffusion process does not require energy. There are specialized carriers for the transport of specific compounds such as amino acids, glucose, peptides, anions, cations, nucleosides, and others. Structurally related compounds can be transported by the same carrier system and these compounds can compete for the same carrier system. So some drugs can competitively inhibit the absorption of other drugs or compounds if they are absorbed by the same carrier system.

Drugs that are absorbed by carrier-mediated transport usually include some structure features that make them resemble endogenous compounds which are substrates for a particular transport system. The carrier-mediated absorption is more important for hydrophilic drugs. This is because if a hydrophilic drug is absorbed by a carrier, this will be its major absorption mechanisms since hydrophilic drugs are less likely to be absorbed by passive diffusion, while lipophilic drugs that are absorbed by a carrier-mediated mechanism can also be absorbed by passive diffusion because of their lipid solubility.

6.3.3 PARACELLULAR

Small drug molecules can cross the membrane via the paracellular route through the junction gap between the epithelial cells. The molecular size is the main factor determining the ability of the molecule to be absorbed by this route. The paracellular absorption is passive, meaning it does not require energy since the drug is usually absorbed from the higher concentration to the lower concentration with the concentration gradient.

6.3.4 OTHER MECHANISMS

Other mechanisms include endocytosis when a small cavity is formed on the surface of the membrane after binding of a drug molecule to a specific receptor on the surface of the membrane. This cavity which surrounds the drug molecule is gradually enclosed by membrane movement and finally taken within the cell. Pinocytosis is a type of endocytosis, which is not specific for the molecule it transports. It occurs spontaneously and brings the molecules inside the cell suspended in small amounts of the extracellular fluid within a small vesicle. Potocytosis is another type of endocytosis where drugs are transported across the cell membrane by caveolae. Phagocytosis occurs when a particle is engulfed inside the cell. First, the particle adheres to the surface of the cell, and then the cell membrane gradually extends over it until it is completely internalized to form a vacuole within the cell. Presorption is a mechanism of drug absorption from the GIT membrane that does not involve the cell membrane. During digestion, cells on the villus may be lost leaving a temporary intercellular gap that may allow large particles to enter the circulation.

6.4   PHYSIOLOGICAL FACTORS AFFECTING DRUG ABSORPTION AFTER PARENTERAL DRUG ADMINISTRATION

Parenteral administration in general involves direct introduction of the drug formulation into the body using a hypodermic needle. However, the fate of the administered drug depends on the site of drug injection. Except for the IV and intra-arterial drug administration, where the drug is directly introduced to the systemic circulation, drugs administered by all other parenteral routes of administration will have to be absorbed to the systemic circulation to exert their therapeutic effects. The rate and extent of drug absorption after parenteral administration depend on the characteristics of the site of administration. Besides IV and intra-arterial administration, drugs can be administered by intramuscular (IM) or subcutaneous (SC) injections to produce their systemic effects. Other sites of drug injections can be used to produce local effect such as the intrathecal injections used to deliver the drug to the central nervous system (CNS) and the intraarticular injections used to treat local joint conditions.

6.4.1   Intramuscular

Intramuscular administration involves injection of the drug into a muscle where the drug can mix and dissolve in the interstitial fluid. The drug can then get absorbed to the systemic circulation by the blood that perfuses the muscles. The rate of absorption after IM drug administration depends on the drug formulation and on the blood perfusion to the site of injection. Drug absorption from highly perfused sites is usually faster than the rate of absorption from poorly perfused sites.

The IM route of administration can be used to administer the drugs when the oral route is not possible, either because the patient cannot swallow the medication or the drug cannot be administered orally. The advantage of the IM route is that it is possible to administer a wide range of formulations including aqueous solution, aqueous suspension, oily solution, emulsions, oily suspension, or solid implants which can have wide range of drug release rate. The choice of the formulation usually depends on the desired rate of absorption.

6.4.2   Subcutaneous

The skin consists of three layers, an outer epidermis layer, followed by the dermis, and then a connective tissue layer. Subcutaneous drug administration involves injection of the drug into the connective tissue underneath the dermis layer. This connective tissue layer has significant interstitial fluid where the drug can distribute before it is absorbed. Drug administered via the SC route can get to the systemic circulation either by absorption directly to the blood capillaries or by the lymph capillaries which drain into the local lymph node then to the systemic circulation. The rate of drug absorption after SC administration is usually slow, providing prolonged drug effect. The intradermal drug administration involves drug administration between the epidermis and dermis layers, and it is usually used to administer vaccines. In the epidermis layer, the volume of the interstitial fluid and the blood perfusion are much lower than the site for SC drug administration which explains the slower rate of drug absorption after intradermal administration.

6.5 PHYSIOLOGICAL FACTORS AFFECTING DRUG ABSORPTION AFTER ORAL DRUG ADMINISTRATION

The major components of the GIT are the buccal cavity, esophagus, stomach, small intestine, large intestine (colon), and the rectum. These GIT segments differ from each other with respect to the anatomical structure, transit time, secretions, and pH. Understanding the physiological nature of the different GIT regions can help in developing strategies to control the rate and extent of drug absorption.

6.5.1 BUCCAL CAVITY

All orally administered drug formulations are taken by the mouth and have to pass through the buccal cavity. The buccal cavity has many advantages as a site of drug absorption. Drugs absorbed from the oral mucosa escape the first-pass hepatic metabolism since they enter the systemic circulation directly through the jugular vein, without going through the portal vein to the liver. Also, the oral cavity is very rich in blood supply so drugs can be absorbed very rapidly, achieving high blood drug concentration and producing rapid onset of action. However, the buccal cavity is not a major site for drug absorption because of its short transit time and its relatively small surface area.

The epithelial layer in the oral cavity acts as a lipoidal barrier to drug absorption. Drugs are absorbed in the buccal cavity mainly by passive diffusion with little paracellular absorption, active transport, and endocytosis. So polar drugs have limited buccal absorption, while lipophilic drugs that are soluble in saliva can be absorbed from the buccal cavity [5]. However, lipophilic drugs have limited solubility in the aqueous medium of the salivary secretion (pH 6.2–7.4), leading to swallowing of the majority of the dose. Specialized dosage forms can be designed to improve the buccal drug absorption by increasing the retention of the dosage form in the buccal cavity.

6.5.2 ESOPHAGUS

The esophagus is about a 25 cm long muscular tube that connects the pharynx to the stomach. The pH of the lumen of the esophagus is about 6–7, and the typical transit time for most pharmaceutical dosage forms in the esophagus is about 15 s. Drugs administered orally are not absorbed from the esophagus because of its very short transit time, very thick mucosal lining, and very small surface area.

6.5.3 STOMACH

The stomach is located in the left upper part of the abdomen attached to the esophagus by the gastro-esophageal sphincter known as the cardia, and attached to the duodenum by the pylorus. The stomach secretes about 1.5 L/day of gastric secretions which are rich in hydrochloric acid and enzymes. The average gastric pH is about 1–3, which usually varies during the day and is different in the different parts of the stomach [6]. It depends on the acid secretion and the gastric contents, with food usually raising the gastric pH due to its buffering and neutralizing effects. Other factors affecting the gastric pH include gender with females having slightly higher gastric pH compared to men [7]. Also, the gastric secretion was found to be higher and the gastric pH is lower in older individuals (mean age 51 versus 33 years) [8].

The stomach has a relatively small surface area compared to the small intestine and relatively short transit time when the drug is administered on an empty stomach. These two factors explain the limited role of the stomach in the absorption of drugs. However, the gastric pH is a very important factor in the absorption of orally administered drugs. The acidic pH of the stomach can cause decomposition of many acid labile drugs such as insulin and penicillin G. Also, basic drugs undergo faster dissolution in the acidic pH of the stomach making them ready to be absorbed once they leave the stomach and reach the small intestine. Furthermore, the acidic pH of the stomach makes it suitable for the absorption of weak acids which are usually present in the unionized form in this pH.

The gastric emptying rate is an important factor in determining the rate at which the drug reaches the small intestine, the major site of absorption for most orally administered drugs. This makes the gastric emptying rate the main factor in determining the rate of absorption for most drugs. In the fasting state, the stomach undergoes a multi-phase cycle which is repeated every 2 h to empty all the gastric contents to the duodenum. However, food usually causes delay in the gastric emptying rate. The delay in the gastric emptying is dependent on the food consistency, food composition, and meal size. In general, the larger the amount of food ingested, the longer it takes to empty the stomach [9]. Also, meals with higher calories per volume slow the gastric emptying rate more than meals with lower calories per volume. Furthermore, food rich in triglycerides and fatty acids delays the gastric emptying rate. Moreover, fluids and low-viscosity meals are emptied from the stomach much faster than meals with higher viscosity [10].

Other important factors that can affect the gastric emptying rate are the effect of drugs and diseases. Narcotic analgesics and drugs with anticholinergic effect such as atropine propantheline, tricyclic antidepressants, and phenothiazenes can significantly decrease the gastric emptying rate while prokinetic drugs such as metoclopramide can significantly speed the gastric emptying rate. This indicates that the effect on the gastric emptying rate is one of the mechanisms by which a drug can affect the rate of absorption of another drug leading to delayed onset of effect. Also, diseases such as pyloric stenosis, gastroenteritis, and gastroesophageal reflux can also slow the gastric emptying rate.

The dosage form in the stomach faces varying environment of pH and food content. The gastric emptying of the dosage form depends on the dosage form characteristics and the gastric contents. Enteric-coated tablets are designed to stay intact in the acidic medium of the stomach until it is emptied from the stomach as one unit with the indigestible materials, while capsules and tablets can disintegrate to granules and particles which can partially dissolve and gradually emptied from the stomach with food. The factors described earlier that can affect the gastric emptying rate also affect the rate of drug absorption to the systemic circulation. Some specialized dosage forms are designed to be retained in the stomach and gradually release the drug over a long period of time to slow the rate of drug absorption.

6.5.4 SMALL INTESTINE

The small intestine is about 6 m in length and it is divided into three parts which are different in their absorptive capacity. The first 20–30 cm is the duodenum, the next 2.5 m constitute the jejunum, and the rest of the small intestine is the ileum. The small intestine is formed of several layers stars with the serosa which is the outer most layer followed by two longitudinal and circular layers of muscles which are very important in the peristaltic movement of the small intestine. Then the submucosa, which is mainly connective tissue, and the mucosa, which consists of several layers, end with the epithelium. The epithelium is the inner most layer which consists mainly of a single layer of columnar epithelial cells and other types of cells that secrete mucous, hormones, peptides, and other secretions. The surface area of the intestinal mucosa is about 600 times that of a simple cylinder with similar dimensions which makes the small intestine the main site of absorption for most drugs. This increase in surface area is due to the folds of Kerckring, villi, and microvilli. The folds of Kerckring extend circularly most of the way around the intestine and protrude into the lumen. The villi are finger-like structures which are present all over the small intestine, while the microvilli are minute projections on the apical surface of the epithelial cells directed toward the lumen of the intestine. Figure 6.3 represents the different structure features of the small intestine that lead to the increase in its surface area per unit length. The jejunum and ileum are supplied by branches from the superior mesenteric artery and drain to the portal vain which take the blood to the liver. The small intestine is also supplied by the lymphatic system which is important in the absorption of many compounds especially fats and highly lipophilic compounds [11].

The intestinal transit time is an important factor that affects the absorption of drugs from different dosage forms. The average mouth to colon transit time is about 6–8 h, which depends greatly on the presence of food, pathological conditions, drugs, and the dosage from characteristics [12]. During fasting the dosage forms pass rapidly through the small intestine, compared to the fed state. Some conditions such as diarrhea and irritable bowel syndrome can shorten the transit time, while constipation, intestinal obstruction, and autonomic neuropathy usually prolong the intestinal transit time. Prokinetic drugs such as metoclopramide can shorten

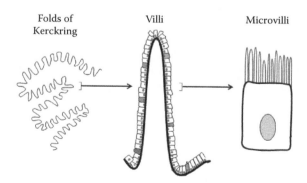

FIGURE 6.3   Different structure features that increase the surface area of the drug absorption surface in the small intestine.

the intestinal transit time, while narcotic analgesics and drugs with anticholinergic activity prolong the intestinal transit time. When the dosage forms are designed to release the drug over 12 h, drug absorption and drug stability in the large intestine are necessary for complete drug absorption.

The effect of intestinal transit time on drug absorption also depends on the characteristics of the dosage forms. The absorption of drugs from dosage forms designed to reach the small intestine as a single unit will start when the drugs reach the small intestine and start dissolving. These dosage forms reach the small intestine faster in the fasting state, while they will empty erratically and will have large variability in their absorption in the fed state. Drug absorption from dosage forms that reach the small intestine as particles or pellets depends on the dissolution of drug in the different intestinal regions and the dispersion of the formulation over the small intestine especially in case of poorly soluble drugs and slowly transported drugs. For this reason drug absorption from particulate dosage forms is more predictable and reproducible when administered with food because the particles are mixed with food and will have more spread over the length of the small intestine.

The permeability of the epithelium layer to small ions and water soluble molecules is greater in the duodenum and jejunum compared to the ileum. This is due to the presence of plenty of larger aqueous pores in the upper part of the small intestine compared to the lower part of the small intestine. Also, the proximal segment of the small intestine has more surface area per unit length, and has more carrier-mediated transport systems compared to the distal segment. Moreover, the ileum contains more commensal bacteria compared to the duodenum and jejunum. The pH of the small intestine ranges from 6 to 6.5 in the duodenum to 7 to 8 in the rest of the small intestine [13]. Studying the microenvironment in the mucosal fluid adjacent to the intestinal epithelium showed pH of 4.5–6.0, which can explain the absorption of weak acids from the small intestine. However, this should suggest poor absorption of weak bases which is not the case.

The small intestine also has high expression of the p-glycoprotein (P-gp) transport system which can transport a wide variety of drugs outside the cells. The P-gp transport system is localized on the apical side of the epithelial cells and can cause efflux of the drug outside the epithelial cell back to the intestinal lumen. Drugs that are substrates for this transport system have lower bioavailability because P-gp acts as a barrier for their absorption. Administration of P-gp inhibitors can also affect the bioavailability of the drugs that are substrates for this transport system. The small intestine also contains different cytochrome P450 (CYP) enzymes specifically CYP 34A which can metabolize a variety of drugs during their absorption reducing the extent of their absorption. Administration of drugs that can inhibit CYP 3A4 can also affect the extent of absorption of many drugs especially those that undergo extensive presystemic metabolism by CYP 3A4 [14].

6.5.5 LARGE INTESTINE

The large intestine is approximately 130 cm in length with diameter longer than that of the small intestine. It consists of the cecum, ascending, transverse, descending, sigmoid colon, rectum, and anus. Although the rectum is part of the large intestine, it will be discussed separately in the following section. The mucosa of the large intestine is histologically similar to that of the small intestine; however, it does not have villi which makes the surface area per unit length of the large intestine much less than that of the small intestine. This decrease in the mucosal surface area in the colon also decreases the metabolic activity in the colonic wall. The pH in the large intestine is approximately 6.5 [15]. The large intestine is characterized by the presence of many aerobic and anaerobic bacteria which have digestive and metabolic functions, and can cause drug degradation. The blood supply to the large intestine is through the superior and inferior mesenteric arteries, and the venous return goes to the portal circulation except for the lower part of the rectum.

Drug absorption from the large intestine is mainly through transmucosal passive diffusion and via the aqueous pores with bulk water absorption because there is no documented active transport system for nutrients in the large intestine. The reduced surface area of the large intestine is balanced by the prolonged transit time which can lead to significant drug absorption. The average transit time in the large intestine is about 14 h, which can vary greatly due to many factors [16]. High dietary fiber intake increases the fecal bulk and shortens the colonic transit time. Also, larger particles move faster in the colon compared to smaller particles. Furthermore, drugs that slow the bowel movement such as codeine, morphine, and anticholinergic drugs can prolong the transit time. The cecum and the ascending colon are the main areas with the favorable environment for drug absorption in the large intestine. This is because going further in the large intestine, the absorption of water increases the viscosity of its contents that can lead to less mixing, slower solubility, and lower chance for the drug to come in contact with the absorption surface. So drug delivery to the colon will have to target the proximal colon.

6.6 PHYSIOLOGICAL FACTORS AFFECTING DRUG ABSORPTION AFTER RECTAL DRUG ADMINISTRATION

The rectum is the last 15–20 cm of the large intestine which can be used for rectal drug administration in the form of suppositories. Rectal drug administration has several advantages including bypassing the half-pass hepatic metabolism if the drug is administered to the lower part of the rectum since the venous return form of this part of the rectum does not go through the portal circulation [17]. Also, this route allows administration of large dosage forms safely to young and old patients. Furthermore, the administered drug is not diluted because the rectum is generally empty and has very limited amount of fluids. Moreover, it is suitable for drug administration when oral administration is not possible and parenteral dosage forms are not available. Drugs are administered rectally in the form of suppositories or enemas and are usually absorbed by passive diffusion or through the aqueous pores.

6.7 PHYSIOLOGICAL FACTORS AFFECTING DRUG ABSORPTION AFTER INTRANASAL DRUG ADMINISTRATION

The nasal cavity starts with the nostrils which open at the back into the nasopharynx and lead to the trachea and esophagus. The main functions of the nose are filtration, warming, and moistening the inspired air. Warming the inspired air is assisted by the rich blood supply to the nasal cavity, while humidification occurs by the fluid secreted by the glands and cells lining the nasal cavity. Also, the nasal cavity is covered with moist mucous membrane with projections known as the cilia that can filter the air and collect debris. The average pH of secretions in the nasal cavity is about 6.2–6.4, which can change due to air temperature, sleep, emotions, and diseases [11].

The mucosal lining of the nasal civility varies in thickness and vascularity and is covered by an epithelial cell layer which is covered by microvilli. These microvilli significantly increase the surface available for absorption. The extensive lymphatic system supplying the nasal cavity plays an important part in the absorption of compounds deposited in the nasal mucosa. The mucosa is covered by a thin layer of mucus secreted by the cells and glands in the mucosa and submucosa and is renewed approximately every 10 min. The anterior end of the nasal septum and part of the interior nose are covered by ciliated epithelial cells which together with the mucus layer play an important roll in clearing particles deposited in the nasal cavity. The ciliary action clears the mucus to the nasopharynx where it can be swallowed or move the mucus forward to be removed by sneezing. This mucociliary effect is important because it can clear drugs administered to the nasal cavity [11].

Drugs administered for their local effect in the nasal cavity can produce significant systemic effects, suggesting that the nasal route can be utilized to deliver systemically acting drugs. The rate of mucus flow and the drug retention in the nasal cavity are important factors that affect drug absorption from the nasal cavity. Slow rate of mucus flow leads to longer retention of the drug in the nasal cavity which leads to more drug absorption. Also, formulation factors such as volume, drug concentration, density, viscosity, pH, and tonicity can affect the nasal drug absorption. Drugs can be absorbed across the nasal mucosa by passive diffusion and through the aqueous pores, while some amino acids can be absorbed by active transport. The advantage of nasal drug delivery is that drugs can be absorbed very rapidly achieving high plasma drug concentration and the absorbed drugs bypass the hepatic first-pass metabolism.

6.8 PHYSIOLOGICAL FACTORS AFFECTING DRUG ABSORPTION AFTER PULMONARY DRUG ADMINISTRATION

The external opening of the respiratory system is the nose with the mouth also involved in the passage of air in and out of the respiratory system under stress. The rest of the respiratory system includes the pharynx, larynx, trachea, bronchi, bronchioles, and ends up with the alveoli. The main function of the respiratory system is the oxygenation of the blood and the removal of carbon dioxide. The function of the components of the respiratory system change from passage of air to gas exchange which occurs mainly in the pulmonary parenchyma which constitute the lobules that contain the alveoli.

The upper respiratory tract and the bronchi are covered by a ciliated epithelial layer and goblet cells that secrete mucus. The bronchioles are also covered by ciliated epithelial cells and contain a layer of smooth muscles which can control the size of the airways. Contraction can stimulate the ciliary action causing expulsion of any foreign substance. The alveoli are covered with a thin epithelial layer that allows gas exchange across the alveolar capillary membrane. The presence of cilia and mucous in the respiratory tract provides an efficient cleansing mechanism to protect the lung from any inhaled foreign materials. The alveolar epithelium and the capillary endothelium are highly permeable to water, most gases, and lipophilic compounds. However, they are impermeable to hydrophilic substances, ionized compounds, and large molecular weight molecules. The large surface area and the high blood flow allow rapid absorption of any substance which can permeate the alveoli-capillary membrane [11].

Drugs are usually delivered to the pulmonary system in the form of aerosols which consist of very fine liquid or solid particles. Administered drugs can be absorbed from the site of their deposition including the upper and lower parts of the respiratory tract. Lipophilic drugs are absorbed better than the hydrophilic drugs. In order for these drugs to be effective, they have to reach their site of action in sufficient quantity. Many factors can affect the site of deposition of the aerosol particles including physical characters of the aerosol and physiological factors. Larger particle size droplets can collide with the upper airway mucus layer and rapidly removed by the mucociliary clearance. Droplets in the range from 0.5 to 5 µm can travel longer distances down the respiratory tract. Other factors related to the characters of the aerosol include the speed of delivery, particle charge, and density [18]. Physiological factors affecting the site of droplet deposition include the rate of respiration with the rapid rate of respiration causing premature deposition and slow rate of respiration allows more time for particles to deposit in distal sites of the lung. Also, obstructive airway diseases cause redistribution of flow to the nonobstructive areas and increase the rate of airflow which decreases drug disposition in distal sites.

Pulmonary drug delivery can be used for the local and the systemic effects of drugs. Drugs administered for their local effect on the respiratory system have the advantage of fewer systemic adverse effects, rapid onset of action, and the use of smaller doses of the drugs. Examples of drugs administered by inhalation for their local effects are beta-agonists and corticosteroids for the management of bronchial asthma. Pulmonary drug delivery can also be used for the systemic effect of drugs. In this case, the drugs are absorbed directly to the systemic circulation and bypass the hepatic first-pass metabolism. Examples of these drugs include inhalation general anesthetics which are usually administered via this route. A fraction of the dose administered by inhalation usually reaches to the GIT after swallowing the drug deposited in the mouth or the esophagus during the inhalation process. Also, part of the dose which is deposited in the respiratory tract and expelled by the mucociliary system can be swallowed and absorbed from the GIT [19].

6.9 PHYSIOLOGICAL FACTORS AFFECTING DRUG ABSORPTION AFTER TRANSDERMAL DRUG ADMINISTRATION

The main function of the skin is to provide sensation and protection from the surrounding environment. The skin consists of three layers: the outer epidermis layer, followed by the dermis and the inner subcutaneous fat layer. The epidermis is a dry and tough layer that constitutes a barrier for the penetration of substance from the environment into the body and also prevents the loss of water, electrolytes, and nutrients from the body. The outer layer of the epidermis is the stratum corneum which is formed of layers of keratinized dead cells and provides the main barrier for drug absorption across the skin. The second layer in the epithelium is the stratum germinativum which grows from the base upward to renew the stratum corneum layer. In this layer, the keratinocytes form hydrophilic units surrounded by lipoid matrix preventing direct contact between these cells. The lipoid matrix forms continuous lipophilic path or channel through the stratum corneum layer. The dermis is a fibrous layer that provides support for the epidermis and is supplied by blood vessels, lymph vessels, and nerves, and contains hair follicles and sweat and sebum glands. The fat layer provides an insulation layer and provides storage area for fat and nutrients [11].

Drug application on the skin has been used to treat local dermatological conditions. However, the slow drug absorption after topical application has been shown to provide therapeutic blood concentrations over an extended period of time for some drugs. Also, the direct absorption to the systemic circulation and avoidance of the first-pass metabolism has made the transdermal delivery of drugs an attractive route for systemic delivery of potent drugs. Drug absorption after application of a transdermal delivery systems goes through a series of barriers starting from drug release from the delivery system, then diffusion across the stratum corneum, epidermis, and dermis where it can be absorbed by the existing capillary network. However, it has been well documented that the stratum corneum is the major barrier for drug absorption from the skin.

Drugs applied to the skin can be absorbed through the lipoid channels or the hydrophilic keratinized cells. Lipophilic drugs are absorbed mainly through the lipoid channel. Hydration of the skin can increase the penetration of polar compounds more than nonpolar compounds. The effect of hydration can be due to hydration and wetting of the lipoid channel and also the keratinized cells. An additional minor route of drug absorption from the skin is through the hair follicles and sebaceous glands. After diffusion through the epithelium, the drug has to diffuse through the dermis to get absorbed by the capillary network supplying this layer. Lipophilic drugs can diffuse slowly through the dermis since this layer is more hydrophilic in nature. This indicates that drugs with optimal penetration characteristics across the skin should not be highly hydrophilic or highly lipophilic [20,21]. Figure 6.4 represents a schematic presentation of the different skin layers and the different pathways for transdermal drug absorption.

Transdermal drug delivery has many advantages including suitability for drug administration when the oral route is not possible, avoidance of the first-pass metabolism, improving patient compliance, achievement of sustained plasma drug concentrations for extended period of time, and suitability for drugs with short half-life. However, transdermal delivery also has several drawbacks including irritation of the site of application, immunological sensitization, suitability for potent drugs only, and the high cost compared to the conventional dosage forms.

When transdermal delivery systems are used, it is important to consider the factors that can affect the rate of drug absorption across the skin. These factors include the surface area of the delivery system, with larger surface area producing proportional increase in the drug absorption rate. Also, the site of application is important because the skin in different parts of the body have different thickness with the highly keratinized sites providing strong barrier for drug absorption. Furthermore,

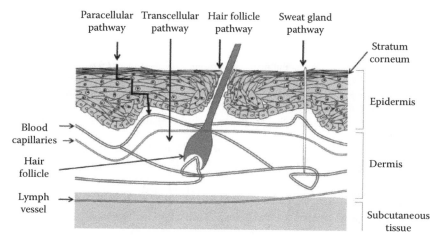

FIGURE 6.4 Schematic presentation of the different skin layer showing the different drug transport mechanisms across the skin.

the stratum corneum in neonates is not well developed and allows much higher rate of drug absorption after topical application compared to older patients who have thick and dry stratum corneum. Moreover, occlusion of the skin which increases skin hydration can increase drug permeability across the stratum corneum especially for polar drugs. Additionally, the integrity of the skin in the application site is important in determining the rate of drug absorption because damaged, broken, or exposed skin usually have compromised barrier function causing higher drug absorption [11].

6.10 SUMMARY

The absorption of drugs administered by any of the extravascular routes is affected by the physiological conditions at the site of drug administration. The drugs have to overcome the absorption barriers before they can be absorbed to the systemic circulation. These physiological conditions and absorption barriers are different for the different routes of administration and can be favorable for the absorption of some drugs and prohibiting for the absorption of others. For example, the lipophilic nature of the biological membranes in general allows lipophilic drugs to cross the biological membranes by passive diffusion while constituting a strong barrier for the diffusion of hydrophilic drugs. Also, the acidic condition in the stomach can destroy acid-labile drugs like peptides while increasing the rate of dissolution of basic drugs. Besides, the bacterial flora in the GIT can metabolize and degrade some drugs while liberating the active drug moieties from prodrugs. Furthermore, intramuscular administration of water soluble drugs can lead to rapid and almost complete absorption while lipophilic drugs may precipitate and slowly absorbed over long time. Moreover, the transdermal delivery systems are designed to allow slow absorption of potent drugs across the skin to achieve effective plasma drug concentration for a long period of time. So the biological and physiological factors that can influence the absorption of drugs should be considered in conjunction with the properties of the drug itself and the dosage form characteristics.

REFERENCES

1. Singer SJ and Nicholson GL (1972) The fluid mosaic model of the structure of cell membrane. *Science* 153:1010–1012.
2. Diamond JM (1977) Epithelial junction: Bridge, gate and fence. *Physiologist* 20:10–18.
3. Higuchi WI and Ho NFH (1988) Membrane transfer of drugs. *Int J Pharm* 2:10–15.
4. Oh DM, Han HK, and Amidon GL (1999) Drug transport and targeting: Intestinal transport. *Pharm Biotechnol* 12:59–88.
5. Squier CA and Johnson NW (1975) Permeability of the oral mucosa. *Br Med Bull* 31:169–175.
6. McLaughlan G, Fullarton GM, Crean GP, and McColl KEL (1989) Comparison of gastric body and antral pH: A 24 hour ambulatory study in healthy volunteers. *Gut* 30:573–578.
7. Feldman M and Barnett C (1991) Fasting gastric pH and its relationship to true hypochlorhydria in humans. *Dig Dis Sci* 36:866–869.
8. Goldschmiedt M, Barnett C, and Schwartz BE (1991) Effect of age on gastric acid secretion and serum gastric concentration in healthy men and women. *Gastroenterology* 101:977–990.
9. Feldman M, Smith HJ, and Simon TR (1984) Gastric emptying of solid radiopaque markers: Studies in healthy subjects and diabetes patients. *Gastroenterology* 87:895–902.
10. Hunt NJ and Knox MT (1968) A relation between the chain length of fatty acids and the slowing of gastric emptying. *J Physiol* 194:327–336.
11. Washington N, Washington C, and Wilson CG (2001) *Physiological Pharmaceutics, Barriers to Drug Absorption*, 2nd edn., Taylor & Francis, New York.
12. Davis SS, Hardy JG, and Fara JW (1986) Transit of pharmaceutical dosage forms through the small intestine. *Gut* 27:886–892.
13. Hardy JG, Evans DF, Zaki I, Clark AG, Tennesen HH, and Gamst ON (1987) Evaluation of an enteric-coated naproxen tablet using gamma scintigraphy and pH monitoring. *Int J Pharmaceut* 37:245–250.
14. Watkins P (1997) The barrier function of CYP3A4 and P-glycoprotein in the small bowel. *Adv Drug Deliv Rev* 27:161–170.
15. Evans DF, Pye G, Bramley R, Clark AG, Dyson TJ, and Hardcastle JD (1988) Measurement of gastrointestinal pH profiles in normal ambulant human subjects. *Gut* 29:1035–1041.
16. Metcalf AM, Phillips SF, Zinsmeister AR, MacCarty RL, Beart RW, and Wolff BG (1987) Simplified assessment of segmental colonic transit. *Gastroenterology* 92:40–47.
17. DeBoer AG, Breimer DD, Pronk FJ, and Gubbens-Stibbe JM (1980) Rectal bioavailability of lidocaine in rats: Absence of significant first-pass elimination. *J Pharm Sci* 69:804–807.
18. Gonda I (1981) A semi-empirical model of aerosol deposition in the human respiratory tract for mouth inhalation. *J Pharm Pharmacol* 33:692–696.
19. Walker SR, Evans ME, Richards AJ, and Paterson JW (1972) The clinical pharmacology of oral and inhaled salbutamol. *Clin Pharmacol Ther* 13:861–867.
20. Carmichael AJ (1994) Skin sensitivity and transdermal drug delivery. A review of the problem. *Drug Safety* 10:151–159.
21. Katz M and Poulsen BJ (1971) Absorption of drugs through the skin, in Brodie BB and Gilette JR (Eds.) *Handbook of Experimental Pharmacology*, New Series 28, Part 1, Springer-Verlag, Berlin, Germany.

7 Drug Absorption Following Extravascular Administration
Molecular and Physicochemical Considerations

OBJECTIVES

After completing this chapter you should be able to

- Describe the different molecular features that can affect drug absorption
- Discuss the effect of pH on drug solubility and drug absorption
- Describe the different bulk solid properties that can affect drug solubility and drug absorption
- Enumerate the different factors that can affect the drug dissolution rate and strategies for enhancing drug solubility
- Discuss the importance of drug stability for drug absorption
- Predict the drug absorption behavior based on the biopharmaceutics classification system
- Predict the drug absorption and disposition characteristics and the potential for drug–drug interactions based on the biopharmaceutics drug disposition classification system

7.1 INTRODUCTION

The physiological environment at the site of drug administration and the drug physicochemical properties are important factors in determining the rate and extent of drug absorption after extravascular drug administration. The drugs have to be in solution before diffusing across the biological membrane and reaching the systemic circulation. Different drugs have different dissolution rates and different abilities to cross biological membranes, which lead to different absorption characteristics. Hydrophilic drugs, in general, have faster rate of dissolution in the aqueous physiological environment and lower diffusivity through the lipophilic biological membranes, whereas lipophilic drugs have lower aqueous solubility and higher membrane diffusivity. Since most drugs are either weak acids or weak bases, the drug solubility is usually affected by the pH of the surrounding environment. Basic drugs can dissolve faster and are mostly ionized in the acidic pH of the stomach, while their dissolution is slower and are mostly unionized in the alkaline pH of the small intestine. The reverse can be observed for acidic drugs: slower dissolution and mostly unionized in the stomach, whilst faster dissolution and mostly ionized in the small intestine. All properties that can affect drug solubility, dissolution rate, stability, and diffusivity across the biological membrane under the physiological conditions can affect the rate and extent of drug absorption. These include the molecular structure features that can affect the drug physicochemical properties as well as the drug properties in the bulk powder form.

7.2 MOLECULAR STRUCTURE FEATURES AFFECTING DRUG ABSORPTION

The correlation of the oral absorption characteristics of drugs and some molecular properties described by Lipinski et al. have introduced what has been known as the "rule of 5" [1]. They have shown that there are some structure features that have been associated with poor drug absorption after oral administration. These include molecular weight more than 500, log P over 5, hydrogen bond donors more than 5, and hydrogen bond acceptor more than 10. Other researchers investigated additional molecular features that can affect drug absorption such as polar surface area and molecular flexibility [2]. In these investigations, the absorption characteristics and the molecular properties for a large number of drugs were determined experimentally or obtained from the literature. Then the correlation between the absorption characteristics and each of the molecular features were examined. This is usually a complicated task because some of the molecular properties are highly correlated and it is very difficult to investigate the effect of each feature separately. For example, the increase in molecular weight is usually accompanied by increasing the H-bond numbers, the polar surface area, and the number of rotatable bond. So it is not possible to separate the effect of these correlated properties on drug absorption. Identification of the molecular-level properties that are important to achieve the optimal drug absorption characteristics provides a useful guide for pharmaceutical chemists while designing new lead compounds.

7.2.1 MOLECULAR WEIGHT

The diffusion coefficient is inversely proportional to the radius (or diameter) of the diffusing molecule according to the Stokes–Einstein relationship. It is the size and the shape of the molecule rather than its molecular weight that determine the diffusion coefficient and the rate of diffusion of a compound across the biological membranes. So a linear molecule usually diffuses across biological membranes slower than a spherical molecule with the same molecular weight. Assuming spherical molecules for simplicity, for a given concentration gradient, molecules with higher molecular weight have larger molecular size and slower diffusion rate. In general, over a wide range of molecular weight, drugs with larger molecular weight have lower ability to diffuse effectively across the biological membranes.

7.2.2 Log P

Log P is the n-octanol/water (o/w) partition coefficient, and it is the logarithm of the concentration ratio of the drug in n-octanol to that in water at equilibrium. Hence, it is a measure of the differential solubility of the drug between the two solvents:

$$\log P = \log \left[\frac{\text{Drug concentration in n-octanol}}{\text{Drug concentration in water}} \right] \tag{7.1}$$

A drug with log P of 2 partitioning between n-octanol and water will have concentration in n-octanol that is 100 times more than that in water at equilibrium. The o/w partition coefficient is a measure of the hydrophilicity/lipophilicity of compounds. Lipophilic drugs with high o/w partition coefficient can easily diffuse across the biological membranes. However, extremely lipophilic drugs can get trapped in the lipid bilayer of the membrane, and their solubility in the physiological aqueous environment is very low. On the other hand, hydrophilic drugs with low o/w partition coefficient have high solubility in the physiological aqueous environment, but their ability to cross the lipoid biological membranes is very limited. Optimal absorption can be achieved when there is a balance between the hydrophilicity and lipophilicity. As stated by Lipinski, drugs with log P higher than 5 that are highly lipophilic will have poor absorption [3].

7.2.3 Hydrogen-Bond Donor/Acceptor

A hydrogen atom attached to a relatively electronegative atom such as oxygen, nitrogen, or fluorine is considered a hydrogen bond donor, while electronegative atoms are regarded as hydrogen bond acceptors. The electronegative atom attracts the electron cloud from around the hydrogen nucleus and by decentralizing the cloud leaves the atom with a partial positive charge. Because of the small size of hydrogen relative to other atoms and molecules, this represents a large charge density. Hydrogen bond is formed when this strong positive charge density attracts a lone pair of electrons on another oxygen or nitrogen atom and becomes the hydrogen-bond acceptor.

It has been found that the total ability of a compound to form H-bonds is a very good predictor for drug absorption. According to Lipinski's Rule of 5, the presence of more than 5 H-bond donors and more than 10 H-bond acceptors is associated with poor absorption across the biological membrane. Studies have shown that molecules with less than 10 H-bonds can be absorbed completely, while molecules with more than 20 H-bonds have very limited membrane permeability. In this case, the energy required to break the large number of H-bonds between the molecule and the surrounding water molecules or between the drug molecule and the function groups on the membrane itself becomes very high.

7.2.4 POLAR SURFACE AREA

The polar surface area is defined as a sum of surface area of nitrogen and oxygen atoms in a molecule plus the surface of the hydrogen atoms attached to these heteroatoms. It is a useful parameter for prediction of drug permeability across biological membranes. It has been shown to be correlated with the results of in vivo and in vitro models for drug absorption and membrane permeability. Molecules with high polar surface area usually have lower permeability across biological membranes by passive diffusion. Different methods have been used to calculate the polar surface area for a molecule by summation of the surface contributions of the polar fragments of the molecules. Molecules with polar surface area over 140 Å^2 are poorly absorbed from the gastrointestinal tract (GIT), whereas molecules with polar surface area below 60 Å^2 are lipophilic enough to penetrate the blood brain barrier (BBB).

7.2.5 NUMBER OF ROTATABLE BONDS

Molecular flexibility depends on the number of rotatable bonds in the structure of the molecule. It is determined from the count of the nonterminal, noncyclic single bonds except the amide C–N bond because of its high rotational energy barrier. The relationship between the number of rotatable bond and the drug bioavailability is dependent on the drug molecular weight. Molecules with molecular weight above 400 have shown to have reduced oral bioavailability with the increase in the number of rotatable bonds; however, this relationship was not clear in molecules with molecular weight below 400.

7.2.6 CHIRALITY

A chiral drug is a drug that has at least one carbon atom that has four different substitutions. Most of the chiral drugs are marketed as the racemates of equal amounts of the two enantiomers, although the therapeutic effect of the drug is mainly produced by one of the enantiomers. Chiral drugs with one chiral center have two enantiomers that are identical in their physicochemical properties. So the enantiomers usually have similar solubility and permeability and hence similar absorption characteristics if it occurs by passive diffusion. However, the absorption process becomes stereoselective, meaning that the absorption of the two enantiomers is different when the absorption process involves a carrier transport system. Also, when chiral additives are included in the formulation, a stereoselective release of the enantiomers from the dosage form may occur. Furthermore, chiral drugs that undergo stereoselective first-pass metabolism can have stereoselective bioavailability, meaning the bioavailability of one of the enantiomers is higher than the bioavailability of the other. Marketing of chiral drugs as a single enantiomer is necessary only when one of the enantiomers produces serious undesired effects.

7.3 PHYSICOCHEMICAL DRUG PROPERTIES

Drugs administered by any of the extravascular routes will have to dissolve at the site of drug administration and stay stable until they are absorbed across the absorption barriers. The solubility and dissolution rate of the drug at the site of administration that depend on its physicochemical properties can affect the rate and extent absorption. This is because fast dissolving drugs are usually absorbed fas slow dissolving drugs. Also, slow dissolving drugs may not be completely absorbed if their transit time at the absorption site is shorter than the time required for their complete dissolution. The stability of the drug at the site of administration is another factor that depends on the chemical properties of the drug and can influence the extent of drug absorption. The drug lipophilicity that is determined from its physicochemical properties is important in determining the drug ability to penetrate the biological membrane. So the physical and chemical properties of drugs are very important in determining the drug absorption characteristics.

7.3.1 pH-Partition Theory

An important factor that can influence drug absorption after extravascular drug administration is the pH-partition theory. This theory describes the relationship between the drug pK_a, the pH at the absorption site, and the lipid solubility of the drug. The physiological pH in blood and the extracellular fluid is between 6.8 and 7.2, while the pH of the GIT varies from 6.2 to 7.4 in the buccal cavity, 1 to 3 in the stomach, 6 to 8 in the small intestine, 6.5 to 7.5 in the large intestine, and 6.5 to 7.5 in the rectum. The pH of the other sites of drug administration is also different and can differ from 6.2 to 6.4 in the intranasal cavity, 4.2 to 5.6 on the surface of the skin, and 6 to 7.5 in the tracheal secretion [4]. The percentage of the drug molecules ionized and unionized are different at the different sites of drug absorption depending on the pH at the site and the pK_a of the drug. For example, weak acids are mainly unionized in the acidic pH of the stomach, while weak bases are mainly unionized in the alkaline pH of the small intestine. Since the unionized form of the drug can cross the biological membranes much better than the ionized form of the drug, drug absorption is affected by the degree of drug ionization. The relationship between the pK_a of the drug and the percentage of drug ionized and unionized at different pH is described by the Henderson-Hasselbalch equation (Equations 7.2 through 7.5):

For weak acids,

$$pK_a - pH = \log \frac{(HA)}{(A^-)} \qquad (7.2)$$

$$pK_a - pH = \log \frac{(unionized)}{(ionized)} \qquad (7.3)$$

For weak bases,

$$pK_a - pH = \log \frac{(HB^+)}{(B)} \qquad (7.4)$$

$$pK_a - pH = \log \frac{(ionized)}{(unionized)} \qquad (7.5)$$

Examining these equations, it is clear that when the pH of the medium is equal to the pK_a of the drug, 50% of the drug will be in the ionized form and 50% in the unionized form. When a weak acid is dissolved in a medium that has pH one unit lower than the pK_a of the drug, 90% of the drug will be in the unionized form and 10% in the ionized form. Similarly, when a weak base is dissolved in a medium that has pH one unit lower than the pK_a of the drug, 90% of the drug will be in the ionized form and 10% in the unionized form. This discussion suggests that weak acids are absorbed better from the acidic environment, while weak bases are absorbed better from the alkaline environment. However, there are many other factors that need to be considered when trying to study the drug absorption process from different sites of administration. For example, the very large surface area of the small intestine makes the small intestine the major site of drug absorption after oral administration for most drugs including weak acids. Also, there are many other factors that make application of the pH-partition theory in describing or predicting the absorption of drugs not an easy task. These factors include the absorption of ionized molecules, the pH at the microenvironment of the absorption site, and the presence of the stagnant layer at the surface of the membrane. So it is important to understand that the aforementioned discussion is a very simple description of a very complex process.

7.3.2 DRUG SOLUBILITY

The drug molecules have to be in solution before they can be absorbed from the site of drug administration to the systemic circulation. The saturation solubility of the drug is the maximum mass of the drug that can dissolve in a certain mass or volume of the solvent. This is a constant for each drug in a certain solvent at a specific temperature [1]. The saturation solubility is the drug concentration in solution when excess drug is dissolved in the solvent until equilibrium between the drug in solution and in the solid state is achieved. The drug solubility in the aqueous physiological environment is dependent mainly on the physicochemical properties of the drug and the pH of environment. The process of solubility involves breaking the solute-solute bonds and the solvent-solvent bonds that require energy and the formation of new solute-solvent association forces that liberate energy. The net energy gained or librated during the solubility of a solute in a solvent is known as the heat of solution. The heat of solution is the change in the enthalpy (the energy of the system) due to the dissolution of a solute in a solvent and is denoted as ΔH of solution. When the heat of solution is negative, it means that the energy librated from the strong interaction between the solute and the solvent molecules is larger than the energy required for breaking the solute-solute bonds and the solvent-solvent bonds. In this case, the solute-solvent attraction is favored and solute dissolution occurs spontaneously. However, when the heat of solution is positive, this means that the solute-solvent attraction is weak and the energy librated is lower than the energy needed to break the solute-solute and the solvent-solvent attractions, leading to limited solubility [5,6].

Hydrophilic drug molecules can form strong bonds with water molecules librating energy that exceeds the energy required for separation of the drug molecule from the bulk solid particles and breaking the hydrogen bonds between the water molecules. This explains the good water solubility of polar drugs. On the contrary, lipophilic drug molecules do not like to interact with water making it difficult to provide the energy required to separate the solute molecules from the drug particles and to break the hydrogen bond between the water molecules, which explains the poor water solubility of these drugs. The solubility of a drug in a certain solvent or dissolution medium is usually constant at constant temperature. However, there are several approaches that can be followed to increase the solubility and hence the absorption of the active drug moiety in pharmaceutical dosage forms. The following are some of the factors that can affect drug solubility from pharmaceutical dosage forms.

7.3.2.1   pH Effect on Drug Solubility

Most drugs are either weak acids or weak bases, so the solubility of most drugs is dependent on the pH. In general, weak acids are more soluble in alkaline medium because they form soluble salts, while in acidic medium these drugs are present mainly in the less soluble unionized form. Also, weak bases are more soluble in acidic medium and less soluble in alkaline medium. According to Henderson-Hasselbalch equation and as shown in Equations 7.2 through 7.5, the degree of ionization of acidic and basic drugs in solution is dependent on the pH of the dissolution medium and the pK_a of the drug. Since the ionized and unionized forms of the drugs have different solubility, the drug solubility (ionized and unionized forms) is different at different pHs specially in the pH range close to the drug pK_a.

For example, the solubility of a weak acid in an aqueous acidic medium that has 2 pH units lower than the drug pK_a is the lowest solubility of this drug, because the drug at this pH is mostly (about 99%) in the less soluble, unionized form. As the pH increases, more of the drug molecules become ionized and the drug solubility increases. At pH equal to the pK_a of the drug, 50% of the drug is ionized and 50% is unionized, while at higher pH, more drug is ionized and the solubility increases progressively. At any pH, the total solubility of the drug is the sum of the solubility of the ionized and unionized species. At pH lower than the pK_a, the solubility of the drug is limited by the solubility of the unionized form of the drug, while at pH higher than the pK_a of the drug, the solubility is limited by the solubility of the ionized form of the drug. The concentration in a saturated solution of the drug at a given pH is the sum of the solubility of one of the species and the concentration of the other species necessary to satisfy the mass balance in the drug dissociation equation [7,8]. The pH-solubility profile is a curve that describes the solubility of a compound at different pH. The effect of pH on drug solubility can be very useful in formulation design because acidic or alkaline additives can be included in the formulations to enhance the drug solubility. Also, drug formulations can be designed to have higher or lower solubility at the site of administration depending on the pH of the site.

7.3.2.2   Drug Salts

Most of the drugs are either weak acids or weak bases, so they are used in pharmaceutical formulations in the form of the free acid/base or in the form of the salt of these acids or bases. For example, the nonsteroidal anti-inflammatory drug, diclofenac, is the drug in its free acid form, while diclofenac sodium and diclofenac potassium are the salts of the drug. Also, quinidine is the free base of the drug, while quinidine sulfate and quinidine phosphate are the salts of the same drug. Whether the drug is administered as the free acid/base or as the salt, once absorbed to the systemic circulation equilibrium is established between the ionized and unionized forms of the drug depending on its pK_a and the physiological pH. The choice of using the free acid/base or the salt in pharmaceutical products depends on the properties of all the available forms of the drug, the procedures used during the manufacturing processes, and the desired properties of the finished drug products. In general, salts are usually more soluble than the free acid/base of the same drug, and different salts of the same drug can have different solubility. For this reason, salts can be used in the pharmaceutical formulations to enhance drug solubility and the absorption characteristics specially for poorly soluble drugs. The choice of the salt of the drug used in the drug formulation can affect the rate and extent of absorption of the active drug moiety to the systemic circulation.

7.3.2.3   Drug Crystal Form

Drugs in the solid state are present either in the crystalline form where the molecules are arranged in a fixed geometric pattern known as the crystal lattice or the amorphous form where the molecules are arranged in a random manner. When the drug is present in only one crystalline or amorphous form, the only choice will be to use this form in drug formulations. However, many drugs exhibit a property known as polymorphism, which means that the drug can exist in more than one crystalline form. Although the chemical nature of the drug is similar in the different crystalline forms, these different crystalline forms can have substantially different physical properties including different solubility [4,9]. Also, drug solubility is usually higher when the drug exists in the amorphous form compared to the crystalline form. This is because the process of drug solubility involves breaking the intermolecular bonds that form the crystal lattice, and these intermolecular bonds are different for the different forms of the same chemical entity. Chloramphenicol palmitate that is used in the formulation of the liquid formulations of this antibiotic exists in different crystal forms with the β-form being the more soluble form of this drug. The solubility and hence the absorption of this antibiotic are much better after administration of formulations that contain the β-crystal form, which result in achieving higher blood drug concentrations. So the choice of the crystal form of the drug can significantly affect the solubility characteristics of the drug that can affect the rate and extent of drug absorption to the systemic circulation.

7.3.2.4   Drug Complexation

The solubility of some drugs can be enhanced by using suitable complexing agents that can form a complex with the dissolved drug molecules, allowing more drug molecules to dissolve. Cyclodextrins have been used to increase the solubility of poorly soluble drugs by the formation of inclusion complexes [10]. This approach has been used to increase the rate and extent of absorption of some drugs. Complexation can enhance the drug solubility only if the formed complex has higher solubility than the drug itself. This is because there are examples where the formed complex is not soluble like the complex formed between the antibiotic tetracycline and calcium.

7.3.3 DRUG DISSOLUTION

The drug solubility is the maximum mass of the drug that can dissolve in a certain volume of the solvent at a specific temperature, while the drug dissolution is the process by which the drug molecules dissolve in the solvent. For drugs with limited aqueous solubility, the rate of drug dissolution is the slowest process involved in drug absorption, and the absorption of the drug will be dissolution-rate limited. In other words, the rate of drug dissolution will be controlling the rate of the overall absorption process. Noyes and Whitney described the dissolution rate of a solid drug that was described by the rate of change of the drug concentration in the bulk solution (dc/dt). In this dissolution model, it was assumed that the drug is present in the form of solid particles with total surface area equal to S, and the solid particles are surrounded by an unstirred (stagnant) layer of the solvent. The thickness of the unstirred layer is h, and the diffusion coefficient of the drug in this unstirred layer is equal to D. The drug concentration on the surface of the solid particles is equal to the saturation solubility of the drug C_s and the drug concentration in the bulk solvent is C.

The drug dissolves in the solvent right on the surface of the particles. The dissolved drug molecules then diffuse through the unstirred layer to reach the bulk solution. The driving force of this diffusion process is the concentration gradient across the unstirred layer ($C_s - C$). As the process continues, more drug molecules dissolve from the surface of the particles, and the drug concentration increases in the bulk solution [11]. This process is presented in Figure 7.1 and can be described by Noyes and Whitney equation:

$$\frac{dc}{dt} = \frac{DS}{h}(C_s - C) \tag{7.6}$$

This equation includes the parameters that affect the rate of drug dissolution. Studying these parameters is important to determine how the rate of drug dissolution can be modified. The following are the factors that can affect the rate of drug dissolution.

7.3.3.1 Surface Area

The rate of drug dissolution increases with the increase in the surface area of the solid particles. The surface area can be increased by particle size reduction. The solubility of poorly soluble drugs can be increased by using micronized forms of

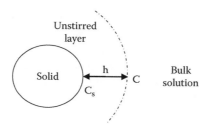

FIGURE 7.1 Model that describes the dissolution of drug from a spherical particle.

the drug [12]. It is well documented that the dissolution rate, the absorption rate, and the amount of the drug absorbed can be increased when the drug used in formulation has very small particle size such as in case of the antifungal drug, griseofulvin.

7.3.3.2   Diffusion Coefficient

The diffusion coefficient of the drug through the dissolution medium is inversely related to the viscosity of the dissolution medium. So the dissolution rate of the drug is inversely related to the viscosity of the dissolution medium. Food, food consistency, and food composition are some of the factors that can affect the viscosity of GIT contents and hence the drug dissolution rate after oral administration.

7.3.3.3   Thickness of the Unstirred Layer

The thickness of the unstirred layer inversely affects the dissolution rate of the drug. Agitation can disturb the unstirred layer resulting in reduction of its thickness and increase the dissolution rate. The viscosity of the GIT contents can affect the rate of mixing of the drug particles with the GIT contents that can affect the thickness of the unstirred layer and the rate of drug dissolution.

7.3.3.4   Drug Solubility at the Site of Absorption

The factors discussed in Section 7.3.2 of this chapter can affect the drug dissolution and can be modified to improve the drug solubility. Some of the factors that can affect the drug solubility and the rate of drug dissolution can be modified. So it is important to modify these factors to achieve the most favorable drug dissolution rate and drug solubility to ensure the optimal rate and extent of drug absorption.

7.3.4   DRUG STABILITY

The stability of drugs at the site of drug administration is an important factor affecting the extent of their absorption. Some drug products are subjected to chemical and enzymatic degradation of the active drug moiety leading to reduction in the drug amount available to be absorbed. The chemical classes of drugs that are susceptible to degradation include esters, amides, lactones, and lactams that can undergo chemical reactions such as hydrolysis, oxidation, or reduction. A common example of chemical degradation of drugs is the effect of the acidic pH of the stomach on the acid-labile drugs such as penicillin G, insulin, and nitroglycerin. Also, drugs such as atropine, digoxin, and sulfinpyrazone undergo enzymatic biotransformation by the intestinal flora decreasing the extent of absorption of the intact molecule.

Studying the stability of drugs after different routes of administration and the factors that affect the stability of drugs is important for dosage form design and selecting the suitable route of drug administration. For example, acid-labile drugs that are unstable in the stomach, such as the proton pump inhibitor, omeprazole, can be formulated as enteric coated tablets that remain intact in the stomach and release their contents in the small intestine. Some other acid-labile drugs such as nitroglycerin are formulated as buccal or sublingual tablets where the drugs are released and absorbed before they reach the stomach. When the drugs are not stable in the acidic pH of the stomach and the alkaline, enzyme-rich environment of the small intestine such as insulin, they cannot be administered by the oral route and should be administered by injections. In some cases, unstable drugs such as dopamine can be administered orally as the prodrug L-dopa, which is a stable chemical derivative of the parent drug that can be absorbed and then releases dopamine in the systemic circulation and the brain. It is important to note that drug stability is an important factor for formulation design and the selection of the suitable route of administration; however, all the other physicochemical drug properties have to be considered.

7.4 INTEGRATION OF THE PHYSICAL, CHEMICAL, AND PHYSIOLOGICAL FACTORS AFFECTING DRUG ABSORPTION

The physicochemical drug properties that can influence the absorption process have to be considered in conjunction with the physiological conditions at the different sites of drug administration. This is important because high aqueous solubility of the drug makes the drug available to be absorbed shortly after drug administration; however, these drugs usually have limited membrane permeability. Similarly lipophilic drugs have limited solubility in the aqueous physiological environment; however, they can easily cross the lipoidal biological membranes. Attempts have been made to utilize the drug physicochemical properties and physiological behavior to classify the drugs to different classes that can have similar in vivo oral absorption characteristics. These efforts resulted in the development of the biopharmaceutics classification system (BCS) and the biopharmaceutics drug disposition classification system (BDDCS).

7.4.1 BIOPHARMACEUTICS CLASSIFICATION SYSTEM

Drug absorption from the GIT by passive diffusion is dependent primarily on the solubility of the drug in the GIT lumen and the ability of the dissolved drug to pass across the GIT membrane. Based on this fact the BCS was proposed in 1995 by Amidon et al., which utilizes information about drug solubility and permeability to predict the in vivo absorption characteristics of the drug after administration in the form of immediate release solid oral dosage forms [13,14]. The BCS categorizes the drug solubility and permeability as either high or low to produce four different categories as presented in Figure 7.2.

The drug is considered highly soluble if the highest strength of the fast release drug product is soluble in 250 mL or less of aqueous media in the entire pH range of 1.0–7.5. Otherwise, the drug is considered poorly soluble. The volume of 250 mL is derived from the typical bioequivalence study protocol that prescribes drug administration to volunteers with a glass (8 oz) of water. Strict categorization of the drug permeability is not possible because of the many factors that affect the process. The drug is considered highly permeable if its extent of absorption is ≥90% of the administered dose and poorly permeable if its extent of absorption is <90%. The extent of drug absorption can be determined directly by measuring the extent of mass transfer across the human intestinal membrane. Alternatively, animal models such as the rat perfusion model or in vitro models such as the epithelial cell culture models (e.g., Caco-2 cell monolayer model) can be used to predict drug absorption

	High solubility	Low solubility
High permeability	Class I High solubility High permeability	Class II Low solubility High Permeability
Low permeability	Class III High solubility Low permeability	Class IV Low solubility Low permeability

FIGURE 7.2 Biopharmaceutical classification system as described by Amidon et al. based on the drug solubility and permeability.

in humans. Metoprolol that has been categorized as a highly permeable drug since it is known to be 95% absorbed from the GIT is used as a reference standard for the high-/low-permeability boundary. Drugs with n-octanol/water partition coefficient value greater than that of metoprolol (log P = 1.72) are considered highly permeable. An immediate release product is considered rapidly dissolving when at least 85% of the labeled amount of the drug substance dissolves within 30 min using standard dissolution apparatus in simulated gastric fluid, in pH 4.5 buffer, and in simulated intestinal fluid.

The BCS has been adopted by the U.S. Food and Drug Administration (FDA) to allow waiver of the in vivo bioequivalence testing for immediate release rapidly dissolving solid oral dosage forms of BCS class I drugs. The in vivo bioequivalence study is a study performed in normal volunteers to compare the rate and extent of drug absorption from the test drug product under investigation and an approved therapeutically effective product that contains the same active drug. Different immediate release products for BCS class I drugs should have rapid in vivo drug dissolution and high drug permeability, which should lead to similar rate and extent of drug absorption, that is, the products are bioequivalent. Thus, the rate and extent of absorption of this class of drugs from immediate release formulations is unlikely to be dependent on the formulation characteristics. This justifies why it is unnecessary to demonstrate bioequivalence for immediate release solid oral formulations of BCS class I drugs.

Also, different immediate release formulations of BCS class III drugs are expected to have rapid in vivo drug dissolution and the drug absorption will be limited by the low permeability of the drug. This indicates that the absorption of BCS class III drugs is unlikely to be affected by the formulation characteristics unless the formulation contains additives that can affect the drug permeability across the membrane. Based on this information, some scientists suggested that it may not be necessary to test for bioequivalence for immediate release solid oral dosage forms of BCS class III drugs when certain formulation conditions are met. These suggestions have not been adopted by any of the regulatory agencies yet.

The BCS has been used extensively by the pharmaceutical industry throughout the drug discovery and development processes. This is because this categorization system allows the assessment of the effect of formulation factors on the rate and extent of drug absorption after oral administration of immediate release formulation. Drugs that fall in BCS class I are highly soluble and highly permeable in the entire pH range and their absorption after rapidly dissolving dosage forms should not be sensitive to formulation factors, while drugs in the BCS class III are highly soluble and their absorption is limited by the permeability across the membrane. This makes BCS class III drugs also not sensitive to formulation factors unless permeability enhancers are included in the formulation. Conversely, drugs in BCS class II and class IV that have low solubility have greater potential for the effect of formulation factors that can affect the drug dissolution rate, with BCS class IV drugs showing more variable absorption due to their low permeability. So, immediate release dosage forms of BCS class I drugs usually do not require novel drug delivery techniques, while BCS class IV drugs require formulation strategies that can overcome the solubility and permeability limitations to improve drug absorption.

7.4.2 BIOPHARMACEUTICS DRUG DISPOSITION CLASSIFICATION SYSTEM

The objective of the BCS, as described earlier, is to use estimates for the drug solubility and permeability to predict the in vivo absorption behavior of drugs administered in the form of immediate release oral solid dosage forms. The BDDCS is a modification of the BCS that utilizes the drug solubility and the extent of drug metabolism as a tool to predict the absorption and disposition characteristics and the drug–drug interaction potential of the drug. In 2005, Wu and Benet reviewed a large number of drugs that were classified in the literature according to the four BCS categories. They recognized that the major route of elimination for the high-permeability class I and class II drugs in human is via enzymatic metabolism, while the major route of elimination for the low-permeability class III and class IV drugs is through the renal and biliary excretion of the unchanged drugs. Since the extent of drug metabolism can be characterized better than the extent of drug absorption, it was proposed in the BDDCS that drugs can be categorized according to their extent of metabolism and solubility rather than the permeability and solubility used by the BCS as in Figure 7.3 [15,16]. This new classification according to the extent of drug metabolism

	High solubility	Low solubility
Extensive metabolism	Class I High solubility Extensive metabolism	Class II Low solubility Extensive metabolism
Poor metabolism	Class III High solubility Poor metabolism	Class IV Low solubility Poor metabolism

FIGURE 7.3 Biopharmaceutical drug disposition classification system as described by Wu and Benet based on the drug solubility and extent of drug metabolism.

and solubility can decrease the number of drugs classified in more than one class due to the uncertainty of permeability determination using different techniques.

The correlation between the extent of drug metabolism and the drug permeability arise from the ability of the highly permeable drugs to cross the biological membranes and get access to the metabolizing enzymes, while low-permeability drugs usually have limited access to the metabolizing enzymes and are excreted unchanged from the body. Extensive metabolism was first defined as $\geq 70\%$ metabolism. It was later recommended that regulatory agencies can use $\geq 90\%$ metabolism as an alternative predictor for the $\geq 90\%$ absorption for defining class I drugs that are eligible for waiver of the in vivo bioequivalence study. The definition of $\geq 90\%$ metabolism means that after a single oral administration of the highest drug strength, a mass balance study can account for $\geq 90\%$ of the administered dose in the form of metabolites in urine and feces. The European Medicines Agency (EMA) revised the guidelines for investigation of bioequivalence to include extensive metabolism as a predictor of high permeability in class I biowaiver.

The broader objective of the BDDCS of predicting the drug disposition and the potential for drug–drug interactions has been explored. The BDDCS has been applied to predict the role of transporters in the gut and liver in drug disposition following oral administration. Class I drugs are highly soluble, highly permeable, and extensively metabolized. These drugs dissolve rapidly in the GIT, have easy access to the metabolizing enzymes because of their high permeability, and then undergo extensive metabolism. So the transporters do not have a significant role in the disposition of these drugs in the intestine and liver. However, the disposition of these drugs may be influenced by the transporters in other organs such as the BBB and kidney. On the contrary, class II drugs have low solubility, are highly permeable, and are extensively metabolized. The amount of these drugs available in the GIT for absorption is limited by their low solubility. However, once in solution they can readily cross the gut membrane because of their high permeability. The drug in the enterocytes can be metabolized, effluxed back to the gut lumen by the transporter, or cross the basolateral membrane and reach the portal circulation. The drug molecules that are effluxed to the gut lumen can get absorbed again and will have another chance to get metabolized, which demonstrates the interplay between the transporters and the metabolizing enzymes. So manipulation of the transporter activity can affect the extent of drug metabolism in the intestinal wall. The transporters that control the drug uptake and efflux in the liver can have similar effect on the extent of hepatic drug metabolism. So for class II drugs, the role of efflux transporter dominates the drug disposition in the intestine, but both uptake and efflux transporters can affect the drug disposition in the liver. Whereas in class III and class IV drugs, which have low permeability and poor metabolism, the uptake transporters play an important role in the intestinal absorption and also liver entry of these poorly permeable drugs. Once inside the cells, the efflux transporters can also affect the disposition of these drugs. So both uptake and efflux transporters can play a significant role in the disposition of these drugs.

Also, the BDDCS has been applied to predict the drug–drug interaction potential for the different drug categories. The disposition of class I drugs are expected to be affected significantly by metabolic interactions in the intestine and liver, while the disposition of class II drugs are most likely affected by metabolic, efflux transporter, and efflux transporter-enzyme interplay drug interactions in the intestine. Class II drugs can also be affected by metabolic, uptake transporter, efflux transporter, and transporter-enzyme interplay drug interactions in the liver. Whereas the disposition of class III and class IV drugs are likely affected by drug interactions that involve the uptake transporter, efflux transporter, and uptake-efflux transporter interplay. The BDDCS cannot predict the significant drug–drug interactions for all drugs; however, it can point out the important drug–drug interactions that should be investigated further.

REFERENCES

1. Lipinski CA, Lombardo F, Dominy BW, and Feeney PJ (1997) Experimental and computational approaches to estimate solubility and permeability in drug discovery and development settings. *Adv Drug Deliv Rev* 23:4–25.
2. Veber DF, Johnson SR, Cheng HY, Smith BR, Ward KW, and Kopple KD (2002) Molecular properties that influence the oral bioavailability of drug candidate. *J Med Chem* 45:2615–2623.
3. Ishii K, Katayama Y, Itai S, Ito Y, and Hayashi H (1995) A new pharmacokinetic model including in vivo dissolution and gastrointestinal transit parameters. *Biol Pharm Bull* 18:882–886.
4. Washington N, Washington C, and Wilson CG (2001) *Physiological Pharmaceutics, Barriers to Drug Absorption*, 2nd edn., Taylor & Francis Group, New York.
5. Grant DJW and Highuchi T (1990) *Solubility Behavior of Organic Compounds*, Wiley, New York.
6. Flynn GL (1984) Solubility concepts and their applications to the formulation of pharmaceutical systems. Part I. theoretical foundations. *J Parenter Sci Technol* 38:202–209.
7. Li SF, Wong SM, Sethia S, Almoazen H, Joshi Y, and Serajuddin ATM (2005) Investigation of solubility and dissolution of a free base and two different salt forms as a function of pH. *Pharm Res* 22:628–635.
8. Tong WQ (2000) Preformulation aspects of insoluble compounds, in Liu R (Ed.) *Water Insoluble Drug Formulation*, Interpharm Press, Denver, CO.
9. Singhal D and Curatolo W (2004) Drug polymorphism and dosage form design: A practical perspective. *Adv Drug Deliv Rev* 56:335–347.
10. Laza-Knoerr AL, Gref R, and Couvreur P (2010) Cyclodextrins for drug delivery. *J Drug Target* 18:645–656.
11. Horter D and Dressman JB (1997) Influence of physicochemical properties on dissolution of drugs in the gastrointestinal tract. *Adv Drug Deliv Rev* 25:3–14.
12. Johnson KC and Swindell AC (1996) Guidance in the setting of drug particle size specifications to minimize variability in absorption. *Pharm Res* 13:1795–1798.
13. Amidon GL, Lennernas H, Shah VP, and Crison JR (1995) A theoretical basis for a biopharmaceutic drug classification: The correlation of in vitro drug product dissolution and in vivo bioavailability. *Pharm Res* 12:413–420.
14. Dahan A, Miller JM, and Amidon GL (2009) Prediction of solubility and permeability class membership: Provisional BCS classification of the world's top oral drugs. *AAPS J* 11:740–746.
15. Wu C-Y and Benet LZ (2005) Predicting drug disposition via application of BCS: Transport/absorption/elimination interplay and development of a biopharmaceutics drug disposition classification system. *Pharm Res* 22:11–23.
16. Benet LZ (2009) Predicting drug disposition via application of a biopharmaceutics drug disposition classification system. *Basic Clin Pharmacol Toxicol* 106:162–167.

8 Drug Absorption Following Extravascular Administration
Formulation Factors

OBJECTIVES

After completing this chapter you should be able to

- Describe the general drug absorption characteristics after administration of solutions, suspensions, capsules, and tablets
- Explain the rationale for performing the dissolution tests for oral solid dosage forms
- Differentiate between the dissolution tests for quality control and for predicting the product in vivo performance
- Describe the requirements for in vivo in vitro correlation in dissolution testing
- Discuss the different strategies used for preparing site-specific drug release solid dosage forms
- Discuss the different formulation approaches to control the rate of drug release from solid dosage forms
- Describe the different factors that can enhance drug absorption after intranasal and transdermal drug administration
- State the advantages and disadvantages of drug delivery via the intranasal, pulmonary, and transdermal routes

8.1 INTRODUCTION

Drugs are usually administered as formulated pharmaceutical preparations. The physicochemical properties of the drug and the physiological factors related to the intended site of drug administration should be considered while developing the pharmaceutical formulation. These formulations should be carefully designed and manufactured using rigorous procedures to produce high-quality products that have the desired specifications. This is important to ensure drug stability, dose uniformity,

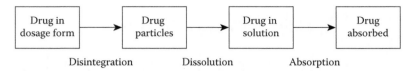

FIGURE 8.1   Processes involved in the absorption of drugs administered as solid dosage forms.

suitability for the route of administration, consistency in the drug absorption behavior, and patient acceptability.

After extravascular administration of any pharmaceutical formulation, the drug has to be released from the formulation and then dissolved at the site of absorption before it can cross the biological membrane to reach the systemic circulation. For example, solid dosage forms such as tablets administered by the oral route have to disintegrate to small granules and fine powder first. Then the drug particles have to dissolve in the gastrointestinal (GIT) secretions before the drug is absorbed to the systemic circulation as described in the scheme presented in Figure 8.1. The rate of overall drug absorption after administration of a dosage form is dependent on the rate of disintegration, dissolution, and absorption, which are influenced by the formulation characteristics. Similarly, the extent of drug absorption to the systemic circulation can be affected by the formulation characteristics because if the drug is not released completely at the site of absorption, the absorption will not be complete. So different formulations for the same active drug from different manufacturers can have different rates and extents of drug absorption. This is true for all extravascular routes of administration; the formulation characteristics can significantly affect the rate and extent of drug absorption.

When the absorption process involves multiple steps such as disintegration, dissolution, and absorption after administration of a solid dosage, the rate of the overall absorption process is determined by the rate of the slowest step. The slowest step in a series of steps is called the rate determining step. For a drug with poor aqueous solubility, the dissolution rate of the drug is usually very slow and the absorption rate of such a drug is dependent on the dissolution rate of the drug. On the other hand, the rate limiting step for the absorption of drugs with high aqueous solubility is the rate of permeation across the biological membrane because it is usually the slowest step. This principle can be applied in formulation design to control one of the steps involved in the drug absorption process, which in turn can control the rate of the overall absorption process. For example, the rate of drug absorption after administration of controlled-release dosage forms can be controlled by controlling the rate of release of the drug from the dosage form. Also, the rate of drug absorption in transdermal batches is determined from the rate of drug release from these batches. Furthermore, some drugs can be formulated in the form of pellets that can release the drug over an extended period of time that can be months or years. The rate of drug absorption after subcutaneous insertion of these pellets usually follows the rate of drug release from the pellets, resulting in slow absorption of the drug over an extended period of time.

8.2 FORMULATION FACTORS AFFECTING DRUG ABSORPTION AFTER PARENTERAL DRUG ADMINISTRATION

Drugs administered intravenously are introduced directly to the systemic circulation, so there is no absorption step involved. Formulations administered by this route have to be water miscible, should not contain particles larger than 5 μm, in addition to the general requirements of sterility, isotonicity, and pH. Once administered, the drugs are distributed via the systemic circulation to all parts of the body including the site of drug action and to eliminating organs where drugs can be eliminated from the body. The kinetics of the drug distribution and elimination processes depends on the drug properties; however, specialized formulations have been developed to modify the distribution characteristics and the elimination rate to improve the therapeutic effect of the drug. Examples of such formulations include the liposomal formulations and the drug-antibody conjugates that can be used for drug targeting to specific organs [1].

A wide range of formulations can be administered intramuscularly including aqueous solutions and suspensions, oily solutions and suspensions, oil-in-water and water-in-oil emulsions, and solid dispersion implants. These formulations are mentioned in the order of their general drug release rate, which can affect the rate of drug absorption after their administration [2]. Drugs administered as aqueous solutions are absorbed completely in few minutes, while drugs administered in oil suspensions may be absorbed over a period of several days, whereas the absorption of drugs administered as solid implants may take several months. The extent of drug absorption is also different for the different formulations; however, this mainly depends on the stability of the drug at the site of administration before it is absorbed. Drugs administered by subcutaneous injection are absorbed directly to the blood capillary and also by the lymphatic system. So in addition to the aqueous solution, formulations that contain particles such as liposomes or suspensions can be administered subcutaneously where they can be absorbed via the lymphatic system.

8.3 FORMULATION FACTORS AFFECTING DRUG ABSORPTION AFTER ORAL DRUG ADMINISTRATION

It is estimated that approximately 90% of drug use is through the oral route since it is the most convenient route especially for drugs used in the management of chronic diseases. A wide range of formulations can be administered by the oral route including liquid and solid dosage forms. These formulations include conventional dosage forms that are formulated to release the active drug in the GIT directly after administration without controlling the site or the rate of drug release. Also, modified-release oral formulations can be formulated to release the active drug at a specific site of the GIT and/or to control the release rate of the active drug.

8.3.1 CONVENTION ORAL FORMULATIONS

Drugs administered in the form of solution are ready to be absorbed once they reach the site of their absorption, while drugs administered in the form of suspension have to dissolve first before they can be absorbed. Also, solid dosage forms such as tablets and capsules have to disintegrate to granules or small particles first before the drug can dissolve and become available for the absorption process. So it is generally acceptable that the rate of drug absorption is usually faster from solution > suspension > capsules > tablets. Although this is the general rule, there are situations when this rule does not apply. So the characteristics of the dosage forms are important in determining the rate and the extent of drug absorption.

8.3.1.1 Solutions

Formulations administered as solutions include aqueous solutions, elixirs, and syrups that have the active drug and other ingredient completely dissolved in the vehicle. In general, the rate determining step in drug absorption after administration of solutions is the rate at which the drug reaches the site of absorption or the rate of permeation across the biological membrane. Drug solutions are emptied from the stomach very rapidly, especially when administered on an empty stomach, to reach the small intestine, which is the main site of absorption for most drugs. This makes the absorption from solution formulations faster than the absorption from other formulations for the same drug. Sometimes the dissolved drugs may precipitate in the GIT due to unfavorable conditions that may affect the drug solubility. For example, weak acids administered as solutions may precipitate once they reach the stomach due to the acidic pH that decreases the solubility of most weak acids. In most cases, the precipitated drug will usually dissolve again without causing any absorption problems.

8.3.1.2 Suspensions

Suspensions contain the drug in the form of fine particles dispersed in the formulation vehicle with the aid of a suspending agent. The dispersed particles have to dissolve first before the drug can be absorbed. Drug absorption from suspensions is usually slower than drug absorption from solutions because of the additional dissolution step involved, while drug absorption from suspension is usually faster than drug absorption from solid dosage forms that need to disintegrate before the drug can be dissolved and then absorbed. Some of the formulation factors that can affect the rate and extent of drug absorption administered in the form of suspension include the particle size of the suspended particles, crystal form, and viscosity of the finished product, all of which affect the rate of drug dissolution.

8.3.1.3 Capsules

The hard gelatin capsules contain the uncompressed drug and additives inside the capsule shell. Once the capsule shell is disrupted by the aqueous environment of the GIT, the capsule contents are released and the drug starts to dissolve. The capsule contents are dispersed and mixed rapidly with the GIT contents and start to dissolve. This makes the rate of drug absorption, after administration in the form of capsules, faster than its absorption from tablets.

8.3.1.4 Tablets

Tablets usually contain the active drug ingredient(s) in addition to many other additives compressed together into a single dosage unit. These additives include diluents, disintegrating agent, granulating agents, lubricants, coloring agents, and others.

After oral administration of a drug in the form of tablets, the drug dissolution is usually slow because of the small surface area of the intact tablets. Then the tablets disintegrate to small granules causing significant increase in the surface area, which increases the rate of drug dissolution. The surface area and hence the drug dissolution rate increase further with the disintegration of the granules to fine particles. Although tablet disintegration is important in the sequence of steps leading to drug absorption, it is unlikely to be the rate-determining step in the absorption of drugs administered as conventional tablets. This is because the disintegration of conventional tablets is usually faster than the drug dissolution rate. So the dissolution rate of the active drug ingredient after administration of conventional tablets is the important factor in determining the rate and extent of drug absorption.

In general, the rate of drug absorption after administration of tablets that have rapid dissolution rate is faster than the rate of drug absorption from tablets that have slow dissolution rate. The effect of the rate of dissolution on the extent of absorption depends on the drug characteristics and the drug absorption mechanisms. For example, drugs absorbed by a saturable mechanism or drugs with site-specific absorption usually have lower extent of absorption after administration of rapidly dissolving tablets compared to after administration of slowly dissolving tablets. Also, drugs that are not stable in the acidic pH of the stomach usually have lower extent of absorption when administered as rapidly dissolving tablets that release the drug in the stomach compared to slowly dissolving tablets that release the majority of the drug in the small intestine. Since tablet disintegration and dissolution rates are dependent on the tablet additives and the manufacturing procedures, different tablets for the same active drug moiety marketed by different drug manufacturers can have different rate and extent of drug absorption. So manufactured tablets are usually subjected to dissolution tests as part of the quality control and to predict the in vivo absorption behavior of the drug after administration of the dosage form.

8.3.1.4.1   In Vitro Dissolution Test

In vitro tablet dissolution test can be utilized as a quality control tool to evaluate the product quality and also to predict the in vivo product performance. The conditions of the dissolution test for different products differ from each other in the choice of the dissolution apparatus, dissolution medium and testing conditions that include the volume of the dissolution medium, and agitation rate. Ideally the same dissolution test conditions can be used for evaluation of the product quality and for predicting the product in vivo performance. However, this is not possible because the conditions of the dissolution test used as a quality control tool are selected to be sensitive to predict formulation and manufacturing changes, while the dissolution test used for predicting the in vivo product performance is designed to simulate the in vivo environment where the drug is expected to be released.

Dissolution testing as a quality control tool: There are several compendial dissolution apparatuses that can be used for dissolution testing with the basket method (USP Apparatus I) and the paddle method (USP Apparatus II) being the most commonly used methods for dissolution testing of conventional tablets. Aqueous dissolution media that have pH that reflects the GIT environment are usually used.

The dissolution media can have pH in the range of 1.2–6.8 that reflects the gastric and intestinal conditions. Surfactants such as sodium lauryl sulfate and tween can be included in the dissolution medium used for poorly soluble drugs. The volume of the dissolution medium can range from 500 to 1000 mL. The common stirring speed for apparatus I is between 50 and 100 rpm, while for apparatus II is between 50 and 75 rpm. The dissolution test is usually performed at 37°C for a period between 15 and 60 min [3]. The reproducibility of the dissolution rate of tablets using these dissolution test conditions is usually used to evaluate the product quality. The major shortcoming of this dissolution testing is that it cannot predict the in vivo performance of the drug product so it does not have any clinical relevance.

Dissolution testing to predict the in vivo product performance: The development of this dissolution testing, also known as biorelevant dissolution testing, should consider the in vivo environment at the site where most of the drug is released from the formulation. This includes the pH, contents, volume, motility, hemodynamics, transit time, and pathological conditions. All the available compendial dissolution apparatuses and different composition of the dissolution media can be used to develop the biorelevant dissolution testing that can simulate the in vivo conditions [4]. For example, the immediate-release tablets of highly soluble drugs are expected to release the active drug in the stomach. The dissolution medium used for such tablets usually has pH between 1.5 and 2.5 and includes surfactants and enzymes such as pepsin to simulate the in vivo conditions of the stomach. On the contrary, conventional tablets that contain drugs with low solubility are expected to release the active drug in the small intestine. The dissolution medium used for such tablets usually has pH between 5.5 and 7.5 and includes bile salts, phospholipids and may include digestive enzymes such as lipase, peptidase, amylase, and protease to simulate the in vivo conditions in the small intestine. Also, the dissolution medium can be modified to study the effect of food on the drug dissolution rate in vivo. In this case, buffers with high buffering capacity are used to mimic the buffering effect of food; dissolution media with higher osmolarity and higher concentration of bile salts and lecithin can be used to imitate the higher bile acid secretion in response to food intake [5]. The development of biorelevant dissolution testing procedures is not an easy task because of the complexity of the conditions needed to be simulated.

8.3.1.4.2   Dissolution Requirements
The dissolution requirement for a solid dosage form is usually expressed as the percent of the labeled amount of the drug (Q) that dissolves over a certain period of time. The Q and the time period specified in the drug monograph will have to be met for the drug product to pass the dissolution testing. The United States Pharmacopoeia (USP) specifies a three-step dissolution testing and the criteria for accepting the results [6].

Step one: The dissolution test results are accepted if the percent dissolved during the specified time for each of six tablets is not less than Q + 5%. If these criteria are not met, go to step two.

Step two: The dissolution test results are accepted if the average percent dissolved during the specified time for 12 tablets (6 from step one + 6 additional tablets) is equal or greater than Q and no one tablet is less than Q − 15%. If these criteria are not met, go to step three.

Step three: The dissolution test results are accepted if the average percent dissolved during the specified time for 24 tablets (6 from step one + 6 from step two + 12 additional tablets) is equal or greater than Q and no more than two tablets are less than Q − 15% and no one tablet is less than Q − 25%. If these criteria are not met, this means that dissolution test failed.

8.3.1.4.3 In Vivo–In Vitro Correlation

The issue of in vivo–in vitro correlation (IVIVC) has been of great importance for pharmaceutical industry, academics, and regulatory agencies. The FDA defines the IVIVC as the correlation between an in vitro property of a dosage form and a relevant in vivo response [7]. Usually the in vitro property is the rate and extent of drug dissolution and the in vivo response is the amount of drug absorbed or the plasma drug concentration–time profile. Pharmaceutical manufacturers usually attempt to develop and optimize the conditions of in vitro dissolution testing procedures for a particular formulation that can predict the in vivo performance of that formulation. When this is achieved and IVIVC is established, the in vitro dissolution testing data only can be used to prove that changes in formulation composition, manufacturing process, suppliers, equipment, and batch size do not affect the in vivo drug absorption. Without the establishment of the IVIVC, minor formulation changes will require in vivo studies in human volunteers to prove that the modified formulation has the same rate and extent of drug absorption as the original formulation, that is, new and old formulations are bioequivalent. Although the IVIVC is discussed in this section under conventional tablets, this concept has a wide range of applications in controlled-release tablets.

Development of a correlation begins with formulation research to develop a drug formulation that can achieve a therapeutically desirable drug concentration–time profile when administered in normal volunteers in pilot pharmacokinetic studies. This is usually followed by extensive in vitro characterization of the formulation by studying the rate and extent of drug dissolution under different conditions of pH, media, and apparatuses. The in vivo performance of the formulation is determined from pharmacokinetic studies performed in normal volunteers. The amount of drug released in vitro from the formulation at different time points under the different dissolution test conditions is compared with the rate and extent of drug absorption in vivo. When good correlation exists between a certain in vitro dissolution test performed under specific conditions and the in vivo rate and extent of drug absorption, this indicates that good IVIVC is established between this specific dissolution test and the in vivo performance of the formulation under investigation. The FDA defines four levels of correlations between the in vitro dissolution test results and the in vivo rate and extent of drug absorption as follows [7]:

Level A: This is the highest degree of correlation and represents point-to-point relationship between the in vitro dissolution rate and the in vivo absorption rate from the dosage form.

Level B: In this level, the mean in vitro dissolution time ($MDT_{in\ vitro}$) is correlated with the in vivo mean residence time (MRT) or mean in vivo dissolution time ($MDT_{in\ vivo}$).

This cannot be considered good correlation because different drug dissolution rate profiles can have the same $MDT_{in\ vitro}$ and different plasma drug concentration–time profiles can have the same MRT.

Level C: In this level, one dissolution time point such as time for 50% or 90% dissolution is compared with one mean pharmacokinetic parameter such as AUC, t_{max}, or C_{max}. Again, this is not a good correlation because it represents a single point correlation that does not reflect the entire plasma drug concentration–time profile.

Multiple-level C: In this level a correlation is established between one or more pharmacokinetic parameters such as AUC, t_{max}, or C_{max} and the amount of drug dissolved at multiple time points that covers the entire dissolution profile. When multiple-level C correlation is achievable, it is possible to achieve level A correlation.

When level A correlation between the formulation in vitro dissolution profile and the in vivo drug absorption is established, the in vitro dissolution testing data only without any additional in vivo data can be used to prove that minor formulation changes do not affect the in vivo absorption of the drug. Level B and level C correlation are usually not accepted by regulatory authorities as a justification for using the in vitro dissolution testing to predict the in vivo absorption of the drug.

The biopharmaceutics classification system (BCS) classifies drugs according to their solubility and permeability and allows regulatory authorities to waive the in vivo bioequivalence testing for immediate release rapidly dissolving solid oral dosage forms for drugs with high solubility and high permeability. This classification system also provides a guideline for determining the conditions under which IVIVC is expected [8]. For BCS class I drugs that have high solubility and high permeability, the rate determining step for drug absorption is likely to be drug dissolution and gastric emptying rate. The IVIVC for BCS class I drugs is expected if the dissolution rate of the formulation is slower than the gastric emptying rate. On the contrary, for BCS class II drugs that have low solubility and high permeability, the rate determining step for drug absorption is the dissolution rate. The IVIVC for BCS class II drugs is expected when the in vitro drug dissolution rate is similar to the in vivo drug dissolution rate [9]. Whereas the BCS class III and class IV drugs have poor permeability and the rate determining step for drug absorption is most likely to be the permeability across the GIT membrane. So the IVIVC is not expected for BCS class III and class IV.

8.3.2 MODIFIED-RELEASE ORAL FORMULATIONS

Modified-release formulations are defined by the USP as the formulations whose time course of drug release and the location of drug release are chosen to accomplish therapeutic or convenient objectives that cannot be offered by conventional formulations. The rational for using modified-release formulations is that these formulations usually have slow rate of drug release that slows the rate of drug absorption. So when the proper dose of the drug is used, therapeutic drug concentrations can be maintained for extended period of time with minimal fluctuations in the drug concentrations during repeated administration. This is important to maintain steady therapeutic effect all the time, especially for drugs that have direct relationship between plasma drug concentration and effect. Also, these formulations can be administered less frequently, which can improve patient compliance. However, not all drugs are suitable for modified-release formulations. The formulation GIT transit time can limit the maximum time over which the drug can be absorbed, and the cost of these formulations is usually higher than the cost of conventional formulations.

8.3.2.1 Formulations with Site-Specific Drug Release

Sublingual and buccal formulations: Drugs can be absorbed rapidly through the buccal mucosa to reach the systemic circulation bypassing the hepatic first-pass metabolism. Because of the limited surface area and the short transit time of the mouth cavity, formulations designed for buccal drug delivery have to dissolve rapidly and have to be retained in the mouth cavity for a period of time to ensure maximum drug absorption. Sublingual tablets are rapidly dissolving tablets that are placed under the tongue to achieve fast rate of drug absorption. This fast rate of drug absorption makes sublingual tablets suitable for drug administration when fast onset of drug effect is required. Formulations designed for buccal drug delivery include fast-dissolving tablets that are usually taken without water and are expected to disperse and dissolve once placed in the tongue allowing large fractions of the administered dose to be absorbed from the buccal cavity. Also, the incorporation of drugs in chewing gums has been used to slowly release the drug during chewing, and the released drug is then absorbed from the buccal cavity. Furthermore, bioadhesive formulations usually utilize polymer such as hydrocolloids and hydrogels to prepare dosage forms that can adhere to the mucosal surface of the buccal cavity and release the drug over an extended period of time [10].

Gastric retentive formulations: Gastric retention of dosage forms has been used as an approach for developing controlled-release formulations when the formulation is intended to deliver the drug to the stomach such as in the treatment of *Helicobacter pylori* infection. Also, this approach can be used to develop controlled-release formulations for acid soluble drugs or for drugs with site-specific absorption from the upper part of the small intestine to increase the extent of their absorption. Gastric retention can be achieved using floating systems that are low-density formulations that absorb water and swell when they come in contact with the gastric secretions. The swelled floating formulations have low density so they float above the gastric contents delaying their gastric emptying [11]. Mucoadhesion is another technique used to increase the formulation gastric retention [12]. Furthermore, formulations that can expand or unfold in the stomach to become too large to exit through the pylorus have been tried to increase the formulation retention in the stomach. The effect of increasing the gastric transit time on the extent of drug absorption depends on the drug properties such as the drug stability and the mechanism of drug absorption whether it is passive or active.

Enteric-coated formulations: Acid labile drugs can be degraded by the acidic environment of the stomach when administered orally in the form of conventional formulations. Enteric coating has been used to deliver acid labile drugs to the small intestine by coating the formulation with an acid-resistant coat that can protect the formulation from the acidic pH of the stomach. Once in the alkaline environment of the small intestine, the coat dissolves releasing the drug in the small intestine.

Drug absorption in this case is delayed depending on the gastric emptying rate of the formulation. This delay in drug absorption, which is also known as the lag time for drug absorption, can be short when the drug is administered in the fasted state or long when the drug is administered after meal.

Colonic delivery formulations: Drug delivery to the colon can be for the local effect of the drug in the colon such as in the treatment of inflammatory diseases and infections or for the systemic effect of drugs that can be absorbed from the colon. Strategies used for delivering drugs to the colon have to protect the formulation from digestion and absorption from the stomach and small intestine and release the drug in the ascending colon. The use of acid resistance coating can keep the formulation intact until it reaches the alkaline pH of the intestine. Controlling the dissolution rate of the formulation allows the delivery of the drug to the ascending colon. Also, the use of timed-release formulation that are designed to release the drug about four hours after leaving the stomach can allow releasing the drug about the same time when the formulation reaches the base of the ascending colon [13]. Additionally, formulations that take advantage of the colonic bacteria have been used to deliver the drug to the colon. The formulation may contain a prodrug that can be hydrolyzed by the colonic bacteria to liberate the active drug in the colon such as the use of salicylazosulfapyridine for the treatment of inflammatory bowel disease [14]. Moreover, coating of the formulations with polymers that undergo degradation by the colonic bacteria can release the drug in the colon. Drug absorption following administration of formulations intended for colonic delivery is usually delayed similar to the enteric-coated formulations but in this case the delay in absorption depends on the gastric and intestinal transit time.

8.3.2.2   Formulations with Controlled Rate of Drug Release
Controlled-release formulations are usually developed to have a slow and constant rate of drug release over an extended period of time. This slow rate of drug release from the formulation results in slow rate of drug absorption to the systemic circulation. The most common controlled-release delivery systems include the matrix systems, the membrane-controlled systems, and the osmotic pump systems [15].

The matrix systems: The matrix-controlled-release drug delivery systems are prepared by dispersing the drug particles in a water soluble matrix. After administration of these drug delivery systems, the drug is released from the delivery system when the matrix dissolves in the GIT contents. Different water soluble matrices that dissolve at different rates can be used in these formulations and can produce different rates of drug release from the delivery systems. Also, the drug particles may be dispersed in an insoluble matrix. The drug is released from these delivery systems when the aqueous fluids in the GIT contents penetrate the matrix, dissolve the drug particles and the drug solution diffuse back out of the delivery system. The water penetration rate through the water insoluble matrix is different for the different matrices. Since water penetration through the matrix is responsible for the drug dissolution and release from these delivery systems, the rate of drug release can be controlled by the choice of the matrix.

Membrane-controlled systems: In the membrane-controlled systems, the tablets or pellets that act as drug reservoirs are coated with a membrane that controls the diffusion of the drug out of the dosage form. The membrane that covers the dosage form becomes permeable by hydration when it comes in contact with the GIT contents or by the drug being soluble in the membrane components. Water diffuses through the membrane into the delivery system and dissolves the drug. The dissolved drug is released out of the delivery system by diffusion across the membrane. The choice of the membrane composition can control the rate of drug release from the delivery system. The drug can be loaded in the membrane to produce an initial fast rate of drug release from the membrane that is followed by slow rate of drug release by diffusion across the membrane.

Osmotic pump systems: The osmotic pump systems are similar to the membrane-controlled systems since they contain a tablet that contains the drug in the core of the system. The tablet is usually coated with a membrane that allows water to pass to the core and dissolves the tablet contents. As the tablet contents dissolve, the hydrostatic pressure increases inside the tablet and forces the dissolved material to be released from the system through a hole drilled in the membrane during manufacturing. The rate of drug release from the tablet can be controlled by controlling the rate of water diffusion across the membrane into the core or by controlling the viscosity of the solution formed inside the system.

The rate and extent of drug absorption following the administration of the modified-release oral formulations is affected by the rate of release of the active drug from the formulation. Consequently, the plasma drug concentration–time profile can be affected by the drug release rate from the formulation. Thus, modified-release formulations are subjected to in vitro dissolution testing as a quality control tool and also to predict the in vivo performance similar to what was discussed under conventional formulations. Establishment of IVIVC is also important for modified-release formulations.

8.4 FORMULATION FACTORS AFFECTING DRUG ABSORPTION AFTER RECTAL DRUG ADMINISTRATION

The rectal route of drug administration is usually more convenient in some patient populations such as elderly and children and in unconscious patients when the oral route is not possible and parenteral formulations are not available. Also, drugs that undergo extensive first-pass metabolism by the liver after oral administration can be administered by the rectal route to bypass the liver first-pass metabolism. Formulations administered by the rectal route include suppositories formulated in the form of solid suspension or solid emulsion and enemas in the form of solutions or suspensions. The rate of drug absorption after rectal drug administration is dependent on the rate of drug release from the dosage form.

Rapid rate of drug release from the rectal formulations is usually preferred because of the short rectal transit time, the limited surface area of the rectum, and the limited spreading of the rectally administered drugs to the colon. Also, the high drug concentration produced in the rectum after the rapid drug release is the driving force for drug absorption, which is mainly by passive diffusion. The solubility of the drug in the base of the dosage form is an important factor in determining the rate of drug release and hence the rate drug absorption. Lipophilic drugs are released faster from hydrophilic vehicles and slower from lipophilic vehicles. This is because lipophilic drugs will partition more into the lipophilic vehicles slowing their rate of release. Similarly, hydrophilic drugs are released faster from lipophilic vehicles and slower from hydrophilic vehicles [16].

The solubility of the released drug in the aqueous environment of the rectum is another important factor affecting the rate of drug absorption in the rectum. Balanced hydrophilic and lipophilic drug properties are important for rectal drug absorption. Highly lipophilic drugs have low solubility in the limited volume of water in the rectum, and highly hydrophilic drugs have limited membrane diffusivity. The drug particle size in formulations administered as liquid or solid suspensions is an important factor in determining the drug dissolution rate. Also, the surface properties of the drug particles and the drug load per unit dose can cause particle agglomeration that slows the drug dissolution rate and may cause unequal drug distribution in the dosage forms. Formulations intended for rectal administration are subjected to in vitro release and dissolution tests that are useful for quality control purposes but have limited predictive value for the formulation in vivo performance. The human in vivo studies remain the most reliable method to determine the rate and extent of drug absorption from rectally administered formulations.

8.5 FORMULATION FACTORS AFFECTING DRUG ABSORPTION AFTER INTRANASAL DRUG ADMINISTRATION

Formulations administered into the nasal cavity contain the drug in the form of solution, suspension, emulsion, and dry powder. Drugs are administered to the nasal cavity for their local effect such as nasal decongestants and for their systemic effects where the drugs have to be absorbed to the systemic circulation to produce their systemic effect. Drugs with small molecular weight have relatively good systemic absorption with the absorption rate decreasing sharply when the molecular weight exceeds 1000 Da. The absorption of drugs after intranasal administration can be enhanced by modification of the pH, the use of penetration enhancer, and prolongation of the nasal residence time [17,18].

The average pH in the nasal cavity is about 6.2–6.4. This pH can affect the absorption of ionizable drugs since the unionized form of the drug can be absorbed better than the ionized form. It is possible to buffer the drug formulation to target the optimal pH required for drug absorption across the nasal epithelium. Also the use of penetration enhancer such as bile salts has been used to decrease the viscosity of the nasal mucus secretions and to transiently form aqueous pores in the epithelium layer where the drugs can be absorbed. Other penetration enhancers such as EDTA and fatty acid salts can increase paracellular absorption by removal of luminal calcium. Furthermore, since most liquid formulations are cleared from the nose within 30 min, increasing the nasal transit time of the nasal formulations can enhance the absorption of drugs. Increasing the nasal transit time can be achieved by increasing the viscosity of the formulation or by using bioadhesive formulations. Both of these techniques can increase the transit time in the nasal cavity allowing more time for drug absorption.

Animal models have been used to evaluate the different strategies for enhancing the nasal delivery of drugs and to compare different formulations. However, drug absorption after administration of intranasal formulations has to be evaluated by in vivo pharmacokinetic studies in humans. Characterization of the drug concentration–time profile after intranasal drug administration can be used for bioequivalence testing for generic formulations and to determine the onset and the expected duration of drug effect if the drug concentration-effect relationship is well defined. In some instances, the plasma drug concentration–time profile cannot be characterized after intranasal administration because the plasma drug concentration is very low, which can complicate the evaluation process. In this case, evaluating the in vivo performance of different formulations should be based on comparing the observed therapeutic effect of the drug after intranasal administration to patients. Normal healthy volunteers can be used in evaluating the intranasal formulation evaluation if the drug effect can be observed in healthy individuals.

8.6 FORMULATION FACTORS AFFECTING DRUG ABSORPTION AFTER PULMONARY DRUG ADMINISTRATION

Different types of inhalation devices are used for drug administration by inhalation including metered-dose inhalers, dry powder inhalers, and nebulizers. In the metered dose inhaler, the drug is dissolved or suspended in the propellant with the other excipients that are filled under pressure in a canister fitted with a metered valve. When the valve is released, the propellant expands quickly to become a gas at atmospheric pressure leaving the drug as fine droplets or fine particles. The high speed gas flow helps in moving the drug down the respiratory tract, while in the dry powder inhaler the drug is inhaled as fine particles. The drug powder is preloaded in the device or included in a capsule that can be loaded to the device before use. Whereas in nebulizers, the drug solution or suspension is converted to spray that can be inhaled with normal breathing with the aid of a mouth piece or a mask.

The inhaled drugs can be absorbed to reach the systemic circulation from the site of their deposition in the upper and lower parts of the respiratory tract. Generally, lipophilic drugs are absorbed better than hydrophilic drugs. Many formulation factors can affect the site of deposition of the aerosol particles in the respiratory tract. Studying the relationship between the inhaled drug particle characteristics and the distance traveled by the drug particles can be used to optimize the inhaler properties. However, these studies cannot be used to predict and compare the in vivo performance of different inhalation devices. Pharmacokinetic studies in humans are usually required to determine the rate and extent of drug absorption after pulmonary drug administration.

Pharmacokinetic evaluation of the rate and extent of drug absorption after inhalation therapy is the most acceptable method for comparing different inhalation delivery systems, as well as for evaluating the bioequivalence of generic drug formulations. Characterization of drug absorption from the lungs can be used to evaluate the expected drug effect after inhalation based on the plasma drug concentration-effect relationship [19]. When the plasma drug concentration–time profile cannot be characterized after drug administration by inhalation, the in vivo performance of the inhalation formulations can be evaluated by monitoring the drug therapeutic effect in humans as discussed for the intranasal drug administration. Drugs may be administered by inhalation for their local effects in the respiratory system to decrease the drug systemic exposure that decreases the drug adverse effects. An example of such drugs is beclomethasone, which is a corticosteroid derivative used by inhalation in the treatment of bronchial asthma. Studying the absorption of beclomethasone to the systemic circulation after using different inhalers is important to compare the systemic exposure to beclomethasone that produces the drug adverse effects. The inhalers with the least systemic exposure (i.e., least absorption) are usually the preferred devices when the drug is used for its local effect in the respiratory system.

8.7 FORMULATION FACTORS AFFECTING DRUG ABSORPTION AFTER TRANSDERMAL DRUG ADMINISTRATION

Pharmaceutical formulations have been used for long time for topical drug administration. This includes medicated ointment, creams, lotions, and gels; however, these formulations are suitable for systemic delivery of controlled amounts of the drug. This is because the rate and extent of drug absorption after topical administration depend on the diffusion rate of the drug from the formulation, the penetration of the drug across the skin, and the area of application on the skin, all of which cannot be controlled by these conventional formulations. Transdermal drug delivery systems have been developed that can produce a controlled rate of drug absorption after application on the skin. The general features of these transdermal delivery systems include a drug reservoir that contains the drug and a mechanism that controls the rate of drug release from a constant area of the delivery system.

The transdermal delivery systems are designed to have slow rate of drug release from the system, so the release rate becomes the rate limiting step in the drug absorption process. This will limit the effect of the physiological variables on the drug absorption rate. So good drug candidates for transdermal delivery are potent drugs that need to be delivered to the body over an extended period of time. Since transdermal absorption of drugs is a slow process, several formulation strategies have been used to improve the absorption of the drugs applied to the skin [20]. These include hydration of the stratum corneum, which is an important factor in the skin penetration rate for most drugs and can be achieved by using occlusive devices such as patches or by using moisturizing additives. Also, transdermal drug absorption can be enhanced by using penetration enhancers that are excipients included in the formulations that can temporarily increase the skin permeability to drugs. Another strategy is the use of prodrugs that can be absorbed better than the active drugs, and after their absorption they can be hydrolyzed to liberate the active drug in vivo.

Numerous experimental techniques can be used to study drug diffusion through the skin. This includes in vitro techniques that investigate the rate of drug transport through an excised skin sample placed between the donor and receptor compartments of a diffusion cell. This technique can utilize animal skin, human skin, or artificial membranes. Also, in vivo studies can be performed in experimental animals to study the skin penetration of drugs. Because of the difference in the nature of the human skin and the animal skin, the in vitro techniques and animal studies can be used in screening for topical agents, comparing the partition coefficient and diffusion coefficient of drugs, studying the formulation factors affecting skin penetration of drugs, and studying the skin penetration mechanisms. However, these techniques cannot substitute the pharmacokinetic studies that are usually performed in humans to determine the rate and extent of drug absorption after transdermal application.

In vivo evaluation of drug absorption to the systemic circulation after application of transdermal drug delivery systems such as transdermal patches has to be performed in humans. This usually includes a single-dose pharmacokinetic study to characterize the plasma drug concentration–time profile produced after application of the patch. This is used to determine the lag time for the drug therapeutic effect, the steady state plateau, and the decline phase after a single application of the patch. Additional in vivo pharmacokinetic studies include application of different sizes of the patch to determine the relationship between the absorbed dose and the patch surface area. Also, pharmacokinetic studies after application of the patch to different skin sites to ensure that the rate determining step in drug absorption is the drug release from the patch and that application to different sites produce the same therapeutic effect. Furthermore, pharmacokinetic studies during repeated patch applications are performed, and the relationship between the plasma drug concentration and therapeutic effect is determined.

REFERENCES

1. Woodle MC, Storm G, Newman MS, Jekot JJ, Collins LR, Martin FJ, and Szoka FC Jr. (1992) Prolonged systemic delivery of peptide drugs by long-circulating liposomes: Illustration with vasopressin in the Brattleboro rat. *Pharm Res* 9:260–265.
2. Washington N, Washington C, and Wilson CG (2001) *Physiological Pharmaceutics, Barriers to Drug Absorption*, 2nd edn., Taylor & Francis Group, New York.
3. Center for Drug Evaluation and Research, U.S. Food and Drug Administration (1997) Guidance for industry: Dissolution testing of immediate release solid oral dosage forms.
4. Dressman JB, Amidon GL, Reppas C, and Shah VP (1998) Dissolution testing as a prognostic tool for oral drug absorption: Immediate release dosage forms. *Pharm Res* 15:11–22.
5. Efentakis M and Dressman JB (1998) Gastric juice as a dissolution medium: Surface tension and pH. *Eur J Drug Metab Pharmacokinet* 23:97–102.
6. United States Pharmacopeia (2011) *34th Rev. and the National Formulary*, 29th edn., United States Pharmacopeial Convention, Rockville, MD.
7. Center for Drug Evaluation and Research, U.S. Food and Drug Administration (1997) Guidance for industry: Extended release oral dosage forms: Development, evaluation and application of in vitro/in vivo correlations.
8. Amidon GL, Lennernas H, Shah VP, and Crison JR (1995) A theoretical basis for a biopharmaceutic drug classification: The correlation of in vitro drug product dissolution and in vivo bioavailability. *Pharm Res* 12:413–420.
9. Dahan A, Miller JM, and Amidon GL (2009) Prediction of solubility and permeability class membership: Provisional BCS classification of the world's top oral drugs. *AAPS J* 11:740–746.
10. Nagai T and Konishi R (1987) Buccal/gingival drug delivery systems. *J Control Rel* 6:353–360.
11. Ingani HM, Timmermans J, and Moes AJ Concept and in vivo investigation of peroral sustained release floating dosage forms with enhanced gastrointestinal transit. *Int J Pharm* 35:157–164.

12. Burton S, Washington N, Steele RJC, Musson R, and Feely L (1995) Intragastric distribution of ion-exchange resins: A drug delivery system for the topical treatment of the gastric mucosa. *J Pharm Pharmacol* 47:901–906.

13. Dew MJ, Hughes PJ, Lee MG, Evans BK, and Rhodes J (1982) An oral preparation to release drugs in the human colon. *Br J Clin Pharmacol* 14:405–408.

14. Rubinstein A (1990) Microbially controlled drug delivery to the colon. *Biopharm Drug Dispos* 11:465–487.

15. Collett JH and Moreton RC (2007) Modified-release peroral dosage forms, in Aulton ME (Ed.) *Aulton's Pharmacetics, the Design and Manufacture of Medicines*, 3rd edn., Elsevier, Edinburgh, U.K.

16. DeBoer AG, Moolenaar F, deLeede LGJ, and Breimer DD (1982) Rectal drug administration: Clinical pharmacokinetic considerations. *Clin Pharmacokinet* 7:285–311.

17. Chien YW, Su KSE, and Chang S (1989) Nasal systemic drug delivery, in Chien YW (Ed.) *Drugs and the Pharmaceutical Sciences*, Marcel Dekker, New York.

18. Merkus FW, Verhoef JC, Marttin E, Romeijn SG, van der Kuy PH, Hermens WA, and Schipper NG (1999) Cyclodextrins in nasal drug delivery. *Adv Drug Deliv Rev* 36:41–57.

19. Walker SR, Evans ME, Richards AJ, and Paterson JW (1972) The clinical pharmacology of oral and inhaled salbutamol. *Clin Pharmacol Ther* 13:861–867.

20. Ranade VV (1991) Drug delivery systems: 6. Transdermal drug delivery. *J Clin Pharmacol* 31:401–418.

9 Drug Pharmacokinetics Following Single Oral Drug Administration
The Rate of Drug Absorption

OBJECTIVES

After completing this chapter you should be able to

- Describe the general characteristics of the plasma drug concentration–time profile after a single oral dose
- Describe how the rate and the extent of drug absorption after oral administration affect the onset and the duration of drug effect
- Evaluate the rate of drug absorption by comparing the plasma drug concentration–time profiles
- Calculate the drug pharmacokinetic parameters after oral drug administration
- Analyze how the change in the absorption rate constant affects the plasma concentration–time profile after a single oral administration
- Estimate the absorption rate constant utilizing the method of residuals
- Estimate the absorption rate constant using the Wagner–Nelson method

9.1   INTRODUCTION

Administration of the drug by any route that does not involve direct introduction into the systemic circulation is called extravascular drug administration. This includes intramuscular, subcutaneous, intradermal, oral, buccal, sublingual, rectal, intranasal, pulmonary, transdermal, ocular, and other routes. The oral route is the most common route of extravascular drug administration because it is the most convenient route, especially when the drug has to be administered repeatedly. Some drugs are administered orally for their local effect in the gastrointestinal tract (GIT) such as in the treatment of hyperacidity or GIT infections. In this case, the drug does not have to be absorbed from the GIT. However, the majority of the drugs administered orally are intended to produce a systemic effect such as to relieve pain, to control blood pressure, or to lower blood sugar, etc. Drugs administered to produce a systemic effect have to be absorbed from the site of administration to the systemic circulation and then distributed to all parts of the body to produce their therapeutic effects.

The rate and extent of drug absorption are very important parameters that have to be determined for any extravascular administration of drugs given their systemic effects. The rate of absorption affects the rate at which the drug appears in the systemic circulation after administration and is determined from the rate constant for the absorption process, while the extent of drug absorption represents the fraction of the administered dose that reaches the systemic circulation and is a measure of the drug bioavailability. In our discussion of the kinetics of drug absorption, the oral route will be used as an example of the extravascular routes of drug administration; however, the same principles can be applied to drug absorption from the other extravascular routes. In this chapter, the rate of drug absorption will be discussed, while the extent of drug absorption will be discussed in the next chapter.

The rate and extent of drug absorption to the systemic circulation after a single oral drug administration determine the plasma drug concentration–time profile and hence the onset and the intensity of drug effect for most drugs as illustrated in Figure 9.1. The assumption is that the plasma drug concentration has to exceed the minimum effective concentration (MEC) in order to produce the effect, and the intensity of the effect is related to the plasma drug concentration. After a single oral administration, the rate of drug absorption affects the onset of drug effect with rapidly absorbed drugs having faster onset of effect. Also, the extent of drug absorption affects the plasma drug concentration, with larger extent of drug absorption producing higher plasma drug concentration and more intense effect. Furthermore, the period of time the plasma drug concentration stays above the MEC, which is determined from the entire drug concentration–time profile, is important in determining the duration of drug effect.

After administration of a solid dosage form, the drug has to be in solution before it can be absorbed to the systemic circulation. So tablets and capsules have to disintegrate to granules, then to fine powder, and the drug has to dissolve before it can cross the GIT membrane to reach the systemic circulation. Once the drug is in the systemic circulation, it is distributed to all parts of the body including the site of

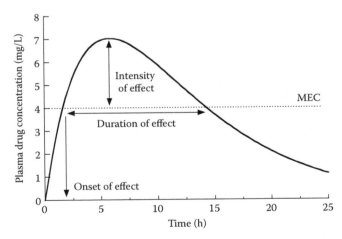

FIGURE 9.1 Relationship between the plasma concentration–time profile and the onset, intensity, and duration of the drug effect.

action and also the eliminating organs. The rate constant that reflects the rate of disintegration, dissolution, and absorption processes and describes the rate of the overall absorption process is the absorption rate constant (k_a). The absorption rate constant after administration of different dosage forms for the same active drug can be different because of differences in the formulation characteristics.

9.2 DRUG ABSORPTION AFTER ORAL ADMINISTRATION

The absorption of most drugs follows first-order kinetics; however, the absorption of some drugs follows zero-order kinetics.

9.2.1 ZERO-ORDER DRUG ABSORPTION

The rate of a zero-order process is constant and is independent of the concentration or amount of the drug available for the process. When the rate of drug absorption follows zero-order kinetics, the rate of drug absorption is constant and is independent of the administered dose. This usually occurs when the drug is absorbed by a specific carrier system and the drug concentration at the site of absorption is high enough to saturate the carrier system. When carrier-mediated transport is the only mechanism for drug absorption and the carrier system is saturated, the rate of drug absorption becomes constant and independent of the drug concentration at the site of drug absorption, that is, zero-order absorption. Also, modified-release formulations can be designed to release the drug at a constant rate over an extended period of time. When the rate of drug release from the dosage form is the rate determining step for the absorption process, the rate of drug absorption will be constant, that is, zero-order absorption, as long as the drug is released from the dosage form at a constant rate. The zero-order absorption rate constant has units of amount/time. After administration of a single dose of a drug that has zero-order absorption and first-order elimination, the plasma drug concentration–time profile starts with a slow rise in the drug concentration due to the slow rate of drug absorption. Then a relatively constant drug concentration is achieved during the period of drug absorption, followed by a slow decline in the drug concentration when the absorption process is complete.

9.2.2 FIRST-ORDER DRUG ABSORPTION

The absorption process for most drugs after oral administration follows first-order kinetics. After oral administration, the drug is introduced to the GIT and it is assumed that all the administered dose is ready for the absorption process. The amount of drug in the GIT (A_i) after oral administration declines exponentially at a rate dependent on the absorption rate constant, k_a, when the absorption process follows first-order kinetics as in Figure 9.2. The amount of the drug in the GIT at any time can be described by Equation 9.1, assuming that the decline in drug amount in the GIT is only due to drug absorption that follows first-order kinetics. The first-order absorption rate constant has units of time^{-1}:

$$A_i = Dose\, e^{-k_a t}$$

(9.1)

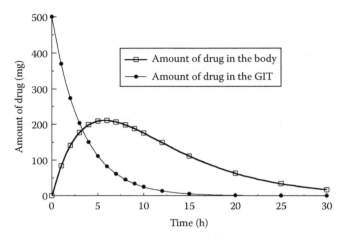

FIGURE 9.2 Drug amount-time profile in the GIT and inside the body after a single oral administration of a drug with first-order absorption and elimination.

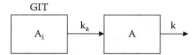

FIGURE 9.3 Diagram representing the pharmacokinetic model that describes the drug absorption from the GIT. A_i is the amount of the drug in the GIT, A is the amount of the absorbed drug in the body, k_a is the first-order absorption rate constant, and k is the first-order elimination rate constant.

The block diagram in Figure 9.3 represents the pharmacokinetic model for oral drug administration with first-order absorption and elimination. The rate of change of the amount of the absorbed drug in the body (A) depends on the rate of drug absorption (k_aA_i) and the rate of drug elimination (kA) as in Equation 9.2:

$$\frac{dA}{dt} = k_aA_i - kA \tag{9.2}$$

Equation 9.2 indicates that the amount of the drug in the body increases if the rate of drug absorption is larger than the rate of drug elimination and decreases if the rate of drug elimination is larger than the rate of drug absorption.

Initially, the rate of drug absorption is at its highest rate because the total dose is in the GIT and then decreases with time because of the decrease in the amount of the drug remaining to be absorbed, while the rate of drug elimination is at its lowest rate initially because no drug is in the body at the time of drug administration, then increases with time due to the increase in drug amount in the body after drug absorption. So after drug administration, the amount of the drug in the body increases because the rate of drug absorption is larger than the rate of drug elimination. When the rate of drug absorption becomes equal to the rate of drug elimination, a transient plateau is achieved for a brief moment. After that the amount of the drug in the body decreases because the rate of elimination becomes larger than the rate of absorption. So after administration of a single oral dose of a drug with first-order absorption and elimination, the drug amount-time profile in the body increases initially and then decreases as in Figure 9.2.

Integrating Equation 9.2 yields the following biexponential equation:

$$A = \frac{A_{i0}k_a}{k_a - k}(e^{-kt} - e^{-k_a t}) \qquad (9.3)$$

where A_{i0} is the initial amount of the drug in the GIT that is equal to the dose of the drug D. Also, the orally administered dose is not always absorbed completely, so the term (F) can be included in the equation to account for the fraction of administered dose that will be absorbed. So, Equation 9.3 can be written as follows:

$$A = \frac{FDk_a}{k_a - k}(e^{-kt} - e^{-k_a t}) \qquad (9.4)$$

Dividing Equation 9.4 by the Vd gives the general equation that describes the plasma drug concentration–time profile after administration of a single oral dose as in Equation 9.5:

$$Cp = \frac{FDk_a}{Vd(k_a - k)}(e^{-kt} - e^{-k_a t}) \qquad (9.5)$$

This equation has two exponents: one includes the rate constant for the absorption process and the other includes the rate constant for the elimination process, indicating that the plasma concentration–time profile for the drug after oral administration is dependent on the absorption and elimination processes.

9.3 PLASMA CONCENTRATION–TIME PROFILE AFTER A SINGLE ORAL DOSE

Figure 9.4 is a representative example of the plasma drug concentration–time profile after a single oral drug administration. The profile includes an absorption phase when the plasma drug concentration is increasing because the rate of drug absorption is larger than the rate of drug elimination. A maximum value for the plasma drug concentration (C_{max}) is reached when the rate of drug absorption is equal to the rate of drug elimination. The time when C_{max} is achieved is called the t_{max}. The t_{max} reflects the rate of drug absorption with shorter t_{max} indicating faster drug absorption. After the C_{max}, drug absorption continues but the plasma drug concentration decreases because the rate of drug elimination is larger than the rate of drug absorption. When the absorption process is completed, the plasma drug concentration decreases at a rate dependent on the rate of the elimination process. The decline phase of the plasma drug concentration is called the elimination phase. The initial phase in the drug concentration profile after oral administration is called the absorption phase;

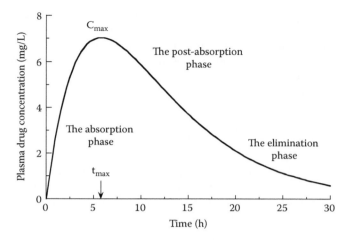

FIGURE 9.4 Plasma drug concentration–time profile after administration of a single oral dose of the drug.

however, both absorption and elimination occur simultaneously during this time, whereas during the elimination phase the absorption process is completed, so the plasma drug concentration is affected only by the drug elimination rate.

At C_{max}, there is a transient steady drug concentration achieved for a brief moment, so the rate of change of the plasma drug concentration is equal to zero at this particular time. The rate of change in plasma drug concentration can be obtained by differentiating Equation 9.5 and the result of the differentiation is equal to zero at this specific time, t_{max}. This allows getting an expression for t_{max} as follows:

$$\frac{dCp}{dt} = \frac{d}{dt}\left(\frac{FDk_a}{Vd(k_a - k)}\left(e^{-kt_{max}} - e^{-k_a t_{max}}\right)\right) = 0 \qquad (9.6)$$

This can be simplified to

$$-ke^{-kt_{max}} + k_a e^{-k_a t_{max}} = 0 \qquad (9.7)$$

$$ke^{-kt_{max}} = k_a e^{-k_a t_{max}} \qquad (9.8)$$

$$\ln k - kt_{max} = \ln k_a - k_a t_{max} \qquad (9.9)$$

$$t_{max} = \frac{\ln k_a - \ln k}{k_a - k} = \frac{\ln(k_a/k)}{k_a - k} = \frac{2.303\log(k_a/k)}{k_a - k} \qquad (9.10)$$

So the time to achieve the maximum plasma drug concentration, t_{max}, is dependent on both k_a and k. The C_{max} can be calculated by substituting time in Equation 9.5 by t_{max}:

$$C_{max} = \frac{FDk_a}{Vd(k_a - k)}\left(e^{-kt_{max}} - e^{-k_a t_{max}}\right) \qquad (9.11)$$

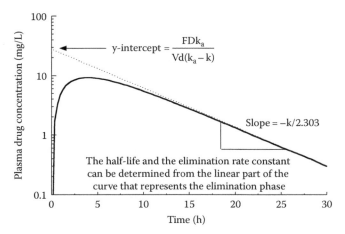

FIGURE 9.5 Plasma drug concentration–time profile after administration of a single oral dose of the drug plotted on the semilog scale. The half-life and the first-order elimination rate constant can be calculated during the elimination phase of the drug.

The time to achieve maximum concentration, t_{max}, is dependent on both k_a and k. Larger k_a that indicates faster rate of absorption will result in shorter t_{max} and higher C_{max} if the other parameters (k and Vd) were kept constant, while larger k that indicates faster rate of elimination will result in shorter t_{max} and lower C_{max} if the other parameters such as k_a and Vd were kept constant.

When the plasma drug concentration–time curve is plotted on semilog graph paper, the elimination phase of the profile will be linear because the plasma drug concentration decreases at a rate dependent on the elimination rate constant as in Figure 9.5. The elimination rate constant and the half-life can be determined from the elimination phase of the plasma drug concentration–time profile plotted on the semilog scale. However, this is only possible when the absorption process is completed and the drug concentration declines due to the elimination process. When the drug concentration declines linearly on the semilog scale, this indicates that the absorption process is completed. The elimination rate constant can be determined from the slope of the linear part of the elimination phase of the drug concentration–time profile on the semilog scale. The slope of the line is equal to $-k/2.303$. The half-life of the drug can also be determined by measuring the time required for any drug concentration in the linear part of the profile to decrease by 50%. When the linear part of the curve is back extrapolated to the y-axis as in Figure 9.5, the y-intercept is equal to the coefficient in the general equation for the drug concentration–time profile after oral administration as in Equation 9.12:

$$\text{y-Intercept} = \frac{FDk_a}{Vd(k_a - k)} \tag{9.12}$$

The value of the y-intercept can be determined graphically from the plasma drug concentration–time plot on the semilog scale. So the y-intercept value can be used to calculate the pharmacokinetic parameters such as Vd, for example, if the other parameters, F, D, k, and k_a are known.

The AUC after a single oral drug administration can be expressed in terms of the other pharmacokinetic parameters as in IV drug administration. However, after oral administration the fraction of dose that reaches the systemic circulation should be considered when calculating the AUC from the other pharmacokinetic parameters. Here the AUC from time zero to infinity after a single oral dose can be expressed as

$$\left.\mathrm{AUC_{oral}}\right|_{t=\infty}^{t=0} = \frac{FD}{kVd} = \frac{F\,\mathrm{Dose}}{CL_T} \tag{9.13}$$

where CL_T is the total body clearance of the drug. Experimentally, the AUC can be calculated from serial drug concentrations determined after drug administration using the trapezoidal rule, which will be discussed in detail in the following chapter. Knowing the AUC and dose, the CL_T can be determined only if the fraction of dose that reaches the systemic circulation, F, is known. Otherwise, the combined term CL_T/F that is referred to as the oral clearance of the drug is obtained.

9.4   DETERMINATION OF THE ABSORPTION RATE CONSTANT

Determination of the absorption rate constant is important because it governs the rate of drug absorption after oral administration. Evaluation of the clinical usefulness of a dosage form has to include the rate of drug absorption. This is because faster drug absorption is usually preferred for treating acute symptoms or emergency condition, while slower rate of drug absorption is favored during multiple drug administration for the management of chronic diseases. There are several graphical methods that can be used to calculate k_a, the drug absorption rate constant. These methods differ in the conditions when each method can be applied.

9.4.1   METHOD OF RESIDUALS

The method of residuals is a graphical method used to determine the drug absorption rate constant and has the following assumptions:

1. The absorption rate constant is larger than the elimination rate constant, that is, $k_a > k$.
2. Both drug absorption and elimination follow first-order kinetics.
3. The drug pharmacokinetics follow one-compartment model.

If any of these three assumptions is not met, the method of residuals cannot be applied and other methods should be used to calculate k_a. The idea of the method of residuals is to characterize the drug elimination rate from the terminal elimination phase of the plasma drug concentration–time profile after a single oral administration. Then the contribution of the drug absorption rate and the drug elimination rate of the drug to the plasma concentration–time profile during the absorption phase is separated. This allows determination of the rate of drug absorption and the estimation of the first-order absorption rate constant.

The plasma drug concentration–time profile after oral administration is described by a biexponential equation that describes the absorption and the elimination processes, Equation 9.5. After drug administration, as the time (t) gets longer, the values for the two exponential terms $e^{-k_a t}$ and e^{-kt} in Equation 9.5 decrease because the power in both terms has a negative sign. However, the exponential term $e^{-k_a t}$ decreases faster than e^{-kt}, because $k_a > k$ from the assumptions of the method. As time gets longer, the term $e^{-k_a t}$ approaches zero indicating that the absorption process is complete, and Equation 9.5 is reduced to

$$Cp = \frac{FDk_a}{Vd(k_a - k)} e^{-kt} \qquad (9.14)$$

Equation 9.14 is a monoexponential equation that includes k only. This means that when the absorption process is completed, the plasma drug concentration declines at a rate dependent only on k. This represents the elimination phase of the drug concentration–time profile after oral administration. The drug $t_{1/2}$ can be calculated from the elimination phase of the curve as illustrated in Figure 9.6. Also, k can be calculated from the slope of the linear elimination phase on the semilog scale where the slope is equal to $-k/2.303$.

If the linear part of the plasma drug concentration–time curve that represents the elimination phase is identified and back extrapolated to time zero, the y-intercept is equal to $FDk_a/Vd(k_a-k)$ as mentioned in Equation 9.12 and as illustrated in Figure 9.6. During the absorption phase, the absorption and elimination processes occur simultaneously. The contribution of the absorption rate and elimination rate of the drug on the plasma concentration–time profile during the absorption rate is separated by calculating the residuals. The residuals are calculated from the difference between the y-coordinate values on the extrapolated line from the elimination phase and the y-coordinate values on the plasma drug concentration–time profile (the measured drug concentration) at the same time points as follows:

$$\text{Residuals} = \frac{FDk_a}{Vd(k_a - k)} e^{-kt} - Cp \qquad (9.15)$$

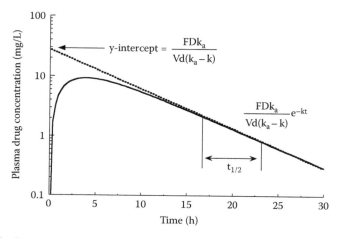

FIGURE 9.6 Plasma drug concentration–time profile during the elimination phase after administration of a single oral dose declines at a rate dependent on the first-order elimination rate constant.

$$\text{Residuals} = \frac{FDk_a}{Vd(k_a - k)}e^{-kt} - \frac{FDk_a}{Vd(k_a - k)}(e^{-kt} - e^{-k_a t}) \qquad (9.16)$$

$$\text{Residuals} = \frac{FDk_a}{Vd(k_a - k)}e^{-k_a t} \qquad (9.17)$$

This means that the plot of the residuals versus time on the semilog scale declines at a rate dependent on the absorption rate constant, k_a. The absorption rate constant can be determined from the slope of the residuals versus time plot (slope $= -k_a/2.303$). Since the slope of this plot is always negative, k_a always has a positive value. The first-order absorption rate constant can be determined using the method of residuals as illustrated in Figure 9.7 by the following steps:

- The plasma drug concentration is plotted against their corresponding time values on the semilog scale.
- The plasma drug concentrations that decline linearly during the elimination phase are identified and the best line that goes through these points is drawn and is back extrapolated to the y-axis.
- The slope of the line that represents the elimination phase is calculated. The slope of this line is equal to $-k/2.303$.
- At least three points on the extrapolated line at three different time values during the absorption phase of the drug are taken. Vertical lines from the points on the extrapolated line are dropped to determine the corresponding points (at the same time values) on the plasma drug concentration–time curve.
- The differences between the y-coordinate values of the points on the extrapolated line and corresponding y-coordinate values on the plasma drug concentration–time curve are calculated. The values of these differences are the residuals.

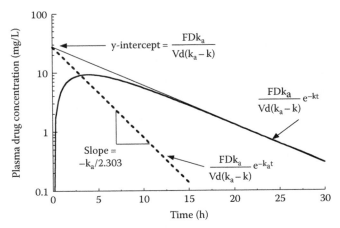

FIGURE 9.7 Method of residuals: The residuals versus time plot on the semilog scale (the dashed line) declines at a rate dependent on the first-order absorption rate constant. The first-order absorption rate constant is calculated from the slope of this plot, slope $= -k_a/2.303$.

- The values of the residuals are plotted versus their corresponding time values for each residual on the same graph. A straight line should be obtained with a slope of $-k_a/2.303$.
- The extrapolated line representing the elimination phase and the residuals versus time line should have the same y-intercept as in Figure 9.7. This is because the equations that describe the two lines have the same coefficient, so substituting time by zero in the two equations should give the same term.

9.4.1.1 Lag Time

Under some conditions, the absorption of drugs after oral administration does not start immediately due to some physiological factors such as delayed gastric emptying or formulation factors as delay in tablet disintegration. This delay time before starting drug absorption is known as the lag time. In some instances, the lag time for drug absorption can be short and does not significantly affect the plasma drug concentration–time profile. However, the lag time can be long such as after administration of enteric coated formulations. In this case, the dosage form disintegration, drug dissolution, and drug absorption start after the dosage form reaches the small intestine, which can take hours, especially if the drug is administered with food. The plasma drug concentration–time profile will be shifted to the right on the time scale because no drug will be detected in plasma before the start of drug absorption as in Figure 9.8. The plasma drug concentration–time profile after single dose of an oral dosage form that has a lag time can be described by Equation 9.18:

$$Cp = \frac{FDk_a}{Vd(k_a - k)}\left(e^{-k(t-t_0)} - e^{-k_a(t-t_0)}\right) \tag{9.18}$$

where
    t is the time of drug administration
    t_0 is the lag time for drug absorption

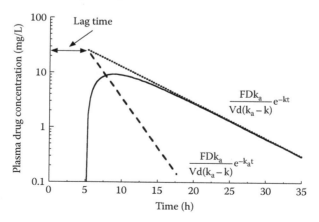

FIGURE 9.8 Method of residuals when there is lag time for drug absorption after oral administration. The lag time is calculated from the x-coordinate of the point of intersection of the two lines representing the elimination and absorption.

In Equation 9.18, t_0 is equal to t during the lag time (when $t \leq t_0$), while t_0 stays constant when $t \geq t_0$. So the plasma drug concentration will be zero during the lag time and starts to rise after the lag time. When the method of residuals is applied to estimate k_a in presence of absorption lag time, the extrapolated line representing drug elimination and the residual versus time line have to intersect at a point with x-coordinate value more than zero. The x-coordinate value of the point of intersection of the two lines in the method of residuals is equal to the lag time for drug absorption as in Figure 9.8.

9.4.1.2 Flip-Flop of k_a and k

One of the assumptions of the method of residuals is that $k_a > k$. In this case, the terminal elimination phase represents the elimination process and the residuals versus time line represents the absorption process. However, when $k_a < k$, the terminal elimination phase will represent the slower process (drug absorption), while the residuals versus time line will represent the elimination process. This behavior is known as flip-flop of k_a and k. The existence of this behavior will make the calculated k after oral drug administration to be different from that determined after IV administration. Figure 9.9 has simulation of the plasma drug concentration–time profile for a drug that has elimination rate constant of $0.4\,h^{-1}$ when administered in the form of two different formulations that have different rates of absorption. When k is $0.4\,h^{-1}$ and k_a is $0.6\,h^{-1}$ ($k_a > k$), the terminal elimination phase will reflect the elimination rate of the drug and the residuals versus time line will reflect its rate of absorption, while when k is $0.4\,h^{-1}$ and k_a is $0.2\,h^{-1}$ ($k_a < k$), the terminal elimination phase will reflect the absorption rate of the drug and the residuals versus time line will reflect its rate of elimination. The flip-flop of k_a and k is usually suspected for drugs that have short elimination half-life (large k) and also after administration of extended release drug products that usually have slow rate of drug absorption (small k_a).

Example

After oral administration of a single dose of an antibiotic, the following concentrations were measured:

Time (h)	Drug Concentration (mg/L)
0	0
0.2	88
0.5	185
1.0	277
2.0	321
2.5	311
4.0	246
6.0	161
8.0	102

Calculate the first-order absorption rate constant.

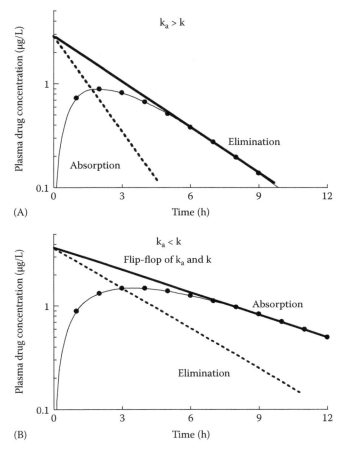

(A)

(B)

FIGURE 9.9 Simulation of the plasma drug concentration–time profiles for a drug that has k of $0.4\,h^{-1}$ when (A) k_a is $0.6\,h^{-1}$ and when (B) k_a is $0.2\,h^{-1}$. In plot A when $k_a > k$, the rate of decline in the terminal phase represents drug elimination and the rate of decline in the residual versus time plot represents drug absorption, while in plot B when $k_a < k$, the rate of decline in the terminal phase represents the slower process, drug absorption and the rate of decline in the residual versus time plot represents drug absorption, flip-flop of k_a and k.

Answer
- Plot the plasma concentration–time profile and follow the procedures for the method of residuals as in Figure 9.10.
- Calculate the residuals.

Time (h)	Residuals (mg/L)
0.2	660 − 88 = 572
0.5	560 − 185 = 375
1.0	420 − 277 = 143

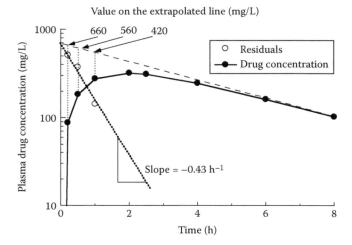

FIGURE 9.10 Method of residuals to calculate the first-order absorption rate constant.

The line resulting from plotting the residuals versus time has slope of $-0.43\,h^{-1}$.

$$\text{Slope} = -0.43\,h^{-1} = \frac{-k_a}{2.303}$$

$$k_a = 0.99\,h^{-1}$$

9.4.2 WAGNER–NELSON METHOD

One of the assumptions for the method of residuals is that the absorption process follows first-order kinetics and that the drug follows one-compartment pharmaco-kinetic model. However, the absorption of drugs does not always follow first-order kinetics specially when administered in the form of extended release formulations. The Wagner–Nelson method is a method that can be used to determine the absorption rate constant for drugs when their absorption follows zero-order kinetics or first-order kinetics [1,2]. The requirement for this method is that the drug follows one-compartment pharmacokinetic model and linear kinetics. A modification of this method, the Loo-Reigelman method, can be used to determine the absorption rate constant when the drug pharmacokinetics follows two-compartment model [3]. The Wagner–Nelson method is one of the deconvolution methods used for the determination of the drug absorption rate constant. It is based on the concept that the observed drug concentrations obtained after oral drug administration are the result of the drug input function presented by absorption and the drug output function presented by elimination. When information about the drug elimination is obtained after IV administration, the drug input function, the absorption process, can be characterized using deconvolution.

The Wagner–Nelson method uses the relationship between the fractions of the administered dose remaining to be absorbed at different time points to determine the absorption rate constant. A mass balance equation can be written to determine the amount of the drug absorbed as follows:

The amount of drug absorbed up to time t (A_{at})

= Amount of drug in the body (at time t) + Amount of drug excreted (up to time t)

$$(9.19)$$

where

$$\text{Amount of the drug in the body (t)} = Cp_t Vd$$

$$\text{Amount of drug excreted (up to t)} = kVd \int_{t=0}^{t=t} Cp\, dt$$

So

$$A_{at} = Cp_t Vd + kVd \int_{t=0}^{t=t} Cp\, dt \qquad (9.20)$$

The total amount of drug absorbed up to time ∞ ($A_{a\infty}$)

= 0 + Total amount of drug excreted (up to time ∞) (9.21)

where

$$\text{Amount of the drug in the body } (t = \infty) = 0$$

$$\text{Amount of the drug excreted } (t = \infty) = kVd \int_{t=0}^{t=\infty} Cp\, dt$$

So

$$A_{a\infty} = kVd \int_{t=0}^{t=\infty} Cp\, dt \qquad (9.22)$$

This means that the fraction of the administered dose already absorbed at any time is determined by dividing Equation 9.20 by Equation 9.22:

$$\text{Fraction of dose absorbed (t)} = \frac{Cp_t Vd + kVd \int_{t=0}^{t=t} Cp\,dt}{kVd \int_{t=0}^{t=\infty} Cp\,dt} \qquad (9.23)$$

Dividing both sides of the equation by Vd yields Equation 9.24:

$$\text{Fraction of dose absorbed (t)} = \frac{A_{at}}{A_{a\infty}} = \frac{Cp_t + k \int_{t=0}^{t=t} Cp\,dt}{k \int_{t=0}^{t=\infty} Cp\,dt} \qquad (9.24)$$

The fraction of the administered dose remaining to be absorbed can be determined by

$$\text{Fraction of dose remaining to be absorbed (at time t)} = 1 - \frac{A_{at}}{A_{a\infty}} \qquad (9.25)$$

The change in the fraction of dose remaining to be absorbed at different time points can be used to determine if the absorption process follows zero-order or first-order kinetics and also can be used to determine the rate constant for the absorption process. After drug administration, the drug is absorbed and the fraction of dose remaining to be absorbed decreases with time. If the decline in the fraction of dose remaining to be absorbed with time is exponential, this means that the absorption process follows first-order kinetics, while if the rate of decline is constant, this means that the absorption process follows zero-order kinetics. The rate of decline in the fraction of dose remaining to be absorbed can be used to calculate the absorption rate constant. If the absorption process is first order, a plot of the fraction remaining to be absorbed versus time should give a straight line on the semilog scale, as in Figure 9.11A. The slope of this line is equal to $-k_a/2.303$. On the contrary, if the absorption process is zero order, a plot of the fraction remaining to be absorbed versus time should give straight line on the Cartesian scale as in Figure 9.11B. The slope of this line is equal to $-k_a$ expressed as the fraction remaining to be absorbed per time. The fraction remaining to be absorbed can be expressed as percent remaining to be absorbed by multiplying the fraction by 100.

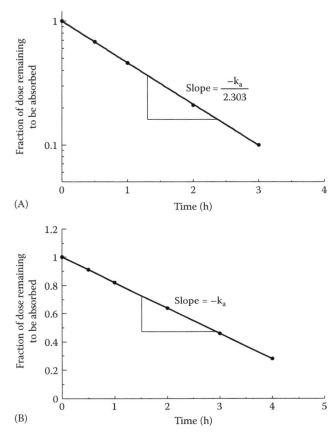

FIGURE 9.11 Fraction of dose remaining to be absorbed versus time plots (A) when the drug absorption follows first-order kinetics and (B) when the drug absorption follows zero-order kinetics.

9.4.2.1 Application of the Wagner–Nelson Method

The absorption rate constant can be determined using the Wagner–Nelson method by going through the following steps:

- Plot the plasma drug concentration–time data to calculate the elimination rate constant, k.
- Construct a table (similar to the table in the following solved example) to calculate all the necessary information to calculate the fraction of the drug remaining to be absorbed in a step-wise fashion.
- Use the plasma drug concentration at different time points to calculate the AUC between each pair of plasma concentrations, partial AUC $\left(\left.\mathrm{AUC}\right|_{t=n-1}^{t=n}\right)$.
- Calculate the cumulative AUC from time zero to time t, for each time point $\left(\left.\mathrm{AUC}\right|_{t=0}^{t=t}\right)$.

- Multiply each cumulative AUC value by the elimination rate constant $\left(k\ AUC\big|_{t=0}^{t=t}\right)$.
- Add the value of the plasma drug concentration to the product of k and the cumulative AUC at each time point $\left(Cp + k\ AUC\big|_{t=0}^{t=t}\right)$. This is the amount of the drug absorbed up to time t divided by Vd. The last value in this column when the plasma drug concentration is not detected is the total amount of drug absorbed up to $t = \infty$ divided by Vd.
- Calculate the fraction of dose absorbed at each time point by dividing the amount absorbed at each time point by the amount absorbed at $t = \infty$, $(A_{at}/A_{a\infty})$.
- Calculate the fraction of dose remaining to be absorbed at each time point $[1 - (A_{at}/A_{a\infty})]$.
- Plot the fraction of dose remaining to be absorbed at different time points on the linear and semilog scales to determine the absorption rate constant.

Example

When applying the Wagner–Nelson method to determine the absorption rate constant for an oral hypoglycemic drug the following data were obtained:

Time (h)	Fraction Remaining to be Absorbed
1	0.63
2	0.40
3	0.25
5	0.10

a. What is the order of the absorption process of this oral hypoglycemic drug?
b. Calculate the absorption rate constant.

Answer

Plot the fraction remaining to be absorbed on Cartesian and semilog graph paper as in Figure 9.12A and B. The relationship is linear on a semilog graph paper indicating first-order absorption.

$$Slope = -0.2h^{-1} = \frac{-k_a}{2.303}$$

$$k_a = 0.46h^{-1}$$

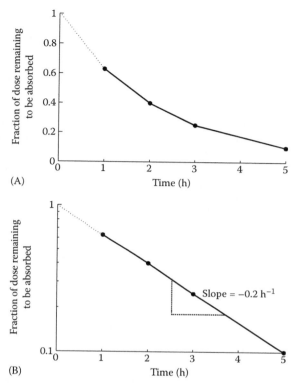

FIGURE 9.12 Fraction of dose remaining to be absorbed versus time is not linear on the Cartesian scale (A) and is linear on the semilog scale (B).

Example

The following plasma concentration–time data were obtained after a single oral dose of 1000 mg of a drug. Using the Wagner–Nelson method, determine the order of the drug absorption of the process and estimate the absorption rate constant, if the first-order elimination rate constant is $0.33\,h^{-1}$.

Time (h)	Concentration (mg/L)
0	0
0.2	10.0
0.5	21.5
1.0	33.4
2.0	40.7
3.0	37.6
4.0	31.1
5.0	24.5
8.0	10.2
12.0	2.9
20.0	0.2

TABLE 9.1
Calculation of the Fraction of Dose Remaining to Be Absorbed

Time (h)	Concentration (mg/L)	$\text{AUC}\vert_{t=n-1}^{t=n}$	$\text{AUC}\vert_{t=0}^{t=t}$	$k\,\text{AUC}\vert_{t=0}^{t=t}$	$\text{Cp}+k\,\text{AUC}\vert_{t=0}^{t=t}$	$A_{at}/A_{a\infty}$	$1-(A_{at}/A_{a\infty})$
0	0	0	0	0	0	0	1
0.2	10.0	1.0	1.0	0.33	10.33	0.1137	0.8863
0.5	21.5	4.73	5.73	1.89	23.39	0.2576	0.7424
1.0	33.4	13.7	19.43	6.41	39.81	0.4384	0.5616
2.0	40.7	37.0	56.43	18.62	59.32	0.6533	0.3467
3.0	37.6	39.2	95.63	31.56	69.16	0.7616	0.2384
4.0	31.1	34.4	130.03	42.9	74.0		
5.0	24.5	27.8	157.83	52.1	76.6		
8.0	10.2	52.0	209.83	69.24	79.44		
12.0	2.9	42.4	262.23	86.54	89.44		
20.0	0.2	12.4	274.63	90.6	90.8		
		0.6	275.23	90.8	$90.8 = A_{a\infty}$		

Answer

Use the drug concentration–time data to construct the table that allows calcula-tion of the fraction of dose remaining to be absorbed as described earlier. Table 9.1 includes the stepwise calculation of the information needed to calculate the fraction of dose remaining to be absorbed.

a. A plot of the fraction remaining to be absorbed versus time on the semilog scale is linear indicating that the absorption of the drug follows first-order kinetics (Figure 9.13).
b. The slope of the line on the semilog scale = $-0.2076\,\text{h}^{-1}$.

$$\text{Slope} = -\frac{k_a}{2.303}, \quad \text{so} \quad k_a = 0.478\,\text{h}^{-1}$$

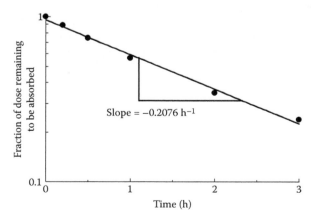

FIGURE 9.13 Plot of the fraction of dose remaining to be absorbed versus time on the semilog scale.

9.5 CLINICAL IMPORTANCE OF THE ABSORPTION RATE CONSTANT

The rate of drug absorption from different drug products for the same active drug may be different depending on the formulation characteristics. The absorption rate constant determines the rate of drug absorption from the site of administration and the rate of its appearance in the systemic circulation. In general, during single use of the drug, faster drug absorption produces faster onset of drug effect. So faster drug absorption is usually required when immediate therapeutic effect is desired such as in case of the treatment of acute symptoms or emergency cases. However, rapid drug absorption is not always required such as in the management of chronic diseases. Sustained release drug products are designed to release the active drug from the dosage form very slowly, which results in slow drug absorption. The slow release and slow absorption of the active drug from the sustained release products usually produce effective plasma drug concentration for longer time after drug administration, leading to prolongation of the therapeutic effect of the drug. Also, the use of slowly absorbed formulations decreases the fluctuations in the plasma drug concentration during multiple drug administration, which produces stable therapeutic effect between drug administrations.

9.6 PHARMACOKINETIC SIMULATION EXERCISE

Simulate the plasma concentration–time profile after administration of a single oral dose of drug with first-order absorption and first-order elimination by choosing a value for each parameter. Repeat the simulation by choosing different values for k_a while keeping all the other parameters constants on the linear scale. Examine how the change in k_a affects the drug concentration–time profile and also the effect on the other parameters, such as t_{max}, C_{max}, AUC, and k. The simulations can be repeated by choosing different values of k while keeping the other parameters constant. Examine the effect of changing k on t_{max}, C_{max}, and AUC. The plotting exercise of the absorption rate constant module in the basic pharmacokinetic concept section of the companion CD to this textbook can be used to run these simulations.

9.7 SUMMARY

- The first-order absorption rate constant is the rate constant that determines the rate of drug absorption from the site of administration. Larger absorption rate constant means faster rate of drug absorption.
- The absorption rate constant determined after drug administration is an operative rate constant that accounts for all the necessary steps required for drug absorption into the systemic circulation including disintegration, dissolution, and absorption.
- The first-order absorption rate constant has units of time^{-1}.

PRACTICE PROBLEMS

9.1   The plasma drug concentration in a patient who had received a single oral dose
of a drug (10 mg/kg) was determined as follows:

Time (h)	Drug Concentration (mg/L)
0	0
1	84
2	141
3	177
4	199
6	207
8	188
10	176
15	111
20	63
25	33.5
30	17.3

Plot the plasma concentration–time profile on a semilog graph paper and then
find the following parameters directly from the graph. (Do not use the method
of residuals.)
a.   The elimination rate constant and the elimination half-life
b.   The t_{max}
c.   The C_{max}

9.2   Two drugs have the following pharmacokinetic parameters, after a single oral
dose of 500 mg. Both drugs are completely absorbed.

Drug	k_a (h^{-1})	k (h^{-1})	Vd (L)
A	1.0	0.2	10
B	0.2	1.0	20

a.   Calculate t_{max} for each drug.
b.   Calculate C_{max} for each drug.

9.3   The plasma concentration–time profile after a single oral dose can be expressed as

$$Cp = \frac{FDk_a}{Vd(k_a - k)}(e^{-kt} - e^{-k_a t})$$

After administration of a single 500 mg oral dose of a drug, the plasma concentration time profile can be expressed as

$$Cp = 75 \, mg/L \, (e^{-0.1t} - e^{-0.9t})$$

where
    Cp is in mg/L
    t is in h

and

$$\frac{FDk_a}{Vd(k_a - k)} = 75\,mg/L$$

a. Calculate the t_{max} after administration of the 500 mg oral dose.
b. Calculate the C_{max} after administration of the 500 mg oral dose.
c. Do you expect t_{max} and C_{max} to be different if the dose was 100 mg?

9.4 A single dose of 500 mg of an antibiotic was given to a 70 kg patient as an oral tablet. The plasma concentration time profile can be described by the following equation:

$$Cp = 21\ mg/L\ (e^{-0.115t} - e^{-0.624t})$$

where
   Cp is in mg/L
   t is in h

The drug has 100% bioavailability (F = 1).
a. Calculate the plasma concentration 6 h after drug administration.
b. Calculate the elimination half-life of this drug.
c. Calculate the first-order absorption rate constant of this drug.
d. Calculate the volume of distribution of this drug.
e. Calculate t_{max}.
f. Calculate C_{max}.
g. What is the slope of the terminal elimination phase for the plasma concentration–time plot (on semilog scale) after administration of the 500 mg dose?

9.5 A single dose of 500 mg of an antibiotic was given to a 70 kg patient as an oral tablet. The plasma concentration time profile can be described by the following equation:

$$Cp = 10\ (e^{-0.154t} - e^{-0.954t})$$

where
   Cp is in mg/L
   t is in h

and the drug is completely absorbed.
a. Calculate the elimination half-life of this drug.
b. Calculate the volume of distribution of this drug.
c. Calculate the total body clearance of this drug.
d. Calculate t_{max} and C_{max}.
e. Calculate the AUC after administration of 500 mg oral dose.

9.6 A patient received a single oral dose of 5 mg of a bronchodilator that is completely absorbed after oral administration. The following plasma concentrations time data were obtained:

Time (h)	Concentration (ng/mL)	Time (h)	Concentration (ng/mL)
0.0	0.00	4.0	31.1
0.2	10.0	6.0	18.6
0.5	21.5	8.0	10.2
1.0	33.4	10.0	5.44
2.0	40.7	14.0	1.47
3.0	37.6		

a. Plot the plasma concentration time curve and determine the absorption rate constant using the method of residuals.
b. What is the equation that describes the plasma concentration time profile of this drug after oral administration?
c. Calculate t_{max} and C_{max} for this drug after administration of a single 5 mg dose.

9.7 The following results were obtained when the Wagner–Nelson method was used to calculate the absorption rate constant after an oral administration.

Time (h)	Fraction Remaining to be Absorbed
1	0.7
2	0.5
3	0.35
5	0.17

a. What is the order of absorption of this drug?
b. Calculate the absorption rate constant.

9.8 A 60 kg patient received a single oral dose of 25 mg of an antibiotic that is completely absorbed after oral administration. Serial samples were drawn and the drug plasma concentration was determined using a sensitive analytical method. The plasma concentrations were as follows:

Time (h)	Concentration (ng/mL)	Time (h)	Concentration (ng/mL)
0.0	0.00	4.0	246.1
0.2	88.5	6.0	161.0
0.5	184.9	8.0	102.2
1.0	276.9	10.0	64.5
2.0	321.6	12.0	40.66
3.0	292.8	14.0	25.61

a. Calculate the absorption rate constant of this drug using the method of residuals.
b. Calculate the half-life and the volume of distribution of this drug.

REFERENCES

1. Wagner JG and Nelson E (1964) Kinetic analysis of blood levels and urinary excretion in the absorptive phase after single doses of drug. *J Pharm Sci* 53:1392–1403.
2. Wagner JG and Nelson E (1963) Percent absorbed time plots derived from blood level and/or urinary excretion data. *J Pharm Sci* 52:610–611.
3. Loo JCK and Riegelman S (1968) New method for calculating the intrinsic absorption rate of drugs. *J Pharm Sci* 57:918–928.

10 Drug Pharmacokinetics Following Single Oral Drug Administration
The Extent of Drug Absorption

OBJECTIVES

After completing this chapter you should be able to

- Define the bioavailability (BA) and the bioequivalence (BE) of drug products
- Describe the different factors contributing to the "first-pass effect" after oral drug administration
- Describe the importance of drug transporters in the drug absorption process
- Discuss the regulatory requirements for performing the in vivo BA studies
- Determine the absolute BA and the relative BA of oral drug products
- Calculate the area under the curve using the trapezoidal rule
- State the general guidelines for performing the in vivo BA studies
- Analyze the effect of changing the drug pharmacokinetic parameters on the plasma drug concentration–time profile after a single oral drug administration

10.1 INTRODUCTION

Drugs administered for their systemic effect have to be absorbed to the systemic circulation and become available at the site of action before they can produce their therapeutic effect. This means that the amount of the drug absorbed to the systemic circulation, rather than the labeled amount of the drug, is what produces the therapeutic effect. The concept of BA, which is a measure of the extent of drug absorption to the systemic circulation, is important in the drug development process and also in evaluating pharmaceutical products. The physiological, physicochemical, and formulation factors that can affect the rate and extent of drug absorption after extravascular drug administration have been discussed in previous chapters. So it is possible that multisource drug products, meaning different drug products for the same active drug manufactured by different manufacturers, can produce different degrees of disease control. The cause of this difference in therapeutic effect can be due to variation of the extent of drug absorption to the systemic circulation and the rate at which the drug reaches the systemic circulation after administration of the different products. This has added a new dimension to the issue of quality of drug products, which should include the BA and BE of drug products. Inclusion of BA determination and proof of BE as regulatory requirements are important to ensure efficacy of drug products and stability of the therapeutic effect when the patient switch between products for the same active drug.

According to U.S. drug regulatory authorities (21 Code of Federal Regulations, 2010), drug BA is defined as "the rate and extent to which the active ingredient or active moiety is absorbed from a drug product and becomes available at the site of action," while BE is defined as "the absence of a significant difference in the rate and extent to which the active ingredient in pharmaceutical equivalents (identical active drug ingredient, same strength, and same dosage form) becomes available at the site of drug action when administered under similar conditions in an appropriately designed study" [1]. The following discussion will focus on BA, while BE will be covered in the next chapter.

10.2 CAUSES OF INCOMPLETE DRUG BIOAVAILABILITY

The IV route of drug administration is the only route that guarantees that the entire dose reaches the systemic circulation, that is, 100% BA. Most of the drugs administered by the extravascular routes usually have incomplete BA. Generally, this can result from the loss of the intact drug molecule during the absorption process and the inability of the drug to cross the biological membrane. Chapters 7 through 9 cover the physiological, physicochemical, and formulation factors that can affect drug absorption after extravascular administration in detail. In this chapter, the focus will be on the effect of the first-pass metabolism and the gastrointestinal tract (GIT) drug transporters. The importance of first-pass metabolism and the GIT drug transporters arise from their direct effect on the oral BA of many drugs and because their modulation can lead to serious clinical consequences.

10.2.1 PHYSIOLOGICAL, PHYSICOCHEMICAL, AND FORMULATION FACTORS

As discussed in the previous chapters, many factors can affect the rate and extent of drug absorption after oral administration. These include factors related to the physiological nature of the site of drug administration, physicochemical properties of the drugs, and formulation-related factors. Studying these factors is important in determining the causes of incomplete drug BA for specific drugs. This is also useful for finding strategies to formulate drug products with optimal BA. For example, the oral BA of acid labile drugs can be improved when formulated as enteric-coated tablets. Also, the water solubility, dissolution rate, and hence the oral BA of highly lipophilic drugs can be improved if a water soluble salt of the drug is used in the formulation. Furthermore, the BA of very hydrophilic drugs with limited membrane permeability can be improved by using more lipophilic derivative with higher membrane permeability that can release the active drug in the systemic circulation after absorption. Besides, gastroretentive formulations can improve the BA of drugs that are actively absorbed from a specific site in the duodenum. These are just few examples to show that optimization of drug BA of orally administered drugs requires thorough knowledge of the obstacles for drug absorption and the means to overcome them.

10.2.2 First-Pass Effect

Drug absorption from the GIT involves passage of the drug from the GIT lumen through the gut wall to reach the hepatic portal vein. The absorbed drug is then delivered via the portal vein to the liver before it can reach the systemic circulation. During the absorption process, a portion of the drug dose may be lost in the GIT lumen by degradation, metabolism, or excretion in the feces due to inability of the drug to cross the GIT membrane, leaving only a fraction of the dose (F_F) permeating across the gut wall. The gut wall contains metabolizing enzymes and transporters that can allow only a fraction of the drug amount that reaches the gut wall to get into the portal vein ($F_F \times F_G$). The drug is delivered to the liver via the portal vein where it can be metabolized by the hepatic metabolizing enzymes or excreted in bile, permitting only a fraction of the drug delivered to the liver to reach the systemic circulation ($F_F \times F_G \times F_H$) [2]. This means that the overall BA (F), which is the fraction of dose that reaches the systemic circulation, can be expressed as in Equation 10.1:

$$F = F_F \times F_G \times F_H \qquad (10.1)$$

The loss of the drug during the sequence of steps involved in the absorption process is known as the first-pass effect, which can be illustrated in the diagram in Figure 10.1. Based on this, it is clear that the BA of the drug is affected by the different processes that can decrease the amount of the drug that reaches the systemic circulation. These include nonenzymatic processes such as chemical hydrolysis of the drug in the stomach, complexation that lead to the formation of nonabsorbable complex, adsorption to nonabsorbable compound, and inability of the drug to cross the GIT membrane due to poor solubility or poor permeability. Efflux transporters can also decrease the absorption of drugs from the GIT. Enzymatic processes can also decrease the drug BA by metabolism of the drug during the absorption process in the gut lumen, in the gut wall, and in the liver. Metabolic reactions including hydrolysis, oxidation, reduction, and conjugation result in the formation of the metabolites that are chemical entities different from the parent drug. These metabolic reactions are catalyzed mainly by the cytochrome P450 (CYP450) and other metabolizing enzymes present in the gut wall and the liver. In addition to drug metabolism in the liver, some drugs can be excreted in bile as the parent drugs or as metabolites. The loss of the drug during the absorption process before it reaches the systemic circulation is also known as presystemic elimination.

The first-pass effect can be very small when the drug is well absorbed from the GIT, and the absorbed drug does not undergo significant metabolism in the gut wall or in the liver leading to high drug BA. When the drug is extensively metabolized

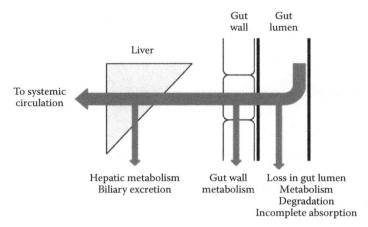

FIGURE 10.1 Diagram illustrating the different causes of loss of the drug during drug absorption after oral administration. The bioavailable drug is the amount of drug that escapes degradation and metabolism in the gut lumen, gut wall metabolism, hepatic metabolism, and biliary excretion and reaches the systemic circulation.

in the gut wall and/or the liver, the first-pass effect becomes large and the drug usually has very limited BA. Changes in the gut and/or hepatic metabolic activity due to drug interactions or change in the hepatic function can cause significant changes in the BA of the drugs that undergo extensive first-pass effect. For example, the BA of the drugs that undergo 90% elimination by the first-pass metabolism is only 10%. If the metabolic activity decreases to a level that will make only 80% of the drug eliminated by first-pass metabolism, the drug BA will increase to 20%. This means that the amount of the drug that reaches the systemic circulation increases by 100%, which can cause significant clinical consequences [3].

Another important factor that can significantly affect the drug BA is the saturable first-pass metabolism. Drugs that are extensively metabolized in the gut wall and liver can saturate the metabolizing enzymes when administered at larger doses resulting in dose dependent BA. This means that the fraction of the dose that reached the systemic circulation is larger after administration of larger doses of the drugs that have saturable first-pass metabolism. Propranolol and verapamil are examples of the drugs that show saturable first-pass metabolism. The rate of drug absorption is an important factor in observing the saturable first-pass metabolism. When the drug is rapidly absorbed, a large quantity of the drug is delivered to the metabolizing enzymes at the same time increasing the chance of enzyme saturation. However, when the drug is administered in the form of a slowly absorbed controlled-release formulation, a small amount of the drug is delivered to the metabolizing enzymes over extended period of time, which decreases the chance of enzyme saturation.

10.2.3 GIT Drug Transporters

The role of the GIT transporters in the drug absorption and oral BA of many drugs has been well recognized. Drug transporters in general are integral cellular proteins that can mediate the influx or efflux of drug molecules across the transcellular membrane by facilitated diffusion or energy-dependent mechanisms. These transporters are expressed in various organs and tissues throughout the body; however, our discussion will focus on the transporters that can affect drug absorption from the GIT. There are several classes of transporters that have been identified. They are different in their distribution pattern, substrate specificity, capacity, and cellular expression pattern. In the GIT, some transporters are expressed on the apical side of the membrane facing the lumen, while others are expressed on the basolateral membrane facing the blood capillaries. The function of the transporters is either to efflux the drug molecules out of the epithelial cells or to influx the drug molecules inside the epithelial cells. So at the apical side of the membrane, efflux transporters promote removal of the absorbed molecules hindering the absorption process, while the influx transporters facilitate the absorption of drug molecules to the epithelial cells, whereas, at the basolateral side of the membrane, the efflux transporters promote drug absorption to the blood, while influx transporters can be involved in removal of drug molecules from the blood for further excretion in the gut lumen. Figure 10.2 includes a diagram that represents the function of drug transporters in epithelial layer of the intestinal mucosa.

There are numerous classes of the transporters that have been identified in the GIT. The two major superfamilies of transporters that play a significant role in drug transport in the body are the ATP-binding cassette (ABC) transporters and the solute carrier transporters (SLCs). The ABC superfamily includes several subfamilies; some of them can influence drug absorption such as P-glycoprotein (P-gp, ABCB1), multidrug resistance associated protein (MRP, ABCC), and the breast cancer resistance protein (BCRP, ABCG2). The SLC superfamily include over 300 members with several subfamilies involved in drug absorption such as the proton dependent oligopeptide transporters (POTs, SLC15A), the organic anion transporters (OATs, SLC21A), the organic cation transporters (OCTs, SLC22A), the nucleoside transporters (CNTs, SLC28A and ENT, SLC29A), and the monocarboxylate transporters (MCTs, SLC16A) [4]. The following discussion covers two representative examples of drug transporters that have been well investigated and have been shown to affect the BA of orally administered drugs. This includes an example of efflux transporter and influx transporter to illustrate the differences in their effect on the drug BA.

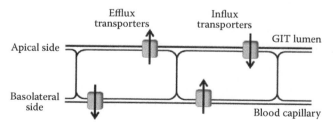

FIGURE 10.2 Schematic presentation of the function of the influx and efflux transporters on the epithelial layer of the intestinal mucosa. The diagram shows the influx transporter in one cell and the efflux transporter in another cell; however, the same epithelial cell can have both influx and efflux transporters.

10.2.3.1   P-Glycoprotein

P-gp is one of the ABC transporters that is expressed in different organs including the kidney, small intestine, liver, lungs, colon, and blood brain barrier. In the small intestine, P-gp is localized in the apical surface of intestinal epithelial mucosa with the primary function of promoting the removal of toxic compounds by active efflux back to the intestinal lumen. Substrates for P-gp include many anticancer drugs, antibiotics, antivirals, calcium channel blockers, and immunosuppressive agents. The absorption of P-gp substrates from the GIT is reduced by the efflux function of this transporter leading to reduction of their systemic BA. Modulation of the P-gp function can lead to changes in the BA of the drugs that are P-gp substrates.

Investigations have shown that P-gp can be inhibited or induced, which can lead to significant clinical consequences. Drugs like rifampicin, steroid hormones, some anticancer drugs, retinoic acid, sodium butyrate, and natural products such as St John's Wort can upregulate the expression of P-gp in animal models, in vitro models, and some human studies. Increased P-gp expression will augment the efflux function of this transport protein leading to lower absorption of P-gp substrates and hence reducing their BA. Also, several drugs can inhibit P-gp activity such as calcium channel blockers, immunosuppressive agents, natural products such as grape fruit juice, and some compounds developed specifically as specific inhibitors of P-gp. Concomitant administration of P-gp inhibitors with P-gp substrates can lead to reduction of the efflux effect of the transporter leading to increase in the absorption and BA of the P-gp substrates. These drug–drug interactions can lead to significant change in the drug therapeutic effect [5]. For example, when the calcium channel blocker valspodar is administered with digoxin, there is significant increase in the plasma digoxin concentrations and adverse effect is observed. An additional P-gp property with significant clinical importance is the existence of P-gp polymorphism meaning that different individuals may have different expression of the transporters, which can cause large variability in the BA of some P-gp substrates.

The P-gp is distributed on the apical surface of the intestinal epithelium to efflux P-gp substrates back to the intestinal lumen, while CYP3A4 that is responsible for the majority of the intestinal first-pass metabolism is localized intracellularly. Since many of the P-gp substrates are also CYP3A4 substrates, drug molecules that enter the enterocytes and are not metabolized by CYP3A4 can be effluxed to the gut lumen by the P-gp. These drug molecules can be absorbed again and get another chance to get metabolized by the intestinal enzymes leading to reduction in the drug overall BA. The interplay between P-gp and CYP3A4 and the difference in their expression between individuals contribute to the variability in drug absorption and BA [6].

10.2.3.2   Oligopeptide Transporters

The peptide transporters are influx transporters that provide good opportunity to design prodrugs that can be recognized and transported to increase drug absorption and BA. This strategy has been utilized to prepare a prodrug for acyclovir, which is an antiviral drug with oral BA of about 20% due to its hydrophilicity. Valacyclovir is the L-valine ester of acyclovir that has been shown to have about 55% BA. This prodrug is a good substrate for one of the peptide transporters (PepT1), which significantly increases its absorption. During the absorption process, the prodrug is hydrolyzed by the esterase enzymes in the liver liberating acyclovir into the systemic circulation, which increases its BA [7]. Other prodrugs that have been shown to be PepT substrates are angiotensin converting enzyme (ACE) inhibitors such as enalapril.

10.2.4 INTESTINAL DRUG METABOLISM

The involvement of the intestine in the first-pass metabolism has been well recognized for many drugs. However, it was generally assumed that the liver played the dominant role in the presystemic metabolism. This was until the discovery of the CYP3A4 in the human intestinal mucosa and liver and the recognition that this enzyme system is involved in the metabolism of many orally administered drugs. The CYP3A4 makes up about 80% of the total CYP450s present in the small intestine, with CYP2C9 comprising the second most abundant CYP450 enzyme. A number of UDP-glucuronosyltransferase and sulfotransferases conjugation enzymes are also expressed in the small intestine and are involved in the presystemic metabolism of numerous drugs. The CYP3A4 is not expressed uniformly in the small intestine with the highest expression being in the proximal region that declines distally. Also, high variability in the CYP3A4 intestinal expression level between individuals is observed [6,8].

The total amount of the CYP3A4 expressed in the small intestine is about 1% of the estimated hepatic level of this enzyme system. The contribution of the intestinal CYP3A4 to the presystemic metabolism of many orally administered drugs is significant despite the low intestinal to hepatic expression ratio. There have been several suggestions to explain the significant intestinal metabolism. The low blood flow rate to the intestinal mucosa can increase the efficiency of the intestinal enzymes in metabolizing the drug by several folds. Also, the intestinal CYP3A4 is affected by induction and inhibition more than the hepatic enzymes. Furthermore, many of the CYP3A4 substrates are also substrates for the P-gp efflux transport protein present in the apical surface of the mucosal membrane. For these mutual CYP3A4 and P-gp substrates, when the drug crosses the epithelial membrane it can be removed back to the intestinal lumen by P-gp, be metabolized by the CYP3A4, or cross the basolateral epithelial membrane to reach the blood. The drug molecules that are removed to the gut lumen by the P-gp can be reabsorbed and become exposed to the CYP3A4 again, which increases the chance for the drug to be metabolized [9].

10.3 REGULATORY REQUIREMENT FOR BIOAVAILABILITY

Evaluation of the drug BA by determining the fraction of dose that reaches the systemic circulation can be very useful in all stages of drug development. During the early stage of development, the drug BA is one of the key factors in making the decision to terminate or to continue the drug development process especially for drugs intended for use in the management of chronic diseases in presence of effective oral alternatives. Also, the results of BA studies can be used in formulation optimization by comparing the fraction of dose absorbed after administration of the different formulations. In addition to the utility of BA information by drug developers, regulatory authorities have specific requirements for the determination of the drug BA to ensure the quality of the marketed drug products. The following discussion will utilize the U.S. Food and Drug Administration (FDA) requirements for the in vivo BA determination as an example; however, the European, Japanese, and all other drug regulatory authorities have similar requirements.

Determination of the in vivo BA is required by the drug regulatory authorities in the following situations (21 CFR, Sec. 320.21, 2010) [1]:

1. All new drug applications for approving a new drug entity for sale and marketing shall include evidence of measuring the in vivo BA of the drug product that is the subject of the application. The new drug application should include detailed information to prove that the drug under consideration is safe and effective and in these studies, the in vivo BA should be determined.

2. All supplemental application should include evidence of measuring the in vivo BA of the approved drug product that is the subject of the application. This is required if the supplemental application proposes changes in the manufacturing site, change in the manufacturing process, change in product formulation, change in dosage strength, change in the labeling to provide for a new indication if clinical studies are required, change in the labeling to provide for a new dosage regimen, or an additional dosage regimen for a special patient population.

3. Any drug manufacturer holding approved drug application should submit supplemental application containing new evidence of measuring the in vivo BA of the drug product that is the subject of the application if notified by the regulatory authorities that
   a. There are data demonstrating that the dosage regimen in the labeling is based on incorrect assumptions or facts regarding the pharmacokinetics of the drug product and that following this dosage regimen could potentially result in subtherapeutic or toxic levels.
   b. There are data measuring significant intra-batch and batch-to-batch variability, for example, ±25%, in the BA of the drug product.

For all the conditions that require determination of the in vivo BA, if the characteristics of the drug product meet at least one of the criteria that allow waiver of the in vivo BA determination, the drug BA is not measured. Instead, the application should contain information to prove that the drug product under consideration falls in one of the categories that do not require measuring the in vivo BA. The criteria for waiving the BA determination requirements are similar to those for waiving the in vivo BE demonstration (21 CFR, Sec. 320.22, 2010) [1]. This issue will be discussed in the next chapter that deals with BE.

10.4   DETERMINATION OF THE DRUG IN VIVO BIOAVAILABILITY

Similar approaches are used to calculate the drug BA after oral and any other extravascular route of administration. The most acceptable approach is to measure the active drug concentration as a function of time in the systemic circulation after drug

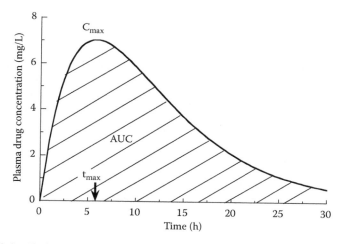

FIGURE 10.3 Typical plasma concentration–time profile after administration of a single oral dose of the drug.

administration. The plasma concentration–time profile shown in Figure 10.3 represents the typical profile obtained after a single oral drug administration. Three important parameters are determined from the drug concentration–time profile that can reflect the rate and extent of drug absorption. The C_{max} represents the highest drug concentration in the systemic circulation achieved after drug administration. Higher C_{max} indicates faster rate and/or higher extent of drug absorption, while t_{max} represents the length of time required to achieve C_{max}. Shorter t_{max} indicates faster rate of drug absorption. The t_{max} is not affected by the extent of drug absorption, whereas the AUC is directly proportional to the amount of the administered drug, which reaches the systemic circulation (assuming constant CL_T). So the AUC is used to compare the extent of drug absorption after oral administration. The AUC is not affected by the rate of drug absorption.

10.4.1 Drug Bioavailability

There are two types of drug BA.

10.4.1.1 Absolute Bioavailability

It is the fraction of the administered dose that reaches the systemic circulation after oral administration, and it is a measure of the extent of drug absorption. The absolute BA is determined by comparing the amount of drug that reaches the systemic circulation after oral administration and after IV administration of the same dose of the same drug. This is because after IV administration the entire dose reaches the systemic circulation. The absolute BA can have values between zero and one. When the drug is not absorbed at all after oral administration, the absolute BA is equal to zero, while when the entire oral dose reaches the systemic circulation, the absolute BA is equal to one. The absolute BA can also be expressed in terms of percentage (0%–100%).

10.4.1.2   Relative Bioavailability

It is the absolute BA of the active drug moiety from a drug product relative to the absolute BA of the same active drug moiety from a second drug product. The relative BA is determined by comparing the amount of the drug that reaches the systemic circulation after administration of two different oral drug products (test product and reference product), which contain the same active drug moiety. The relative BA can have any positive value and can be more than one when the drug BA from the test product is higher than that of the reference product.

10.4.2   Calculation of the Drug Bioavailability

When the drug elimination follows first-order kinetics (most drugs do), then the AUC after IV administration of a single dose of the drug is given by

$$AUC_{IV} = \frac{Dose}{kVd} \tag{10.2}$$

The AUC after oral administration of a single dose of the same drug is given by

$$AUC_{oral} = \frac{F\,Dose}{kVd} \tag{10.3}$$

where F is the absolute BA of the oral dosage form that is the fraction of the oral dose that reaches the systemic circulation. If the same dose of the drug is used for the oral and IV administration, and because the drug CL_T (kVd) is independent of the route of the drug administration, dividing Equation 10.3 by Equation 10.2 yields

$$\frac{AUC_{oral}}{AUC_{IV}} = \frac{F\,Dose_{oral}/kVd}{Dose_{IV}/kVd} = F \tag{10.4}$$

This means that the drug absolute BA can be determined from the ratio of the AUC after oral administration to that after IV administration of the same drug to the same individual (to ensure similar CL_T). Equation 10.5 is the general equation that can be used to calculate the absolute BA of the drug after oral administration even if the oral and IV doses are different:

$$F = \frac{AUC_{oral}}{AUC_{IV}}\,\frac{Dose_{IV}}{Dose_{oral}} \tag{10.5}$$

Similarly, the relative BA for different formulations or products of the same active drug moiety can be determined by comparing the AUCs after administration of these products to the same individuals. Usually the new oral product under investigation is called the test product and the oral product used to compare with is called the reference product:

$$AUC_{test} = \frac{F_{test}\,Dose_{test}}{kVd} \tag{10.6}$$

$$AUC_{standard} = \frac{F_{standard} \, Dose_{standard}}{kVd} \tag{10.7}$$

where

F_{test} is the absolute BA of the drug from the test drug product
$F_{standard}$ is the absolute BA of the drug from the standard drug product

If the same dose of the two drug products is administered, and because the drug CL_T (kVd) is independent of the drug formulation, dividing Equation 10.6 by Equation 10.7 yields

$$\frac{AUC_{test}}{AUC_{standard}} = \frac{F_{test} \, Dose/kVd}{F_{standard} \, Dose/kVd} = \frac{F_{test}}{F_{standard}} \tag{10.8}$$

This means that the drug BA from the test drug product relative to the drug BA from the standard drug product can be determined from the ratio of the calculated AUC after administration of the two products to the same individuals, as in the following general equation:

$$F_{relative} = \frac{F_{test}}{F_{standard}} = \frac{AUC_{test}}{AUC_{standard}} \frac{Dose_{standard}}{Dose_{test}} \tag{10.9}$$

where the relative BA ($F_{test}/F_{standard}$) is the absolute BA of the test product relative to the absolute BA of the standard product. Calculating the relative BA does not give the value of the absolute BA for the individual products but it gives the ratio of the absolute BA for the two products. For example, assume that the BA of product A relative to the BA of product B is 0.8. This means that the ratio of the absolute BA of product A to that of product B is 0.8 without providing the value of the absolute BA of the two products. It can be any combination of the absolute BA that has a ratio of 0.8 (e.g., 0.8/1.0, 0.6/0.75, 0.4/0.5, 0.2/0.25, etc.).

10.4.3 CALCULATION OF THE DRUG BIOAVAILABILITY FROM THE DRUG URINARY EXCRETION DATA

The drug that reaches the systemic circulation is excreted by one or more elimination pathways such as metabolism and urinary excretion. The fraction of the drug in the systemic circulation that is excreted by each pathway is usually constant for a particular drug in an individual patient. So for a drug that is partially excreted unchanged in urine, administration of larger doses to the same individual results in proportional increase in the amount of the drug recovered unchanged in urine when the drug is completely eliminated from the body. Based on this, it is possible to use the drug urinary excretion information after drug administration to calculate the drug BA.

For example, if the total amount of a drug recovered unchanged in urine is 60 mg after administration of a single IV dose of 100 mg, this means that 60% of the drug that reaches the systemic circulation of this drug is excreted unchanged in urine. Assume that the same dose of this drug is administered orally to the same individual and the total amount of the drug excreted in urine is 30 mg. This means that the 30 mg of the drug excreted in urine after the oral dose represents 60% of the amount of the drug that reached the systemic circulation, indicating that only 50 mg of the drug reached the systemic circulation after oral administration. The absolute oral BA of this drug is 50%.

The use of urinary excretion data to calculate the drug BA requires that significant amount of the drug is excreted unchanged in urine after IV and oral administration. A single IV and a single oral dose of the drug are administered to the same individual or group of individuals, and then urine is collected and added together until all the drug is completely excreted, that is, no more drug remaining in the body. The total amount of the drug excreted in urine ($A_{e\infty}$) is determined from the volume of the total urine sample and the concentration of the drug in the total urine sample as follows:

$$A_{e\infty} = \text{Volume of sample} \times \text{Drug concentration in sample} \qquad (10.10)$$

The absolute BA can be calculated as follows:

$$F = \frac{A_{e\infty\,oral}}{A_{e\infty\,IV}} \frac{\text{Dose}_{IV}}{\text{Dose}_{oral}} \qquad (10.11)$$

Similarly, the relative BA can be determined from the urinary excretion data after administration of two oral products for the same drug, a test product and a reference product.

$$F_{relative} = \frac{A_{e\infty\,test}}{A_{e\infty\,reference}} \frac{\text{Dose}_{reference}}{\text{Dose}_{test}} \qquad (10.12)$$

10.5   GUIDELINES FOR CONDUCTING IN VIVO BIOAVAILABILITY STUDY

10.5.1   GUIDING PRINCIPLES

The in vivo BA study is generally performed in normal adult volunteers under standardized conditions (21 CFR, Sec. 320.25, 2010). However, in some situations, in vivo BA studies may be performed in patients.

10.5.2   BASIC STUDY DESIGN

The reason for performing the in vivo BA study usually determines the basic design and the choice of the reference product with which the product of interest will be compared. BA studies may be performed to determine the absolute BA for a new dosage form, the BA after different routes of administration, or the BA for different formulations, etc. In all these situations, the study involves administration of both the drug product under investigation and an appropriate reference product to the study participants in two different occasions in a crossover experimental design. The choice of the reference products can be different in the different studies. The drug product under investigation and the reference product shall meet all compendial standards of identity, strength, quality, and purity, including potency, and where applicable, content uniformity, disintegration times, and dissolution rates.

10.5.2.1   For New Active Drug Moieties That Have Never Been Previously Marketed

Determination of the absolute BA for the new active drug moiety requires administration of the solution of the active drug ingredient intravenously and the drug formulation proposed for marketing. Then the absolute BA can be determined from the calculated AUCs as described before. Additional studies can be performed to establish the essential pharmacokinetic characteristics of the active drug ingredient such as the rate of absorption, the extent of absorption, the half-life of the therapeutic moiety in vivo, the rate of excretion and/or metabolism, and dose proportionality. The formulation used to obtain the general drug pharmacokinetic characteristics should be a solution or suspension of the drug and can be compared with the formulation proposed for marketing.

10.5.2.2   For New Formulations of an Approved Active Drug Ingredient

The BA study is conducted for the new dosage form or the new formulation of the approved active ingredient and should involve characterization of the pharmacokinetic parameters of the new formulation. The reference product should be one of the approved drug products to compare the new formulation with the currently marketed drug product.

10.5.2.3   For Extended-Release Formulations

The BA study is conducted to determine if the drug product meets the extended-release claims made for it and to rule out the occurrence of any dose dumping. Also, studies are performed to prove that the drug product's steady-state performance is equivalent to the currently marketed immediate-release or extended-release drug product that contains the same active drug ingredient. The reference products for such BA study can be a solution or suspension of the active drug ingredient or currently marketed immediate-release or extended-release drug products containing the same active drug ingredient.

10.5.2.4   For Combination Drug Products

The rate and extent of absorption of each active drug ingredient or therapeutic moiety in the combination drug product have to be compared to the rate and extent of absorption of each active drug ingredient administered concurrently in separate single-ingredient product. In this case, the reference products can be two or more currently marketed, single-ingredient drug products each of which contains one of the active drug ingredients in the combination product. Under some circumstances, the reference products can be an approved combination drug product that contains the same drug combination as the product under investigation. The BA study may involve determination of the rate and extent of selected, but not all, active ingredient of the combination drug product. This is permitted when the therapeutic effect of the drug combination is due to one of the active ingredients, for example, ampicillin in ampicillin-probenecid combination product.

10.6 CLINICAL IMPORTANCE OF BIOAVAILABILITY

The plasma drug concentration–time profile observed after administration of a single oral dose is dependent on the rate and extent of drug absorption. Administration of drug products with lower BA results in decreasing the amount of the drug that reaches the systemic circulation. The drug C_{max} will be lower and the AUC will be smaller after administration of a single dose of drug products with lower BA as illustrated in Figure 10.4. During repeated use of the drug, shifting to products with lower BA will decrease the steady-state drug concentration. This means that drug products with lower BA can decrease the intensity and possibly the duration of therapeutic effect after a single dose administration. Also, switching to drug products with lower oral BA may decrease the disease control during multiple drug administration for the management of chronic disease. This illustrates the importance of the determination of the BA of the drug from the different products. Also, it is important to enforce strict regulatory requirements for demonstrating BE for the different drug products for the same active drug to enable switching between products for the same active drug without affecting the therapeutic response.

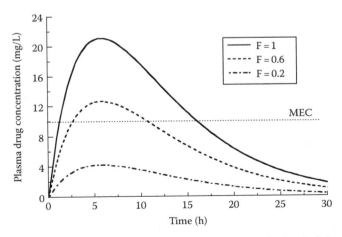

FIGURE 10.4 Plasma drug concentration–time profiles after a single administration of the same dose of a drug from different drug products that have different absolute BA.

10.7 CALCULATION OF THE AUC (THE LINEAR TRAPEZOIDAL RULE)

The principle of the linear trapezoidal rule for calculating the AUC is based on dividing the plasma drug concentration–time profile to a number of trapezoids. The area of each trapezoid can be calculated as in Figure 10.5 and it is equal to

$$\text{Area} = \left(\frac{a+b}{2}\right) W \tag{10.13}$$

Then the total AUC can be calculated from the sum of the areas of these trapezoids in addition to the area under the tail of the curve as in Figure 10.6. The area of each trapezoid is calculated as

$$\text{Area} = \left(\frac{C_n + C_{n+1}}{2}\right)(t_{n+1} - t_n) \tag{10.14}$$

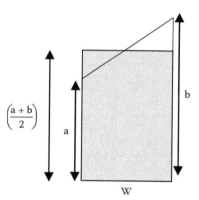

FIGURE 10.5   Calculation of the area of a trapezoid.

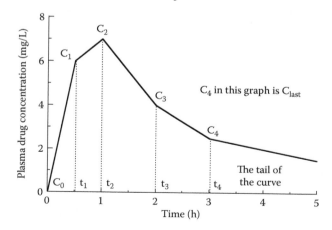

FIGURE 10.6   AUC is the sum of the area of all trapezoids and the area under the tail of the curve.

and the area of the tail is

$$\text{Area of the tail} = \frac{C_{last}}{k} \qquad (10.15)$$

or

$$\text{Area of the tail} = \frac{C_{last}t_{1/2}}{0.693} = 1.44C_{last}t_{1/2} \qquad (10.16)$$

where
C_{last} is the last measured concentration
k is the first-order elimination rate constant

The total AUC is the sum of all trapezoids plus the area of the tail:

$$\text{AUC} = \left(\frac{1}{2}\right)(C_0 + C_1)(t_1 - t_0) + \left(\frac{1}{2}\right)(C_1 + C_2)(t_2 - t_1) + \cdots + \text{area of tail} \qquad (10.17)$$

Example

In a study to evaluate the BA of an antibiotic, a patient received a single 250 mg IV bolus dose, a single 500 mg dose in the form of an oral suspension, and a single 500 mg in the form of an oral capsule on three separate occasions, and the following plasma concentrations were obtained:

Time (h)	IV Bolus (250 mg) Concentration (mg/L)	Oral Suspension (500 mg) Concentration (mg/L)	Oral Capsule (500 mg) Concentration (mg/L)
1	6.3	5.0	3.1
2	5.0	7.0	4.7
3	4.0	7.4	5.2
4	3.2	7.0	5.3
6	2.0	5.4	4.5
8	1.3	3.7	3.4
12	0.5	1.6	1.7

The half-life of this antibiotic is 3 h and the absorption process is complete after 12 h of oral administration.

- a. Calculate the absolute BA of the oral suspension and the oral capsule of this antibiotic.
- b. Calculate the BA of the oral capsule relative to the oral suspension of this antibiotic.

Answer

a. To calculate the absolute BA of the oral suspension and the capsule, we need to calculate the AUC after administration of the IV and the oral formulations.

Calculation of the AUC after administration of 250 mg IV:
Plot the plasma concentration–time profile after IV administration on the semilog scale and back extrapolate the resulting line to calculate the initial plasma concentration Cp_0. The Cp_0 is 8 mg/L and the first-order elimination rate constant (k) is 0.693/3 h = 0.231 h^{-1}.

$$AUC_{IV} = \frac{Cp_0}{k} = \frac{8\,mg/L}{0.231\,h^{-1}} = 34.63\,mg\,h/L$$

Calculation of the AUC after administration of 500 mg oral suspension by the trapezoidal rule:

$$\text{Area of a trapezoid} = \left(\frac{C_n + C_{n+1}}{2}\right) \cdot (t_{n+1} - t_n)$$

Please note that after oral administration the drug concentration at time zero is equal to zero, and the 0,0 point should be used in calculating the AUC after oral administration.

$$\text{Area of trapezoid 1} = \left(\frac{0+5}{2}\right) \cdot (1-0) = 2.5\,mg\,h/L$$

$$\text{Area of trapezoid 2} = \left(\frac{5+7}{2}\right) \cdot (2-1) = 6\,mg\,h/L$$

$$\text{Area of trapezoid 3} = \left(\frac{7+7.4}{2}\right) \cdot (3-2) = 7.2\,mg\,h/L$$

$$\text{Area of trapezoid 4} = \left(\frac{7.4+7}{2}\right) \cdot (4-3) = 7.2\,mg\,h/L$$

$$\text{Area of trapezoid 5} = \left(\frac{7+5.4}{2}\right) \cdot (6-4) = 12.4\,mg\,h/L$$

$$\text{Area of trapezoid 6} = \left(\frac{5.4+3.7}{2}\right) \cdot (8-6) = 9.1\,mg\,h/L$$

$$\text{Area of trapezoid 7} = \left(\frac{3.7+1.6}{2}\right) \cdot (12-8) = 10.6\,mg\,h/L$$

$$\text{Area of the tail} = \frac{C_{last}}{k} = \frac{1.6\,mg/L}{0.231\,h^{-1}} = 6.93\,mg\,h/L$$

Total AUC = 2.5 + 6.0 + 7.2 + 7.2 + 12.4 + 9.1 + 10.6 + 6.93 = 61.93 mg h/L

Calculation of the AUC after administration of 500 mg oral capsule by the trapezoidal rule:

$$\text{Area of trapezoid } 1 = \left(\frac{0+3.1}{2}\right) \cdot (1-0) = 1.55 \, \text{mg h/L}$$

$$\text{Area of trapezoid } 2 = \left(\frac{3.1+4.7}{2}\right) \cdot (2-1) = 3.9 \, \text{mg h/L}$$

$$\text{Area of trapezoid } 3 = \left(\frac{4.7+5.2}{2}\right) \cdot (3-2) = 4.95 \, \text{mg h/L}$$

$$\text{Area of trapezoid } 4 = \left(\frac{5.2+5.3}{2}\right) \cdot (4-3) = 5.25 \, \text{mg h/L}$$

$$\text{Area of trapezoid } 5 = \left(\frac{5.3+4.5}{2}\right) \cdot (6-4) = 9.8 \, \text{mg h/L}$$

$$\text{Area of trapezoid } 6 = \left(\frac{4.5+3.4}{2}\right) \cdot (8-6) = 7.9 \, \text{mg h/L}$$

$$\text{Area of trapezoid } 7 = \left(\frac{3.4+1.7}{2}\right) \cdot (12-8) = 10.2 \, \text{mg h/L}$$

$$\text{Area of the tail} = \frac{C_{last}}{k} = \frac{1.7 \, \text{mg/L}}{0.231 \, \text{h}^{-1}} = 7.36 \, \text{mg h/L}$$

Total AUC $= 1.55 + 3.9 + 4.95 + 5.25 + 9.8 + 7.9 + 10.2 + 7.36 = 50.9 \, \text{mg h/L}$

The absolute BA of the suspension (note that the doses for the IV and the oral suspension are different):

$$F_{suspension} = \frac{AUC_{suspension}}{AUC_{IV}} \times \frac{Dose_{IV}}{Dose_{suspension}} = \frac{61.93 \, \text{mg h/L}}{34.63 \, \text{mg h/L}} \times \frac{250 \, \text{mg}}{500 \, \text{mg}} = 0.89$$

The absolute BA of the capsule (Note that the doses for the IV and the oral capsule are different):

$$F_{capsule} = \frac{AUC_{capsule}}{AUC_{IV}} \times \frac{Dose_{IV}}{Dose_{capsule}} = \frac{50.9 \, \text{mg h/L}}{34.63 \, \text{mg h/L}} \times \frac{250 \, \text{mg}}{500 \, \text{mg}} = 0.73$$

b. The BA of the capsule relative to the suspension (the dose is similar):

$$F_{relative} = \frac{AUC_{capsule}}{AUC_{suspension}} \times \frac{Dose_{suspension}}{Dose_{capsule}} = \frac{50.9 \, \text{mg h/L}}{61.93 \, \text{mg h/L}} \times \frac{500 \, \text{mg}}{500 \, \text{mg}} = 0.82$$

The relative BA can also be determined from the ratio of the absolute BA of the two oral products:

$$F_{relative} = \frac{F_{capsule}}{F_{suspension}} = \frac{0.73}{0.89} = 0.82$$

10.8 FACTORS AFFECTING THE PLASMA DRUG CONCENTRATION–TIME PROFILE AFTER A SINGLE ORAL DOSE

After administration of a single oral dose, the plasma drug concentration–time profile depends on the dose, F, CL_T, Vd, and the k_a of the drug. The CL_T and the Vd are constants for a given drug in a given patient and are independent of the route of administration and the formulation characteristics. However, F and k_a are dependent on the characteristics of the formulation and different products for the same active drug from different drug manufacturers can have different F and k_a.

The plasma drug concentration increases after administration of a single oral dose and the rate of increase in drug concentration is dependant on the rate of drug absorption. The drug concentration reaches a maximum value at t_{max}, which reflects the rate of drug absorption. After t_{max}, the drug concentrations start to decline. During the terminal elimination phase, and if the elimination process follows first-order kinetics, the plasma concentration–time profile declines at a rate dependent on k. The time course of the therapeutic effect of the drug including the intensity of the effect and the duration of effect is related to the plasma drug concentration–time profile. Changes in the plasma drug concentration–time profile usually cause modification of the therapeutic effect of the drug. So it is important to examine how the change in each of the pharmacokinetic parameters affects the plasma drug concentration–time profile. Pharmacokinetic simulations can be very useful for this purpose.

10.8.1 PHARMACOKINETIC SIMULATION EXERCISE

Pharmacokinetic simulations can be used to examine how each of the parameters included in the equation that describes the drug plasma concentration–time profile after a single oral dose affects the drug profile. The drug plasma concentration–time profile is simulated using an average value of each of the pharmacokinetic parameters. Then the pharmacokinetic parameters are changed one parameter at a time while keeping all the other parameters constant and the simulation is repeated. The resulting drug concentration–time profile is examined to see how the change affects the drug profile. The plotting exercise of the oral administration module in the basic pharmacokinetic concept section and the pharmacokinetic simulations section of the companion CD to this textbook can be used to run these simulations.

10.8.1.1 Dose

Administration of increasing oral doses to the same individual causes proportional increase in C_{max} and AUC due to the increase in the amount of the drug that reaches the systemic circulation (F Dose). However, changing the dose does not affect k, Vd, CL_T, F, and t_{max} if the drug elimination follows first-order kinetics. Higher doses produce higher plasma drug concentrations and increase the systemic exposure to the drug that augments the therapeutic drug effect and increases the chance of producing toxicity at higher doses. Also, administration of larger oral doses of the drug produces drug concentrations-time profile that stay above the drug minimum effective concentration for longer duration of time, resulting in prolongation of the drug effect.

10.8.1.2 Bioavailability

Administration of the same dose of the same drug in the form of drug products that have similar rate of drug absorption but different BA should produce different C_{max} and AUC. This is because the amount of the drug that reaches the systemic circulation is larger for the products with higher BA. Products with higher BA should produce proportionally higher C_{max} and AUC without affecting CL_T, Vd, k_a, and k.

10.8.1.3 Total Body Clearance

Administration of the same dose of a drug from the same product (same F and k_a) to a group of patients who have different CL_T, for example, patients with different degree of eliminating organ dysfunction, results in different rates of decline of the blood drug concentration during the elimination phase, if the Vd of the drug is similar in these patients. Assuming similar Vd of the drug, patients with higher CL_T will have faster rate of drug elimination during the elimination phase (larger k and shorter $t_{1/2}$), while patients with lower CL_T will have slower rate of drug elimination (smaller k and longer $t_{1/2}$). This is because k and $t_{1/2}$ depend on both CL_T and Vd. The AUC will be smaller in the patients with higher CL_T and larger in the patients with lower CL_T. This is because the AUC is inversely proportional to CL_T.

10.8.1.4 Volume of Distribution

Administration of the same dose of a drug from the same product (same F and k_a) to a group of patients who have different Vd, for example, patients with different body weight, but have similar CL_T will cause change in the rate of decline in the drug concentration during the elimination phase without affecting the AUC. This is because the AUC is directly proportional to the bioavailable dose (FD) and inversely proportional to the CL_T and both were assumed to be constant. However, since k and $t_{1/2}$ depend on both CL_T and Vd, the rate of decline in the drug concentration will be different in patients with the same CL_T but different Vd.

Assuming similar CL_T, patients with smaller Vd will eliminate the drug at a faster rate (larger k and shorter $t_{1/2}$), while patients with larger Vd will eliminate the drug at slower rate (smaller k and longer $t_{1/2}$). In this discussion, we assumed that the change is only in Vd while CL_T is constant. It is important to note that the change in Vd does not cause change in CL_T since the Vd and CL_T are independent pharmacokinetic parameters. However, it is possible that the change in Vd is accompanied by change in CL_T. For example, patients with small body weight usually have lower Vd, and the lower body weight may be accompanied by lower eliminating organ weight, which may be reflected by lower CL_T. So it is a condition that caused both CL_T and Vd to change rather than the change in one parameter is caused by change in the other parameter. When both CL_T and Vd are different, the effect on the drug concentration–time profile will depend on the relative change in each parameter.

10.8.1.5 Absorption Rate Constant

Larger absorption rate constant results in faster drug absorption, which is usually reflected in shorter t_{max}. Also, faster drug absorption produces higher C_{max} if the elimination rate does not change (similar CL_T and Vd). The change in the rate of drug absorption (different k_a) does not usually affect CL_T, Vd, F, AUC, and k when the drug elimination follows first-order kinetics.

10.9 SUMMARY

- Orally administered drugs may not be absorbed completely to the systemic circulation because of many physiological, physicochemical, and formulation factors, which can all contribute to the presystemic drug elimination.
- The absolute BA is the fraction of the administered dose that reaches the systemic circulation, while the relative BA is the BA of an oral product relative to the BA of a second oral drug product for the same active drug.
- The drug BA can be determined by comparing the AUCs calculated after oral and IV drug administration in the same individuals in case of absolute BA, while the relative BA is determined from the comparison of AUCs calculated after administration of the two products under investigation.
- The use of drug products with lower BA results in reduction of the bioavailable dose of the drug that may reduce the intensity and the duration of therapeutic effect after single drug administration and can decrease the therapeutic effect during multiple drug administration.

PRACTICE PROBLEMS

10.1 After administration of a single IV bolus dose of acyclovir 300 mg to a patient, the total AUC was 16 mg h/L, and the elimination half-life was 2.4 h, while after oral administration of a 300 mg tablet to the same patient, the following plasma concentrations were obtained:

Time (h)	Drug Concentration (mg/L)
0	0
1	0.364
3	0.716
5	0.787
7	0.730
10	0.569
15	0.318
20	0.162

    a. Calculate the absolute BA of acyclovir in this patient.

10.2 Different formulations of the same drug were administered to the same individuals and the following data were obtained:
- After IV bolus administration of 10 mg the AUC was 5 mg h/L
- After intramuscular (IM) administration of 20 mg, the AUC was 9 mg h/L

- After oral administration of 50 mg capsule, the AUC was 10 mg h/L
- After oral administration of 20 mg oral suspension, the AUC was 5 mg h/L
  a. Calculate the absolute BA of the drug from the capsules.
  b. Calculate the absolute BA of the drug after IM administration.
  c. Calculate the BA of the oral suspension relative to the capsules.
  d. Other than the IV solution, which formulation has the highest absolute BA?

10.3 A group of volunteers received a single oral dose of two different formulations of an oral hypoglycemic drug. Each tablet from the two formulations contains 500 mg of the drug. The average plasma drug concentrations obtained at different time points after administration of the two formulations are tabulated in the following:

	Formulation A	Formulation B
Time (h)	Concentration (mg/L)	Concentration (mg/L)
0	0	0
1	12.9	6.89
2	18.6	11.9
4	20.9	17.7
6	18.8	19.8
8	15.9	19.8
10	13.2	18.6
12	10.8	16.8
20	4.87	9.36
30	1.79	3.78

  a. Which formulation is absorbed faster? Why?
  b. What is the BA of formulation A relative to the BA of formulation B? How can you interpret this result?

10.4 Different formulations of the same drug were administered to a group of individuals and the plasma concentrations were measured after administration of each formulation. The results are tabulated in the following:

	Concentration (mg/L)			
Dose	200 mg	500 mg	500 mg	500 mg
Time (h)	IV	Syrup	Capsule	Tablet
0		0	0	0
1	7.40	9.22	6.0	4.22
2	5.5	11.9	8.14	5.99
3	4.56	11.6	8.25	6.32
5	2.23	8.32	6.35	5.27
7	1.22	5.16	4.15	3.70
10	0.50	2.27	1.94	1.89
15	0.111	0.527	0.475	0.518
20	0.0245	0.119	0.11	0.129

   a. Calculate the half-life and volume of distribution of this drug.
   b. Which oral formulation has the fastest absorption rate?
   c. Calculate the absolute BA of the three oral formulations.
   d. Calculate the BA of the oral capsule relative to the syrup.
   e. Calculate the BA of the tablet relative to the BA of the capsule.

10.5 The following plasma concentrations were obtained after administration of a single 500 mg tablet of an antihypertensive drug to a patient.

Time (h)	Concentration (mg/L)
1	3.75
3	6.1
6	5.2
10	3.14
15	1.32
20	0.56
26	0.197

When a single IV bolus dose of 250 mg was administered to the same patient, the total AUC was 60 mg h/L.

   a. What is the half-life of this drug in this patient?
   b. What is the total AUC of the drug after administration of 500 mg oral dose in this patient?
   c. What is the BA of the oral tablet in this patient?
   d. What are the CL_T and the Vd of this drug in this patient?

10.6 A patient received a single 300 mg IV bolus dose and a single 500 mg oral dose of an antibiotic on two separate occasions, and the following plasma concentrations were obtained:

IV Administration		Oral Administration	
Time (h)	Concentration (mg/L)	Time (h)	Concentration (mg/L)
2	12.86	0	0
6	9.45	1	2.24
12	5.95	3	4.69
24	2.36	5	5.54
		7	5.58
		10	5.0
		15	3.68
		20	2.57
		30	1.20

   a. Calculate the half-life and the volume of distribution of this drug in this patient.
   b. Calculate the fraction of the drug absorbed after oral administration.

10.7 After oral administration of a single 500 mg tablet of an antihypertensive drug to a normal volunteer, the total calculated AUC was 70 mg h/L. After an IV bolus administration of the same drug to the same volunteer, the drug half-life was 3 h and the volume of distribution was 25 L.

   a. Calculate the BA of this oral tablet in this volunteer.

   b. What is the expected AUC after administration of a single IV bolus dose of 250 mg of this drug to the same volunteer?

REFERENCES

1. U.S. Code of Federal Regulations (April 2010) Title 21-Food and Drugs, Chapter I, Food and Drug Administration, Department of Health and Human Services, Sub-Chapter D, Drugs for Human Use, Part 320, Bioavailability and Bioequivalence Requirements.
2. Rowland M, Benet LZ, and Graham GG (1973) Clearance concepts in pharmacokinetics. *J Pharmacokinet Biopharm* 1:123–136.
3. Lilja JJ, Neuvonen M, and Neuvonen PJ (2004) Effect of regular consumption of grapefruit juice on the pharmacokinetics of simvastatin. *Br J Clin Pharmacol* 58:56–60.
4. Goole J, Lindley DJ, Roth W, Carl SM, Amighi K, Kauffman JM, and Knipp GT (2010) The effect of excipients on transporter mediated absorption. *Int J Pharm* 393:17–31.
5. Kunta JR and Sinko PJ (2004) Intestinal drug transporters: In vivo function and clinical importance. *Curr Drug Metab* 5:109–124.
6. Watkin PB (1997) The barrier function of CYP3A4 and P-glycoprotein in the small bowel. *Adv Drug Deliv Rev* 27:161–170.
7. Sugawara M, Huang W, Fie YJ, Leibach FH, Ganapathy V, and Ganapathy ME (2000) Transport of valganciclovir, a ganciclovir prodrug via peptide transporters PEPT1 and PEPT2. *J Pharm Sci* 89:781–789.
8. Wacher VJ, Silverman JA, Zhang Y, and Benet LZ (1997) Role of P-glycoprotein in cyclosporine P450 3Ain limiting oral absorption of peptide and peptidomimetics. *J Pharm Sci* 87:1322–1330.
9. Benet LZ and Cummins CL (2001) The drug efflux-metabolism alliance: Biochemical aspects. *Adv Drug Deliv Rev* 50(Suppl. 1):S3–S11.

11 Bioequivalence

OBJECTIVES

After completing this chapter you should be able to

- Define bioavailability, bioequivalence, pharmaceutical equivalence, and therapeutic equivalence
- Discuss the situations when bioequivalence determination is required
- Discuss the situations when bioequivalence determination can be waived
- Describe the different approaches that can be used to demonstrate bio-equivalence of drug products
- Describe the general guidelines for study design, study execution, and data analysis of in vivo bioequivalence studies
- State the different components of the analytical assay validation
- Explain the different approaches to modify the in vivo bioequivalence studies to handle special conditions such as the presence of active metabolites, highly variable drugs, endogenous compounds, and long half-life drugs

11.1   INTRODUCTION

The requirements for drug approval may differ from one country to another; however, the approval process usually goes through the same general steps. In the United States, the Food and Drug Administration (FDA) requires that the pharmaceutical company files a new drug application (NDA) for the approval of a new molecular entity that has never been marketed in the United States before. In the NDA, the company should provide comprehensive drug information and results of investigations that prove that the new drug is safe and effective. If the NDA is approved, the drug can be marketed in the United States as "innovator product" exclusively by that drug company for the remaining of the patent period. When the drug patent expires, other pharmaceutical companies can request marketing "generic products" for the same active drug. A generic drug product is the same as the innovator drug product in dosage form, route of administration, strength, quality, performance, and intended use. For marketing generic products, companies have to file abbreviated new drug application (ANDA). The ANDA is not required to include evidence of drug safety and effectiveness; however, it should include evidence of bioequivalence (BE), that is, a proof that the performance of the generic product in vivo is similar to that of the innovator product. Once approved, applicant(s) can manufacture and market the generic drug product to provide safe, effective, and low-cost alternative drug products. Supplemental applications are usually filed whenever changes are introduced to the manufacturing process, formulation, or indications of approved drugs to prove that all the qualities originally set for the product are still met.

The primary objective of the ANDA is to demonstrate that the safety and efficacy of the generic drug product is comparable to that of the innovator drug product. This should allow patient switching from the innovator product to the generic product without compromising the safety and therapeutic efficacy. The in vivo BE studies are usually the bases for evaluating the "interchangeability" between the generic and innovator products. Regulatory drug authorities around the world including the U.S. FDA, the European Medicines Agency (EMA) in the European Union, Japan's National Institute of Health, Division of Drugs, and the World Health Organization (WHO) develop guidance for pharmaceutical industry for the design, execution, data analysis, data reporting, and submission of BE study results. This helped in the standardization of the approaches used to evaluate the BE of pharmaceutical products and resulted in the approval of large number of generic drug products every year.

11.2 GENERAL DEFINITIONS

Drug products: The finished dosage form, for example, tablet, capsule, or solution that contains the active drug ingredient with or without inactive ingredients.

Pharmaceutical alternatives: Drug products that contain the same therapeutic moiety but differ in dosage form, strength, salt or ester of the active therapeutic moiety.

Pharmaceutical equivalents: Drug products that contain the exact active ingredient (i.e., the same salt or ester of the therapeutic moiety), identical strength, the same dosage form for the same route of administration, but differ in shape, release mechanism, labeling, scoring, and excipients including color, flavor, and preservative.

Bioequivalent products: Pharmaceutical equivalent products with no significant difference in the rate and extent to which the active ingredient becomes available at the site of action when administered under similar conditions in an appropriately designed study.

Therapeutic equivalents: Drug products for the same active ingredient that can be substituted with the full expectation that the substituted product will produce the same clinical effect and safety profile as the prescribed product. Drug products are considered to be therapeutically equivalent if they are pharmaceutical equivalents and bioequivalents.

Reference listed drug products: It is the listed approved drug products identified by regulatory authorities as the drug products upon which new generic versions are compared to prove that they are bioequivalent. By designating a single reference listed drug as the standard to which all generic versions must be shown to be bioequivalent, regulatory authorities hope to avoid possible significant variations among generic drugs and their brand name counterparts.

11.3 REGULATORY REQUIREMENT FOR BIOEQUIVALENCE

As defined earlier, two drug products for the same active ingredient are considered bioequivalent if the rate and extent to which the active drug becomes available at the site of action are similar. This can be attained only if similar drug concentration–time profiles in the systemic circulation are achieved after administration of the two products. Similar drug profiles in the body can be achieved only when the rate and extent of drug absorption are similar. So testing for BE can be based on comparing the rate and extent of drug absorption after administration of the two products. Pharmaceutical companies are required to prove that generic drug products are bioequivalent before marketing. This is to ensure that the marketed generic products for the same active drug produce similar therapeutic effect. The following discussion will utilize the U.S. FDA requirements for the in vivo BE determination as an example; however, the European, Japanese, and all other drug regulatory authorities have similar requirements.

Determination of the in vivo BE is required by the drug regulatory authorities in the following situations (21CFR 320.21, 2010) [1]:

1. All ANDA requesting approval of a generic drug product shall include evidence demonstrating that the drug product that is the subject of the ANDA is bioequivalent to the reference listed drug. A complete study report must be submitted for the in vivo BE study upon which the applicant relies for approval.
2. All supplemental applications should include evidence demonstrating that the approved generic drug product that is the subject of the supplemental application is bioequivalent to the reference listed drug. This is required if the supplemental application proposes changes in the manufacturing site, change in the manufacturing process, change in product formulation, change in dosage strength, change in the labeling to provide for a new indication if clinical studies are required, change in the labeling to provide for a new dosage regimen, or an additional dosage regimen for a special patient population.
3. Pharmaceutical companies holding approved ANDA should submit supplemental application containing new evidence demonstrating the in vivo BE of the drug product that is the subject of the application if notified by the drug regulatory authorities that
   a. There are data demonstrating that the dosage regimen in the labeling is based on incorrect assumptions or facts regarding the pharmacokinetics of the drug product and that following this dosage regimen could potentially result in subtherapeutic or toxic levels
   b. There are data showing significant intra-batch and batch-to-batch variability, for example, $\pm 25\%$, in the bioavailability (BA) of the drug product

The in vivo BE study is not performed in the aforementioned situations, if the characteristics of the drug product meet at least one of the criteria that permit waiver of demonstrating in vivo BE. Instead, the application should contain evidences to prove that the drug product under consideration falls in one of the product categories that do not require in vivo BE determination.

11.4 CRITERIA FOR WAIVER OF THE BIOAVAILABILITY OR BIOEQUIVALENCE DETERMINATION REQUIREMENTS

Under certain circumstances when there is sufficient evidences that in vivo BA or in vivo BE studies are not required for a particular product, the drug manufacturer may apply for waiver of the BA or BE determination requirements. The drug manufacturer has to submit evidences that the product meet at least one of the criteria that allow granting waiver of the in vivo BA or BE determination. The following are the criteria for waiver of the evidence of in vivo BA or BE (21CFR 320.22, 2010) [1]:

1. Drug products when the BA and BE are self-evident. A drug product's in vivo BA or BE is considered self-evident if the product meets one of the following criteria:
   a. Parenteral solutions intended solely for administration by injection or ophthalmic or otic solutions that contain the same active and inactive ingredients in the same concentration as an approved drug product.
   b. Products administered by inhalation as a gas, for example, an inhalation anesthetic, that contain the same active ingredient in the same dosage form as an approved drug product.
   c. Solutions for application to the skin, oral solutions, elixirs, syrups, tinctures, solutions for aerosolization or nebulization, nasal solutions, or similar other solubilized form that contain an active drug ingredient in the same concentration and dosage form as an approved drug product and contain no inactive ingredient that can affect the in vivo BA of the active ingredients.
2. Drug products when the BA may be measured or BE may be demonstrated by evidences obtained in vitro, as described in the following:
   a. The drug product in the same dosage form, but in a different strength, and is proportionally similar in its active and inactive ingredients to another approved drug product for the same manufacturer. Providing that approval of the original product is based on measuring in vivo BA, both drug products meet the appropriate in vitro tests, and the applicant supply evidences showing that both drug products are proportionally similar in their active and inactive ingredients. This condition does not apply to delayed-release or extended-release products.
   b. The drug product is a reformulated product that is identical to another drug product for which the same manufacturer has obtained approval, except for a different color, flavor, or preservative that could not affect the BA of the reformulated product. Providing that the approval of the original product was based on measuring the in vivo BA and both drug products meet the appropriate approved in vitro tests.

c. The drug product is, on the basis of scientific evidence submitted in the application, shown to meet an in vitro test that has been correlated with in vivo product performance. For example, immediate-release solid dosage forms of the biopharmaceutics classification system (BCS) class I drugs (highly soluble, highly permeable) have rapid and similar in vitro dissolution characteristics. Rapid dissolution means at least 85% dissolution in 30 min in 900 mL at pHs 1.2, 4.5, and 6.8, while similar dissolution profile can be evaluated by comparing the similarity factor (f_2) at the three pHs. Comparing the dissolution profile is not necessary if the dissolution is 85% in less than 15 min.

Calculation of the similarity factor is used to compare the test and standard products' dissolution profiles, which can be more accurate than relying on a single-point dissolution test. This has been advocated for comparing product dissolution for purposes of biowaivers and investigating the effect of post-approval changes. The similarity factor can be calculated according to Equation 11.1:

$$f_2 = 50 \log \left\{ \frac{100}{\sqrt{1 + (1/n) \sum_{t=1}^{n} (R_t - T_t)^2}} \right\} \qquad (11.1)$$

where R_t and T_t are the cumulative percentage dissolved from the reference and test products, respectively, at each of the n sampling time points during the dissolution experiment. When the dissolution profiles for the reference test products are identical, f_2 will be equal to 100, while when the difference is 10% at each time point, f_2 will be equal to 50. So values for f_2 in the range of 50–100 indicate that the two dissolution profiles are similar [2].

11.5 APPROACHES FOR DEMONSTRATING PRODUCT BIOEQUIVALENCE

The most acceptable approach for determining the BE for systemically acting orally administered drugs in humans involves measuring the active drug concentration as a function of time in the systemic circulation. Characterization and comparison of the drug concentration–time profiles in the systemic circulation have been shown to be the most accurate, sensitive, and reproducible methods for demonstrating BE. This is because if two products for the same active drug have similar rate and extent of drug absorption, the drug concentration–time profile in the systemic circulation after administration of a single dose of each product in two different occasions should be comparable. Also, drug products that produce similar drug concentration–time profiles are expected to produce similar therapeutic effects. The pharmacokinetic-based approach for demonstrating BE will be discussed in detail in the next section. However, there are other approaches that can be used to demonstrate product bioequivalency including acute pharmacodynamic effects, clinical trials, and in vitro testing (21CFR 320.24, 2010) [1].

11.5.1 ACUTE PHARMACODYNAMIC EFFECT

Studies that use acute pharmacodynamic measures to establish BE for two drug products can be used when the drug and/or metabolite concentration in biological fluids cannot be determined with sufficient accuracy. Also, when the drug concentration in the systemic circulation is not correlated with the drug therapeutic effect, such as in case of topically applied drugs that are not intended to produce systemic effects. When the drug pharmacodynamic effect is used to demonstrate BE, several important issues should be considered. The pharmacodynamic effect measured should be relevant to the efficacy and/or safety of the drug, and the approach used for measurement should be validated for accuracy, precision, specificity, and reproducibility. Also, the effect produced after administration of the test and reference products should not reach the maximum effect to allow the detection of formulation differences. Besides, the drug effect should be evaluated under double blind conditions, meaning that neither the subject nor the evaluator knows which product is being evaluated to eliminate personal bias. Furthermore, the experiment should be performed using the crossover experimental design if possible, and if a placebo effect can occur, a placebo treatment can be added as a third phase in the study design. Additionally, when measuring the drug effect in patients, the underlying disease state and the natural history of the condition should be considered in the study design. Moreover, when the effect changes with time, the effect-time profile can be constructed by repeating the measurement at different time points. The statistical analysis of the obtained drug effect after administration of the two products can be performed similar to the general BE guidelines but the acceptance limits can be determined based on the nature of the pharmacodynamic effect measured.

11.5.2 CLINICAL STUDIES

In some instances when measuring the drug in the systemic circulation is not possible and when there is no meaningful acute drug effect that can be measured, clinical trials can be used to compare different products and to demonstrate BE. In this case, several important issues should be considered. The target parameter should be a relevant clinical endpoint from which the intensity and onset of response can be defined. Also, a placebo treatment should be included as a third phase in the study protocol. If possible, a safety endpoint should be included in the final comparative assessment. Appropriate statistical procedures should be used to compare the study results. The acceptance limit has to be defined on a case-by-case basis depending on variability in the target endpoint and the specific clinical condition.

11.5.3 IN VITRO DISSOLUTION TESTING

Under certain conditions, BE can be demonstrated using in vitro approaches. Such as in the case of rapidly dissolving oral drug products for drugs that are highly soluble and highly permeable (BCS class I drugs). In this case, documentation of BE using in vitro approaches is appropriate. Evidences of the drug high solubility, high permeability, and the rapidly dissolving product as defined by regulatory authority should be included as part of the study report [3,4].

11.6 PHARMACOKINETIC APPROACH TO DEMONSTRATE PRODUCT BIOEQUIVALENCE

A number of regulatory guidance documents have been developed through the joint efforts of scientists in regulatory authorities, pharmaceutical companies, and academic institutions. These documents outline the general requirements for the design, execution, and reporting of the in vivo BE studies. The primary objective of these guidance documents is to help the pharmaceutical companies to fulfill all the requirements for performing in vivo BE studies and increase the likelihood of their acceptance and approval. These general guidelines are applicable for performing in vivo BE studies for most of the orally administered drugs. Under certain circumstances, these guidelines have to be modified to accommodate some special drug characteristics. The following discussion covers the general guidelines for performing in vivo BE studies that can be applied for most drugs. The BE study consists of a clinical phase that involves drug product administration to the subjects participating in the study and the laboratory phase that involves sample analysis, data analysis, and preparation of the report. In general, it is required by all regulatory authorities that the principles of good clinical practices (GCP) applied to the clinical phase of the BE study and the principles of good laboratory practices (GLP) applied to all the laboratory activities during the study.

11.6.1 STUDY DESIGN

11.6.1.1 Basic Principles

An in vivo BE study involves a single-dose administration of the test drug product and a suitable reference product on two different occasions to normal adult volunteers in the fasting state, followed by comparing the rate and extent of absorption of the two products [1,5].

11.6.1.2 Study Subjects

Normal healthy male and female volunteers, preferably nonsmokers, between 18 and 50 years of age, within 10% of their ideal body weight are recruited to participate in the BE study. The volunteers should not have any history of serious chronic diseases or adverse reaction to the drug or any other drug in its class. Study participants are subjected to physical examination, routine blood chemistry, hematology, and urinalysis, which are performed to ensure normal renal, hepatic, and hematological functions. The volunteers are not allowed to take any prescription or over-the-counter drugs for 2 weeks before the study and should not use any alcohol, caffeine, or other xanthines containing beverages during the 2 days before the study. Each volunteer is enrolled after signing an informed consent form that contains detailed information about the study including all risks associated with participation in the study and the right to withdraw at any time from the study.

11.6.1.3 Number of Volunteers

The number of volunteers enrolled in the study should be sufficient to ensure adequate statistical results. An initial estimation of the number of volunteers required to participate in the BE study can be made before the study. The number of volunteers required for the BE study depends on the variability in the pharmacokinetic parameters of the drug, the acceptable significance level ($\alpha = 0.05$), and the acceptable deviation level between the products being compared ($\pm 20\%$). Since the variation in the pharmacokinetic parameters for most drugs is <30% coefficient of variation, the number of volunteers needed for most bioequivalent studies is 24. Drugs with larger variability in their pharmacokinetic parameters require larger number of volunteers [6].

11.6.1.4 Ethical Approval

The BE study has to be performed in accordance with the ethical principles included in the current version of the Declaration of Helsinki for involving human subjects in research. An independent review committee has to review the study protocol to confirm that the study complies with the ethical standards for using human subjects in research. The study can be performed only after approval of the study protocol by the ethical committee.

11.6.1.5 Drug Dose and Products

An approved drug product for the same active drug moiety is selected as the reference drug product. The reference drug product is normally the innovator product for which efficacy, safety, and quality have been established. The BE study is usually performed on the highest approved strength and the dose of the test product and the reference product should be similar. A single dose of the drug is administered with sufficient water (250 mL of water) after an overnight fasting (8 h of fasting), and fasting usually continues for at least 4 h after drug administration. The volunteers are monitored clinically throughout the study period and any complains have to be recorded in the clinical data sheet for each volunteer [5].

11.6.1.6 Drug Administration Protocol

A single-dose, two-treatment (two-product), two-period, two-sequence, fasting crossover experimental design is usually used in BE studies. The crossover experimental design involves random assignment of the volunteers participating in the study to one of two groups that will receive the drug products in different sequence [5]. The first group receives the test product first then the reference product, while the second group receives the reference product first then the test product. So each volunteer receives the two products in two different occasions separated by a sufficient period of time between treatments. Figure 11.1 represents the crossover experimental design. The period of time between treatments, known as the washout period, should allow complete elimination of the active drug before administration of the second drug product. The washout period should be at least five times the elimination half-life of the active drug. After each drug administration, blood sampling should continue during the elimination phase for at least three times the elimination half-life of the active drug ingredient.

11.6.1.7 Collection of Blood Samples

Comparison of the test product and the reference product is based on characterization of the blood drug concentration–time curve. Blood samples should be obtained

	Period I	Period II
Sequence I	Test product	Reference product
Sequence II	Reference product	Test product

FIGURE 11.1 Diagram illustrating the crossover experimental design.

with sufficient frequency over a period of at least three times the half-life of the active drug ingredient to permit good estimation of the C_{max} and the total AUC. The sampling schedule is usually determined from a pilot study performed before the actual BE study or from the available literature information available about the pharmacokinetic behavior of the drug. After administration of the test and reference drug products, the sampling times should be identical. Samples are stored frozen until analysis by a suitable analytical technique.

11.6.2 ANALYSIS OF BE STUDY SAMPLES

The samples obtained after drug administration are analyzed for the concentration of the active drug or its metabolite using a validated analytical method. The analytical method used in the analysis of samples has to be selective, sensitive, and accurate since the outcome of the BE study is solely dependent on the measured drug concentrations. Also, all the analytical procedures used have to be documented in written standard operating procedures (SOPs).

11.6.2.1 Analytical Method Validation

Analytical method validation includes all the procedures used to demonstrate that the method used for quantitative measurement of the concentration of a given analyte in a biological matrix is reliable and reproducible for the intended use. The main parameters for validation include selectivity, accuracy, precision, sensitivity, reproducibility, and stability [7].

11.6.2.1.1 Selectivity

It is the ability of the analytical method to differentiate and quantify the analyte in the presence of other compounds in the samples. For selectivity, blank samples from the biological matrix being analyzed are obtained from different sources and each blank sample should be tested for interference with the analysis of the analyte of interest.

11.6.2.1.2 Accuracy

Accuracy of an analytical method is the closeness of the mean test results obtained by the analytical method and the true value of the analyte concentration. It is determined by the analysis of replicate samples containing known concentration of the analyte and then comparing the measured concentration with the nominal concentration. Accuracy is usually determined by measuring at least five different samples for each concentration. A minimum of three different concentrations that cover the range of expected concentrations (low, medium, and high) is recommended. The mean value for the five different determinations for each concentration should be within 15% of the nominal concentration. At the lower limit of quantitation, the deviation from the nominal value can be up to 20%.

11.6.2.1.3 Precision

Precision is the closeness of individual measurements when several aliquots of the same sample are analyzed repeatedly. It is usually determined using five different replicates for the same concentration. A minimum of three different concentrations that cover the expected range of concentrations (low, medium, and high) is recommended. The precision measured as the coefficient of variation of the detector response determined at each concentration should not exceed 15%, except for at the lower limit of quantitation where it should not exceed 20%. Precision can be within-run precision or between-run precision. For within-run precision, the five samples for each concentration are analyzed on the same run, while for between-run precision five samples for each concentration are analyzed on five different runs.

11.6.2.1.4 Extraction Efficiency or Recovery

The recovery is the amount of the analyte extracted from the sample compared to the total amount of the analyte in the sample. The extraction efficiency does not have to be 100% but it has to be constant, precise, and reproducible at different analyte concentrations. However, when the extraction efficiency is low, this indicates the possibility for improving the extraction that can increase the sensitivity of the analytical method. The extraction efficiency experiment is performed by measuring the analyte concentration in extracted samples and unextracted samples at three different concentrations (low, medium, and high).

11.6.2.1.5 Calibration Curve

The calibration curve is constructed from the relationship between the detector response and the analyte concentration. It should be constructed in the same biological matrix as in the samples. The analyte concentrations used in the calibration curve depend on the expected range of concentrations for a particular study. The samples used to construct the calibration curve should include a blank matrix sample, a blank matrix sample spiked with the internal standard, and 6–8 additional samples covering the range of the expected concentrations including the lower limit of quantitation.

11.6.2.1.6 Stability

Drug stability in biological matrix during sample handling, sample preparation, sample storage should be evaluated. For example, analyte stability is determined at three different concentrations after three freeze and thaw cycles to make sure that the analyte remains stable while freezing. Also, stability of the processed samples at room temperature should be determined for a period of time equivalent to the time required to finish the analysis on one batch of samples to make sure that the analyte remains stable after processing at room temperature while waiting to be analyzed. Furthermore, the stability of the analyte for a period of time equivalent to the time between the first collected samples and the last analyzed samples should be determined to ensure that the analyte remains stable during storage.

11.6.2.2 Determination of the Drug Concentration in the BE Study Samples

Once the analytical method is validated, the BE study samples are analyzed using the same procedures utilized during the validation. Standard samples containing 6–8 different drug concentrations in the same matrix as the study samples and covering the entire range of expected drug concentrations are also analyzed. The relationship between the detector response and the drug concentration for each standard sample is used to construct the standard curve and the mathematical equation that describes this relationship is determined. The detector response of the unknown study sample is used to estimate the drug concentration in the sample utilizing the mathematical equation that describes the relationship between the drug concentration and the detector response for the standard sample. Quality control (QC) samples that contain three different analyte concentrations (low, medium, and high) are prepared before the start of sample analysis by spiking the blank matrix with the drug. At least two different QC samples at each concentration (total of six samples, and can be increased according to the run size) are included with each run and the analysis of these QC samples is used to accept or reject the run. The measured concentrations in at least four out of six QC samples should be within 15% of the nominal concentrations. The two QC samples outside this acceptance limit should not have the same analyte concentration.

11.6.3 Pharmacokinetic Parameter Determination

The BE of two different products for the same active drug is demonstrated if the rate and extent of drug absorption after administration of the two products is comparable.

11.6.3.1 Extent of Drug Absorption

The extent of drug absorption is generally determined from the AUC. The AUC is calculated using the trapezoidal rule until the last measured concentration (AUC_{0-t}), then extrapolated to calculate the total area ($AUC_{0-\infty}$). Enough samples should be obtained to make AUC_{0-t} covers at least 80% of the total $AUC_{0-\infty}$.

11.6.3.2 Rate of Drug Absorption

The rate of drug absorption is determined from C_{max} and t_{max}. The C_{max} is the highest drug concentration measured after drug administration, and t_{max} is the time of the sample that has the highest concentration. Other pharmacokinetic parameters such as the terminal elimination rate constant and the elimination half-life are calculated and they are used in the extrapolation of the AUC.

11.6.4 Statistical Analysis

The analysis of variance (ANOVA) is usually performed on the pharmacokinetic parameters that reflect the rate and extent of drug absorption, AUC, C_{max}, and t_{max}.

Appropriate statistical model relevant to the study design is applied. The statistical model includes factors that explain the different sources of errors in the calculated pharmacokinetic parameters including

- Sequence effect (order effect)
- Subjects nested in sequence
- Period effect (phase effect)
- Treatment effect (product effect)

All these effects that contribute to the variation in the calculated parameters are analyzed by the ANOVA to test the assumptions of the study design [6]. However, the decision about product BE is not usually made based on the ANOVA results.

The statistical method commonly used to test for BE is the two one-sided t-test procedures [8]. These procedures are based on calculation of the 90% confidence interval for the ratio (or difference) of the average log-transformed pharmacokinetic parameters for the test and reference products. The log-transformed values of AUC and C_{max} are used because these parameters are not normally distributed around their mean value, but the log transformed values are normally distributed (log-normal distribution). To establish BE the calculated 90% confidence intervals for the ratio of the average log-transformed AUC and C_{max} should fall within the BE limit of 80%–125%. Products with confidence intervals that fall outside this range are not considered bioequivalent.

11.6.5   IN VITRO TESTING OF STUDY PRODUCTS

In addition to the vivo BE study, the test and the reference drug products undergo in vitro evaluation. This includes physical description, dimension, mean weight, weight uniformity, content uniformity, and dissolution testing. The in vitro dissolution testing is an essential part of BE assessment for generic drug products. The comparative dissolution profile of the test and reference drug products is examined. The dissolution testing is performed using an approved method and the test drug product must pass the test specifications. For extended-release products, the dissolution method and specifications are developed for each drug product and the specifications are applied to that drug product to ensure its quality. All the results of the in vitro evaluation are included in the final BE report.

11.6.6   DOCUMENTATION AND REPORTING

All information related to the BE study has to be documented and included in the BE study report. This includes information about the drugs under investigation, volunteers, study design, analytical technique, pharmacokinetic analysis, in vitro testing, and statistical analysis. Also, the detailed results of the measured drug concentrations, the estimated pharmacokinetic parameters, analytical technique validation report, statistical analysis report, examples of the analytical instrument output, for example, chromatograms for the analysis of BE samples, and BE decision based on the obtained results should be included in the report [9].

11.7 SPECIAL ISSUES RELATED TO BE DETERMINATION

The general guidelines for conducting in vivo BE studies can be applied to the BE studies used for the majority of drugs. However, under certain circumstances, modification of these general guidelines may be necessary to demonstrate BE of drug products. These modifications can be as simple as the change in the acceptance limit for BE, or can be significant modification such as using different study design. The following discussion covers some suggested modifications of the general guidelines used in BE studies to address specials issues related to BE determination. The applicability of these suggestions has to be evaluated for each particular drug.

11.7.1 MULTIPLE-DOSE BE STUDIES

BE studies can be conducted to compare the performance of the test and reference drug products during multiple administration. Multiple-dose BE studies are performed when there is a difference in the rate of absorption but not in the extent of absorption of the study products, when there is excessive inter-subject variability in the BA, when the concentration of the active drug ingredient in the blood resulting from a single dose is too low for accurate determination by the analytical method, and for extended-release dosage forms. The crossover experimental design is usually used in multiple-dose BE studies. Whenever a multiple-dose study is conducted, sufficient doses of the test product and reference product should be administered to achieve steady state. Samples should be obtained to completely characterize the blood concentration–time profile during one dosing interval at steady state. The pharmacokinetic parameters calculated in multiple-dose BE study are

$AUC_{0-\tau}$: The AUC during one dosing interval at steady state.

$C_{max\,ss}$: The maximum drug concentration at steady state. It is the highest measured concentration during one dosing interval at steady state.

$C_{min\,ss}$: The minimum drug concentration at steady state. It is the drug concentration just before drug administration at steady state.

$C_{average\,ss}$: The average drug concentration at steady state. It is calculated as

$$C_{average\,ss} = \frac{AUC_{0-\tau}}{\tau} \tag{11.2}$$

where τ is the length of the dosing interval.

$t_{max\,ss}$: The time to achieve the maximum drug concentration within the dosing interval at steady state.

% Swing: $100\,(C_{max\,ss} - C_{min\,ss})/C_{min\,ss}$

% Fluctuation: $100\,(C_{max\,ss} - C_{min\,ss})/C_{average\,ss}$

Both % swing and % fluctuation are measures of the variation in the drug concentrations during repeated drug administration at steady state.

In multiple-dose BE studies, $C_{max\,ss}$, $C_{min\,ss}$, and $t_{max\,ss}$ are determined directly from the drug concentrations, $AUC_{0-\tau}$ is estimated by the trapezoidal rule, and % swing and

% fluctuation are calculated as mentioned earlier. In these studies, the % swing and % fluctuation are used as the primary parameters that describe the rate of drug absorption, while $AUC_{0-\tau}$ is used as a measure of the extent of drug absorption. The decision regarding bioequivalency is based on the results of the statistical comparison of the parameters calculated for the test and reference products.

11.7.2 FOOD-EFFECT BE STUDIES

Coadministration of food with oral products can affect the rate and extent of absorption of the active drug ingredient. This can be due to many factors including delay in gastric emptying, change in GIT pH, stimulation of bile secretion, change in luminal drug metabolism, and direct interaction between the food constituents and the drug. So studying the effect of food on the rate and extent of drug absorption may be necessary. Performing BE studies in fed subjects is usually recommended for immediate-release dosage forms that contain drugs with narrow therapeutic range, drugs that exhibit nonlinear pharmacokinetic behavior, drugs recommended to be given with food, and for all modified-release oral dosage forms. The food-effect BE study is usually performed using single-dose, two-treatment, two-period, two-sequence crossover experimental design. The highest strength of the drug product is administered within 5 min after completion of a meal that is expected to produce the maximum effect on the drug absorption. A high fat containing high-calorie breakfast is usually used as the test meal for the food effect BE study. All the study procedures and data analysis are similar to the fasting BE study.

11.7.3 DRUGS WITH LONG HALF-LIVES

BE studies for oral products of drugs that have long half-lives should involve prolonged period of sampling to ensure adequate characterization of the terminal elimination half-life. For these drugs the crossover experimental design may not be practical because of the prolonged washout period required to ensure complete elimination of the drug. In this case, the parallel experimental design may be used [5]. So the test drug product and the reference drug product are administered to two different groups of volunteers. After each drug administration, samples should be obtained for at least 2–3 days to make sure that the drug in the GIT is completely absorbed and to obtain good estimates for C_{max} and t_{max}. For drugs with long half-lives that have low intrasubject variability, the use of AUC truncated at 72 h can be used in the data analysis to test for BE.

11.7.4 DETERMINATION OF BE FROM THE DRUG URINARY EXCRETION DATA

When significant amount of the drug is excreted unchanged in urine, the BE study can be performed utilizing urinary excretion data to test for BE. Single oral doses of the test drug product and the reference drug product are administered to the volunteers enrolled in the study on two different occasions. Urine samples are collected after drug administration at a predetermined time intervals until the drug is completely eliminated from the body. The urinary excretion rate during each urine collection interval is calculated (see Chapter 14). The urinary excretion rate versus time profile should have the same shape as the plasma drug concentration–time profile. The highest value on the urinary excretion rate–time profile is proportional to C_{max}, and the interval when this highest urinary excretion rate is obtained reflects the t_{max}. However, because frequent urine samples cannot be obtained, the urinary excretion rate data cannot be used to detect small changes in the rate of drug absorption after administration of different products. Nevertheless, the total amount of the drug excreted unchanged in urine ($A_{e\infty}$) is a good measure of the extent of drug absorption after oral drug administration. So $A_{e\infty}$ can be used to compare the extent of drug absorption from different products. In BE studies, the BA of the drug from the test product relative to that of the reference products can be determined as follows:

$$F_{relative} = \frac{A_{e\infty test}}{A_{e\infty reference}} \frac{Dose_{reference}}{Dose_{test}} \qquad (11.3)$$

11.7.5 Fixed Dose Combination

Fixed dose combination (FDC) are products that contain fixed amounts of multiple active drugs that are used in the treatments of a specific disease state. For example, FDC for the treatment of tuberculosis (TB) contains rifampicin, isoniazid, ethambutol, and pyrazinamide. Also, FDC for the treatment of human immunodeficiency virus (HIV) usually contains two drugs from the nucleoside reverse transcriptase inhibitor class and one drug from either the nonnucleoside reverse transcriptase inhibitor class or the protease inhibitor class. The rationale is that these diseases have to be managed using combination therapy, so having these combination of drugs in one product should improve the patient compliance, and hence the therapeutic outcome.

However, having this combination of drugs in the same dosage form makes it challenging to select additives and use manufacturing procedures that are compatible with and maintain the stability of the drugs in the combination. BE testing is required for FDC. The study is performed by single-dose, two-formulation, and two-period crossover study. The volunteers receive the FDC as the test product and the single drug products for all the drugs in the combination administered together as the reference product, with suitable washout period between treatments. The pharmacokinetic parameters AUC and C_{max} obtained for each drug after administration of the FDC and the individual drug products are compared to determine if they are BE. All the drugs in the FDC have to be BE to the drug products for the individual drugs [10].

11.7.6 Measuring Drug Metabolites in BE Studies

Measuring the parent drug released from the dosage form is generally recommended in the BE studies since the parent drug concentration in the systemic circulation is more sensitive to change in formulation performance. However, measuring the metabolite is preferred when the parent drug concentrations are too low and measuring the drug concentration in biological fluids for adequate period of time is not possible. In this case, the metabolite C_{max} and AUC are calculated and the confidence interval approach is used to demonstrate BE. Also, when the metabolite contributes significantly to the therapeutic and/or adverse effects of the drug, it is recommended that both the parent drug and the metabolite should be measured [5]. In this case, the pharmacokinetic parameters of the parent drug should be analyzed by the confidence limit approach, while the metabolite data can be used to provide evidence of comparable therapeutic activity.

11.7.7   HIGHLY VARIABLE DRUGS

Highly variable drugs are those that exhibit within-subject variability of 30% coefficient of variation (CV) or greater in the AUC and/or C_{max}. Volunteers receiving products for highly variable drugs can have different pharmacokinetic parameters when they receive the same product in more than one occasion. This makes it possible for a test drug product, which is truly therapeutically equivalent to the reference product, not to meet the BE acceptance criteria. This is because the width of the 90% confidence interval for the ratio of the averages of AUC and C_{max} for the test and reference products is proportional to the estimated variability in the pharmacokinetic parameters and is inversely proportional to the number of the volunteers participating in the study. So to improve the power of the BE study for highly variable drugs using the two-treatment crossover design, the number of volunteers has to increase to 72 or even 120, depending on the within-subject variability. The use of this large number of volunteers may not be justified especially if they may develop adverse effects after taking the drug [11].

Several approaches have been suggested to help in testing the BE of products for highly variable drugs without the need for using large number of volunteers. These approaches include the expansion of the BE acceptance limit for the 90% confidence intervals to an arbitrary wider limit [12]. For example, increasing the 90% confidence limit from 80%–125% to 70%–143% when testing the BE of highly variable drugs. Based on this new wider acceptance limit the number of volunteers needed to be enrolled in the study will be smaller. Another approach involves expansion of the BE acceptance limit to the limit that will make using 24 volunteers in the BE study sufficient to demonstrate BE. An additional approach involves expansion of the acceptance limit based on the within-subject variability of the reference product. In this case, a replicate study design is used where each volunteer receives the reference drug product twice at two different periods in addition to the test product that is administered once or twice at different periods. This replicate design allows calculation of the within-subject variability that is used to calculate a new wider acceptance limit.

11.7.8   DRUGS EXHIBITING NONLINEAR PHARMACOKINETICS

Drugs are considered exhibiting nonlinear pharmacokinetics when the change in dose causes disproportional change in AUC after a single dose or disproportional change in steady-state concentration during multiple dosing. These drugs can be treated as those following linear pharmacokinetics if the dose normalized AUC deviates (increase or decrease) by less than 25%. The in vivo BE studies should be performed in the fed and fasted states except if taking the drug on the fed or the fasted states is contraindicated. Also, if there are evidences that nonlinearity occurs after the drug reaches the systemic circulation, BE study in the fed state may not be performed.

When the increase in dose results in more than proportional increase in the AUC, such as in the case of nonlinear elimination, the BE study should be performed using the highest strength of the drug product, while if the nonlinearity is observed only during multiple drug administration, multiple-dose studies using the highest strength or steady-state studies in the nonlinear range should be performed. When multiple-dose studies are performed single-dose studies are not required. For drugs that exhibit nonlinear absorption, the increase in dose results in less than proportional increase in the AUC. In this case, the BE study should be performed using the lowest strength of the drug product [13].

11.7.9 ENDOGENOUS SUBSTANCES

Drug products whose active ingredients are naturally occurring in the body represent a challenge for BE evaluation. Examples of these products include potassium supplement, iron salts, some steroid formulations, insulin, etc. This is because after administration of these products the measured blood concentrations represent the endogenous concentration in addition to the increase in concentration due to product administration. The protocol for the BE study can be modified according to the product under investigation. For example, insulin products can be evaluated by measuring the effect on the blood sugar concentration, while iron products can be evaluated by pharmacokinetic studies or clinical trials, whereas potassium salts can be evaluated by determination of the urinary potassium excretion under controlled conditions.

For example, determination of the BE for slow-release potassium chloride tablets or capsules can be performed by comparing the urinary excretion of potassium after administration of the potassium containing products [14]. In these studies, the volunteers receive standardized diet containing standard amounts of sodium, potassium, calories, and fluids for 5 days and the physical activity is restricted to avoid excessive potassium loss with sweating. During the last 2 days of this diet, equilibration period urine is collected daily to determine the baseline potassium excretion. On the sixth day, the dose of the test product or the standard product for potassium chloride is administered while the standardize diet is continued. Urine is collected to measure the change in urinary potassium excretion due to potassium product administration. The study is repeated for the second arm of the crossover study; 3 days of diet equilibration, followed by 2 days of potassium base line excretion, and on the sixth day the test or reference product is administered and urine is collected to determine the urinary potassium excretion. Comparison of the potassium urinary excretion after administration of the test drug product and the reference drug product, under controlled dietary intake, is used to evaluate the BE of potassium products.

11.7.10 ENANTIOMERS VERSUS RACEMATES

It is well documented that the different enantiomers of the same optically active drug can differ in their therapeutic effect and also in their pharmacokinetic characteristics. However, because of the difficulties associated with separation of individual enantiomers, the majority of the optically active drugs are marketed as the racemate mixture of the individual enantiomers. The BE studies for optically active drugs are usually performed using the racemate mixture of the drug. However, measuring the individual enantiomers in BE studies is recommended only when the enantiomers have different pharmacological activity, the enantiomers have different pharmacokinetic characteristics, the primary safety and activity resides with the minor enantiomer, and at least one of the enantiomers exhibits nonlinear absorption. All these conditions have to be met for recommending the measurement of the individual enantiomers in BE studies for optically active drugs [5].

11.7.11 NARROW THERAPEUTIC RANGE DRUG

Narrow therapeutic range drugs are drugs that have small differences between their minimum effective concentration and minimum toxic concentration. So these drugs are usually subjected to therapeutic drug monitoring. It is recommended that drug manufacturers should consider additional testing and/or control for the quality of drug products containing narrow therapeutic range drugs. This additional testing should provide increased assurance of interchangeability of these products. The usual acceptance BE limit of 80%–125% is applied for the products that contain narrow therapeutic range drugs [5].

11.7.12 ORAL PRODUCTS INTENDED FOR THE LOCAL EFFECT OF THE DRUG

BE studies to compare oral drug products that are intended to produce local GIT effect should be based on clinical efficacy and safety endpoints. In these studies, the clinical effect observed after administration of the two products is compared. Also, studies can be designed to compare the degree of systemic exposure that occurs following administration of the drug products intended for local action in the GIT. Other locally acting drugs may not require in vivo testing of their clinical efficacy, and in vitro testing may be sufficient [5]. For example, cholestyramine is a bile acid sequestering antilipemic agent. After oral administration, cholestyramine releases chloride ion and adsorbs anions of bile acid conjugates in the intestine forming a nonabsorbable complex that is excreted with cholestyramine in the feces. In vivo BE studies are not required to document BE of cholestyramine formulations. Equilibrium and kinetic in vitro bile acid salt binding studies are recommended to demonstrate BE between generic and innovator products.

11.7.13 FIRST POINT C_{max}

The first measured drug concentration in the BE study is sometimes the highest drug concentration, which raises questions regarding the accuracy of estimating

C_{max} due to insufficient early sampling. A pilot study can help in determining the approximate time for achieving the highest concentration. Extensive sampling during the early time after drug administration (e.g., 5 and 15 min) may be sufficient to determine C_{max} even if the highest concentration occurs in the first measured sample [5].

11.8 SUMMARY

- Bioequivalent drug products are products containing the same active drug, the same strength, and the same dosage form for the same route of administration that have the same rate and extent to which the active ingredient becomes available at the site of action.
- Manufacturers of generic drug products have to demonstrate that their drug products are bioequivalent with the innovator products for the same active drugs. This is important to ensure that switching from the innovator product to the generic product does not compromise the drug therapeutic efficacy and safety.
- The design, execution, data handling and reporting of in vivo BE studies have to follow the general guidelines developed by the drug regulatory authorities. It is required that the principles of good clinical practices be applied to the clinical phase of the bioequivalence study and the principles of good laboratory practices be applied to all the laboratory activities during the study.

REFERENCES

1. U.S. Code of Federal Regulations (April 2010) Title 21-Food and Drugs, Chapter I, Food and Drug Administration, Department of Health and Human Services, Sub-chapter D, Drugs for human use, Part 320, Bioavailability and Bioequivalence Requirements.
2. Shah VP, Tsong Y, and Sathe P (1998) In vitro dissolution profile comparison: Statistics and analysis of the similarity factor, f_2. *Pharm Res* 15:889–896.
3. Amidon GL, Lennernas H, Shah VP, and Crison JR (1995) A theoretical basis for a biopharmaceutic drug classification: The correlation of in vitro drug product dissolution and in vivo bioavailability. *Pharm Res* 12:413–420.
4. Center for Drug Evaluation and Research, U.S. Food and Drug Administration (2001) Guidance for industry: Waiver of in vivo bioavailability and bioequivalence studies for immediate release solid oral dosage forms based on biopharmaceutical classification system.
5. Center for Drug Evaluation and Research, U.S. Food and Drug Administration (2003) Guidance for industry: Bioavailability and bioequivalence studies for orally administered drug products-general considerations.
6. Center for Drug Evaluation and Research, U.S. Food and Drug Administration (2001) Guidance for industry: Statistical approaches to establish bioequivalence.
7. Center for Drug Evaluation and Research, U.S. Food and Drug Administration (2001) Guidance for industry: Bioanalytical method validation.
8. Schuirmann DJ (1987) A comparison of the two one-sided tests procedure and the power approach for assessing the equivalence of average bioavailability. *Pharmacokinet Biopharm* 15:657–680.
9. Henney JE (1999) Review of generic bioequivalence studies. *JAMA* 282:1995.

10. Center for Drug Evaluation and Research, U.S. Food and Drug Administration (2006) Guidance for industry: Fixed dose combinations, co-packaged drug products, and single-entity versions of previously approved antiretrovirals for the treatment of HIV.
11. Shah VP, Yacobi A, Barr WH et al. (1996) Evaluation of orally administered highly variable drugs and drug formulation. *Pharm Res* 13:1590–1594.
12. Boody AW, Snikeris FC, Kringle RO, Wei GC, Oppermann JA, and Midha KK (1995) An approach for widening the bioequivalence acceptance limits in the case of highly variable drugs. *Pharm Res* 12:1865–1868.
13. Therapeutic Product Directorate, Health Canada (2003) Report of expert advisory committee on bioavailability and bioequivalence, Bioequivalence requirements: Drugs exhibiting nonlinear pharmacokinetics, Ottawa, Ontario.
14. Center for Drug Evaluation and Research, U.S. Food and Drug Administration (2002) Guidance for industry: Potassium chloride modified release tablets/capsules: In vivo bioequivalence and in vitro dissolution testing.

12 Drug Pharmacokinetics during Constant Rate IV Infusion
The Steady-State Principle

OBJECTIVES

After completing this chapter you should be able to

- Define the steady state during constant rate IV infusion
- State the factors that affect the steady-state plasma concentration during constant rate IV infusion
- Estimate the steady-state drug concentrations and the pharmacokinetic parameters during constant rate IV infusion
- Analyze the effect of changing the pharmacokinetic parameters on the steady-state plasma concentration during constant rate IV infusion
- Recommend an appropriate IV loading dose and IV infusion rate to achieve specific steady-state plasma concentrations

12.1 INTRODUCTION

Drugs are administered as a single dose usually for the management of acute medical conditions or transient symptoms. If rapid drug action is required such as in case of emergency or if the patient is unconscious, the drug can be administered intravenously. When the drug is administered orally, the rate of drug absorption usually determines the onset of drug effect. Due to drug elimination from the body, the effect of drugs administered as single dose subsides with time and repeated drug administration may be required if the symptoms persist. The plasma drug concentration fluctuates up and down during repeated intravenous (IV) or oral drug administration, which can lead to change in symptoms control when direct relationship exists between the drug effect and plasma drug concentration. So to maintain constant plasma drug concentration, the drug has to be administered as constant rate IV infusion.

Constant rate IV infusion involves direct administration of the drug into the systemic circulation continuously at a constant rate with the aid of an infusion pump. The drug solution for IV administration is prepared to include a suitable drug concentration (amount/volume) depending on the drug solubility, the average drug dose, and the volume of fluids that can be administered to the patient. Then, the infusion rate of the IV solution (volume/time) is selected to administer the drug at a constant rate (amount/time). This mode of drug administration should maintain the plasma drug concentration relatively constant as long as the drug administration continues. The rate of drug administration can be changed by increasing or decreasing the rate of infusion. The major drawback of this route of drug administration is that it can only be used in hospitalized patients because of the need for an infusion pump and the special precautions needed for the preparation and administration of the IV solution. Many drugs can be administered by this route of administration such as heparin, vasodilators, bronchodilators, inotropic agents, and general anesthetics. The therapeutic effect of these drugs is highly correlated with their concentrations in the body. So the rate of infusion can be titrated up and down to achieve the drug concentration that produces the desired effect.

12.2 STEADY STATE

Drug administration during the constant rate IV infusion is constant, which means that the rate of drug administration is zero order. If drug elimination follows first-order kinetics, the rate of drug elimination is dependent on the amount of the drug in the body. Initially, there is no drug in the body before starting the infusion. Once the IV infusion starts, the amount of the drug in the body increases because the rate of drug administration is larger than the rate of drug elimination. As the IV infusion continues, the rate of drug elimination increases because the amount of the drug in the body increases. The rate of drug elimination continues to increase until it becomes equal to the rate of drug administration. At this point, the rate of drug administration is equal to the rate of drug elimination and the drug amount and plasma drug concentration remain constant while the drug is administered continuously as illustrated in Figure 12.1. The state when the rate of drug administration is equal to the rate of drug elimination is known as the steady state.

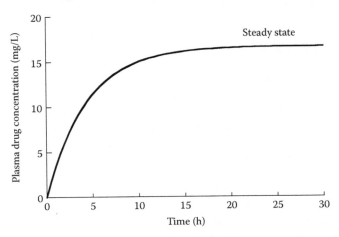

FIGURE 12.1 Drug plasma concentration–time profile after the start of the constant rate IV drug infusion.

Mathematically, the rate of change of the amount of the drug in the body at any time is the difference between the rate of drug administration and the rate of drug elimination as expressed in the following differential equations:

$$\frac{dA}{dt} = \text{Rate of drug administration} - \text{Rate of drug elimination} \qquad (12.1)$$

$$\frac{dA}{dt} = K_0 - kA \qquad (12.2)$$

where
   A is the amount of the drug in the body
   K_0 is the rate of drug administration (amount/time)
   k is the first-order elimination rate constant

Integrating Equation 12.2 and dividing by the drug Vd, the equation for the plasma drug concentration at any time during the infusion is obtained:

$$Cp = \frac{K_0}{kVd}(1 - e^{-kt}) \qquad (12.3)$$

where t is the time after the start of the infusion. Equation 12.3 indicates that after starting the IV infusion, the plasma drug concentration increases and exponentially approaches the steady-state concentration. The steady state is achieved after administration of the IV infusion for a period of time, so substituting time in Equation 12.3 by a large value, an equation for the steady-state concentration is obtained:

$$Cp_{ss} = \frac{K_0}{kVd} \qquad (12.4)$$

Examining Equation 12.4 shows that the plasma drug concentration at steady state is directly proportional to the rate of the drug infusion and inversely proportional to the drug CL_T. This means that if a patient is receiving a drug as a constant rate IV infusion, changing the rate of drug infusion leads to a proportional change in the steady-state drug concentration as in Figure 12.2. This illustrates the ease of changing the drug infusion rate up and down until the desired plasma drug concentration and hence the desired therapeutic effect is obtained. Also, during IV infusion of the same drug at the same rate to two different patients who have different CL_T, the drug steady-state drug concentration will be higher in the patient with the lower clearance as in Figure 12.3. This is important in clinical practice because to achieve the same steady-state concentration of drugs, patients with eliminating organ dysfunction require lower infusion rate compared to patients with normal eliminating organ function. This illustrates the importance of adjusting the rate of drug administration based on the patient's specific characteristics.

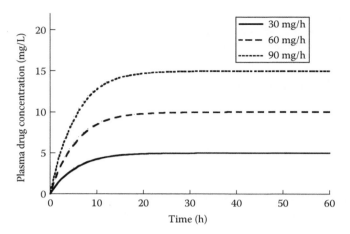

FIGURE 12.2 Steady-state drug concentration is proportional to the infusion rate if the total body clearance is similar.

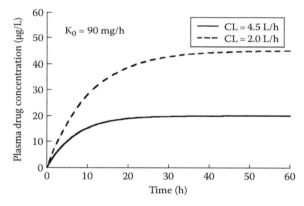

FIGURE 12.3 Steady-state drug concentration is inversely proportional to the total body clearance of the drug if the drug is administered at the same infusion rate.

12.3   TIME REQUIRED TO ACHIEVE STEADY STATE

During constant rate IV infusion, the drug plasma concentration increases gradually until it reaches the steady state as in Figure 12.1. The drug infusion rate is usually selected to achieve the desired plasma drug concentration at steady state. So before reaching steady state, the drug is not expected to produce its full therapeutic effect, which makes it important to determine the time required to achieve steady state. Equation 12.3 describes the plasma drug concentration at any time during the infusion, which indicates that the drug concentration exponentially approaches the steady state after the start of the infusion. So theoretically it should take very long time for the plasma concentration to reach the steady-state concentration. Practically, it can be assumed that steady state is achieved when the drug concentration is about 98% of the true steady-state concentration. So Equation 12.3 can be rewritten as

$$Cp = 0.98Cp_{ss} = \frac{K_0}{kVd}(1-e^{-kt_{ss}})$$ (12.5)

Substitution for Cp_{ss} from Equation 12.4 yields

$$0.98\frac{K_0}{kVd} = \frac{K_0}{kVd}(1-e^{-kt_{ss}})$$ (12.6)

where t_{ss} is the time to achieve steady state. The time needed to achieve steady state is determined by solving for t_{ss}:

$$0.98 = (1-e^{-kt_{ss}})$$ (12.7)

$$t_{ss} = \frac{3.91}{k} = 5.6\,t_{1/2}$$ (12.8)

This means that the time required to achieve steady state is dependent on the half-life of the drug. It takes about 5.6 times the drug half-life of continuous infusion to achieve drug concentration about 98% of the true steady-state concentration. Generally, it takes five to six elimination half-lives of continuous IV infusion of the drug to reach steady state. The longer the drug half-life the longer it takes to reach steady state. Figure 12.4 shows the time required to achieve steady state during administration of different drugs that have different half-lives. Administration of the

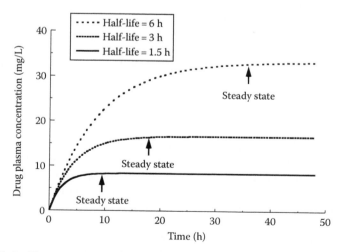

FIGURE 12.4 Time required to achieve steady state during continuous IV infusion is dependent on the half-life of the drug. The longer the half-life the longer it takes to achieve steady state.

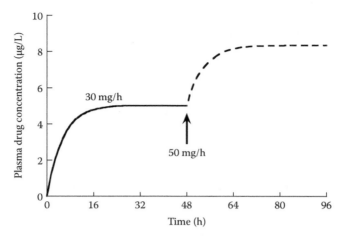

FIGURE 12.5   Change in the IV infusion rate results in the change in the plasma drug concentration until the new steady state is achieved.

same drug to the same patient at different infusion rates should achieve steady-state concentration that are proportional to the IV infusion rate as in Figure 12.2, and the time to achieve the steady state will be the same since the drug half-life is similar.

12.3.1   CHANGING THE DRUG INFUSION RATE

As mentioned previously, one of the advantages of using the constant rate IV infusion as a route of drug administration is the ease of changing the drug infusion rate until the desired therapeutic effect is achieved. So if the patient is at steady state while receiving a drug as a constant rate IV infusion and the infusion rate is changed, a new steady-state drug concentration is achieved. The new steady-state concentration is not achieved immediately, but the drug concentration changes to exponentially approach the new steady state. When the drug infusion rate is changed, it takes five to six half-lives of continuous drug infusion for the drug concentration to achieve the new steady-state concentration as illustrated in Figure 12.5.

12.4   LOADING DOSE

During constant rate IV administration, the drug accumulates until steady state is achieved after five to six half-lives. This can constitute a problem when immediate drug effect is required and immediate achievement of therapeutic drug concentrations is necessary such as in emergency situations. In this case, administration of a loading dose will be necessary. The loading dose is an IV bolus dose administered at the time of starting the IV infusion to achieve faster approach to steady state. So administration of an IV loading dose and starting the constant rate IV infusion simultaneously can rapidly produce therapeutic drug concentration. The loading dose is chosen to produce plasma concentration similar or close to the desired plasma concentration that will be achieved by the IV infusion at steady state. In this case,

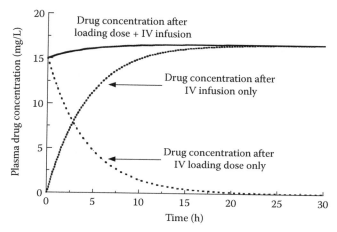

FIGURE 12.6 Plasma drug concentration–time profile after administration of a bolus IV loading dose and constant rate IV infusion simultaneously.

the plasma drug concentration at any time will be the sum of the drug concentration resulting from the IV infusion, and the drug concentration remaining from the IV bolus dose as illustrated in Figure 12.6. The drug concentration resulting from the IV infusion increases and exponentially approaches the steady state, and the drug concentration remaining from IV bolus loading dose declines exponentially. So, when the proper loading dose is administered at the time of starting the IV infusion, drug concentration very close to the steady-state drug concentration is achieved immediately after the start of drug administration.

$$Cp \text{ total} = Cp \text{ from infusion} + Cp \text{ from IV bolus} \qquad (12.9)$$

The steady-state plasma drug concentration is dependent only on the infusion rate and the drug CL_T as indicated from Equation 12.4. So the loading dose does not affect the steady-state concentration. If the loading dose produces initial plasma concentration higher than the steady-state concentration that should be achieved by the infusion, the drug concentration will decline slowly to reach the steady state, while if the loading dose produces initial plasma concentration lower than the steady-state concentration that should be achieved by the infusion, the drug concentration will increase slowly to reach the steady state. It takes five to six half-lives for the initial drug concentration produced by the loading dose to reach steady state. So administration of the right loading dose is important to achieve drug plasma concentration very close to the steady-state concentration immediately after the start of drug administration as in Figure 12.7. The IV loading dose required to achieve a certain concentration can be calculated from the relationship between the dose, Vd, and drug concentration as in Equation 12.10:

$$\text{Loading dose (IV bolus)} = \text{Desired } Cp \times Vd \qquad (12.10)$$

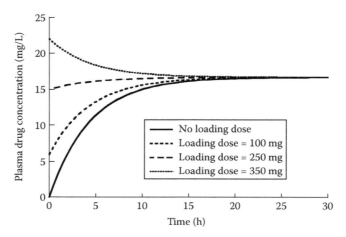

FIGURE 12.7 Plasma drug concentration–time profile after administration of different loading doses followed immediately by the same continuous IV infusion rate of the drug.

12.5 TERMINATION OF THE CONSTANT RATE IV INFUSION

Drug administration by constant rate IV infusion is usually used in hospitalized patients to produce the drug therapeutic effect for a period of time such as in the case of anesthetic drugs or to stabilize the patient condition such as in the case of vasodilators, bronchodilators, or inotropic drugs. If the drug administration continues for more than five to six times the drug elimination half-life, steady state is achieved. Once the desired therapeutic outcome of the drug use is accomplished, the IV infusion is terminated. After termination of the IV infusion at any time whether steady state is achieved or not, the drug concentration declines at a rate dependent on the elimination rate constant of the drug as illustrated in Figure 12.8. When the

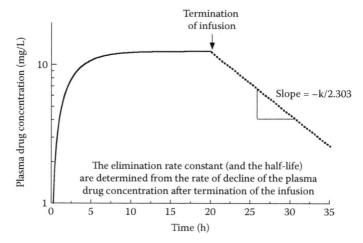

FIGURE 12.8 Plasma drug concentration–time profile during and after termination of the continuous IV infusion of the drug.

drug elimination follows first-order kinetics, the plasma drug concentration after termination of the infusion declines exponentially on the linear scale and linearly on the semilog scale. The drug elimination rate constant and half-life can be estimated from the post-infusion drug concentration–time profile.

12.6 DETERMINATION OF THE PHARMACOKINETIC PARAMETERS

12.6.1 TOTAL BODY CLEARANCE

The CL_T of the drug can be determined from the IV infusion rate and the steady-state concentration by rearrangement of Equation 12.4:

$$CL_T = \frac{K_0}{Cp_{ss}} \tag{12.11}$$

The steady-state plasma concentration is determined by measuring the plasma drug concentration during the IV infusion at steady state or can be estimated from the plasma concentrations during the post-infusion phase. In this case, the plasma concentrations measured after termination of the IV infusion are plotted on the semilog scale. The post-infusion plasma concentration–time profile is back extrapolated to determine the plasma concentration at the time of termination of the IV infusion, which is equal to the steady-state concentration.

12.6.2 ELIMINATION RATE CONSTANT

The first-order elimination rate constant, k, can be determined from the post-infusion plasma drug concentration–time profile plotted on the semilog scale:

$$\text{Slope} = \frac{-k}{2.303} \tag{12.12}$$

The drug half-life can be determined from k (half-life = 0.693/k). Also, the half-life can be determined graphically from the post-infusion drug concentration–time profile by determining the time required for any concentration during the post-infusion phase to decline by 50%.

12.6.3 VOLUME OF DISTRIBUTION

The volume of distribution is determined from CL_T and k:

$$Vd = \frac{CL_T}{k} \tag{12.13}$$

Example

A patient is receiving an antiarrhythmic drug as a constant rate IV infusion of 24 mg/h. After 3 days, the drug infusion is terminated and three plasma samples are obtained.

Time after the End of Infusion (h)	Drug Concentration (mg/L)
1	3.3
3	2.2
6	1.2

a. Calculate the CL_T and Vd of this drug in this patient.
b. The patient experienced irregular heart rhythm again and the physician wanted to start this antiarrhythmic again. Recommend an IV loading dose and a constant rate IV infusion that should achieve steady state of 10 mg/L.

Answer

a. The steady-state drug plasma concentration and the half-life (or the elimination rate constant) from the plot of the plasma drug concentrations are obtained after termination of the infusion versus time on semilog scale as in Figure 12.9.

　　Time zero represents the time when the infusion was terminated, so the y-intercept is equal to the steady-state drug concentration:

$$Cp_{ss} = 4\,mg/L$$

$$Cp_{ss} = \frac{K_0}{CL_T}$$

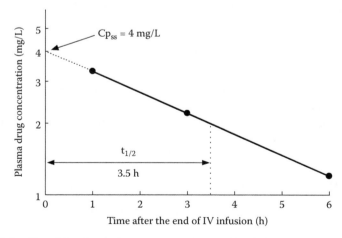

FIGURE 12.9 Plot of the plasma drug concentrations obtained after termination of the infusion versus time on the semilog scale. The y-intercept is equal to the steady-state concentration and the half-life can be calculated graphically.

$$CL_T = \frac{24\,mg/h}{4\,mg/L} = 6\,L/h$$

$$t_{1/2} = 3.5\,h \quad k = 0.198\,h^{-1}$$

$$Vd = \frac{CL_T}{k} = \frac{6\,L/h}{0.198\,h^{-1}} = 30.3\,L$$

b. $LD = Cp \times Vd = 10\,mg/L \times 30.3\,L = 303\,mg$

$$K_0 = Cp_{ss} \times CL_T = 10\,mg/L \times 6\,L/h = 60\,mg/h$$

Recommendation: 300 mg administered as an IV bolus dose (loading dose) followed immediately by 60 mg/h as a constant rate IV infusion. This regimen should achieve steady-state concentration of 10 mg/L.

12.7 DOSAGE FORMS WITH ZERO-ORDER INPUT RATE

The advantage gained from the steady drug plasma concentration and the stable therapeutic effect achieved during constant rate IV drug administration prompted scientists to develop dosage forms for extravascular administration that can deliver the drug at a constant rate. The most common strategy utilized to achieve this goal is to design dosage forms that can release the drug at a slow zero-order rate. If the drug release rate from the dosage form becomes the rate determining step in the drug absorption process, the drug is delivered to the systemic circulation at a constant rate. In this case, the systemic drug concentration is maintained relatively constant for a period of time and the therapeutic effect achieved is usually stable.

Examples of these dosage forms include modified-release oral dosage forms that can release the drug at zero-order rate over 12–24 h. Also, transdermal patches have been developed to release the drug at a constant rate over a period of days such as clonidine and scopolamine patches. Besides, intramuscular injections of sustained-release formulations have been developed to deliver the drug at a relatively constant rate for weeks such as in some hormonal injections. Furthermore, subcutaneous implants have been developed to deliver the drugs at a constant rate over a period of months such as in case of contraceptive implants. Additionally, medicated devices have been developed to release therapeutic agents included in the components of the device over a period of few years such as the progesterone-medicated intrauterine devices. The plasma drug concentration achieved after using these extravascular dosage forms with zero-order release rate is not identical to the profile achieved during administration of constant rate IV infusion. This is because of many factors related to the formulation design and the complex nature of the absorption process. However, many well-designed dosage forms have been shown to maintain relatively constant plasma drug concentration and produce steady therapeutic effect over the manufacturer claimed period of time.

12.8 FACTORS AFFECTING THE STEADY-STATE DRUG PLASMA CONCENTRATION DURING CONSTANT RATE IV INFUSION

During constant rate IV infusion, the plasma drug concentration increases gradually until steady state is achieved. The steady-state drug concentration is dependent on the infusion rate and CL_T of the drug. The time to achieve steady-state concentration is dependent on the half-life of the drug and administration of an IV loading dose can help in faster approach to steady state.

12.8.1 PHARMACOKINETIC SIMULATION EXERCISE

Pharmacokinetic simulations can be used to examine how the pharmacokinetic parameters affect the steady-state concentration achieved during constant rate IV infusion. The plasma drug concentration–time profile during constant rate IV infusion is simulated using average values for the pharmacokinetic parameters, and then the steady-state concentration and the time to achieve steady state are observed. The pharmacokinetic parameters are changed one parameter at a time while keeping all the other parameters constant and repeating the simulation. The resulting plasma drug concentration–time profile is examined to see how the change affects the drug steady-state concentration and the time to achieve steady-state concentration. The plotting exercise of the steady-state during constant rate IV infusion module in the basic pharmacokinetic concept section and the pharmacokinetic simulation section of the companion CD to this textbook can be used to run these simulations.

12.8.1.1 Infusion Rate

The steady-state plasma drug concentration is proportional to the infusion rate of the drug. Increasing the infusion rate of the drug causes proportional increase in the steady-state drug concentration if the total body clearance of the drug is constant. The time to achieve steady state does not change with the change in the infusion rate.

12.8.1.2 Total Body Clearance

The steady-state plasma drug concentration is inversely proportional to the CL_T of the drug. Lower CL_T results in higher steady-state concentration when the infusion rate is kept constant. The same drug can have different CL_T in different individuals due to differences in the function of the eliminating organ(s). Administration of the same infusion rate of the drug to patients with different CL_T produces higher steady-state drug concentration in patients with lower CL_T. When different values for CL_T are used in the simulation while keeping the same Vd, the profile for the higher CL_T reaches steady state faster than the profile for the lower CL_T. This is because higher CL_T means larger k and shorter $t_{1/2}$ when Vd is kept constant.

12.8.1.3 Volume of Distribution

The Vd does not affect the steady-state concentration. The steady-state drug concentration is only dependent on CL_T and the infusion rate. When different values for Vd are used in the simulation while using similar CL_T, the dependent parameters $t_{1/2}$ and k will be different. This is reflected by faster approach to the same steady-state concentration for the drugs with the larger CL_T/Vd ratio (larger k and shorter $t_{1/2}$).

12.8.1.4 Loading Dose

During constant rate IV infusion, the plasma drug concentration increases and exponentially approaches the steady state when no loading dose is administered. Administration of an IV loading dose produces an initial drug concentration that is dependent on the size of the loading dose. When the IV infusion and the IV loading dose are administered simultaneously, the initial drug concentration achieved from the loading dose will gradually approach the steady-state concentration. If the loading dose produces an initial drug concentration close to the steady-state concentration, steady state is achieved immediately. The steady-state concentration achieved does not depend on the loading dose.

PRACTICE PROBLEMS

12.1 A physician asked you to recommend a loading dose and a constant rate IV infusion of a drug to rapidly achieve a steady-state concentration of 15 mg/L. The half-life of this drug is 6 h and the volume of distribution is 30 L. What is your recommendation?

12.2 A patient received an antiasthmatic medication as 200 mg IV loading dose followed immediately by constant rate IV infusion of 70 mg/h. The IV infusion continued for 5 days and after termination of the infusion the half-life was found to be 3 h and the volume of distribution was 30 L.
  a. What is the elimination rate of this drug during the infusion at steady state?
  b. What is the steady-state concentration during the infusion?
  c. What is the elimination rate constant of this drug?
  d. What is the steady-state concentration if a loading dose of 400 mg was administered followed by the 70 mg/h infusion?
  e. What is the time to reach steady state if no loading dose was administered?
  f. What is the steady-state concentration if an infusion rate of 140 mg/h was administered?

12.3 A patient was admitted to the hospital because of cardiac arrhythmia. He received antiarrhythmic drug as an IV loading dose injection followed by constant rate infusion of 30 mg/h. The infusion continued for 3 days and then the physician decided to stop the infusion. Samples were obtained after the end of infusion. A plot of the plasma concentrations obtained after stopping the infusion versus time was linear on the semilog graph paper and had a slope of $-0.043\,h^{-1}$ and an intercept of 7.5 mg/L.
  a. Calculate the half-life and the volume of distribution of the antiarrhythmic drug in this patient.
  b. Recommend an IV loading dose and a constant rate infusion that can achieve steady-state plasma concentration of 12 mg/L.

12.4 A patient received an antiasthmatic medication as 300 mg IV loading dose followed immediately by constant rate IV infusion of 100 mg/h. The IV infusion continued for 5 days, and, after termination of the infusion, three plasma samples were obtained. A plot of the plasma concentrations obtained after termination (stopping) of the infusion has a y-intercept of 16 mg/L and a slope of $-0.06\,h^{-1}$.

a. What is the half-life of this drug?
b. What is the volume of distribution of this drug?
c. What is the steady-state concentration if no loading dose was administered?
d. What is the steady-state drug concentration if the infusion rate was 200 mg/h?

12.5 A patient received an antiasthmatic medication as 300 mg IV loading dose followed immediately by constant rate IV infusion of 100 mg/h. The IV infusion continued for 5 days and after termination (stopping) of the infusion three plasma samples were obtained.

Time after Termination of the Infusion (h)	Plasma Drug Concentration (mg/L)
3	10.6
6	7.0
12	3.0

a. Calculate the plasma drug concentration at steady-state graphically.
b. What is the elimination rate of the drug at steady state?
c. What is the half-life of this drug?
d. What is the steady-state concentration if the loading dose was changed to 600 mg?
e. What is the steady-state drug concentration if the infusion rate was 200 mg/h?

12.6 A 60 kg male was admitted to the hospital with chief complain of shortness of breath. He was diagnosed as having acute bronchial asthma. He received a single IV loading dose of theophylline, followed by a constant rate IV infusion of 60 mg/h of the same drug. On the fourth day after starting the IV infusion, the patient complained of nausea and vomiting, which are the most common adverse effects of this drug. For this reason, the continuous IV infusion was stopped and three plasma samples were obtained 1, 3, and 9 h after termination of the IV infusion.

Time after Termination of the IV Infusion	Concentration (mg/L)
1	18.3
3	15.0
9	8.3

a. What is the rate of elimination of this antiasthmatic drug during the constant rate IV infusion at steady state?
b. Calculate the half-life of this drug graphically.
c. Calculate the volume of distribution of this drug.
d. Recommend an IV loading dose and an IV infusion rate that should achieve steady-state theophylline concentration of 15 mg/L in this patient.

12.7 A patient received an anticancer drug by constant rate IV infusion of 20 mg/h. The IV infusion continued for 3 days and after termination of the infusion the half-life was found to be 6 h and the volume of distribution was 35 L.

a. What is the elimination rate of this drug during the infusion at steady state?
b. What is the steady-state concentration during the infusion?
c. What is the elimination rate constant of this drug?
d. What is the steady-state concentration if a loading dose of 200 mg was administered followed by the 20 mg/h infusion?
e. What is the time to reach steady state if the loading dose was not administered?
f. What is the steady-state concentration if the infusion rate was 40 mg/h?

13 Steady State during Multiple Drug Administration

OBJECTIVES

After completing this chapter you should be able to

- Define the $Cp_{max\,ss}$, $Cp_{min\,ss}$, and $Cp_{average\,ss}$ during multiple drug administration
- State the factors that affect the steady-state plasma concentration during multiple drug administration
- Describe the factors that affect the time to achieve steady state during multiple drug administration and the rationale for administration of a loading dose
- Calculate the steady-state drug concentrations and patients' pharmacokinetic parameters during multiple drug administration
- Analyze the effect of changing the pharmacokinetic parameters on the steady-state plasma concentration during multiple drug administration
- Recommend IV and oral dosing regimen to achieve specific plasma concentrations at steady state in patients
- Evaluate the appropriateness of certain dosing regimens for a particular patient

13.1 INTRODUCTION

Constant rate IV infusion has been used to maintain a relatively constant drug concentration that is important for producing a steady therapeutic effect. However, once the patient's condition is stabilized, the patient is shifted to multiple-dose regimen, which involves administration of a fixed dose of the drug at every fixed dosing interval (τ), when continued disease control is required. Also, multiple-dose regimens are used in patients with medical conditions that require extended period of treatment such as in the management of chronic diseases. These patients can take the drugs either by repeated IV or oral administration.

After initiation of the multiple-dose regimens, the second dose of the drug is usually administered before the first dose is completely eliminated. Subsequent doses are also administered before complete elimination of the previous doses of the drug. This results in drug accumulation in the body during repeated drug administration. When the elimination process follows first-order kinetics, and the rate of drug elimination is proportional to the amount of the drug in the body. So as the drug accumulates in the body during repeated administration, the amount of the drug eliminated during each dosing interval increases with time. This continues until the rate of drug administration becomes equal to the rate of drug elimination during each dosing interval and steady state is achieved. At steady state, the average amount of the drug in the body remains constant during continued drug administration.

13.2 PLASMA DRUG CONCENTRATION–TIME PROFILE DURING MULTIPLE DRUG ADMINISTRATION

At steady state during multiple drug administration, the plasma drug concentrations are changing during each dosing interval. If the drug elimination follows first-order kinetics and the drug is administered intravenously every dosing interval, the plasma drug concentration just before drug administration is the minimum plasma drug concentration at steady state ($Cp_{min\,ss}$), while the plasma drug concentration right after drug administration is the maximum plasma drug concentration at steady state ($Cp_{max\,ss}$). At steady state, the rate of drug administration is equal to the rate of drug elimination, which implies that the amount of the drug eliminated during one dosing interval is equal to the administered IV dose. This means that when the drug dose is administered at the beginning of the dosing interval and the drug concentration increases from $Cp_{min\,ss}$ to $Cp_{max\,ss}$, the drug concentration has to return back to $Cp_{min\,ss}$ at the end of the dosing interval. So the plasma drug concentration–time profile during each dosing interval at steady state is identical during the successive dosing interval as long as the same dose is administered at equally spaced dosing intervals as shown in Figure 13.1.

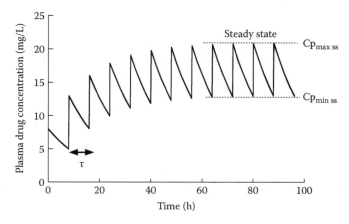

FIGURE 13.1 Plasma drug concentration–time profile during multiple IV administration of a fixed dose of the drug every fixed dosing interval.

For a drug that is eliminated by first-order process, during multiple IV administration of similar doses, D, administered every fixed dosing interval, τ, the amount of drug in the body after administration of the first dose is

$$D$$

The amount of the drug in the body before administration of the second dose is

$$De^{-k\tau}$$

The amount of the drug in the body after administration of the second dose is

$$D + De^{-k\tau}$$

The amount of the drug in the body before administration of the third dose is

$$(D + De^{-k\tau})e^{-k\tau} = De^{-k\tau} + De^{-2k\tau}$$

The amount of the drug in the body after administration of the third dose is

$$D + De^{-k\tau} + De^{-2k\tau}$$

At steady state the amount of the drug in the body after drug administration, $A_{max\,ss}$, is

$$D(1 + e^{-k\tau} + e^{-2k\tau} + e^{-3k\tau} + e^{-4k\tau} + \cdots)$$

This is an infinite series that can be solved as

$$A_{max\,ss} = \frac{D}{(1 - e^{-k\tau})} \tag{13.1}$$

where k is the first-order elimination rate constant. Dividing Equation 13.1 by Vd, the equation for the maximum plasma drug concentration can be obtained:

$$Cp_{max\,ss} = \frac{D}{Vd(1 - e^{-k\tau})} \tag{13.2}$$

Since $Cp_{max\,ss}$ declines to become $Cp_{min\,ss}$ at the end of the dosing interval, the equation for $Cp_{min\,ss}$ can be written as

$$Cp_{min\,ss} = Cp_{max\,ss}e^{-k\tau} \tag{13.3}$$

At steady state, drug administration of the IV dose causes an increase in the plasma drug concentration from $Cp_{min\,ss}$ to $Cp_{max\,ss}$. The change in the plasma drug concentration depends on the dose and Vd:

$$Cp_{max\,ss} - Cp_{min\,ss} = \frac{Dose}{Vd} \tag{13.4}$$

The equations for $Cp_{max\,ss}$ and $Cp_{min\,ss}$ mentioned earlier can be applied only for multiple IV drug administration of a constant dose at equally spaced dosing intervals.

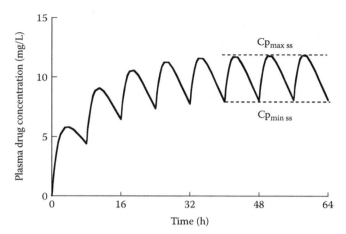

FIGURE 13.2 Plasma drug concentration during multiple administration of a rapidly absorbed drug. At steady state, the $Cp_{max\,ss}$ and $Cp_{min\,ss}$ will be similar during each dosing interval as long as the same dose is administered at fixed dosing intervals.

However, for the drugs that are administered by extravascular administration, and the rate of drug absorption to the systemic circulation is rapid; the same approach can be applied to approximate the relationship between the maximum and the minimum drug concentrations at steady state. Figure 13.2 represents the plasma drug concentration during multiple extravascular administration of a rapidly absorbed drug. Rapid drug absorption after extravascular drug administration allows most of the drug to reach the systemic circulation before significant amount of the drug is eliminated. Also, the time difference between $Cp_{max\,ss}$ and $Cp_{min\,ss}$ is approximately equal to the dosing interval when the drug absorption is rapid. So the drug profile during multiple oral drug administration with rapid absorption approximates the profile after multiple IV bolus administration. However, during oral drug administration, the bioavailability of the drug has to be considered because rapid absorption does not mean complete absorption. So similar group of expressions can be written to relate the maximum and minimum plasma drug concentration at steady state during multiple extravascular drug administration when the drug absorption is rapid:

$$Cp_{max\,ss} = \frac{FD}{Vd(1 - e^{-k\tau})} \qquad (13.5)$$

and

$$Cp_{min\,ss} = Cp_{max\,ss}e^{-k\tau}$$

and

$$Cp_{max\,ss} - Cp_{min\,ss} = \frac{F\,Dose}{Vd} \qquad (13.6)$$

When the drug is not rapidly absorbed, Equations 13.3, 13.5, and 13.6 cannot be used because significant amount of the drug is eliminated during the absorption phase. So the difference in the amount of the drug in the body at $Cp_{max\ ss}$ and $Cp_{min\ ss}$ is not equal to the dose and the time between $Cp_{max\ ss}$ and $Cp_{min\ ss}$ is not equal to τ.

13.3   TIME REQUIRED TO REACH STEADY STATE

During multiple drug administration, the administered dose is called the maintenance dose which is administered to gradually achieve and maintain the steady-state drug concentration. An approach similar to that used for constant rate IV infusion can be used to calculate the time required to achieve steady state during multiple drug administration. The time required to reach steady state is dependent on the half-life of the drug. Generally, it takes five to six times the elimination half-life of the drug to reach steady state. This means that the drug has to be repeatedly administered for a period equal to five to six half-lives to achieve steady state. The longer the drug half-life the longer it takes to reach steady state. Figure 13.3 represents the plasma drug concentration during repeated administration of different drugs that have different elimination half-lives. Administration of larger doses of the same drug will produce higher steady-state drug concentrations; however, the time to achieve steady state is similar as illustrated in Figure 13.4.

13.4   LOADING DOSE

The loading dose is a dose larger than the maintenance dose administered at the initiation of therapy to achieve faster approach to steady state as illustrated in Figure 13.5. Administration of the loading dose is necessary when rapid therapeutic effect is required. In these cases, waiting for five to six half-lives to achieve steady state may not be appropriate. The loading dose can be administered whether the drug

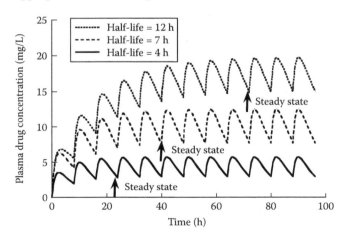

FIGURE 13.3 Plasma drug concentration during repeated administration of different drugs that have different half-lives. Drugs with shorter half-lives will reach steady state faster than the drugs with longer half-lives.

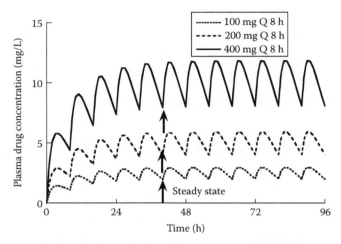

FIGURE 13.4 Administration of different doses of the same drug will achieve steady-state concentrations that are proportional to the administered dose. However, the time to achieve steady state will be the same.

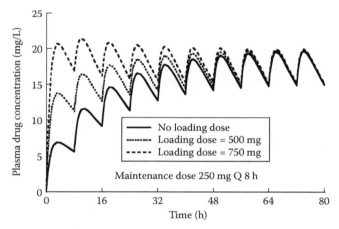

FIGURE 13.5 Plasma drug concentration after administration of different loading doses followed by the same maintenance dose. The steady state is similar because the maintenance dose is similar.

is administered by multiple IV or multiple oral administrations. A classical example of administration of oral loading dose is the rapid digitalization that involves administration of several tablets of digoxin during the first day of initiation of digoxin therapy followed by one tablet a day afterward. Also, the recommendation for starting therapy with some antibiotic is to take two tablets or capsules as the starting dose followed by single tablet or capsule every dosing interval. The idea is to administer a large dose in the beginning of therapy to immediately achieve drug concentration within the therapeutic range. Then, the maintenance dose is chosen to maintain the steady-state concentration within the therapeutic range. The loading dose does not affect the steady-state concentration and similar maintenance dose should achieve similar steady-state concentration whether a loading dose is administered or not as in Figure 13.5.

13.4.1 IV LOADING DOSE

The loading dose is calculated from the desired plasma drug concentration and the Vd of the drug. The desired drug concentration is usually a drug concentration within the therapeutic range:

$$\text{Loading dose} = Cp_{desired} \times Vd \tag{13.7}$$

13.4.2 ORAL LOADING DOSE

Oral loading dose can be calculated similarly; however, the bioavailability of the drug has to be considered:

$$\text{Loading dose} = \frac{Cp_{desired}\,Vd}{F} \tag{13.8}$$

The average steady-state plasma drug concentration is dependent on the dosing rate (FD/τ) and the total body clearance of the drug. Again, the loading dose does not affect the steady-state concentration.

13.5 AVERAGE PLASMA CONCENTRATION AT STEADY STATE

During multiple drug administration, the plasma drug concentrations at steady state and the $Cp_{max\ ss}$ and $Cp_{min\ ss}$ fluctuate around an average drug concentration as in Figure 13.6. The average steady-state concentration is not the arithmetic mean of the maximum and the minimum plasma concentrations at steady state. At steady state, the rate of drug administration is equal to the rate of drug elimination. The rate of

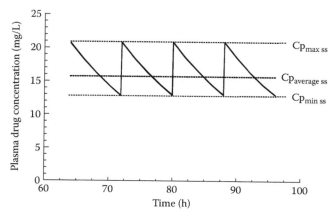

FIGURE 13.6 Plasma drug concentrations fluctuate around the average plasma drug concentration during multiple drug administration at steady state.

drug administration is equal to FD/τ where F is the bioavailability, D is the dose, and τ is the dosing interval. The rate of drug elimination is changing during the dosing interval at steady state because of the change in drug concentration during the dosing interval. However, the average rate of drug elimination during the entire dosing interval can be calculated from the product of the elimination rate constant and the average amount of the drug in the body at steady state, $kA_{\text{average ss}}$. So at steady state, Equation 13.9 can be obtained:

$$\frac{FD}{\tau} = kA_{\text{average ss}} \tag{13.9}$$

$$\frac{FD}{\tau} = kVdCp_{\text{average ss}} \tag{13.10}$$

$$Cp_{\text{average ss}} = \frac{FD}{kVd\tau} \tag{13.11}$$

Hence, the average plasma concentration at steady state is dependent on the dosing rate (FD/τ) and the total body clearance (CL_T, kVd). Different dosing regimens have the same dosing rate if the bioavailability is constant. For example, consider the following dosing regimens:

100 mg Q 4 h
150 mg Q 6 h
200 mg Q 8 h
300 mg Q 12 h

All these dosing regimens provide similar daily dose, that is, the same dosing rate. According to Equation 13.11, the average drug concentration achieved at steady state while administration of any of these regimens should be similar, assuming that the CL_T is constant. Although the average steady-state concentration is similar, the fluctuations in the plasma concentration around this average concentration are different for the different dosing regimens. This means that the maximum and the minimum concentrations at steady state are different for the different dosing regimens. The regimen with the largest dose and longest dosing interval usually has the largest fluctuations in the plasma concentration. Large fluctuations in the drug concentration at steady state produce high drug concentration that may be toxic at the beginning of the dosing interval and low drug concentration that may be subtherapeutic toward the end of the dosing interval. So the appropriate dosing regimen has to maintain the drug concentration within the therapeutic range during the entire dosing interval.

The total AUC observed after administration of a single dose of the drug is dependent on the bioavailable dose (FD) and CL_T as in Equation 13.12:

$$AUC = \frac{FD}{kVd} \tag{13.12}$$

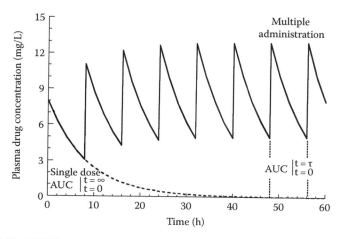

FIGURE 13.7 AUC from time zero to ∞ after administration of a single dose of the drug is equal to the AUC from time zero to τ at steady state during multiple administration of the same dose of the drug.

By substituting the value of AUC in Equation 13.11, an expression for the average drug concentration at steady state is obtained:

$$Cp_{\text{average ss}} = \frac{\text{AUC}}{\tau} \qquad (13.13)$$

After administration of a single dose of a drug, the AUC calculated from time zero to ∞ is equal to the AUC from time 0 to τ during multiple administration of the same dose of the drug at steady state as shown in Figure 13.7, that is,

$$\text{AUC}_{0-\infty} \text{ after a single dose} = \text{AUC}_{0-\tau} \text{ at steady state} \qquad (13.14)$$

This means that the average plasma concentration that should be achieved at steady state can be determined from the AUC calculated after administration of a single dose of the drug.

Example

A patient is receiving 1000 mg of an antibiotic as repeated IV bolus doses every 12 h to treat her lung infection. The maximum and minimum steady-state plasma concentrations of this antibiotic are 48 and 5 mg/L, respectively.

    a. Calculate the volume of distribution and the total body clearance of this antibiotic.

    b. Calculate the average plasma concentration of this antibiotic at steady state while receiving 1000 mg every 12 h.

Answer

a.
$$Cp_{maxss} - Cp_{minss} = \frac{Dose}{Vd}$$

$$48 - 5\,mg/L = \frac{1000\,mg}{Vd}$$

$$Vd = \frac{1000\,mg}{43\,mg/L} = 23.3L$$

$$Cp_{minss} = Cp_{maxss}e^{-k\tau}$$

$$5\,mg/L = 48\,mg/L\,e^{-k12h}$$

$$\ln\frac{5\,mg/L}{48\,mg/L} = -k12h$$

$$-2.262 = -k12h$$

$$k = 0.188h^{-1}$$

$$CL_T = 0.188h^{-1}23.3L = 4.38L/h$$

b.
$$Cp_{average\,ss} = FD/kV\,d\tau$$

$$Cp_{average\,ss} = \frac{1000\,mg}{0.188h^{-1}23.3L12h} = 19\,mg/L$$

13.6   DRUG ACCUMULATION

During multiple drug administration, the drug is accumulated in the body until steady state is achieved. The degree of drug accumulation is different from one drug to the other. Several approaches have been used to describe drug accumulation during multiple drug administration. One of these approaches that can be applied for IV and oral dosing regimens is the calculation of the accumulation ratio (R_{accum}). The accumulation ratio is defined as the amount of drug in the body at steady state relative to the dose of the drug. The larger the accumulation ratio, the higher is the degree of drug accumulation:

$$R_{accum} = \frac{A_{average\,ss}}{FD} \qquad (13.15)$$

$$R_{accum} = \frac{FD/k\tau}{FD} = \frac{1}{k\tau} \tag{13.16}$$

Drugs that are eliminated slowly from the body (small k) and are administered frequently (short τ) usually have large accumulation ratio. In these drugs, the average amount of the drug in the body at steady state is much larger than the dose of the drug, indicating high accumulation. Determination of the degree of accumulation of the drug has important clinical applications. If a patient develops toxicity while receiving repeated doses of a drug that is not accumulated in the body to a large extent, discontinuation of therapy in most cases will be enough for the patient to recover from this toxicity, while for drugs that have high degree of accumulation, development of toxicity indicates that the patient will continue to experience the signs and symptoms of toxicity for prolonged period even after discontinuation of the drug therapy. In most of these cases, additional measures have to be installed to accelerate the rate of drug elimination and hasten the recovery from this toxicity.

Also, missing a dose during multiple drug administration of a drug that has low accumulation leads to elimination of the majority of the drug in the body, which may significantly affect the drug therapeutic effect. In this case, a replacement dose should be administered once the patient remembers that he or she missed the dose. On the other hand, missing a dose of a drug that has high degree of accumulation may not affect the amount of the drug in the body significantly. In this case, the patient can be instructed to take the drug dose at the time of the following dose unless the drug has very narrow therapeutic index.

13.7 CONTROLLED-RELEASE FORMULATIONS

Controlled-released formulations are specially designed formulations that can slowly release the drug from the dosage forms over an extended period of time. The rate of drug absorption from these modified-release formulations usually depends on the drug release rate from the formulation. This means that if the formulation is designed such that it releases the drug at a slow and constant rate over an extended period of time, the rate of drug absorption becomes slow and relatively constant over the drug release period. This slow absorption rate, which usually covers the entire dosing interval, causes slow rise and slow decline in the plasma drug concentration that is reflected in the small fluctuations in the plasma drug concentration during multiple administration at steady state. Controlled-release formulations allow administration of larger doses of the drug less frequently without increasing the fluctuations in the drug concentration during the dosing interval.

Modified-release formulations are ideal for drugs that have relatively short half-life when direct relationship exists between the plasma drug concentration and the drug therapeutic effect. This is because these drugs are usually administered in large doses to decrease the frequency of drug administration. In this case, administration of immediate-release formulations causes rapid increase in the plasma drug concentration followed by rapid decline in the drug concentration and large fluctuations in the plasma drug concentrations occur. These large fluctuations in the plasma drug concentration are reflected in the therapeutic effect when direct plasma concentration-effect

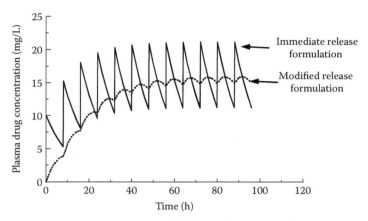

FIGURE 13.8 Plasma concentration–time profile after multiple administration of the same dose of immediate-release and modified-release oral formulations.

relationship exists. However, modified-release formulations produce small fluctuations in the plasma drug concentration and steady therapeutic effect for these drugs. Figure 13.8 is a representative example of the plasma drug concentration during multiple administration of immediate-release and modified-release formulations.

The cost of modified-release products is usually higher than the cost of conventional dosage forms because of the techniques utilized in the formulation and manufacturing of these formulations. For some drugs, modified-release products can be more beneficial to the patient than conventional products that can justify their higher cost. However, modified-release products are not always better than conventional products for all drugs. For example, drugs with long half-life like digoxin usually produce small fluctuations during repeated administration, so modified-release formulations may not be advantageous. Also, comparable therapeutic effect is produced from modified-release and conventional products of drugs that do not have direct plasma concentration-effect relationship such as the oral anticoagulants. Furthermore, drugs with saturable first-pass effect such as propranolol usually have lower oral bioavailability when administered as modified-release formulations compared to immediate-release products. So drugs should be formulated as modified-release formulation only when these formulations are more beneficial to the patient than conventional products.

13.8 EFFECT OF CHANGING THE PHARMACOKINETIC PARAMETERS ON THE STEADY-STATE PLASMA DRUG CONCENTRATION DURING MULTIPLE DRUG ADMINISTRATION

The drug is accumulated in the body during multiple drug administration until steady state is achieved. The average steady-state plasma drug concentration is directly proportional to the administration rate, FD/τ, and inversely proportional to the drug CL_T, while the time required to achieve steady state is dependent on the drug half-life.

13.8.1 Pharmacokinetic Simulation Exercise

Pharmacokinetic simulations can be used to examine how the pharmacokinetic parameters affect the steady-state drug concentration achieved during multiple drug administration. The drug concentration–time profile is simulated using an average value of each of the pharmacokinetic parameters and the steady-state concentration and the time to achieve steady state are observed. Then, the pharmacokinetic parameters are changed one parameter at a time while keeping all the other parameters constant, and the simulation is repeated. The resulting profile is examined to see how the change affects the drug steady-state concentration and the time to achieve steady-state concentration. The plotting exercise of the steady-state during multiple drug administration module in the basic pharmacokinetic concept section and the pharmacokinetic simulation section of the companion CD to this textbook can be used to run these simulations.

13.8.1.1 Dosing Rate

The average steady-state plasma concentration is directly proportional to the dosing rate (FD/τ) according to Equation 13.11. Higher dosing rate is achieved by administration of larger doses, using products with higher bioavailability or administration of the drug more frequently. Increasing the dosing rate causes proportional increase in the average steady-state concentration if the CL_T remains constant. The AUC during each dosing interval at steady state increases with the increase in dose or the increase in bioavailability. Although increasing the dosing rate increases the average steady-state concentration, the time to achieve steady state is not affected.

13.8.1.2 Total Body Clearance

The steady-state plasma concentration is inversely proportional to CL_T. Lower CL_T results in higher steady-state concentration when the dosing rate is kept constant. The same drug can have different CL_T in different individuals due to differences in the function of the drug-eliminating organ(s). Administration of a drug at the same dosing rate to patients with different CL_T should produce higher steady-state drug concentration in patients with lower CL_T. When different values for CL_T are used in the simulation while keeping the same Vd, the profile for the higher CL_T will reach steady state faster than the profile for the lower CL_T. This is because higher CL_T means higher k and shorter $t_{1/2}$ when Vd is kept constant.

13.8.1.3 Volume of Distribution

The Vd does not affect the steady-state concentration if the CL_T and the dosing rate were constant. When Vd is different in patients with similar CL_T, the $t_{1/2}$ and k (the dependent parameters) will be different in these individuals. In these individuals, the steady state will be the same (same CL_T and FD/τ); however, the approach to steady state will be faster in the individuals with larger CL_T/Vd ratios (larger k and shorter half-life).

13.8.1.4 Absorption Rate Constant

The absorption rate of the drug does not affect the average steady-state drug concentration. However, fast rate of drug absorption, large k_a, produces large difference between $Cp_{max\ ss}$ and $Cp_{min\ ss}$, that is, large fluctuations in drug concentrations at steady state, while slow rate of drug absorption produces small fluctuations in drug concentrations at steady state.

13.9 DOSING REGIMEN DESIGN BASED ON DRUG PHARMACOKINETICS

The dosage requirement for different patients is different because of the differences in the patients' characteristics. The design of a dosing regimen involves selection of the appropriate dose and dosing interval for each individual patient. The appropriate dosing regimen is the regimen that maintains the plasma drug concentration within the therapeutic range all the time during the dosing interval.

13.9.1 FACTORS TO BE CONSIDERED

Few factors have to be considered before calculating the dosing regimen. These factors should help in the selection of the proper dosing regimen.

13.9.1.1 Therapeutic Range of the Drug

The therapeutic range of the drug is the range of plasma drug concentrations associated with the maximum probability of producing the desired drug therapeutic effect and the minimum probability of producing adverse effects. This range of concentrations is different for different drugs. Some drugs may have a narrow therapeutic range and others may have a wide therapeutic range. Dosing regimens for drugs with wide therapeutic range are easier to determine because wide range of doses can maintain the plasma concentration within the therapeutic range at steady state. This means that drugs with wide therapeutic range are can be considered relatively safer drugs. However, drugs with narrow therapeutic range require accurate calculation of the appropriate dosing regimen because small change in dose can result in toxic or subtherapeutic effects.

13.9.1.2 Required Onset of Effect

It is important to determine if an immediate drug effect is required or not. Immediate drug effect is usually required in emergency cases and when the patient's condition is severe enough to necessitate instant intervention. In this case, the dosing regimen should include an initial loading dose to achieve faster approach to steady state. On the other hand, when the patient's condition is stable and the dosing regimen is used to initiate the treatment of a chronic condition, administration of loading dose may not be necessary.

13.9.1.3 Drug Product

It is important to consider the availability of modified-release products for the drug of interest and the suitability of these products for the patient's condition. This is because modified-release formulations produce small fluctuations in drug concentration within each dosing interval, while immediate-release formulations produce large fluctuations in drug concentration during multiple administrations. When modified-release products are used, the goal of the dosing regimen design is to maintain the average plasma drug concentration within the therapeutic range, while when immediate-release products are used, the dosing regimen should be selected to ensure that the $Cp_{max\ ss}$ does not exceed the upper limit of the therapeutic range and that the $Cp_{min\ ss}$ does not go below the lower limit of the therapeutic range.

13.9.1.4   Progression of the Patient's Disease State

The progression of the patient's disease state and the response of the patient to the administered drugs have to be considered when selecting the dosing regimens. For example, progression of the renal disease with time may necessitate periodic modification of the dose of the drugs excreted mainly by the kidney. Also, the dose of some drugs is increased gradually after initiation of therapy because of the increase in their metabolic rate such as in the case of carbamazepine autoinduction. So with the initiation of the dosing regimen a plan should be installed to periodically evaluate the dosing regimen and make the necessary modification.

13.9.2   ESTIMATION OF THE PATIENT PHARMACOKINETIC PARAMETERS

The dose of the drug in each patient has to be individualized according to the patient's specific pharmacokinetic parameters. The drug pharmacokinetic parameters can depend on many factors such as age, weight, sex, eliminating organ function, concomitant drugs, genetic factors, and many other factors. So selection of the appropriate dosing regimen for a drug in a particular patient requires knowledge of the drug pharmacokinetic parameters in this particular patient, which can be estimated with different levels of accuracy depending on the available information about the patient.

13.9.2.1   When No Information Is Available about the Patient's Medical History

The average value for the drug pharmacokinetic parameters in the general population is the best estimate for the patient pharmacokinetic parameters when absolutely no information is known about the patient's medical history. These estimates for the pharmacokinetic parameters can be used to calculate the dosing regimen for the patient. The dosing regimen calculated this way has to be used with caution because it is based on an approximate estimate for the patient's pharmacokinetic parameters.

13.9.2.2   When Information Is Available about the Patient's Medical History

The drug pharmacokinetic parameters can be estimated by utilizing the information from the patient's medical history and the factors that can affect the drug pharmacokinetic parameters. In this case, the best estimate for the patient's specific pharmacokinetic parameters is the parameters of a patient population similar to that of the patient with regard to age, weight, gender, organ function, in addition to other medical conditions and other drugs that can affect the pharmacokinetics of the drug of interest. The pharmacokinetic parameters estimated based on the patient's medical conditions provide better approximation of the drug pharmacokinetic parameters in that particular patient compared to using the average population parameters. These estimated pharmacokinetic parameters are used to calculate the dosing regimen for the patient.

13.9.2.3   When the Patient Has a History of Using the Drug under Consideration

The history of using the drug under consideration should be utilized to estimate the patient's specific pharmacokinetic parameters. The previous dose administered, the plasma drug concentration if measured, and the therapeutic outcomes are usually considered to estimate the patient's specific pharmacokinetic parameters and design the new drug dosing regimen. Any changes in the patient's condition that can alter the drug pharmacokinetics should be considered in the design of the new dosing regimen. The availability of information about the history of drug use, especially if the plasma drug concentrations were determined, provides the best estimate for the patient's specific pharmacokinetic parameters. Determination of the patient's specific parameter is very useful for calculation of the appropriate dosing regimen for the patient and for individualization of drug therapy.

13.9.3   SELECTION OF DOSE AND DOSING INTERVAL

The dose and the dosing interval of the drug should maintain plasma drug concentration within the therapeutic range all the time. The selection of dose and dosing interval depends on the drug pharmacokinetic parameters and therapeutic range of the drug. Also, dosing regimens that involve using modified-release formulations are designed to accommodate the dosing intervals recommended by the manufacturer.

13.9.3.1   Modified-Release Oral Formulation

Modified-release formulations are slowly absorbed and produce small fluctuations in the plasma drug concentration at steady state. The choice of the dosing interval of modified-release formulations usually depends on the formulation characteristics and is usually recommended by the product manufacturer. The estimates for the drug pharmacokinetic parameters should be used to calculate the dose required to achieve an average plasma drug concentration within the therapeutic range according to

$$Cp_{average\,ss} = \frac{FD}{kVd\tau}$$

13.9.3.2   Fast-Release Oral Formulations and IV Administration

During repeated administration of IV and immediate-release oral formulations, large fluctuations in plasma concentrations are observed. The dose and dosing intervals should be selected to keep the steady-state maximum and minimum plasma concentrations within the therapeutic range all the time. Usually, the dosing interval is selected based on the expected maximum and minimum plasma drug concentrations and then the dose to achieve the maximum concentration is calculated.

13.9.3.2.1   Selection of the Dosing Interval

The target maximum and minimum plasma drug concentrations are selected to be within the therapeutic range of the drug. Then, the dosing interval is calculated from the time period required for the maximum plasma concentration to decline to the minimum plasma concentration. The target maximum and minimum concentrations and the drug elimination rate constant are substituted in the following equation and solved for the dosing interval:

$$Cp_{min\,ss} = Cp_{max\,ss}e^{-k\tau}$$

The calculated dosing interval should be rounded to the nearest practical dosing interval. The practical dosing interval is the interval that allows drug administration at the same time every day (e.g., 6, 8, 12, and 24 h).

13.9.3.2.2   Selection of Dose

The dose required to achieve the target maximum steady-state drug concentration when given every τ (the rounded τ) can be determined as follows:

$$Cp_{max\,ss} = \frac{FD}{Vd(1-e^{-k\tau})}$$

Again, it may be necessary to round the selected dose to the nearest practical dose.

13.9.4   SELECTION OF THE LOADING DOSE

When immediate effect of the drug is required, the dosing regimen should include a recommendation for a loading dose. The loading dose is calculated from the desired plasma concentration and the drug Vd:

$$Loading\ dose = \frac{Cp_{desired}\,Vd}{F}$$

Example

A patient was admitted to the hospital after experiencing an episode of ventricular arrhythmia. The physician decided to start the patient on IV regimen of an antiarrhythmic drug. The Vd of this antiarrhythmic drug is 45 L, the $t_{1/2}$ is 7 h, and the therapeutic range is 4–12 mg/L.

    a. Recommend an IV loading dose and the IV dosing regimen (dose and dosing interval) that should maintain the drug concentration within the therapeutic range all the time.

    b. The patient was stabilized on the regimen you recommended and she is ready to go home. The physician wanted to shift the patient to oral formulation of the same drug. What will be the dosing regimen (dose and dosing interval) from the oral formulation if the oral formulation of this drug is rapidly absorbed and has bioavailability of 75%.

Answer

    a. The loading dose is the dose that should achieve the maximum plasma concentration:

$$Loading\ dose = Cp_{desired} \times Vd$$

$$LD = 12\,mg/L \times 45L = 540\,mg$$

Dosing interval:

$$4\,mg/L = 12\,mg/L\,e^{-0.099h^{-1}\tau}$$

$$\ln\frac{4\,mg/L}{12\,mg/L} = -0.099h^{-1}\tau$$

$$-1.0986 = -0.099h^{-1}\tau$$

$$\tau = 11h$$

So an appropriate dosing interval will be 12 h.

Selection of dose:

$$Cp_{maxss} = \frac{D}{Vd(1-e^{-k\tau})}$$

$$12\,mg/L = \frac{D}{45L(1-e^{-0.099h^{-1}12h})}$$

Dose = 375 mg.

Recommendation: The patient should receive an IV loading dose of 540 mg and then the maintenance dose is 375 mg IV administered every 12 h.

b. The dosing regimen from the oral formulation.
The dosing interval is dependent on the rate of elimination of the drug, so this rapidly absorbed oral formulation should also be administered every 12 h. However, the dose will be different because of the incomplete bioavailability:

$$Cp_{maxss} = \frac{FD}{Vd(1-e^{-k\tau})}$$

$$12\,mg/L = \frac{0.75D}{45L(1-e^{-0.099h^{-1}12h})}$$

Dose = 500 mg.

Recommendation: 500 mg of the oral formulation every 12 h.

PRACTICE PROBLEMS

13.1 An antibiotic has a volume of distribution of 20 L and an elimination rate constant of 0.1 h^{-1}. This antibiotic is administered by repeated IV bolus doses of 200 mg every 8 h.

a. Calculate the maximum and the minimum plasma drug concentration at steady state.
b. Calculate the average steady-state concentration of this antibiotic.
c. What is the dose that should be given every 8 h to achieve steady-state average plasma drug concentration of 25 mg/L?

13.2 A 72-year-old, 85 kg, male patient was admitted to the hospital for the treatment of severe lung infection. His dosing regimen of the antibiotic was 500 mg daily given at 8 a.m. in the morning by IV bolus administration. At steady state, the maximum and the minimum plasma concentration of this antibiotic were 35 and 10 mg/L, respectively.
   a. Calculate the half-life of this antibiotic in this patient.
   b. Calculate the volume of distribution of this antibiotic in this patient.
   c. Calculate the average steady-state plasma concentration of the drug.

13.3 After a single oral dose of 200 mg theophylline to a 10-year-old patient, the total AUC was 100 mg h/L. (Assume that theophylline is completely absorbed.)
   a. Calculate the average theophylline plasma concentration at steady state if this patient is taking 200 mg theophylline every 6 h.
   b. Calculate the average theophylline plasma concentration at steady state if this patient is shifted to 400 mg every 12 h from a controlled-release formulation.
   c. Calculate the dose of this controlled-release formulation that can achieve an average steady-state concentration of 10 mg/L in this patient.

13.4 An antihypertensive drug is administered as 200 mg daily for a controlled-release formulation that is known to have 75% bioavailability. The drug has a half-life of 24 h and a volume of distribution of 24 L.
   a. Calculate the average steady-state concentration of this drug.
   b. What is the dose required to achieve an average steady-state concentration of 20 mg/L using the same formulation?
   c. What is the daily IV dose required from an IV formulation of the drug to achieve an average steady-state concentration of 20 mg/L?
   d. Calculate the maximum and the minimum plasma drug concentration at steady state while taking the regimen you recommended in (c).

13.5 A patient is receiving his antihypertensive medication as 500 mg every 8 h in the form of an oral capsule. After administration of this oral capsule, only 80% of the active ingredient in the capsule reaches the systemic circulation. The CL_T of this drug in this patient is 2.5 L/h.
   a. What is the average steady-state plasma concentration of this drug in this patient?
   b. What will be the average steady-state plasma concentration if the patient was taking 1000 mg every 8 h from the same oral drug product?
   c. What will be the CL_T of the drug in this patient while taking the 1000 mg every 8 h oral dose?
   d. What will be the oral dose required to achieve an average plasma concentration of 30 mg/L from this drug in this patient?
   e. Because the patient had problems swallowing the oral capsules he was shifted to 500 mg IV every 8 h regimen. What will be the average steady-state concentration of this drug in this patient?

13.6 A patient received a single IV bolus dose of 300 mg of an antibiotic and the following plasma concentrations were obtained.

Time (h)	Drug Concentration (mg/L)
2	12.86
6	9.45
12	5.95
24	2.36

    a. What is the maximum and the minimum steady-state drug concentration in a patient who was taking 250 mg every 12 h from an oral formulation that is rapidly absorbed and has bioavailability of 80%?

    b. What is the average steady-state concentration of this drug in the patient while taking the regimen in (a)?

    c. What will be the maximum and the minimum steady-state drug concentration if the dose was increased to 500 mg every 12 h from this oral formulation?

13.7 A patient is taking 450 mg of an antibiotic every 12 h as IV bolus doses. At steady state, the maximum and minimum plasma antibiotic concentrations were 40 and 10 mg/L, respectively.

    a. Calculate the half-life of this antibiotic in this patient.

    b. Calculate the volume of distribution of this antibiotic in this patient.

    c. Calculate the average steady-state plasma concentration of the drug.

    d. What is the approximate time for this drug to achieve steady state?

    e. What is the amount of the drug eliminated from this antibiotic during one dosing interval at steady state.

13.8 A patient is receiving IV theophylline to control an acute episode of bronchial asthma. The maintenance dose is 320 mg IV bolus of theophylline every 8 h. At steady state, the maximum and minimum theophylline plasma concentrations were 18 and 10 mg/L, respectively.

    a. What is the half-life and the volume of distribution of theophylline in this patient?

    b. What is the daily dose of an oral theophylline preparation that is required to achieve an average plasma theophylline concentration of 18 mg/L? (The bioavailability of the oral preparation is 100%.)

13.9 A patient was admitted to the hospital because of severe attack of ventricular arrhythmia. The patient's acute condition was treated and the physician wanted to start the patient on multiple IV bolus administration on an antiarrhythmic drug. The physician asked you to recommend a loading dose and the dosing regimen that should maintain the maximum and the minimum steady-state drug concentration approximately 20 and 10 mg/L, respectively. This drug has an elimination rate constant of $0.06 \, h^{-1}$ and volume of distribution of 30 L.

    a. What is your recommendation for the IV loading dose that should immediately achieve 20 mg/L?

    b. What is the most appropriate dosing interval for this drug?

    c. What is the appropriate maintenance dose for this drug?

    d. What is the average steady-state concentration of this drug achieved from the regimen you recommended?

    e. The patient was stabilized on the regimen you recommended, and he is ready to go home. The physician asked you to recommend the dosing regimen of the oral formulation of the same drug to achieve the same average steady-state concentration, if this oral formulation is known to have bioavailability of 75%. What is your recommendation?

13.10 The therapeutic range of an antihypertensive drug is 8–25 mg/L. The drug has half-life of 7 h and volume of distribution of 30 L. After oral administration, this drug is rapidly absorbed and only 85% of the dose reaches the systemic circulation.

    a. What is the most appropriate dosing interval for this drug?

    b. What is the appropriate maintenance dose for this drug?

    c. What is the average steady-state concentration achieved from the regimen you recommended?

14 Renal Drug Excretion

OBJECTIVES

After completing this chapter you should be able to

- Discuss the mechanisms of drug excretion in urine
- Describe the importance of studying the drug elimination through a specific pathway
- Estimate the drug pharmacokinetic parameters from the urinary excretion rate data
- Calculate the renal clearance of drugs from the urinary excretion rate data
- Describe the procedures for determining the creatinine clearance
- Analyze the effect of changing the dose, total body clearance, and renal clearance on the urinary excretion of drugs
- Predict the change in the overall elimination rate of drugs due to the change in their renal excretion

14.1   INTRODUCTION

Drugs are eliminated from the body by excretion of the unchanged drug from the body or by metabolism to form one or more metabolites that can then be excreted. The major excretion pathways include renal excretion of drugs in urine, biliary excretion of drugs to the gastrointestinal tract (GIT), lung excretion of volatile drugs during expiration, in addition to other minor excretion pathways such as excretion of drugs in sweat and in milk. Drug metabolism involves enzymatic modification of the drug chemical structure to form the metabolites. Most of the metabolites are pharmacologically inactive; however, few metabolites have pharmacological activity and some metabolites can cause adverse effects.

Most of the drugs are eliminated from the body by one or more elimination pathways. The CL_T is the sum of the clearances associated with each of the drug elimination pathways. For example, if a drug is excreted by renal excretion and hepatic metabolism, the CL_T for this drug is the sum of the renal clearance and the metabolic clearance. When the drug is metabolized by different metabolic pathways to form different metabolites, each of these metabolic pathways has its own clearance. A general relationship can be written as shown in Equation 14.1:

$$CL_T = CL_R + CL_M + CL_L + CL_B + \cdots \qquad (14.1)$$

where
  CL_R is the renal clearance
  CL_M is the metabolic clearance
  CL_L is the lung clearance
  CL_B is the biliary clearance

If a drug is not excreted through a particular pathway, the clearance associated with this pathway becomes equal to zero. For example, if a drug is not excreted by the kidney, the CL_R becomes equal to zero, while if a drug is completely eliminated by a single elimination pathway, the CL_T becomes equal to the clearance associated with this elimination pathway. For example, if a drug is completely eliminated by metabolism to form one metabolite, the CL_T becomes equal to CL_M.

Also when the drug elimination processes follow first-order kinetics, each of the elimination pathways should have a rate constant that is dependent on the clearance of each elimination pathway and the Vd of the drug as in Equations 14.2 and 14.3:

$$\frac{CL_T}{Vd} = \frac{CL_R}{Vd} + \frac{CL_M}{Vd} + \frac{CL_L}{Vd} + \frac{CL_B}{Vd} \cdots \tag{14.2}$$

$$k = k_e + k_m + k_l + k_b \cdots \tag{14.3}$$

where
   k_e is the first-order rate constant for the renal excretion
   k_m is the first-order rate constant for the metabolic process
   k_l is the first-order rate constant for the lung excretion
   k_b is the first-order rate constant for the biliary excretion

This means that the first-order elimination rate constant for the overall elimination process is the sum of the rate constants for the different elimination pathways.

14.2   STUDYING DRUG ELIMINATION THROUGH A SINGLE PATHWAY

In the previous chapters drug elimination was viewed as an overall elimination process that removes the drug from the body. The rate of decline in the plasma drug concentration that reflects the rate of drug elimination by all elimination pathways was used to determine the rate constant and half-life of this overall process. Also, the calculated drug clearance reflected the total body clearance by all elimination pathways. Studying the kinetics of drug elimination through specific elimination pathway requires determination of the rate of drug elimination through this specific elimination pathway.

The contribution of each elimination pathway to the overall elimination process determines how much drug is eliminated by each pathway. This is because the rate of drug elimination through each of the elimination pathways at any time is related to the clearance and the rate constant associated with each of these pathways. Integration of the rate of excretion from time zero to infinity gives the amount of drug excreted by each elimination pathway. This means that the fraction of the administered IV dose of a drug excreted by a specific pathway is determined from the magnitude of the drug clearance or rate constant associated with this specific pathway relative to the CL_T or k, respectively. For example, if the CL_R of a drug is

60% of its CL_T (this means that k_e is 60% of k), 60% of the administered IV dose is excreted unchanged in urine and the rest of the dose is excreted by the other elimination pathways.

Determination of the rate of drug elimination by the different elimination pathways is useful because the change in the function of one of the eliminating organs involved in drug elimination usually causes change in the overall rate of drug elimination. However, the magnitude of the change in the overall drug elimination rate depends on the contribution of the affected organ to the overall elimination process. When significant amount of the drug is eliminated by the affected pathway, significant change occurs in the overall rate of drug elimination, while if the affected pathway represents a minor elimination pathway, small change will occur in the overall rate of drug elimination. For example, the renal elimination of digoxin is approximately 70% of the total drug elimination. The decrease in the renal function causes significant change in the overall elimination rate of digoxin, which necessitates dose reduction in renal failure patients, while the dose of propranolol should not be reduced in renal failure patient since minor fraction of propranolol dose is excreted unchanged in urine.

Also, evaluation of the clinical significance of the interaction of a drug with another agent that affects the drug elimination process requires knowledge of the contribution of the different elimination pathways to the overall drug elimination process. This is because the interacting agent usually affects a specific elimination pathway, such as inhibition of the renal drug excretion or inhibition of drug metabolism by a specific enzyme system. The clinical significance of the drug interaction is dependent on the contribution of the affected pathway to the overall drug elimination. For example, metronidazole, which is an inhibitor of the metabolizing enzymes, can significantly slow the rate of elimination of the oral anticoagulants warfarin because it is eliminated mainly by metabolism. Also, probenecid inhibits the renal active secretion of penicillins leading to significant reduction of penicillins elimination rate because they are eliminated mainly by the kidney.

Studying the rate of drug excretion through a specific elimination pathway is not easy because of the complex experimental settings required to study some of the pathways. The easiest excretion pathway that can be studied is the renal drug excretion, which can be achieved by collection of urine samples and measuring the amount of drug excreted unchanged in urine during a certain period of time. Also, drug metabolism through a specific metabolic pathway can be studied by measuring the rate of metabolite appearance in the systemic circulation after administration of the parent drug. This is because the rate of drug metabolism to a particular metabolite is similar to the rate of formation of this metabolite in the systemic circulation. Furthermore, determination of the rate of lung excretion of drugs can be achieved by collecting all the expired air over some time intervals and measuring the drug concentration in this expired air. Moreover, measuring the rate of biliary drug excretion requires collection of bile over specific time intervals and measuring the drug concentration in the collected bile. Such experiments can only be performed in experimental animals. In this chapter, the kinetics of the renal drug excretion will be discussed, while the kinetics of drug metabolism will be discussed in the next chapter.

14.3 RENAL EXCRETION OF DRUGS

The renal excretory function starts with the filtration of the blood reaching the glomeruli, which occurs normally at a rate of 120 mL/min and ends with urine formation at a rate of 1–2 mL/min. This means that about 98%–99% of the water in the glomerular filtrate is reabsorbed in the renal tubules. When a solute is filtered in the glomeruli, the concentration of that solute in the glomerular filtrate is equal to its concentration in plasma. If the solute is not secreted or reabsorbed in the renal tubules, the concentration of this solute increases as it moves through the renal tubules due to water reabsorption. Water reabsorption makes the solute concentration gradient between the tubular lumen and blood in favor of passive tubular reabsorption if the solute can cross the tubular membrane. Some compounds can undergo carrier-mediated reabsorption from the renal tubules. However, solute secretion from the blood to the renal tubules has to occur by active transport because it is against the concentration gradient. So the three processes involved in the renal excretion of drugs are the glomerular filtration, active tubular secretion, and tubular reabsorption [1].

14.3.1 GLOMERULAR FILTRATION

The blood is filtered in the glomeruli and the rate of this process is called the glomerular filtration rate (GFR). All small molecules with molecular weight below 2000 g/mol can be filtered freely in the glomeruli. However, large protein molecules such as albumin cannot be filtered. Drug molecules that are bound to plasma protein are not filtered and only free drug molecules are filtered. The rate of drug filtration in the glomeruli is the product of the free (unbound) drug concentration in plasma and the GFR (i.e., free drug concentration × GFR). Impaired kidney function is manifested by lower GFR. Also, some diseases (e.g., nephrotic syndrome) can affect the glomerular filtration process and allow the excretion of large protein molecules such as albumin and globulins in urine.

14.3.2 ACTIVE TUBULAR SECRETION

The drug molecules can be actively secreted from the plasma to the lumen of the proximal tubules. There are several transport systems for specific classes of compounds that exist in the renal tubules. These transport systems are saturable, and drugs that belong to these specific chemical classes can be secreted by these transport systems. Different drugs that belong to the same chemical class can compete with each other for the same transport system, and drugs with higher affinity for the transport system can inhibit the secretion of other drugs with lower affinity. For example, probenecid inhibits the active secretion of penicillins in the renal tubules, which can prolong the duration of effect of penicillins. As mentioned previously, the drug cannot be passively secreted from the blood to the renal tubules against the concentration gradient.

14.3.3 TUBULAR REABSORPTION

Drugs and solutes filtered in the glomeruli and actively secreted in the proximal tubules can be reabsorbed throughout the tubules by passive or carrier-mediated reabsorption. Because of the water reabsorption in the renal tubules, the concentration of solutes increases in the renal tubules. Lipophilic molecules can be reabsorbed by passive diffusion from the renal tubules to the blood with the concentration gradient. Also, ionizable molecules can be reabsorbed in the renal tubules when they are in their unionized form. However, hydrophilic and ionized molecules have very limited reabsorption from the renal tubules. So the reabsorption and urinary secretion of ionizable molecules can be manipulated by changing the urinary pH. Some vitamins, amino acids, and glucose can be reabsorbed by a carrier-mediated saturable transport system. The drug that is not reabsorbed moves through the collecting tubules and is collected in the urinary bladder until it is excreted with urine.

The rate of renal excretion of a drug is the sum of the rate of filtration and active secretion minus the rate of reabsorption from the renal tubules:

$$\text{Renal excretion rate} = \text{Rate of filtration} + \text{Rate of active secretion}$$
$$- \text{Rate of reabsorption}$$

14.4 DETERMINATION OF THE RENAL EXCRETION RATE

After a single IV dose of the drug, monitoring the change in the plasma drug concentration with time allows determination of the overall rate of elimination by all elimination pathways. Studying the renal drug excretion requires collecting multiple urine samples at different time points and determination of the rate of drug excretion in each of these urine samples. Because of the nature of urine formation and excretion, the amount of the drug in the urine sample represents the drug excreted during the period of time over which the urine sample was formed. So urine samples are usually collected over predetermined time intervals. The drug concentration in the urine samples does not reflect the amount of the drug excreted during the urine collection intervals because the volume of urine collected during different intervals can be different depending on the hydration state of the individual. So the volume of urine collected over the urine collection interval and the drug concentration in the urine sample are multiplied to calculate the amount of drug excreted in urine over the collection interval. The amount of drug excreted unchanged in urine is divided by the length of the urine collection interval to determine the average renal drug excretion rate over the urine collection interval.

Consider a drug that is eliminated by first-order processes, including renal excretion as in Figure 14.1. The renal excretion rate of the drug at any time is equal to

$$\frac{dA_e}{dt} = k_e A \qquad (14.4)$$

where
A_e is the amount of the drug excreted in urine
k_e is the first-order renal excretion rate constant
A is the amount of the drug in the body

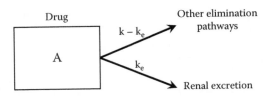

FIGURE 14.1 Diagram representing a drug that is eliminated by renal and nonrenal elimination pathways. A is the amount of the drug in the body, k is the first-order overall elimination rate constant, and k_e is the first-order renal excretion rate constant.

However, as mentioned earlier, urine samples are collected over certain time intervals:

$$\frac{\Delta A_e}{\Delta t} = k_e A_{average} \qquad (14.5)$$

where

ΔA_e is the amount of the drug excreted in urine over a certain urine collection interval Δt

$\Delta A_e/\Delta t$ is the average renal excretion rate over the urine collection interval

k_e is the first-order renal excretion rate constant

$A_{average}$ is the average amount of the drug in the body during the urine collection interval

14.4.1 EXPERIMENTAL DETERMINATION OF THE RENAL EXCRETION RATE

While planning a renal excretion rate experiment for a drug, the total period of sampling and the duration of each urine collection interval have to be specified based on the drug pharmacokinetic characteristics. In general, frequent samples are obtained when the monitored variable is changing rapidly and less frequent samples are obtained when the variable is changing slowly. After a single IV bolus drug administration, frequent samples are obtained initially and then the sampling frequency decreases with time. For example, if the drug has an elimination half-life of 5–6 h, the total sampling duration can be chosen as 18–24 h. This sampling duration represents about three to four elimination half-lives for the drug, which is enough to eliminate more than 90% of the administered drug dose. The urine collection intervals can be chosen as 0–2, 2–4, 4–8, 8–12, 12–18, and 18–24 h. This is an example of the sampling schedule; however, the sampling schedule can be changed as needed to obtain the required information from the study. In human subjects, urine samples obtained over intervals shorter than 1 h cannot be obtained accurately since complete collection of the urine samples is required for correct determination of the renal drug excretion rate. The following steps are usually followed for the determination of the drug renal excretion rate during each urine collection interval after a single drug administration:

1. The subjects are asked to empty their bladder before drug administration. The drug is administered and the time of drug administration is taken as time zero.
2. Urine samples are collected completely at the end of each urine collection interval. When multiple collections are obtained during the collection

interval, which is common during long intervals, a final urine sample is collected at the end of the interval and all the collected urine is combined together as one sample.

3. The volume of the total urine sample collected over the entire interval is determined accurately and recorded. An aliquot of the urine sample is kept for drug analysis.
4. The drug concentration is determined in each urine sample.
5. The total amount of the drug excreted during each urine collection interval is calculated from the drug concentration in the urine sample and the volume of the sample:

$$\text{Amount of drug excreted} = \text{Drug concentration} \times \text{Sample volume} \quad (14.6)$$

6. The average renal excretion rate during each urine collection interval is determined from the amount of drug excreted during each collection interval and the length of the collection interval as follows:

$$\text{Renal excretion rate} = \frac{\text{Amount excreted}}{\text{Time of urine collection}} \quad (14.7)$$

14.4.2 RENAL EXCRETION RATE–TIME PROFILE

The renal excretion rate of the drug at any time is determined from the renal excretion rate constant and the amount of the drug in the body according to Equation 14.4, assuming that the renal excretion process follows first-order kinetics. Since the amount of the drug in the body after a single IV administration decreases with time due to drug elimination, the renal excretion rate of the drug also decreases with time. The rate of decline in the renal excretion rate of the drug after a single IV bolus administration is parallel to the rate of decline of the amount of the drug in the body. The equation that describes the amount of the drug in the body at any time after a single IV bolus dose can be written as

$$A = A_0 e^{-kt} \quad (14.8)$$

where
  A is the amount of the drug in the body
  A_0 is the initial amount of the drug in the body after IV bolus administration, which is equal to the dose
  k is the first-order elimination rate constant

Since the renal excretion rate of the drug at any time is the product of the renal excretion rate constant and the amount of the drug in the body, the drug renal excretion rate ($\Delta A_e / \Delta t$)-time profile after a single IV bolus dose can be described as

$$\frac{\Delta A_e}{\Delta t} = k_e A_0 e^{-kt} \quad (14.9)$$

Equations 14.8 and 14.9 indicate that both the amount of the drug in the body and the renal excretion rate of the drug after a single IV bolus dose decline at a rate dependent on k, the overall elimination rate constant of the drug. To construct the drug renal excretion rate versus time plot, the experimentally determined renal excretion rate for the drug during each urine collection interval is plotted against the time corresponding to the middle of the urine collection interval (t_{mid}). This is because the calculated drug renal excretion rate represents the average rate of renal drug excretion during the urine collection interval. After a single IV bolus drug administration, a plot of the drug renal excretion rate versus time on the semilog scale is a straight line with y-intercept that equals $k_e A_0$ (or k_e dose) and the slope is $-k/2.303$. This means that the elimination rate constant, the half-life, and the renal excretion rate constant of the drug can be determined from the drug renal excretion rate versus time plot as in Figure 14.2.

The renal excretion rate versus time profile is parallel to the drug amount-time profile and the drug concentration–time profile after a single IV administration when the drug elimination follows first-order kinetics. After extravascular drug administration, the drug amount in the body-time profile increases initially during the absorption phase and then declines during the elimination phase. Since the drug renal excretion rate at any time is the product of k_e and the amount of the drug in the body, the drug renal excretion rate–time profile is always parallel to the drug amount-time profile and drug concentration–time profile. So after extravascular drug administration, the drug renal excretion rate–time profile increases initially during the drug absorption phase and then declines during the elimination phase. The drug elimination rate constant and half-life can be determined from the renal excretion rate–time profile during the elimination phase after extravascular drug administration.

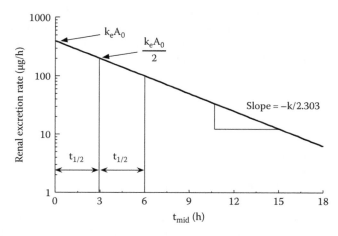

FIGURE 14.2   Slope of the drug renal excretion rate versus time plot on the semilog scale is equal to $-k/2.303$ and the y-intercept is equal to k_e Dose. The elimination rate constant, k, can be determined from the slope of the plot, the elimination half-life can be calculated from k or estimated graphically by determining the time required for any value on the line to decrease by 50%, and k_e can be determined from the y-intercept.

14.5 RENAL CLEARANCE

The CL_R for a drug represents the contribution of the renal excretion pathway to CL_T. The CL_T is defined as the volume of the blood or plasma that is completely cleared of the drug per unit time. Similarly, the CL_R is defined as the volume of the blood or plasma that is completely cleared of the drug per unit time by the kidney. As mentioned previously, the drug renal excretion rate is determined by

$$\frac{\Delta A_e}{\Delta t} = k_e A_{t\text{-mid}} \tag{14.10}$$

where $A_{t\text{-mid}}$ is the amount of drug in the body at the midpoint of the urine collection interval, which is approximately equal to the average amount of the drug during the urine collection interval. Since the amount of drug is the product of the drug concentration and Vd

$$\frac{\Delta A_e}{\Delta t} = k_e VdCp_{t\text{-mid}} \tag{14.11}$$

and

$$\frac{\Delta A_e / \Delta t}{Cp_{t\text{-mid}}} = k_e Vd \tag{14.12}$$

or

$$\frac{\Delta A_e / \Delta t}{Cp_{t\text{-mid}}} = \text{Renal clearance} \tag{14.13}$$

where $Cp_{t\text{-mid}}$ is the drug plasma concentration at the midpoint of the urine collection interval. This means that the drug CL_R can be determined by collecting urine over a certain interval and also obtaining a plasma sample at the middle of the urine collection interval. The drug renal excretion rate is determined as mentioned before and the plasma sample is analyzed for the drug concentration. The CL_R is calculated from the drug renal excretion rate and the plasma drug concentration as in Equation 14.13. Multiple urine collections and plasma samples at the middle of each urine collection can be obtained after a single drug administration to calculate the CL_R during different intervals. When the drug elimination follows first-order kinetics, drug clearance is constant. So the drug CL_R estimated during different intervals should be similar [2].

Equation 14.11 is an equation of a straight line with the y-intercept equal to zero, that is, the line passes through the origin. A plot of the drug renal excretion rate versus the plasma drug concentration at the middle of the urine collection interval on the Cartesian scale is a straight line that passes through the origin, and the slope of the line is equal to the renal clearance as in Figure 14.3. When accurate estimate for the CL_R is required, multiple urine samples and plasma samples are collected

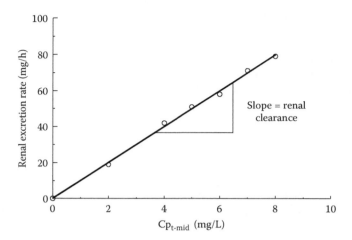

FIGURE 14.3 Drug renal excretion rate versus plasma drug concentration at the middle of the urine collection interval plot. The renal clearance is determined from the slope of the line.

after a single drug administration. The drug renal excretion rate is plotted against the corresponding plasma concentration on the Cartesian scale. The slope of the resulting line is equal to the CL_R.

A similar approach can be used to calculate the CL_R by plotting the renal excretion rate of the drug versus the partial drug AUC (i.e., the area under the curve calculated in plasma during each urine collection interval) on the Cartesian scale. This is because the AUC for the drug during the urine collection interval is correlated with the average plasma drug concentration. A plot of the drug renal excretion rate versus the partial AUC on the Cartesian scale is a straight line that passes through the origin, and the slope of this line is equal to the renal clearance.

The estimated CL_R of the drug can help in determining the mechanism of renal excretion for some drugs. A drug that is not bound to plasma protein and is filtered in the glomeruli and neither secreted nor reabsorbed should have CL_R equal to the GFR. When the estimated drug CL_R is larger than the average GFR, this means that the drug must be actively secreted in the renal tubules, while when the drug CL_R is lower than the average GFR, this means that the drug is filtered in the glomeruli and then reabsorbed in the renal tubules or the drug is filtered in the glomeruli and then secreted and reabsorbed in the renal tubules.

14.5.1 Creatinine Clearance as a Measure of Kidney Function

Creatinine is an endogenous compound that is completely eliminated from the body by the kidney. It is filtered in the glomeruli and neither secreted nor reabsorbed significantly in the renal tubules. So the renal clearance of creatinine represents an accurate measure of the GFR that is correlated with the number of functioning nephrons and the kidney function. The average GFR in a normal adult is 120 mL/min. The creatinine clearance is used as a diagnostic test to evaluate the kidney function. Since the rate of renal creatinine excretion may be affected by physical activity, creatinine clearance is determined in the urine sample collected over a 24 h period to obtain an average estimate for the creatinine renal excretion rate during the day. The creatinine clearance is determined using the following procedures:

1. The patient is asked to collect all the urine over a period of 24 h. All the urine collected is combined to one sample.
2. One plasma sample is obtained to determine the plasma creatinine concentration. Since creatinine plasma concentration is relatively constant, this sample is obtained at any time during the urine collection period and can represent the average creatinine concentration during the urine collection period.
3. The volume of the combined urine sample is determined and the creatinine concentration in the urine sample is measured.
4. The total amount of creatinine excreted during the 24 h collection period is calculated:

Amount of creatinine excreted = Volume of the urine sample
$$\times \text{Urine creatinine concentration}$$

5. The average creatinine renal excretion rate during the 24 h urine collection period is calculated:

$$\text{Renal excretion rate} = \frac{\text{Amount excreted}}{\text{Time of urine collection}} \qquad (14.14)$$

6. The creatinine clearance is calculated from the creatinine renal excretion rate and the plasma creatinine concentration:

$$\text{Creatinine clearance} = \frac{\text{Creatinine excretion rate}}{\text{Creatinine plasma concentration}} \qquad (14.15)$$

14.6 CUMULATIVE AMOUNT OF THE DRUG EXCRETED IN URINE

After a single IV dose of the drug, the renal excretion rate of the drug represents the rate of drug excretion in urine during a certain time interval. If the amount of the drug excreted in urine during each interval is added to the total amount of the drug excreted in urine during the previous intervals, the cumulative amount of the drug excreted in urine is obtained. The cumulative amount of the drug excreted in urine increases exponentially until it reaches a plateau as in Figure 14.4.

The drug renal excretion rate–time profile can be described by Equation 14.9. The total amount of the drug excreted in urine is determined by integrating this equation and substituting time by infinity:

$$\frac{\Delta A_e}{\Delta t} = k_e A_0 e^{-kt}$$

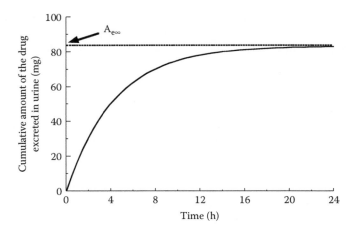

FIGURE 14.4 Cumulative amount of the drug excreted in urine after a single IV dose increases exponentially until it reaches a plateau. The plateau represents the total amount of the drug excreted in urine, $A_{e\infty}$.

$$A_{e\infty} = \frac{k_e}{k} A_0 = \frac{k_e}{k} Dose_{IV} \qquad (14.16)$$

where $A_{e\infty}$ is the total amount of the drug excreted in urine when all the drug is eliminated from the body. This means that after an IV dose of a drug, the total amount of the drug excreted unchanged in urine is a fraction of the administered dose. This fraction (f) is equal to the ratio of the k_e to k and the ratio of the CL_R to CL_T as in Equation 14.18:

$$A_{e\infty} = \frac{k_e Vd}{kVd} Dose_{IV} = \frac{\text{Renal clearance}}{\text{Total body clearance}} Dose_{IV} \qquad (14.17)$$

and

$$f = \frac{A_{e\infty}}{Dose_{IV}} = \frac{k_e}{k} = \frac{CL_R}{CL_T} \qquad (14.18)$$

When the entire dose of the drug is excreted unchanged in urine, this indicates that CL_R is equal to CL_T and k_e is equal to k, while when no drug is excreted unchanged in urine, the CL_R and k_e will be equal to zero. The same principle can be applied for the renal drug excretion after extravascular drug administration. In this case, only a fraction of the administered dose reaches the systemic circulation. For extravascular drug administration, the fraction of the bioavailable dose that is excreted unchanged in urine, f, is equal to the ratio of the k_e to k and the ratio of CL_R to CL_T as in Equation 14.19:

$$f = \frac{A_{e\infty}}{FD} = \frac{k_e}{k} = \frac{CL_R}{CL_T} \qquad (14.19)$$

The fraction of the bioavailable dose excreted unchanged in urine is constant for the same drug in the same patient. So after administration of different products for the same active drug, the cumulative amount of the drug excreted unchanged in urine will be larger for the product with higher bioavailability. This principle is used in the determination of product bioavailability and also in testing for bioequivalence of different drug products.

14.6.1 Determination of the Drug Bioavailability from the Cumulative Amount Excreted in Urine

The fraction of the bioavailable dose excreted unchanged in urine is constant for the same drug in the same patient. So after administration of different products for the same active drug, the cumulative amount of the drug excreted unchanged in urine will be larger for the product with higher bioavailability. The absolute bioavailability can be determined from the ratio of the cumulative amount of the drug excreted unchanged in urine after oral and after IV administration of the same dose of the same drug:

$$F_{absolute} = \frac{A_{e\infty\ oral}}{A_{e\infty\ IV}}$$

(14.20)

Also, the renal excretion rate data can be used to determine the relative bioavailability of different drug products for the same active drug after extravascular administration. This is determined from the ratio of the cumulative amount of the drug excreted unchanged in urine after administration of the test and standard drug products [3]:

$$F_{relative} = \frac{A_{e\infty\ test}}{A_{e\infty\ standard}}$$

(14.21)

14.6.2 Determination of the Renal Clearance from the Cumulative Amount Excreted in Urine

Equation 14.19 indicates that f, which is the fraction of the bioavailable dose excreted unchanged in urine, is determined from the ratio of the CL_R to the CL_T. Since FD/CL_T is equal to the AUC, the renal clearance can be determined from the amount of the drug excreted unchanged in urine and the drug AUC [2]:

$$CL_R = CL_T \frac{A_{e\infty}}{FD} = \frac{A_{e\infty}}{AUC\Big|_0^\infty}$$

(14.22)

This relationship can be applied for both IV and extravascular drug administration since the drug bioavailability affects both the amount excreted unchanged in urine and the AUC to the same extent.

14.7 DETERMINATION OF THE PHARMACOKINETIC PARAMETERS FROM THE RENAL EXCRETION RATE DATA

14.7.1 ELIMINATION RATE CONSTANT AND HALF-LIFE

The elimination rate constant of the drug is determined from the plot of the drug renal excretion rate versus time after a single IV administration on the semilog scale. The slope of the resulting straight line is equal to $-k/2.303$. The half-life of the drug can be determined graphically from the same plot by determining the time required for the renal excretion rate at any time point to decrease by 50%.

14.7.2 RENAL EXCRETION RATE CONSTANT

The renal excretion rate constant, k_e, can be determined from the renal excretion rate versus time plot on the semilog scale. The y-intercept of this plot is equal to $k_e A_0$. Since A_0 is equal to the dose, k_e can be determined from the value of the y-intercept and the dose. Also, k_e can be determined if both CL_R and Vd are known ($CL_R = k_e Vd$). Furthermore, k_e can be determined if the fraction of dose excreted unchanged in urine after IV administration, f and k, are known ($f = k_e/k$).

14.7.3 VOLUME OF DISTRIBUTION

The Vd of the drug cannot be determined from the renal excretion rate versus time plot. Plasma samples after drug administration are required to estimate Vd. The Vd can be determined if CL_R and k_e are known ($CL_R = k_e Vd$).

14.7.4 RENAL CLEARANCE

The CL_R can be determined from k_e and Vd ($CL_R = k_e Vd$). Also, the CL_R during each urine collection interval is determined from the ratio of the renal excretion rate and the average plasma concentration during the urine collection interval. When serial urine and plasma samples are obtained, CL_R can be determined from the slope of the plot of the renal excretion rate versus the plasma concentration at the midpoint of the urine collection interval on the Cartesian scale. Also, a lot of the drug renal excretion rate versus the partial AUC during each urine collection interval on the Cartesian scale has a slope equal to the CL_R. Furthermore, the CL_R can be determined from the total amount of the drug excreted unchanged in urine and the drug AUC ($CL_R = A_{e\infty}/AUC$). Additionally, the CL_R can be calculated if the fraction of the IV dose excreted unchanged in urine and the CL_T are known ($f = CL_R/CL_T$).

14.7.5 FRACTION OF DOSE EXCRETED UNCHANGED IN URINE

The fraction of the bioavailable dose that is excreted unchanged in urine is determined from the ratios of k_e/k, CL_R/CL_T, or $A_{e\infty}/FDose$.

14.7.6 BIOAVAILABILITY

The absolute bioavailability is determined from the ratio of $A_{e\infty}$ after oral and IV administration of the same dose of the drug ($F = A_{e\infty}$ oral/$A_{e\infty}$ IV), while the relative bioavailability is determined from the ratio of $A_{e\infty}$ after administration of the test and standard products.

Example

After an IV injection of 500 mg of a new drug to a patient, the following data were obtained:

Collection Interval (h)	Urine Volume (mL)	Urine Concentration (mg/mL)	$Cp_{t\text{-mid}}$ (mg/L)
0–2	119	0.60	22.3
2–4	81	0.70	17.7
4–8	160	0.50	12.5
8–12	220	0.23	7.88
12–18	284	0.15	4.42
18–24	212	0.10	2.21

a. Estimate the biological half-life of this drug in this patient using the urinary excretion data.
b. Estimate the renal clearance of this drug in this patient.
c. Calculate the fraction of the administered dose excreted unchanged in the urine from the available data.

Answer

Use the following available information to calculate the renal excretion rate:

Collection Interval (h)	Urine Volume (mL)	Urine Concentration (mg/mL)	Amount Excreted (mg/L)	Renal Excretion Rate (mg/h)	$Cp_{t\text{-mid}}$ (mg/L)
0–2	119	0.60	71.4	35.7	22.3
2–4	81	0.70	56.7	28.35	17.7
4–8	160	0.50	80.0	20.00	12.5
8–12	220	0.23	50.6	12.65	7.88
12–18	284	0.15	42.6	7.10	4.42
18–24	212	0.10	21.2	3.53	2.21

a. The half-life can be estimated from the renal excretion rate versus time plot as in Figure 14.5.
The half-life is = 6 h $k = 0.1155 \, h^{-1}$
The elimination rate constant can also be determined from the slope of the line.

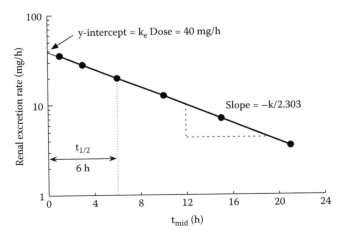

FIGURE 14.5 Half-life and the elimination rate constant are determined from the renal excretion rate versus time plot.

    b. The CL_R can be estimated from the slope of the renal excretion rate versus plasma concentration plot as in Figure 14.6.
       The renal clearance = 1.6 L/h
    c. The fraction excreted unchanged in urine can be calculated from the ratio of the (k_e/k) or (CL_R/CL_T).

The plasma concentration–time data can be used to determine the CL_T. Plot the plasma concentration–time data and calculate the Vd, k, and CL_T:

$$CL_T = 2.31 \text{ L/h}$$

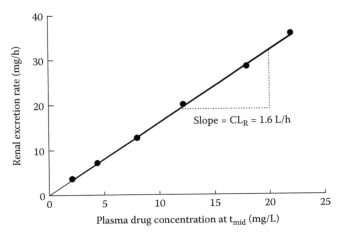

FIGURE 14.6 Renal excretion rate versus drug plasma concentration at the middle of the urine collection interval.

$$\text{Fraction} = \frac{CL_R}{CL_T} = \frac{1.6\,L/h}{2.31\,L/h} = 0.69$$

Also, the renal excretion rate constant can be calculated from the y-intercept of the renal excretion rate–time profile:

$$\text{y-intercept} = k_e\,\text{Dose} = k_e\,500\,mg = 40\,mg/h$$

$$k_e = 0.08\,h^{-1}$$

$$\text{Fraction} = \frac{k_e}{k} = \frac{0.08\,h^{-1}}{0.1155\,h^{-1}} = 0.69$$

14.8 EFFECT OF CHANGING THE PHARMACOKINETIC PARAMETERS ON THE URINARY EXCRETION OF DRUGS

The renal excretion rate–time profile after a single IV dose declines at a rate dependent on the drug elimination rate constant. The y-intercept for the drug renal excretion rate–time profile on the semilog scale is equal to $k_e \times$ Dose, while the fraction of the IV dose excreted unchanged in urine is determined from the ratio of k_e/k and CL_R/CL_T.

14.8.1 Pharmacokinetic Simulation Exercise

Pharmacokinetic simulations can be used to examine how the change in the pharmacokinetic parameters affects the drug renal excretion rate–time profile and the cumulative renal drug excretion. The drug renal excretion rate–time profile is simulated using an average value of each of the pharmacokinetic parameters, and the renal excretion rate–time profile and the cumulative renal drug excretion are observed. Then, the pharmacokinetic parameters are changed one parameter at a time while keeping all the other parameters constant, and the simulation is repeated. The resulting profile is examined to see how the change affects the drug renal excretion rate–time profile and the cumulative renal drug excretion. The plotting exercise of the renal drug elimination module in the basic pharmacokinetic concept section of the companion CD to this textbook can be used to run these simulations.

14.8.1.1 Dose

The renal excretion rate–time plots after administration of increasing doses on the semilog scale are linear with the same slope since k is constant. However, the initial renal excretion rate (y-intercept = $k_e \times$ Dose) after administration of different doses is proportional to the administered dose since k_e is constant. Administration of increasing doses of the drug results in proportional increase in the cumulative (total) amount of the drug excreted unchanged in urine if k_e and k remain constant (the fraction of the dose excreted unchanged in urine is constant).

14.8.1.2 Total Body Clearance

The change in CL_T while CL_R remains constant means that the nonrenal clearance changes. The CL_T can change without affecting the CL_R, for example, in patients with liver dysfunction or in case of inhibition of the metabolizing enzymes that can decrease the metabolic drug clearance and CL_T without affecting CL_R. Assuming that Vd does not change, the rate of decline of the renal excretion rate–time plot on the semilog scale is slower when CL_T is reduced because the slope of this plot is equal to $-k/2.303$ ($k = CL_T/Vd$). Also, enzyme induction increases CL_T without affecting CL_R. In this case if Vd remains constant, the rate of decline of the renal excretion rate–time plot on the semilog scale is faster because the k is larger.

The fraction of the administered dose excreted unchanged in urine is determined from the ratio of CL_R/CL_T. After administration of the same dose, the cumulative amount of the drug excreted unchanged in urine is larger in the case of liver dysfunction and inhibition of the metabolizing enzymes, if the drug is eliminated by renal excretion and hepatic metabolism. However, in the case of enzyme induction, there is a decrease in the ratio of CL_R/CL_T, which makes smaller fraction of the dose excreted unchanged in urine.

14.8.1.3 Renal Clearance

The change in CL_R is usually accompanied by a change in CL_T because the CL_T is the sum of the clearances of all eliminating organs. However, the decrease in CL_R, for example, in the case of a patient with renal dysfunction usually causes less than proportional decrease in the CL_T. This is because the nonrenal clearance is usually not affected by the decrease in kidney function. If the decrease in kidney function does not affect Vd of the drug, the drug renal excretion rate versus time plot declines at slower rate. This is because the slope of this plot depends on k, which decreases due to the reduction in CL_T ($k = CL_T/Vd$).

The fraction of the administered dose excreted unchanged in urine is determined from the ratio of CL_R/CL_T. As mentioned earlier, the decrease in CL_R is usually accompanied by less than proportional decrease in CL_T, so the ratio of CL_R to the CL_T usually decreases in patients with renal dysfunction. So after administration of the same dose, the amount of the drug excreted unchanged in urine is smaller in patients with renal dysfunction. This makes the fraction of dose excreted unchanged in urine to be smaller in patients with renal dysfunction.

PRACTICE PROBLEMS

14.1 The urine was collected in a patient over a 24 h period to determine the creatinine clearance. The total volume of urine collected was 1800 mL and the creatinine concentration in urine was 0.4 mg/mL. If the serum creatinine determined in this patient was 1 mg/dL (1 mg/100 mL)

   a. Calculate the amount of creatinine excreted (eliminated) during the 24 h period.
   b. Calculate the average renal excretion rate of creatinine during the 24 h period.
   c. Calculate the creatinine clearance in this patient.
   d. Calculate the renal clearance of creatinine in this patient.

14.2 A patient received a single 1000 mg IV dose of an antibiotic. Urine and plasma samples were collected and the following results were obtained:

Interval (h)	Urine Volume (mL)	Urine Concentration (µg/mL)	Plasma Concentration $(Cp_{t\text{-mid}})$ (µg/mL)
0–1	67	2.1	Not determined
1–2	70	1.01	Not determined
2–4	100	0.5	0.5 µg/mL at time 3 h
4–8	250	0.05	Very low

a. Calculate the average renal excretion rate of the drug during the first urine collection interval (0–1 h).

b. Calculate the average renal excretion rate of the drug during the third urine collection interval (2–4 h).

c. Calculate the renal clearance of this drug in this patient.

d. What is the slope of the renal excretion rate versus time plot on a semilog graph paper?

14.3 A new antihypertensive drug is rapidly but incompletely absorbed.

• When 800 mg is given intravenously to normal volunteers:
  800 mg is recovered in urine unchanged from time 0 to ∞
  The AUC obtained from time zero to infinity is 400 mg h/L.

• When 400 mg is given orally:
  Only 350 mg of the drug is recovered unchanged in urine from time 0 to ∞
  The elimination half-life is 8 h.

a. What is the bioavailability of this drug after oral administration?

14.4 After an IV injection of 10 mg of a new drug to a patient, the following data were obtained:

Collection Interval (day)	Urine Volume (mL)	Urinary Drug Concentration (µg/mL)	$Cp_{t\text{-mid}}$ (µg/L)
0–1	1250	1.8	16.0
1–2	1500	0.984	10.4
2–3	1750	0.544	6.8
3–4	1380	0.448	4.4
4–5	1630	0.248	2.9
5–7	3130	0.136	1.5

a. Using a graphical method, estimate the biological half-life of this drug in this patient.

b. Calculate the renal clearance and the total body clearance of this drug in this patient.

c. Calculate the fraction of the administered dose excreted unchanged in the urine from the aforementioned data.

d. Estimate how much drug is in the body 5 days after the dose was administered.

e. Assuming that the unexcreted portion of this drug is metabolized, determine its metabolic rate constant (k_m) in this patient.

14.5 After an IV injection of 1000 mg of a new drug to a patient, the following data were obtained:

Collection Interval (h)	Urine Volume (mL)	Urinary Concentration (mg/mL)	$Cp_{t\text{-mid}}$ (mg/L)
0–2	125	1.776	15.9
2–4	150	0.933	10.0
4–6	175	0.504	6.3
6–8	138	0.403	4.97
8–10	163	0.215	2.51
10–14	313	0.112	1.24

a. Using a graphical method, estimate the biological half-life of this drug in this patient.
b. Calculate the renal clearance of this drug in this patient.
c. Calculate the fraction of the administered dose excreted unchanged in the urine from the aforementioned data.
d. Assuming that the unexcreted portion of this drug is metabolized, determine its metabolic rate constant (k_m) in this patient.

REFERENCES

1. Cafruny EJ (1977) Renal tubular handling of drugs. *Am J Med* 62:490–496.
2. Tucker GT (1981) Measurement of the renal clearance of drugs. *Br J Clin Pharm* 12:761–770.
3. U.S. Code of Federal Regulations (April 2010) Title 21-Food and Drugs, Chapter I, Food and Drug Administration, Department of Health and Human Services, Sub-chapter D, Drugs for human use, Part 320, Bioavailability and Bioequivalence Requirements, Sec. 24.

15 Metabolite Pharmacokinetics

OBJECTIVES

After completing this chapter you should be able to

- Discuss the importance of studying metabolite pharmacokinetics after a single and repeated drug administration
- Describe the metabolic pathways involved in the formation of the metabolites after parent drug administration
- Discuss the models that can be used to describe the formation of metabolites after administration of the parent drug
- Identify the factors that affect the metabolite formation after administration of the parent drug
- Calculate the different metabolite pharmacokinetic parameters after IV administration of the parent drug
- Analyze the effect of changing each of the drug and metabolite pharmacokinetic parameters on the drug and metabolite profiles after a single drug administration
- Analyze the effect of changing each of the drug and metabolite pharmacokinetic parameters on the drug and metabolite profiles at steady state during multiple drug administration

15.1   INTRODUCTION

Drug elimination from the body involves excretion of the unchanged drug through various excretion pathways or drug metabolism via the different metabolic pathways. Drug metabolism involves enzymatic or chemical modification of the chemical structure of the drug molecule to form a new chemical entity called metabolite. Studying of the metabolite pharmacokinetics is important because in most cases the effect of the drug disappears when the drug is metabolized to pharmacologically inactive metabolites. However, some of the formed metabolites are pharmacologically active, and some metabolites are reactive and can cause serious adverse effects.

Procainamide is an antiarrhythmic drug metabolized to n-acetyl procainamide (NAPA) that also possesses antiarrhythmic activity similar to the parent drug. So the antiarrhythmic effect observed after administration of procainamide results from both the parent drug and the metabolite. Cocaethylene (CE) is a cocaine metabolite formed only when cocaine is abused simultaneously with alcohol, which is a commonly used combination. This metabolite is more lethal than cocaine with regard to the cardiovascular complications and has central nervous system stimulant activity similar in potency to that of cocaine. Also, the antiepileptic drug carbamazepine is metabolized to carbamazepine epioxide that is responsible for most of the parent drug toxicity. So studying the factors that affect the metabolite formation and elimination and the general pharmacokinetic behavior of the metabolites is necessary for accurate prediction of the therapeutic and the adverse effects produced by the parent drug and its metabolite(s).

15.2   DRUG METABOLIC PATHWAYS

Drug metabolism, also referred to as drug biotransformation or drug detoxification, usually involves enzymatic modification of the chemical structure of a drug to form one or more metabolites. This modification of the drug chemical structure causes change (increase or decrease) in the pharmacological and adverse effects of the drugs. The metabolites are usually more polar than their parent drugs and are excreted rapidly from the body by the different excretion mechanisms. However, there are exceptions to this general rule where the metabolite half-life is longer than that of the parent drug. Drug metabolism is usually mediated by specialized enzyme systems that can be induced or inhibited resulting in modification of the rate of the drug metabolic process. Also, different drugs that are metabolized through the same metabolic pathway can compete for the same enzyme system. The drug with higher affinity to the enzyme slows or inhibits the metabolism of the drug with lower enzyme affinity. Furthermore, many nutritional, environmental, and genetic factors in addition to alcohol and smoking can affect the activity of the drug metabolizing enzymes. So drug metabolism is one of the important mechanisms by which clinically significant drug–drug interactions occurs.

15.2.1   CLASSIFICATION OF THE METABOLIC REACTIONS

The drug metabolic pathways are classified into two major groups of reactions: phase I and phase II metabolic reactions [1].

15.2.1.1   Phase I Metabolic Reactions

These metabolic reactions are also known as functionalization reactions or non-synthetic reactions. They involve the introduction of polar function groups such as hydroxyl group, primary amines, carboxylic acids, etc., to form more polar metabolites. Phase I metabolic reactions do not have to occur before phase II reactions because some drugs are metabolized directly by phase II reactions without going through phase I metabolism. Also, there are examples of some metabolites that are formed by phase II metabolic reactions that undergo further metabolism through phase I metabolic reactions. The most common phase I reactions include oxidation, reduction, and hydrolysis. Oxidation reactions usually involve addition of oxygen or removal of hydrogen such as aliphatic and aromatic hydroxylation, n-dealkylation, o-dealkylation, s-dealkylation, n-oxidation, s-oxidation, deamination, dehalogenation, etc. These oxidation reactions are mediated mainly by the cytochrome P450 (CYP450) monooxygenase enzyme system in addition to other enzyme systems.

TABLE 15.1

Most Common Enzyme Systems Involved in the Different Types of Phase I and Phase II Metabolic Reactions

Phase	Reaction Type	Enzyme System
I	Oxidation	Cytochrome P450 monooxygenase system
		Flavin-containing monooxygenase system
		Alcohol dehydrogenase
		Aldehyde dehydrogenase
		Monoamine oxidase
		Co-oxidation by peroxidases
	Reduction	NADPH-cytochrome P450 reductase
		Reduced cytochrome P450
	Hydrolysis	Esterases
		Amidases
		Epoxide hydrolase
II	Methylation	Methyltransferase
	Sulfation	Glutathione S-transferases
		Sulfotransferases
	Acetylation	N-acetyltransferase
		Amino acid N-acyl transferases
	Glucuronidation	UDP-glucuronosyltransferases

The phase I reduction reactions involve removal of oxygen or addition of hydrogen. Most of the products of the oxidative metabolism are substrates for the reductive reactions causing redox cycling, with the equilibrium between the oxidation and reduction reactions determined by the balance of cofactors and oxygen concentration. The phase I hydrolysis reactions include hydrolysis of esters, hydrolysis of amides including the peptides, and hydration of epoxides. The most common enzyme systems involved in phase I metabolism are listed in Table 15.1.

15.2.1.2 Phase II Metabolic Reactions

These metabolic reactions are also known as conjugation reactions or synthetic reactions. Phase II reactions usually involve formation of conjugates between the drug and other compounds such as glucuronic acid, glutathione, amino acids, and others. The most common sites on the drug chemical structure where conjugation reactions occur include carboxyl, hydroxyl, amino, and sulfhydryl groups. The products of phase II metabolic reactions have increased molecular weight and are usually inactive. The most common enzyme systems involved in phase II metabolism are listed in Table 15.1.

15.2.2 CYTOCHROME P450

CYP450 is a superfamily of metabolizing enzymes that are responsible for approximately 75% of the total drug metabolism in humans. It contains heme cofactors, so it is considered a hemoprotein. The reduced iron in the heme cofactor can produce a colored adduct with carbon monoxide that can absorb light at a wavelength of 450 nm, which gave this superfamily of enzymes the name CYP450. This superfamily of metabolizing enzymes is classified into families and subfamilies depending on the degree of structure similarity of the different enzymes [2,3]. The CYP enzymes in the same family have to share ≥40% of the amino acid identity, while CYP enzymes in the same subfamily must share ≥55% amino acid identity. Individual enzymes within the same subfamily are identified based on their catalytic specificity. The nomenclature of the specific CYP metabolizing enzyme includes its family and the subfamily as follows:

CYP enzymes: CYP
Family: 1–51 and up (Arabic numerals)
Subfamily: A–Z (capital letters)
Individual enzyme within a subfamily: 1 to any number (Arabic numerals)

For example, CYP3C9 is the CYP metabolizing enzyme that belongs to family number 3, subfamily C, and it is the ninth identified enzyme within this subfamily. In humans, most of the drugs are metabolized by CYP families 1, 2, and 3.

The CYP metabolizing enzymes are present in many organs including the liver, kidney, lung, gastrointestinal tract, brain, nasal mucosa, and skin. However, the special importance of the role of hepatic CYP enzymes in drug metabolism arises from the existence of large amount of enzymes in the liver and the high hepatic blood flow, which exposes large amount of the drug in the systemic circulation to the hepatic CYP enzymes, and also the contribution of the hepatic drug metabolism to the presystemic metabolism of orally administered drugs. The different CYP metabolizing enzymes have different specificities for the substrates and the metabolic reaction that they can catalyze. The expression of the different CYP enzymes is different, which results in different capacities for the different metabolic reactions catalyzed by these CYP enzymes. The most abundant CYP in the liver, for example, is the CYP3A subfamily that is involved in the metabolism of approximately 33% of the marketed drugs. The CYP metabolizing enzymes are primarily membrane-associated proteins located in the inner membrane of the mitochondria or in the endoplasmic reticulum of cells. So the drugs have to cross the cell membrane to come in contact with the metabolizing enzymes and get metabolized. This can explain why relatively lipophilic drugs are usually eliminated by metabolism, while hydrophilic drugs that cannot penetrate the cell membrane are mainly excreted unchanged from the body.

The information about the substrates, inducers, and inhibitors for each specific CYP enzyme is continuously collected and updated. Determination of the specific CYP enzymes involved in the metabolism of a particular drug is important in identifying the potential drug interactions for that drug. This is an important component in the new drug development process. Also, the amount of a particular CYP metabolizing enzyme can vary in different individuals resulting in variation in the drug metabolic rate and the overall drug elimination rate in different individuals. The variation in the specific CYP expression can result from normal interindividual variability that causes small variability in the drug metabolic rate in different individuals. However, the variation in the specific CYP expression can be genetically mediated and results in large difference in the expression of specific CYP between individuals. This large variability can cause significant difference in the rate of drug metabolism and drug elimination in different individuals. The variation in the drug metabolic rate that results from genetic factors is termed genetic polymorphism in drug metabolism.

15.3   METABOLITE PHARMACOKINETICS

Drugs can be metabolized through different metabolic pathways to one or more metabolites, and more than one metabolite can be detected simultaneously in the body as in Figure 15.1. Some drugs are metabolized to different metabolites through parallel metabolic pathways. This means that the different metabolites are formed from the parent drug, and the formed metabolites are then eliminated from the body (parallel metabolism). In some other drugs, the formed metabolite is further metabolized to another metabolite, which is then excreted from the body as illustrated in Figure 15.2 (sequential metabolism).

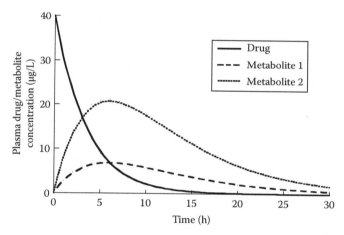

FIGURE 15.1   Plasma drug and metabolite concentration–time profiles after a single IV administration of the drug that is metabolized to two different metabolites.

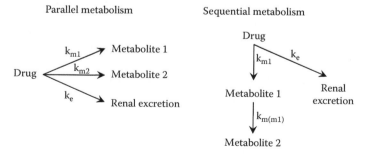

FIGURE 15.2   Schematic presentation of the parallel and sequential drug metabolism. The rate constants k_{m1} and k_{m2} are the drug metabolic rate constants for the formation of metabolite 1 and metabolite 2, respectively, k_e is the drug renal excretion rate constant, and $k_{m(m1)}$ is the metabolic rate constant for metabolite 1 in the sequential metabolism example.

When a drug is eliminated via parallel metabolic pathways, the amount of the drug that is metabolized through each pathway is proportional to the clearance (and the rate constant) associated with each metabolic pathway, assuming first-order elimination. Taking the parallel metabolism example in Figure 15.2, the CL_T is the sum of the metabolic clearance responsible for the formation of metabolite 1, the metabolic clearance responsible for the formation of metabolite 2, and the renal clearance as in Equation 15.1:

$$CL_T = CL_{m1} + CL_{m2} + CL_R \qquad (15.1)$$

Also, the overall elimination rate constant for the drug, k, is the sum of the rate constants associated with the three pathways as in Equation 15.2:

$$k = k_{m1} + k_{m2} + k_e \qquad (15.2)$$

When a drug is eliminated by different pathways including the formation of a metabolite, the rate of drug elimination through the pathway responsible for the formation of the metabolite is the same as the rate of formation of the metabolite if the difference in molecular weight between the drug and the metabolite is considered. So for the parallel metabolism example in Figure 15.2, the rate of drug elimination by the pathway that forms metabolite 1 is the same as the rate of formation of metabolite 1, and the rate of drug elimination through the pathway that forms metabolite 2 is the same as the rate of formation of metabolite 2, if the rates are calculated in terms of mole/time. Since the rate of any first-order process is the product of the first-order rate constant for the process and the amount of the compound available for the process, the rate of each of the three parallel processes in Figure 15.2 can be calculated as follows:

The rate of formation of metabolite $1 = A\,k_{m1}$
The rate of formation of metabolite $2 = A\,k_{m2}$
The rate of urinary excretion $= A\,k_e$

The fraction of the dose of the drug that is metabolized to metabolite 1, f_{m1}, is

$$f_{m1} = \frac{k_{m1}}{k_{m1} + k_{m2} + k_e} = \frac{k_{m1}}{k} \qquad (15.3)$$

while the fraction of dose that is metabolized to metabolite 2, f_{m2}, is

$$f_{m2} = \frac{k_{m2}}{k_{m1} + k_{m2} + k_e} = \frac{k_{m2}}{k} \qquad (15.4)$$

and the fraction of dose excreted unchanged in urine, f, is

$$f = \frac{k_e}{k_{m1} + k_{m2} + k_e} = \frac{k_e}{k} \qquad (15.5)$$

15.4 SIMPLE MODEL FOR METABOLITE PHARMACOKINETICS

The simple pharmacokinetic model for drug metabolism described by the scheme in Figure 15.3 has the following assumptions [4]:

- The drug is administered as a single IV bolus dose.
- The drug is completely metabolized to one metabolite by a first-order process.
- The metabolite is completely excreted in urine by a first-order process.
- The metabolite is not converted back to the parent drug.
- The metabolite and the parent drug follow one-compartment pharmacokinetic model.
- The amount and the concentration of the drug and the metabolite are expressed in moles and moles/volume to account for the difference in molecular weight of the drug and the metabolite.

In this model, the rate of drug elimination is equal to the rate of formation of the metabolite because the drug is eliminated by a single elimination pathway. The rate of metabolite formation and elimination can be expressed as follows:

The rate of metabolite formation = Ak
The rate of metabolite elimination = $A_{(m)}k_{(m)}$

The rate of change of the amount of metabolite in the body is the difference between the rate of metabolite formation and the rate of metabolite elimination:

$$\frac{dA_{(m)}}{dt} = Ak - A_{(m)}k_{(m)} \tag{15.6}$$

By integration of Equation 15.6,

$$A_{(m)} = \frac{kD}{k_{(m)} - k}(e^{-kt} - e^{-k_{(m)}t}) \tag{15.7}$$

In order to obtain an expression that describes the time course for the metabolite concentration in the body, Equation 15.7 can be divided by the volume of distribution of the metabolite $V_{(m)}$:

$$Cp_{(m)} = \frac{kD}{Vd_{(m)}(k_{(m)} - k)}(e^{-kt} - e^{-k_{(m)}t}) \tag{15.8}$$

Equation 15.8 describes the time course for the plasma metabolite concentration at any time (t). This expression is biexponential because it describes two different

$$A \xrightarrow{\;k\;} A_m \xrightarrow{\;k_{(m)}\;} A_{e\,(m)}$$

FIGURE 15.3 Schematic presentation of a simple pharmacokinetic model for drug metabolism. In this model, A is the amount of drug in the body, k is the first-order rate constant for drug elimination, $A_{(m)}$ is the amount of metabolite, and $k_{(m)}$ is the first-order rate constant for the elimination of the metabolite.

processes: the formation and the elimination of the metabolite. The two exponential terms in Equation 15.8 include the drug elimination rate constant, which is the same as the metabolite formation rate constant in the model, and the metabolite elimination rate constant.

At time zero, there is no metabolite in the body and $Cp_{(m)}$ is equal to zero. After drug administration, the amount of metabolite in the body starts to increase because the rate of metabolite formation is more than the rate of its elimination. As time proceeds, the rate of metabolite formation decreases and the rate of metabolite elimination increases. When the metabolite formation rate becomes equal to the metabolite elimination rate, the plasma metabolite concentration reaches a maximum value $C_{max(m)}$. The time when the metabolite plasma concentration is at its maximum value is called $t_{max(m)}$. After $t_{max(m)}$, the rate of metabolite elimination is larger than the rate of metabolite formation and the metabolite plasma concentration decreases. The plasma drug and metabolite concentration–time profiles after IV administration of a single dose of the drug are illustrated in Figure 15.4.

After drug administration, the metabolite formed is a new chemical entity that has pharmacokinetic behavior different from that of the parent drug. The elimination rate constant, half-life, volume of distribution, clearance, and area under the curve for the metabolite are different from the parameters of the parent drug. So the plasma concentration–time profile for the drug and the metabolite are usually different because of the difference in the pharmacokinetic parameters for the drug and metabolite. For example, in the simple model described earlier and after IV drug administration, the molar amount of the metabolite formed in vivo is equal to the molar amount of the drug administered because the model assumes a single elimination pathway. However, the AUC for the drug and the metabolite is always different because the AUC of any compound is dependent on the amount of compound that reaches the systemic circulation and the clearance of that compound.

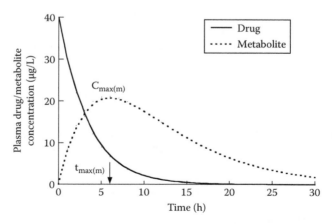

FIGURE 15.4 Plasma drug and metabolite concentration–time profiles after IV administration of a single dose of the drug.

So although the amount of the drug and the metabolite that reaches the systemic circulation is equal on the molar basis, the clearances of the drug and the metabolite are different.

15.4.1 METABOLITE CONCENTRATION–TIME PROFILE

The plasma metabolite concentration–time profile after administration of the parent drug falls into one of two major categories based on the magnitude of the metabolite elimination rate constant relative to the drug elimination rate constant. When the metabolite elimination is slower than the drug elimination, the terminal phase of the metabolite profile depends on the elimination rate of the metabolite, while when the metabolite elimination is faster than the drug elimination, the decline in the metabolite profile depends on the elimination rate of the drug and also on the formation rate of the metabolite [4].

15.4.1.1 Elimination Rate Limitation

When $k_{(m)} < k$: This is the situation when the metabolite is eliminated at a slower rate compared to the parent drug, so the half-life of the metabolite is longer than the half-life of the parent drug. After a single IV dose of the drug, the slope of the terminal phase of the metabolite concentration–time profile on the semilog scale reflects the elimination rate of the metabolite as in Figure 15.5. The metabolite concentration–time profile increases initially and then decreases. When the parent drug is completely eliminated, no more metabolite is formed and the metabolite concentration–time profile declines at a rate dependent on the metabolite elimination rate constant, slope $= -k_{(m)}/2.303$. This is usually observed after five half-lives of the drug when more than 95% of the drug is eliminated and the metabolite formation becomes negligible. The slope of the terminal metabolite concentration–time profile

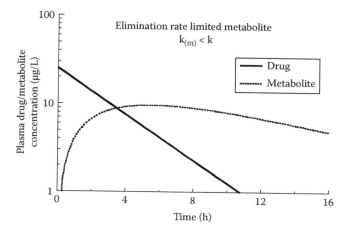

FIGURE 15.5 Plasma drug and metabolite concentration–time profiles after IV administration of a single dose of the drug when the metabolite elimination rate constant is smaller than the drug elimination rate constant.

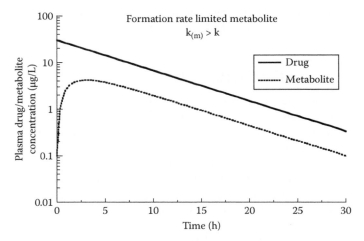

FIGURE 15.6 Drug and metabolite concentration–time profiles after IV administration of a single dose of the drug when the metabolite elimination rate constant is larger than the drug elimination rate constant.

is smaller than the slope of the drug concentration–time profile because $k_{(m)}$ is <k; however, the plasma concentration of the metabolite can be lower or higher than the plasma concentration of the parent drug. The profile of the metabolite in this case is described as elimination rate limited.

15.4.1.2 Formation Rate Limitation

When $k_{(m)} > k$: This is the situation when the metabolite is eliminated faster than the parent drug, so the half-life of the metabolite is shorter than the half-life of the parent drug. After IV bolus dose of the drug, the metabolite concentration–time profile increases initially and then decreases. The slope of the decline phase of the metabolite concentration–time profile on the semilog scale is similar to the slope of the drug concentration–time profile as in Figure 15.6. The slope of the decline phase of the metabolite concentration–time profile does not reflect the rate of metabolite elimination, but it reflects the rate of drug elimination, slope = −k/2.303. Since the rate of drug elimination is the same as the rate of the metabolite formation, the decline in the metabolite profile reflects the metabolite formation rate. The profile of the metabolite in this case is described as formation rate limited.

15.4.2 MATHEMATICAL DESCRIPTION OF THE ELIMINATION RATE AND FORMATION RATE LIMITED METABOLITES

The metabolite plasma concentration–time profile after administration of the parent drug is described by Equation 15.8:

$$Cp_{(m)} = \frac{kD}{Vd_{(m)}(k_{(m)} - k)}(e^{-kt} - e^{-k_{(m)}t})$$

When $k_{(m)} < k$ (i.e., elimination rate limited metabolites), as time increases the term e^{-kt} approaches zero faster than the term $e^{-k_{(m)}t}$. At time longer than five half-lives of the drug, the term e^{-kt} becomes very small and negligible, and Equation 15.8 is reduced to

$$Cp_{(m)} = \frac{kD}{Vd_{(m)}(k_{(m)} - k)} e^{-k_{(m)}t} \tag{15.9}$$

Equation 15.9 indicates that when the drug is completely eliminated and the metabolite formation rate is equal to zero, the decline in metabolite concentration–time profile depends on the elimination rate of the metabolite. The slope of the decline phase of the metabolite concentration–time profile on the semilog scale is equal to $-k_{(m)}/2.303$.

When $k_{(m)} > k$ (i.e., formation rate limited metabolites), as time increases the term $e^{-k_{(m)}t}$ approaches zero faster than the term e^{-kt}. So at time longer than five half-lives of the metabolite, the term $e^{-k_{(m)}t}$ becomes very small and negligible, and Equation 15.8 is reduced to

$$Cp_{(m)} = \frac{kD}{Vd_{(m)}(k_{(m)} - k)} e^{-kt} \tag{15.10}$$

Equation 15.10 indicates that the decline phase of the metabolite concentration–time profile depends on the drug elimination rate that is equal to the metabolite formation rate. The decline in metabolite concentration is parallel to the decline of the parent drug. The slope of the decline phase of the metabolite concentration–time profile on the semilog scale is equal to $-k/2.303$.

15.4.3 TIME TO ACHIEVE THE MAXIMUM METABOLITE CONCENTRATION

The time required to reach the maximum metabolite concentration is determined by differentiation of the equation that describes the metabolite concentration–time profile (Equation 15.8). At $t_{max(m)}$, the rate of change of the metabolite concentration is equal to zero, so the differentiation of Equation 15.8 is equal to zero at $t_{max(m)}$. The time of the maximum metabolite concentration is as follows:

$$t_{max(m)} = \frac{\ln(k_{(m)}/k)}{k_{(m)} - k} \tag{15.11}$$

Equation 15.11 indicates that the time of the maximum metabolite concentration is dependent on the metabolite elimination rate constant and the drug elimination rate constant. The maximum metabolite concentration, $C_{max(m)}$, is determined by substitution for $t_{max(m)}$ in Equation 15.8. As $(k_{(m)}/k)$ increases (i.e., the rate of metabolite elimination is faster than the rate of parent drug elimination), the $C_{max(m)}$ becomes lower and occurs at shorter $t_{max(m)}$.

15.5   GENERAL MODEL FOR METABOLITE KINETICS

The general model for drug metabolism described by the scheme in Figure 15.7 has the following assumptions [4]:

- The drug is administered by a single IV administration.
- A fraction of the drug dose (f_m) is metabolized to one metabolite by a first-order process.
- The metabolite is eliminated by a first-order process.
- The metabolite is not converted back to the parent drug.
- The metabolite and the parent drug follow one-compartment pharmacokinetic model.
- The amount and the concentration of the drug and the metabolite are expressed in moles and moles/volume to account for the difference in molecular weight for the drug and the metabolite.

The difference between the general model and the simple model presented previously is that this general model represents the actual situation in most drugs where only a fraction of the drug is metabolized to the metabolite and the rest of the drug dose is eliminated by other metabolic or nonmetabolic pathways. In this general model, the rate of metabolite formation is not equal to the rate of drug elimination because of the presence of other elimination pathways. The drug metabolism is only a fraction of the overall drug elimination, so the rate of metabolite formation represents a fraction (f_m) of the total rate of elimination of the parent drug.

At any time, the rate of change of the amount of metabolite in the body is the difference between the rate of metabolite formation and the rate of metabolite elimination. Based on the general model presented in Figure 15.7,

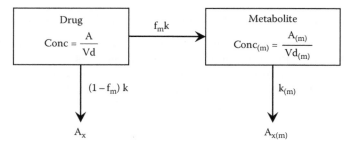

FIGURE 15.7   Schematic presentation of the general model for drug metabolism. Conc and $Conc_{(m)}$ are the plasma drug concentration and metabolite concentration, respectively, A and $A_{(m)}$ are the amount of the parent drug and metabolite, respectively, k is the first-order elimination rate constant for the parent drug, f_m is the fraction of the drug dose that is metabolized to the metabolite of interest, $(1 - f_m)$ is a fraction of the drug dose that is eliminated by the other pathways, Vd and $Vd_{(m)}$ are the volumes of distribution of the drug and the metabolite, respectively, $k_{(m)}$ is the first-order elimination rate constant for the metabolite, A_x is the amount of the parent drug eliminated by pathways other than metabolism, and $A_{x(m)}$ is the amount of metabolite eliminated from the body.

The rate of metabolite formation $= A f_m k$
The rate of metabolite elimination $= A_{(m)} k_{(m)}$

$$\frac{dA_{(m)}}{dt} = f_m k - A_{(m)} k_{(m)} \tag{15.12}$$

By integration of Equation 15.12, the expression that describes the amount of the metabolite in the body at any time after a single IV administration is obtained:

$$A_{(m)} = \frac{f_m k D}{k_{(m)} - k}(e^{-kt} - e^{-k_{(m)}t}) \tag{15.13}$$

Dividing Equation 15.13 by the volume of distribution of the metabolite, $Vd_{(m)}$, gives the expression that describes the plasma metabolite concentration–time profile at any time:

$$Cp_{(m)} = \frac{f_m k D}{Vd_{(m)}(k_{(m)} - k)}(e^{-kt} - e^{-k_{(m)}t}) \tag{15.14}$$

This is the general expression for metabolite concentration after a single IV dose of the drug. This general expression describes the plasma concentration–time profile of the metabolite when only a fraction (f_m) of the administered dose of the parent drug is metabolized and the rest of the dose is excreted by other pathways. Equation 15.8 is a special case of the general expression when all the dose of the parent drug is converted to one metabolite (i.e., $f_m = 1$). In the general model, only a fraction of the parent drug total body clearance becomes responsible for the formation of the metabolite $(f_m CL_T)$. This is the formation clearance of the metabolite. The formed metabolite can have longer or shorter half-life compared to the parent drug. The formed metabolite follows formation rate limitation or elimination rate limitation depending on the relationship between $k_{(m)}$ and k, as described previously.

Integration of the equation that describes the metabolite concentration from time zero to infinity yields the metabolite area under the plasma concentration–time curve, $AUC_{(m)}$. The $AUC_{(m)}$ is dependent on the amount of the metabolite formed in vivo, f_m Dose, and the total body clearance of the metabolite, $CL_{T(m)}$:

$$AUC_{(m)} = \frac{f_m D}{CL_{T(m)}} \tag{15.15}$$

Based on Equation 15.15, when larger amount of the metabolite is formed in vivo, the metabolite AUC is directly proportional to the amount of metabolite formed in vivo and is inversely proportional to the metabolite clearance. The parent drug AUC after IV administration of the parent drug is determined from the dose and CL_T of the drug as follows:

$$AUC = \frac{D}{CL_T} \tag{15.16}$$

Dividing Equation 15.15 by Equation 15.16 gives the ratio of the AUC for the metabolite to that of the parent drug:

$$\frac{AUC_{(m)}}{AUC} = \frac{f_m CL_T}{CL_{T(m)}} \tag{15.17}$$

Equation 15.17 indicates that the ratio of the AUC of the metabolite to that of the parent drug after a single IV dose of the drug is the ratio of the fraction of the total body clearance of the drug responsible for the formation of the metabolite ($f_m CL_T$, metabolite formation clearance) to the total body clearance of the metabolite ($CL_{T(m)}$, metabolite elimination clearance). If the metabolite AUC is larger than the parent drug AUC, this indicates that the metabolite formation clearance is larger than the metabolite elimination clearance.

15.6   ESTIMATION OF THE METABOLITE PHARMACOKINETIC PARAMETERS

When the drug metabolite is pharmacologically active or is responsible for any adverse effect, determination of the metabolite pharmacokinetic parameters becomes very important. Parameters such as the metabolite elimination rate constant, the amount of the metabolite formed, metabolite clearance, and metabolite accumulation during repeated drug administration are very important to characterize the metabolite kinetics. Some metabolite parameters can be determined from administration of the parent drug. However, some other metabolite pharmacokinetic parameters cannot be determined after administration of the parent drug and require administration of the preformed purified metabolite.

15.6.1   METABOLITE ELIMINATION RATE CONSTANT

The method used for the determination of the metabolite elimination rate constant depends on whether the metabolite is elimination rate limited ($k_{(m)} < k$) or formation rate limited ($k_{(m)} > k$).

15.6.1.1   Elimination Rate Limited Metabolites

In this case, $k_{(m)} < k$ and the metabolite half-life ($t_{1/2(m)}$) > the parent drug $t_{1/2}$. So when the parent drug is completely eliminated, the decline in the metabolite profile is dependent on $k_{(m)}$, which can be determined from the slope of the linear part of the metabolite concentration–time profile after drug administration on the semilog scale. Also, $t_{1/2\,(m)}$ can be determined graphically from the same plot:

$$Slope = \frac{-k_{(m)}}{2.303}$$

15.6.1.2   Formation Rate Limited Metabolites

In this case, $k_{(m)} > k$ and $t_{1/2\,(m)} < t_{1/2}$. So the decline in the metabolite profile after administration of the parent drug does not reflect the elimination rate of the metabolite and

$k_{(m)}$ cannot be determined from the elimination phase of the metabolite after drug administration. Indirect methods should be used to determine $k_{(m)}$ after administration of the parent drug. Alternatively, $k_{(m)}$ and $t_{1/2(m)}$ can be determined after administration of the preformed metabolite. This is possible if the metabolite is available in sufficient quantities, and it is safe to administer the preformed metabolite.

15.6.2 FRACTION OF THE PARENT DRUG CONVERTED TO A SPECIFIC METABOLITE

After IV administration of the parent drug, the area under the curve for the metabolite is dependent on the amount of the metabolite formed in vivo and the metabolite total body clearance as in Equation 15.15:

$$AUC_{(m)} = \frac{f_m D}{CL_{T(m)}}$$

Since both f_m and $CL_{T(m)}$ are not known, the amount of metabolite formed after administration of the parent drug cannot be determined just from the information obtained from parent drug administration. For this reason, determination of the amount of metabolite formed after administration of the parent drug or the fraction of parent drug dose converted to a certain metabolite requires knowledge of f_m or $CL_{T(m)}$. The $CL_{T(m)}$ can be determined after IV administration of the preformed purified metabolite as follows:

$$AUC'_{(m)} = \frac{M}{CL'_{T(m)}} \tag{15.18}$$

where
$AUC'_{(m)}$ is the metabolite AUC after metabolite administration
M is the dose of the metabolite
$CL'_{T(m)}$ is the total body clearance of the metabolite after metabolite administration

If equimolar doses of the parent drug and the metabolite are administered (i.e., $D = M$) and because the metabolite clearance should be the same after parent drug administration and metabolite administration (i.e., $CL'_{T(m)} = CL_{T(m)}$), the fraction of the parent drug dose converted to the metabolite can be determined as follows:

$$\frac{AUC_{(m)}}{AUC'_{(m)}} = \frac{f_m D CL'_{T(m)}}{M CL_{T(m)}} = f_m \tag{15.19}$$

The fraction of the parent drug dose converted to the metabolite can be used to calculate the amount of metabolite formed in vivo after administration of the parent drug. If different doses of the metabolite and the parent drug are administered, the metabolite AUC after parent drug administration or after metabolite administration should be normalized for the administered dose. It is necessary to compare the metabolite AUCs resulting from equimolar doses of the parent drug and the metabolite.

Urinary recovery of the metabolite can be used to determine the fraction of parent drug dose converted to a particular metabolite under certain conditions. This is possible only when the formed metabolite is completely excreted unchanged in urine without undergoing sequential metabolism, the metabolite is stable in urine after urinary excretion, and urine is collected completely until all drug and metabolite are completely eliminated.

15.6.3 Metabolite Clearance, $CL_{(m)}$

The total body clearance of the metabolite can be determined after administration of the parent drug only if f_m is known. This is determined by administration of a dose of the parent drug and calculating the $AUC_{(m)}$. When f_m, D, and $AUC_{(m)}$ are known, $CL_{T(m)}$ can be calculated using Equation 15.15. If f_m is not known, administration of the preformed metabolite is necessary for the determination of $CL_{T(m)}$ from Equation 15.18.

15.6.4 Metabolite Volume of Distribution

Determination of the metabolite volume of distribution requires IV administration of the preformed metabolite. The metabolite volume of distribution can be determined as follows:

$$Vd_{(m)} = \frac{M}{Cp_{o(m)}} \tag{15.20}$$

where
    $Vd_{(m)}$ is the metabolite volume of distribution
    M is the dose of the metabolite
    $Cp_{o(m)}$ is the plasma metabolite concentration at time zero

Also, $Vd_{(m)}$ can be determined if $CL_{T(m)}$ and $k_{(m)}$ are known as in Equation 15.21:

$$Vd_{(m)} = \frac{CL_{T(m)}}{k_{(m)}} \tag{15.21}$$

15.6.5 Metabolite Formation Clearance

The metabolite formation clearance is the fraction of the CL_T of the parent drug that is responsible for the formation of a particular metabolite. This can be determined from the CL_T of the parent drug and the fraction of parent drug dose converted to the metabolite as follows:

$$\text{Metabolite formation clearance} = f_m CL_T \tag{15.22}$$

Example

When cocaine (Coc) is administered to human or experimental animals, it is metabolized to two major metabolites, benzoylecgonine (BE) and ecgonine methylester (EME), in addition to several minor metabolites. After concurrent abuse of cocaine and ethanol, CE, which is a pharmacologically active and more toxic metabolite, is formed. Concurrent abuse of cocaine and alcohol has been associated with very high incidence of sudden death. This has been attributed to the effect of ethanol on the rate of cocaine metabolism and the formation of the pharmacologically active and more toxic metabolite, CE.

In an experiment to study the pharmacokinetic interactions between cocaine and ethanol in experimental animals, a group of rats received cocaine, cocaine + ethanol, BE, BE + ethanol, and CE + ethanol by intraperitoneal (IP) administration in a crossover experimental design. The following results were obtained:

Treatment	Dose	AUC	
Coc	100 μmol/kg	Coc	4.2 μmol h/L
		BE	8.15 μmol h/L
		CE	0.0 μmol h/L
BE	50 μmol/kg	BE	9.32 μmol h/L
Coc + ethanol	100 μmol/kg	Coc	6.78 μmol h/L
		BE	4.12 μmol h/L
		CE	0.432 μmol h/L
BE + ethanol	50 μmol/kg	BE	9.93 μmol h/L
CE + ethanol	50 μmol/kg	CE	1.02 μmol h/L

Assuming that the bioavailability of cocaine and its metabolites with and without alcohol after IP administration is equal to 100%, answer the following questions:

a. What is the effect of ethanol administration on cocaine CL_T?
b. What is the fraction of cocaine dose that is metabolized to BE when cocaine is administered alone and in combination with ethanol?
c. What is the fraction of cocaine dose that is metabolized to CE when cocaine is administered with alcohol?
d. What is the formation clearance of BE and CE when cocaine is administered alone and in combination with ethanol?
e. Comment on the effect of ethanol on cocaine metabolic profile.

Answer

a. When cocaine was given alone:

$$CL_{Tcoc} = \frac{F \, Dose}{AUC} = \frac{100 \, \mu mol}{4.2 \, \mu mol \, h/L} = 23.8 \, L/h$$

When cocaine was given with ethanol:

$$CL_{Tcoc} = \frac{F \, Dose}{AUC} = \frac{100 \, \mu mol}{6.78 \, \mu mol \, h/L} = 14.7 \, L/h$$

Ethanol decreased the CL_T of cocaine by approximately 40%.

b. When BE was administered alone:

$$CL_{TBE} = \frac{F\,Dose}{AUC} = \frac{50\,\mu mol}{9.32\,\mu mol\;h/L} = 5.36\,L/h$$

After cocaine administration:

$$AUC_{BE} = \frac{BE(amount)}{CL_{TBE}}$$

$$8.15\,\mu mol\;h/L = \frac{BE(amount)}{5.36\,L/h}$$

BE amount = 43.7 μmol = 43.7% of the cocaine dose

The total body clearance when BE was administered with ethanol:

$$CL_{T\,BE} = \frac{F\,Dose}{AUC} = \frac{50\,\mu mol}{9.93\,\mu mol\;h/L} = 5.035\,L/h$$

After cocaine administration with ethanol:

$$AUC_{BE} = \frac{BE(amount)}{CL_{T\,BE}}$$

$$4.12\,\mu mol\;h/L = \frac{BE(amount)}{5.035\,L/h}$$

BE amount = 20.7 μmol = 20.7% of cocaine dose when given with ethanol

c.
$$CL_{T\,CE} = \frac{F\,Dose}{AUC} = \frac{50\,\mu mol}{1.02\,\mu mol\;h/L} = 49\,L/h$$

After cocaine administration with ethanol:

$$AUC_{CE} = \frac{CE(amount)}{CL_{T\,CE}}$$

$$0.432\,\mu mol\;h/L = \frac{CE(amount)}{49\,L/h}$$

CE amount = 21.2 μmol = 21.2% of cocaine dose when given with ethanol

d. When cocaine administered alone:
Formation clearance of BE = $f_{m\,BE}CL_{T\,coc}$ = (0.437) 23.8 L/h = 10.4 L/h
Formation clearance of CE = $f_{m\,CE}CL_{T\,coc}$ = (0) 23.8 L/h = 0 L/h
When cocaine is administered with ethanol:
Formation clearance of BE = $f_{m\,BE}CL_{T\,coc}$ = (0.207) 14.7 L/h = 3.04 L/h
Formation clearance of CE = $f_{m\,CE}CL_{T\,coc}$ = (0.212) 14.7 L/h = 3.12 L/h

e. Ethanol inhibits the CL_T of cocaine by approximately 40% and results in the formation of a new metabolite, CE. Also, when cocaine is administered with ethanol, the amount of BE formed will be lower than when cocaine is administered alone.

15.7 STEADY-STATE METABOLITE CONCENTRATION DURING REPEATED ADMINISTRATION OF THE PARENT DRUG

The drug concentration in the body increases gradually during multiple drug administration until steady state is achieved. As the drug accumulates, the rate of metabolite formation increases, which increases the metabolite concentration in the body. When the drug steady state is achieved, the rate of metabolite formation becomes constant, and gradually the rate of metabolite formation becomes equal to the rate of metabolite elimination and steady state is achieved. If the steady state for the drug is achieved when the rate of drug administration is equal to the rate of drug elimination, the steady state for the metabolite is achieved when the rate of metabolite formation is equal to the rate of metabolite elimination. So at steady state during multiple drug administration, the metabolite concentration and the metabolite to drug concentration ratio become constant. Monitoring the metabolite concentration in addition to the parent drug concentration during multiple drug administration is important when the metabolite contributes significantly to the drug pharmacological and/or adverse effects.

At steady state, the rate of metabolite formation is determined from the fraction of the drug clearance responsible for metabolite formation and the average drug steady-state concentration ($f_{m}CL_{T}Cp_{ss}$), while the rate of metabolite elimination is determined from the metabolite clearance and the average metabolite steady-state concentration ($CL_{T(m)}Cp_{(m)ss}$). So at steady state,

$$f_{m}CL_{T}Cp_{ss} = CL_{T(m)}Cp_{(m)ss} \qquad (15.23)$$

By rearrangement

$$\frac{Cp_{(m)ss}}{Cp_{ss}} = \frac{f_{m}CL_{T}}{CL_{T(m)}} \qquad (15.24)$$

This indicates that the metabolite to drug concentration ratio at steady state during multiple drug administration is determined from the ratio of the metabolite formation clearance to the metabolite elimination clearance. The metabolite to drug AUC ratio after a single IV dose of the drug is also determined from the ratio of the metabolite formation clearance to the metabolite elimination clearance according to Equation 15.17. From Equations 15.17 and 15.24, the following expression can be obtained:

$$\frac{Cp_{(m)ss}}{Cp_{ss}} = \frac{f_m CL_T}{CL_{T(m)}} = \frac{AUC_{(m)}}{AUC} \tag{15.25}$$

This relationship suggests that the ratio of the average metabolite concentration to the average parent drug concentration at steady state during multiple administration of the parent drug can be predicted from the ratio of metabolite to parent drug AUC measured after a single IV bolus dose of the parent drug. Also, the metabolite to parent drug concentration ratio during constant rate IV infusion of the parent drug can be predicted from the ratio of metabolite to parent drug AUC after a single IV bolus dose of the parent drug.

Example

A drug is eliminated by renal excretion and metabolism to a pharmacologically active metabolite after administration to humans. This metabolite is eliminated in the urine or metabolized to a second metabolite that is completely excreted in urine according to the scheme in Figure 15.8.

After administration of 100 μmol of the parent drug to a normal volunteer, the total amounts of the parent drug, metabolite 1, and metabolite 2 recovered in the urine were 20, 30, and 50 μmol, respectively. The half-life of the parent drug is 4 h and its volume of distribution is 25 L.

a. Calculate the CL_T and the AUC of the parent drug after administration of the 100 μmol dose.
b. What is the renal clearance of the parent drug?
c. What is the fraction of the administered dose of the parent drug that is metabolized to metabolite 1?
d. If the observed AUC of metabolite 1 was 10 μmol h/L, what is the CL_T of metabolite 1?
e. What is the renal clearance of metabolite 1?
f. What is the formation clearance of metabolite 1 and metabolite 2?
g. If a dose of 300 μmol of the parent drug is administered to the same volunteer, what are the expected AUCs of the parent drug and metabolite 1?

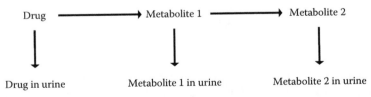

FIGURE 15.8 Schematic presentation for the different pathways involved in the elimination of the parent drug and its two metabolites in the solved example.

h. If 100 µmol of metabolite 1 is administered to the same volunteer, what are the total amounts of metabolite 1 and metabolite 2 that will be excreted in urine?

i. If a constant rate IV infusion of the parent drug is administered to this volunteer, what is the expected ratio of the metabolite concentration to that of the parent drug at steady state?

j. From the information provided earlier, can you determine whether metabolite 1 and metabolite 2 follow formation rate limited of elimination rate limited profile?

Answer

The fraction of the parent drug dose excreted in urine:

$$\text{Fraction (parent drug)} = \frac{\text{Amount excreted in urine}}{\text{Dose of parent drug}} = \frac{20\,\mu mol}{100\,\mu mol} = 0.2$$

a.
$$CL_T = kVd = \frac{0.693}{4h}\,25L = 4.33L/h$$

$$AUC = \frac{100\,\mu mol}{4.33L/h} = 23\,\mu mol\ h/L$$

b. Renal clearance = Fraction excreted unchanged in urine × CL_T

$$CL_R = (0.2)\ 4.33\ L/h = 0.866\ L/h$$

c. Fraction metabolized to metabolite 1 = 1 − 0.2 = 0.8

d.
$$CL_{T(m1)} = \frac{80\,\mu mol}{10\,\mu mol\ h/L} = 8L/h$$

e. Fraction excreted in urine of metabolite 1

$$= \frac{\text{Amount of metabolite 1 excreted in urine}}{\text{Total amount of metabolite 1 formed}}$$

$$\text{Fraction}_{(m1)} = \frac{30\,\mu mol}{80\,\mu mol} = 0.375$$

Renal clearance of metabolite I = fraction excreted in urine × CL_T of metabolite 1

$$CL_{R(m1)} = 0.375 \times 8\ L/h = 3\ L/h$$

f. Formation clearance (metabolite 1) $= f_{m(metabolite\ 1)} \times CL_{T(parent\ drug)}$

$$= 0.8 \times 4.33 \text{ L/h} = 3.46 \text{ L/h}$$

Formation clearance (metabolite 2) $= f_{m(metabolite\ 2)} \times CL_{T(metabolite\ 1)}$

$$= (1 - \text{fraction excreted in urine of metabolite 1}) \times CL_{T(metabolite\ 1)}$$
$$= (1 - 0.375) \times 8 \text{ L/h} = 3.46 \text{ L/h}$$

g. Increasing the dose of the parent drug will cause proportional increase in the drug AUC and the metabolite AUC:

$$AUC_{parent\ drug} = 3 \times 23 \,\mu mol\ h/L = 69 \,\mu mol\ h/L$$

$$AUC_{m1} = 3 \times 10 \,\mu mol\ h/L = 30 \,\mu mol\ h/L$$

h. After administration of 100 μmol of metabolite 1
   Amount of metabolite 1 excreted in urine = (30/80) 100 μmol = 37.5 μmol
   Amount of metabolite 2 excreted in urine = 100 − 37.5 μmol = 62.25 μmol

i.
$$\text{Ratio} = \frac{Cpss_{(m1)}}{Cpss} = \frac{f_{m1}CL_T}{CL_{T(m1)}} = \frac{0.8 \times 4.33 \text{L/h}}{8 \text{L/h}} = 0.433$$

j. No because we do not have any information about the half-life and the excretion rate constant of the parent drug and the metabolites.

15.8 METABOLITE PHARMACOKINETICS AFTER EXTRAVASCULAR ADMINISTRATION OF THE PARENT DRUG

When the parent drug is given as IV bolus, the highest concentration of the drug is achieved immediately after administration. The rate of metabolite formation, which is a function of the amount of the drug in the body and the metabolic rate constant for that particular pathway, is the highest immediately after drug administration when the drug concentration is the highest. Then, the rate of metabolite formation decreases as the amount of drug in the body decreases due to drug elimination.

However, when the parent drug is given by extravascular administration (e.g., oral administration), the amount of the parent drug in the systemic circulation is zero initially. After oral drug administration, the drug plasma concentration increases with time due to drug absorption until it reaches the maximum concentration when the rate of drug absorption is equal to the rate of drug elimination. Beyond this maximum concentration, the drug in the body declines due to drug elimination. Since the rate of metabolite formation is dependent on the amount of the drug in

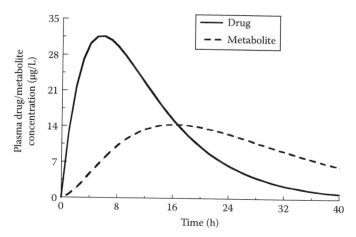

FIGURE 15.9   Drug and metabolite concentration–time profiles after oral administration of a single dose of the drug.

the body, the rate of metabolite formation is very low initially and then increases as the amount of the parent drug in the body increases until the maximum rate of metabolite formation is achieved when the amount of drug in the body is the highest. After this point, the metabolite formation rate decreases. This makes the time to achieve the maximum metabolite concentration ($t_{max(m)}$) usually larger than the time to achieve the maximum drug concentration t_{max}. The parent drug and the metabolite plasma concentration–time profiles after oral administration of the parent drug are illustrated in Figure 15.9.

The metabolite plasma concentration–time profile is described by a triexponential expression. This expression describes three different processes: parent drug absorption, metabolite formation (or parent drug elimination to form the metabolite of interest), and metabolite elimination. The example presented here assumes that during the absorption process, the parent drug does not undergo significant first-pass metabolism. However, in many cases the parent drug can be metabolized during the absorption process. This will usually result in the appearance of the metabolite and the parent drug simultaneously in the systemic circulation. So when the drug undergoes presystemic metabolism, the resulting metabolite concentration–time profile may be different from the profile described earlier.

15.9   KINETICS OF SEQUENTIAL METABOLISM

Sequential metabolism is a process where the parent drug is metabolized to form a metabolite that is further metabolized to form a second metabolite. Many drugs are metabolized by sequential metabolism. Carbamazepine, which is an antiepileptic drug, is eliminated through different pathways: one of them is the formation of its major metabolite carbamazepine epioxide. The epioxide metabolite is further metabolized to carbamazepine diol that is then excreted in the urine.

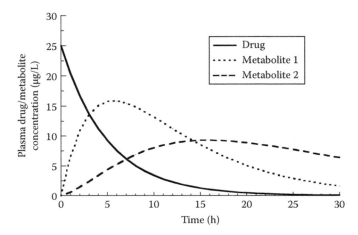

FIGURE 15.10 Drug and metabolite concentration–time profiles after IV administration of a single dose of a drug that is metabolized to metabolite 1, which is then metabolized to metabolite 2.

After IV administration of the parent drug, the amount of metabolite 1 in the body initially increases until it reaches a maximum concentration and then it decreases due to metabolite 1 elimination. The rate of formation of metabolite 2, which is dependent on the amount of the metabolite 1 in the body, is low initially and gradually increases until it reaches its maximum rate of formation when the amount of metabolite 1 is the highest. Beyond this point, the rate of formation of metabolite 2 decreases. This results in the appearance of the maximum concentration of metabolite 2 after the maximum concentration of metabolite 1. The drug and metabolite concentration–time profiles after IV administration of a drug that is sequentially metabolized to two metabolites are illustrated in Figure 15.10. Assuming first-order elimination, the plasma metabolite concentration–time profile of metabolite 2 is described by a triexponential expression. This expression describes three different processes: the formation of metabolite 1 (or the parent drug elimination to form metabolite 1), the elimination of metabolite 1 (or the formation of metabolite 2), and the elimination of metabolite 2.

15.10 EFFECT OF CHANGING THE PHARMACOKINETIC PARAMETERS ON THE DRUG AND METABOLITE CONCENTRATION–TIME PROFILES AFTER A SINGLE IV DRUG ADMINISTRATION AND DURING MULTIPLE DRUG ADMINISTRATION

After IV bolus administration, the plasma drug concentration–time profile depends on the drug pharmacokinetic parameters. The initial plasma drug concentration is dependent on the drug dose and Vd. The rate of decline in the drug concentration is dependent on the drug elimination rate constant, where the slope of the drug concentration–time profile on the semilog scale is equal to $-k/2.303$. The metabolite concentration initially increases after IV drug administration until it reaches a maximum value and then the metabolite concentration decreases with time. The rate of increase in metabolite concentration is dependent on the rate of drug elimination, with rapidly eliminating drugs producing fast increase in metabolite concentration. The rate of decline in the metabolite concentration depends on the metabolite elimination rate constant when $k_{(m)} < k$ (elimination rate limited metabolite), and depends on the drug elimination rate constant when $k_{(m)} > k$ (formation rate limited metabolite). The metabolite to drug AUC ratio after a single IV drug administration and also the metabolite to drug concentration ratio during multiple drug administration are dependent on the ratio of the metabolite formation clearance to the metabolite elimination clearance.

The following discussion deals with the effect of changing the different drug and metabolite pharmacokinetic parameters on the drug and metabolite plasma concentration–time profiles. This discussion is intended to illustrate how each of the drug and metabolite pharmacokinetic parameters affects the drug and metabolite concentration–time profiles. However, in reality the change in one pharmacokinetic parameter may be accompanied by a change in some other parameters. For example, the change in the drug metabolic clearance due to liver dysfunction is usually accompanied by a change in the metabolite clearance when the metabolite is further metabolized to a second metabolite by the liver. Also, the change in the drug volume of distribution due to differences in body weight is usually accompanied by a change in the metabolite volume of distribution.

15.10.1 PHARMACOKINETIC SIMULATION EXERCISE

Pharmacokinetic simulations can be used to examine how the drug and metabolite pharmacokinetic parameters affect the plasma drug and metabolite concentration–time profiles after a single IV dose of the drug. The plasma drug and metabolite concentration–time profiles are simulated using an average value of each of the pharmacokinetic parameters. Then, the drug and metabolite pharmacokinetic parameters are changed one parameter at a time while keeping all the other parameters constant, and the simulation is repeated. The resulting profiles are examined to determine how the change affects the drug and metabolite concentration–time profiles. Also, the drug and metabolite concentration–time profiles during multiple drug administration can be simulated to examine the effect of each of the drug and metabolite pharmacokinetic parameters on the drug steady-state concentration, metabolite steady-state concentration, and the metabolite to drug concentration ratio at steady state. The plotting exercise of the two metabolite kinetics modules in the basic pharmacokinetic concept section of the companion CD to this textbook can be used to run these simulations.

15.10.1.1 Drug Dose

Administration of higher IV doses of the drug results in proportional increase in the initial drug concentration, the slope of the drug concentration–time profile on the semilog scale does not change since the drug elimination rate constant is similar, and the drug AUC increases proportional to the dose. The increase in drug dose causes proportional increase in the amount of metabolite formed in vivo because f_m is constant, which results in a proportional increase in the metabolite AUC. The metabolite to drug AUC ratio after administration of increasing IV doses of the drug remains constant because the metabolite formation clearance and elimination clearance do not change by changing the drug dose. Also, increasing the dose of the drug causes proportional increase in the drug and metabolite steady-state concentrations, and the metabolite to drug concentration ratio at steady state does not change.

15.10.1.2 Drug Total Body Clearance

After administration of the same IV dose of the drug, the change in drug clearance causes change in the rate of drug elimination if Vd is constant. Lower drug clearance results in larger drug AUC, while higher drug clearance results in smaller drug AUC if Vd is constant. The amount of the metabolite formed in vivo is constant as long as f_m is constant. However, high drug clearance causes faster rate of metabolite formation while low drug clearance causes slower rate of metabolite formation. If the metabolite parameters are kept constant, the change in drug clearance does not affect the amount of the metabolite formed in vivo and the metabolite AUC. The change in drug clearance affects the drug AUC and the metabolite formation clearance $f_m CL_T$, and causes change in the metabolite to parent drug AUC ratio. Lower drug clearance decreases the metabolite to drug AUC ratio if the metabolite parameters are kept constant. During multiple drug administration, lower drug clearance increases the drug steady-state concentration without affecting the metabolite steady-state concentration if f_m and the metabolite clearance remain constant. This produces lower metabolite to drug steady-state concentration ratio during multiple drug administration, while higher drug clearance increases the metabolite to drug AUC ratio and increases the metabolite to drug concentration ratio at steady state during multiple drug administration.

15.10.1.3 Drug Volume of Distribution

After administration of the same IV dose of the drug, the change in Vd causes change in the initial drug concentration with larger drug Vd producing lower initial drug concentration and smaller Vd producing higher initial drug concentration. Smaller Vd results in faster rate of drug elimination and larger Vd causes slower rate of drug elimination, if the drug clearance is constant. However, the drug AUC is not affected by the change in the drug Vd because the drug AUC is dependent on the dose and clearance of the drug. The amount of the metabolite formed after administration of the same dose of the drug is not affected by the change in the drug Vd if f_m is kept constant. However, faster rate of drug elimination produces faster rate of metabolite formation and slower rate of drug elimination produces slower rate of metabolite formation. If the metabolite parameters are kept constant, the change in drug Vd does not affect the amount of the metabolite formed in vivo and the metabolite AUC. The change in drug Vd does not affect the metabolite to drug AUC ratio since the metabolite formation clearance and elimination clearance do not change due to the change in drug Vd. During multiple drug administration, the drug and metabolite concentration at steady state and their ratio are not affected by the change in the drug Vd because the clearances for the drug and for the metabolite are not affected by the change in the drug Vd.

15.10.1.4   Fraction of the Drug Dose Converted to Metabolite

After administration of the same dose, the drug concentration–time profile does not change if the drug clearance and Vd are constant. The change in f_m affects the amount of the metabolite formed after administration of the drug; larger f_m results in the formation of more metabolite after administration of the same dose of the drug. If the metabolite parameters are kept constant, the formation of larger amount of the metabolite results in proportional increase in the metabolite AUC. The metabolite to drug AUC ratio after administration of the same dose of the drug increases with the increase in f_m. During multiple drug administration, the change in f_m causes proportional change in the formation clearance of metabolite. Higher f_m produces higher metabolite to drug steady-state concentration ratio, while lower f_m produces lower metabolite to drug steady-state concentration ratio during multiple administration of the drug.

15.10.1.5   Metabolite Total Body Clearance

After administration of the same dose, the drug concentration–time profile and the drug AUC remain constant if the drug CL_T and Vd are constant. The amount of metabolite formed in vivo remains constant if f_m is constant. The change in metabolite clearance produces inversely proportional change in the metabolite AUC. Also, the change in metabolite clearance affects the rate of metabolite elimination rate if the metabolite Vd is constant. The higher metabolite clearance produces faster rate of metabolite elimination and lower metabolite clearance produces slower rate of metabolite elimination, if the metabolite Vd is constant. The metabolite to drug AUC ratio is affected by the change in metabolite clearance, with the higher metabolite clearance producing lower metabolite to drug AUC ratio. During multiple drug administration, lower metabolite clearance increases the metabolite steady-state concentration without affecting the drug steady-state concentration if f_m and drug clearance remain constant. This produces higher metabolite to drug steady-state concentration ratio during multiple drug administration. On the contrary, higher metabolite clearance decreases the metabolite steady-state concentration without affecting the drug steady-state concentration, which results in lower metabolite to drug concentration ratio.

15.10.1.6   Metabolite Volume of Distribution

After administration of the same dose, the drug concentration–time profile and the drug AUC remain constant if the drug CL_T and Vd are constant. The amount of metabolite formed in vivo remains constant if f_m is constant. The change in the metabolite Vd does not affect the metabolite AUC. However, the change in metabolite Vd affects the rate of metabolite elimination rate if the metabolite clearance is kept constant. The larger metabolite Vd produces slower rate of elimination, while smaller metabolite Vd produces faster rate of elimination, if the metabolite clearance is constant. The metabolite to drug AUC after administration of the same dose of the drug is not affected by the change in the metabolite Vd. During multiple drug administration, the drug and metabolite concentration at steady state and their ratio are not affected by the change in the metabolite Vd because the clearances for the drug and the metabolite are not affected by the change in the metabolite Vd.

PRACTICE PROBLEMS

15.1 A drug is metabolized to three different metabolites through three parallel pathways. After administration of 1000 mg of the parent drug, plasma samples were obtained and the concentrations of the parent drug and the metabolites were determined.

Time (h)	Drug (mg/L)	Metabolite I (mg/L)	Metabolite II (mg/L)	Metabolite III (mg/L)
0	50	0	0	0
1	36.6	21.0	25.7	6.43
2	26.8	26.3	42.1	10.5
4	14.4	21.3	56.9	14.2
8	4.1	7.7	54.3	13.5
12	1.2	2.33	40.9	10.2
16	0.34	0.678	28.6	7.1
24	0.03	0.056	13.1	3.28

a. Plot the plasma concentration–time profiles for the parent drug and its metabolites and determine which of the metabolites follow formation rate limited profile and which follow elimination rate limited profile.

15.2 After administration of a drug to humans, it is eliminated by renal excretion and metabolized to two different metabolites that are completely excreted in urine according to the scheme in Figure 15.11.

After administration of 100 μmol of the parent drug to a normal volunteer, the total amounts of the parent drug, metabolite 1, and metabolite 2 recovered in the urine were 20, 30, and 50 μmol, respectively. The half-life of the parent drug is 4 h and its volume of distribution is 25 L.

a. Calculate the CL_T and the AUC of the parent drug after administration of the 100 μmol dose.

b. What is the renal clearance of the parent drug?

c. What is the fraction of the administered dose of the parent drug that is metabolized to metabolite 1?

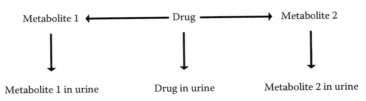

FIGURE 15.11 Schematic presentation for the different pathways involved in the elimination of the parent drug and its two metabolites in Problem 15.2.

d. If the observed AUC of metabolite 1 was 10 μmol h/L, what is the CL_T of metabolite 1?
e. What is the renal clearance of metabolite 1?
f. What is the formation clearance of metabolite 1 and metabolite 2?
g. If a dose of 300 μmol of the parent drug is administered to the same volunteer, what are the expected AUCs of the parent drug and metabolite 1?
h. If 100 μmol of metabolite 1 is administered to the same volunteer, what is the total amount of metabolite 1 and metabolite 2 that will be excreted in urine?
i. If a constant rate IV infusion of the parent drug is administered to this volunteer, what is the expected ratio of the metabolite concentration to that of the parent drug at steady state?
j. From the aforementioned information, can you determine whether metabolite 1 and metabolite 2 follow formation rate limited of elimination rate limited profile?

15.3 One mmol of a drug was administered by IV to a human volunteer and the following data were obtained:

Time (h)	Parent Drug Concentration (μmol/L)	Metabolite Concentration (μmol/L)
0.5	13.0	0.56
1.5	10.8	1.15
3.0	9.5	2.5
5.0	7.5	4.7
7.0	5.6	6.0
9.0	4.5	6.4
12.5	2.8	4.3
17.5	1.5	2.3
23.5	0.74	1.1
30.0	0.32	0.48

On a separate occasion, 2 weeks later, the same volunteer received 1 mmol of the metabolites IV and the following data were obtained:

Time (h)	Metabolite Concentration (μmol/L)
1.0	21
3.5	9.9
6.0	4.5
8.5	2.0
11.0	0.94
16.0	0.2
20.0	0.059
25.0	0.013
32.0	0.0014

a. Calculate the following parameters:
    • Fraction of parent drug converted to the metabolite
    • Total body clearance of the metabolite
    • Volume of distribution of the metabolite
    • Formation clearance and formation rate constant of the metabolite.
b. If the parent drug is to be given as a constant rate infusion at 0.25 mmol/h, what will be the steady-state concentration of the metabolite?
c. What will be the concentration ratio of metabolite to parent drug at steady state during a constant rate infusion of the drug?

15.4 An oral hypoglycemic drug is eliminated from the body by renal excretion or metabolism to a metabolite that is completely excreted in urine. After administration of 1000 mg of this drug to a normal volunteer, plasma samples were obtained and the concentrations of the parent drug and its major metabolite were determined.

Time (h)	Parent Drug Concentration (mg/L)	Metabolite Concentration (mg/L)
1	2.97	0.166
2	5.1	0.61
3	6.87	1.27
4	7.56	1.65
6	8.42	2.44
8	8.37	2.85
10	7.82	2.95
12	7.04	2.85
16	5.34	2.35
20	3.847	1.75
24	2.69	1.24

On a separate occasion, after administration of 1000 mg of the metabolite to the same volunteer, the following concentrations were observed:

Time (h)	Concentration (mg/L)
1	33.5
4	10.1
8	2.04
12	0.411
16	0.083

The bioavailability of this oral hypoglycemic drug is known to be 80% due to incomplete absorption from the GIT. Because the difference in molecular weight between the parent drug and the metabolite is small, assume that the molecular weights are equal. The elimination rate constant of the parent drug is $0.2\,h^{-1}$.

a. Calculate the CL_T and Vd of the metabolite.
b. What is the fraction of the parent drug (in the systemic circulation) that is converted to metabolite?
c. What are the formation clearance and the formation rate constant of the metabolite?
d. What is the total amount of the parent drug and its metabolite excreted in urine after administration of the 1000 mg dose orally?
e. If the parent drug is administered as 1000 mg every 12 h, what will be the average steady-state plasma concentrations of the parent drug and the metabolite?

15.5 After IV administration of an antihypertensive drug, 30% of the administered dose is excreted unchanged in urine and 70% of the dose is metabolized to inactive metabolite that is completely eliminated in the urine. After administration of 50 µmol of this drug, its half-life was 1 h, its volume of distribution was 20 L, and its AUC was 3.6 µmol h/L.

a. What is the renal clearance of the parent drug?
b. What is the metabolic clearance of the parent drug?
c. What is the formation clearance of the metabolite?
d. If the observed metabolite AUC was 5 µmol h/L, what are the metabolite CL_T, metabolic clearance, and renal clearance?
e. If the metabolite volume of distribution is 30 L, determine whether this metabolite follows the formation rate or elimination rate limited behavior.
f. If 120 µmol of the drug is administered, what will be the expected parent drug and metabolite AUCs?
g. If the parent drug is administered by constant rate IV infusion, what will be the steady-state metabolite to parent drug concentration ratio?

REFERENCES

1. Meyer UA (1996) Overview of enzymes of drug metabolism. *J Pharmacokinet Biopharm* 24:449–459.
2. Guengerich FP (2003) Cytochromes p450, drugs, and diseases. *Mol Intervent* 3:194–204.
3. Nelson DR, Koymans L, Kamataki T, Stegeman JJ, Feyereisen R, Waxman DJ, Waterman MR et al. (1996) P450 superfamily: Update on new sequences, gene mapping, accession numbers and nomenclature. *Pharmacogenetics* 6:1–42.
4. Houston JB (1981) Drug metabolite kinetics. *Pharmacol Ther* 15:521–552.

16 Nonlinear Pharmacokinetics

OBJECTIVES

After completing this chapter you should be able to

- Describe the most common causes of nonlinear pharmacokinetic behavior and the common characteristics of nonlinear pharmacokinetics
- Define the Michaelis-Menten pharmacokinetic parameters
- Describe the basic characteristics of Michaelis-Menten pharmacokinetics
- Analyze the effect of changing the Michaelis-Menten pharmacokinetic parameters on the steady-state plasma concentration after a single and multiple drug administration
- Estimate the Michaelis-Menten pharmacokinetic parameters using mathematical and graphical methods
- Recommend the dosing regimen required to achieve therapeutic plasma concentration of drugs that follow nonlinear pharmacokinetics in patients

16.1 INTRODUCTION

In the previous discussion of the pharmacokinetic behavior of drugs after single and multiple drug administration by different routes, it was assumed that the drug absorption, distribution, and elimination processes follow first-order kinetics. In this case, the drug CL_T, Vd, k, and $t_{1/2}$ are constant irrespective of the administered dose, that is, dose independent and concentration independent. After administration of increasing doses of the drug, the plasma drug concentration–time profiles during the elimination phase are parallel when plotted on the semilog scale. Also, the AUC of the drug from 0 to ∞ after a single drug administration is directly proportional to the administered dose, which is known as the principle of superposition. Furthermore, at steady state during multiple drug administration, the AUC from 0 to τ and the average drug concentration are directly proportional to the administered dose. The drug is said to follow linear or dose-independent pharmacokinetics when there is a linear relationship between the dose and AUC after single dose administration and the dose and steady-state concentration during multiple drug administration.

In some drugs, one or more of the absorption, distribution, metabolism, and elimination processes do not follow first-order kinetics. The pharmacokinetic parameters of these drugs can be different after administration of different doses, that is, dose dependent or concentration dependent. The AUC from time 0 to ∞

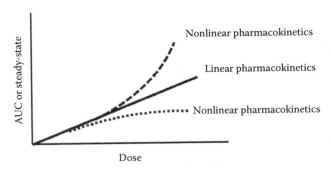

FIGURE 16.1 Relationship between the administered dose and AUC or steady-state concentration for drugs that follow linear and nonlinear pharmacokinetics.

after single dose, the AUC during one dosing interval, and the average steady-state drug concentration during multiple drug administration are disproportional to the administered dose. Drugs with this behavior are considered following nonlinear, dose-dependent, or concentration-dependent pharmacokinetics as in Figure 16.1.

The dose proportionality study that is usually designed to determine whether the drug follows linear or nonlinear pharmacokinetics is an important component of the drug development process. In this study, increasing doses of the drug are administered and the AUCs are calculated to determine whether linear relationship between the dose and AUC exists or not. Linear relationship between the dose and AUC indicates that the drug follows linear pharmacokinetics within the range of doses used in the study. Also, increasing doses can be administered repeatedly until steady state is achieved. Linear relationship between the dose and the steady-state drug concentration indicates that the drug follows linear pharmacokinetics. It is important to specify the range of doses over which linear or nonlinear pharmacokinetic behavior is observed because some drugs can follow linear pharmacokinetics over a certain range of doses and follow nonlinear pharmacokinetics at higher range of doses. For example, theophylline follows linear pharmacokinetics in the range of doses used clinically, while nonlinear pharmacokinetic behavior has been observed in some overdose cases in children.

16.2 CAUSES OF NONLINEAR PHARMACOKINETICS

Drugs with evidence of nonlinear pharmacokinetic behavior, such as nonlinear relationship between dose and AUC or between dose and steady-state concentration, are studied further to determine the cause of this nonlinearity. As mentioned earlier, nonlinear pharmacokinetic behavior occurs when one or more of the absorption, distribution, and elimination processes do not follow first-order kinetics. The following brief discussion covers the dose-dependent absorption, distribution, and/or elimination that can lead to nonlinear pharmacokinetic drug behavior [1,2]. The capacity-limited metabolism, which is the most common cause of nonlinearity in the drugs used clinically, is discussed in detail thereafter.

16.2.1 DOSE-DEPENDENT DRUG ABSORPTION

The extent of absorption of some drugs can be dose dependent leading to nonlinear pharmacokinetic behavior [3]. Dose-dependent absorption may be observed in drugs with limited solubility, drugs absorbed by carrier-mediated transport, and drugs with saturable first-pass metabolism in the gastrointestinal tract (GIT) and/or liver. Drugs with limited aqueous solubility especially those administered in large doses may not be absorbed completely due to incomplete drug dissolution in the GIT. After administration of increasing doses, smaller fractions of the administered doses can dissolve in the GIT, leading to lower extent of absorption if the drug transit time in the GIT does not change. In the case of digoxin, which has very low aqueous solubility, partial dissolution does not represent a major cause of its incomplete bioavailability because its dose is very small. Griseofulvin is an antifungal drug that has an aqueous solubility of about $10 \mu g/mL$ and is administered in doses of $100-600 mg/day$. Administration of increasing doses of the drugs with high dose-to-solubility ratio such as griseofulvin produces less than proportional increase in the AUC. So 100% increase in dose results in less than 100% increase in the drug AUC, indicating lower extent of absorption due to the increase in dose, that is, dose-dependent absorption.

Passive diffusion is the main mechanism of absorption for most drugs. However, some drugs are absorbed from the small intestine via a specific carrier-mediated transport system. The rate of drug transport by the carrier-mediated transport system can be described by Equation 16.1:

$$\text{Transport rate} = \frac{T_{max}C_{GIT}}{K_T + C_{GIT}} \tag{16.1}$$

where
  T_{max} is the maximum rate of drug transport
  C_{GIT} is the drug concentration at the site of transport
  K_T is the constant for the transport process and it is a measure of the affinity of the drug to the transport system

Administration of increasing doses of drugs that are absorbed by a carrier-mediated transport system can saturate the transport system and the rate of drug absorption becomes constant, that is, zero order. So larger doses require longer time for their complete absorption by this transport system. When the drug transit time in the GIT segment containing the transport system is not long enough to allow complete absorption, increasing the dose will decrease the fraction of dose absorbed. So administration of increasing doses that can saturate the transport system responsible for drug absorption leads to less than proportional increase in the drug AUC because of the decrease in the fraction of dose absorbed. Saturation of the transport system after administration of large doses of the drug is more likely when the transport system is localized in a specific site in the GIT, and when the drug is administered in the form of immediate-release formulation. Drugs such as L-dopa, methyldopa, cephalexin, amoxicillin, methotrexate, and cephradine are examples of drugs that are absorbed by carrier-mediated transport from the GIT.

Some drugs that undergo significant first-pass metabolism in the GIT and liver can saturate the drug metabolizing enzymes when administered in large doses. This allows larger fraction of the administered doses to escape the presystemic metabolism and increases the drug bioavailability with the increase in dose. Propranolol is a nonselective beta-adrenergic blocking agent that undergoes saturable first-pass metabolism. Administration of increasing doses of propranolol produces more than proportional increase in propranolol AUC due to the increase in its bioavailability. Saturable first-pass metabolism is more pronounced after administration of rapidly absorbed dosage forms where a large amount of the drug is presented to the metabolizing enzymes over a short time, thereby increasing the chance of enzyme saturation. Examples of other drugs that undergo saturable first-pass effect include nicardipine, omeprazole, verapamil, and atrovastatin. All the discussed conditions that lead to dose-dependent absorption will make the drug follow nonlinear pharmacokinetics even if the distribution and elimination processes follow first-order kinetics.

16.2.2 Dose-Dependent Drug Distribution

The Vd of drugs is dependent on the drug binding to plasma and tissue proteins as discussed previously. The expression that relates the drug Vd and the free fraction of the drug in plasma and tissues is as follows:

$$Vd = V_p + V_t \left(\frac{f_{uP}}{f_{uT}} \right) \tag{16.2}$$

where
  V_p is the volume of the plasma
  V_t is the volume of the tissues
  f_{uP} is the free fraction of the drug in plasma
  f_{uT} is the free fraction of the drug in tissues

This relationship indicates that changes in the drug binding in plasma or tissues can lead to changes in the drug Vd. When similar changes in drug binding occur in the plasma and tissues, Vd is not affected. However, if the drug free fraction in plasma increases due to reduction in plasma protein binding without affecting the tissue binding, the drug Vd increases, while the increase in free fraction in tissues due to reduction in tissue binding without affecting the plasma protein binding decreases the drug Vd.

The extent of drug binding to proteins is determined from the equilibrium between the free unbound drug and the bound drug. Assuming that for each protein molecule there are n number of independent sites (drug binding to one site does not affect the binding to other sites) where the drug can bind, the free fraction of the drug, f_u, can be expressed as

$$f_u = \frac{K_d + D_f}{np_t + K_d + D_f} \tag{16.3}$$

where
  K_d is the drug-protein dissociation constant
  D_f is the free drug concentration
  p_t is the protein concentration
  n is the number of binding sites per protein molecule

Equation 16.3 indicates that the free fraction of the drug, which is a measure of the extent of drug protein binding is affected by the drug concentration, protein concentration which can be affected by some diseases, the number of binding sites, and the dissociation constant which can change when there is more than one drug competing for the same binding sites.

Some drugs have saturable plasma protein binding. This means that the free fractions of these drugs are higher at high plasma drug concentration. The change in the free fraction of the drug in plasma can affect the CL_T of drugs with low intrinsic clearance. The increase in the drug-free fraction increases the free drug concentration in plasma, which increases the chance of the free drug molecules to come in contact with the metabolizing enzymes. This leads to approximately proportional increase in the drug CL_T. So administration of increasing doses in this case results in less than proportional increase in the drug AUC due to the increase in the drug CL_T. Good correlation between the CL_T and the unbound fraction in plasma has been reported for naproxen, disopyramide, warfarin, valproic acid, and tolbutamide. The saturable plasma protein binding in these drugs is the main cause of the change in the CL_T and the nonlinear pharmacokinetic behavior [4].

16.2.3 Dose-Dependent Renal Excretion

Urinary drug excretion involves glomerular filtration, active and passive tubular reabsorption, and active tubular secretion. The renal excretion rate of drugs that are only excreted by glomerular filtration is proportional to the free drug concentration in the plasma. This is because under the normal conditions only the free drug is filtered in the glomeruli. In this case, the drug renal clearance that can be determined from the slope of the plot of the drug renal excretion rate versus plasma drug concentration is constant as in Figure 16.2. The rate of active drug secretion in the renal tubules can be described by an equation in the same form of Equation 16.1 but the concentration term in this case will be the drug concentration in the systemic circulation. The rate of tubular secretion increases proportional to the drug concentration when the drug concentration is very low. The plasma drug concentration achieved after administration of therapeutic doses of most actively secreted drugs is in this range and the rate of active tubular secretion is proportional to the plasma drug concentration. At high drug concentration when the active transport system becomes saturated, the rate of tubular secretion becomes constant, that is, zero order as in Figure 16.2. The renal excretion rate for drugs that are actively secreted in the renal tubules is the sum of the filtration rate and the active secretion rate as in Figure 16.2. Tubular reabsorption for most drugs occurs by passive diffusion where a fraction of the drug in the renal tubules is reabsorbed.

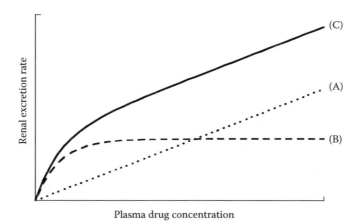

FIGURE 16.2   Renal drug excretion rate versus plasma drug concentration plot: (A) if the drug is excreted only by filtration, (B) for the active tubular secretion, and (C) if the drug is excreted by filtration and active tubular secretion.

The slope of the renal excretion rate versus the plasma drug concentration is a measure of the renal clearance. For drugs that are filtered and actively secreted, the renal clearance is constant at low drug concentration. As the drug concentration increases and the active transport system starts to be saturated, the renal clearance decreases. At very high drug concentration, the renal clearance becomes constant again when the increase in the renal excretion rate is only due to the increase in the rate of filtration because the active secretion is saturated, that is, the rate of active secretion is constant. Drugs that are mainly eliminated by renal excretion and are actively secreted in the renal tubules can follow nonlinear pharmacokinetics when administered in doses that are high enough to saturate the renal tubular secretion. In this case, administration of increasing doses results in more than proportional increase in the drug AUC due to the decrease in the drug clearance such as in the case of dicloxacillin. Examples of drugs that are actively secreted in the renal clearance include ampicillin, cephalexin, enalaprilat, methotrexate, cimetidine, and famotidine; however, all these drugs do not saturate the renal tubular secretion transport system in the range of doses used clinically, so they follow linear pharmacokinetics.

Tubular reabsorption that occurs by a specific carrier system can be saturated also after administration of high doses of the drug. Ascorbic acid is reabsorbed from the renal tubules by an active transport system. Administration of large doses of ascorbic acid can cause saturation of ascorbic acid reabsorption and larger fraction of the dose is excreted in urine. So the renal clearance of ascorbic acid increases after administration of larger doses.

16.2.4   Dose-Dependent Drug Metabolism

Drug metabolism involves enzymatic modification of the drug chemical structure to form one or more metabolites. According to the principles of enzyme kinetics that will be discussed in detail in the rest of this chapter, the metabolic reaction follows first-order kinetics at low drug concentration. However, when the drug concentration is high and/or the metabolizing enzymes have low capacity, the enzymes can be saturated and the metabolic reaction does not follow first-order kinetics. In this case, the drug metabolic clearance becomes dependent on the drug concentration, with higher drug concentration resulting in lower drug clearance. Saturation of the drug metabolizing enzymes leads to nonlinear pharmacokinetic behavior. Administration of increasing doses of the drugs that are eliminated by saturable metabolism leads to more than proportional increase in the drug AUC after single drug administration and the drug steady-state concentration during multiple drug administration. Drugs like ethanol, phenytoin, and salicylate have been shown to have saturable drug metabolism and follow nonlinear pharmacokinetics in the range of doses that are used clinically [5,6].

Some drugs are eliminated by multiple parallel pathways in which one or more of these pathways can be saturated. For example, aspirin is eliminated from the body by five different parallel pathways, and two of these pathways are saturable. Whether the drug will follow clear nonlinear behavior or not depends on the relative contribution of the saturable pathway to the overall elimination of the drug. For example, if the saturable metabolic pathway represents a major elimination pathway, the nonlinear behavior of the drug will be evident. Also, the contribution of the saturable pathway to the overall drug elimination can change with the drug concentration. As the drug concentration increases, the rate of drug elimination by the saturable pathway becomes constant and the clearance for this saturable pathway decreases, while the rate of drug elimination via the first-order pathway increases with the increase in drug concentration and the clearance associated with this pathway remains constant. So as the concentration increases, the contribution of the saturable pathway to the overall elimination of the drug and the total clearance becomes smaller.

16.2.5 OTHER CONDITIONS THAT CAN LEAD TO NONLINEAR PHARMACOKINETICS

Product inhibition occurs when the drug is metabolized to metabolites that can compete with the parent drug for the same metabolizing enzymes [7]. Isosorbide dinitrate that is used in ischemic heart diseases is metabolized by denitration to isosorbide-2-mononitrate and isosorbide-5-mononitrate. These metabolites are further denitrated to isosorbide by the same enzymatic pathway. So the metabolites compete with the parent drug for the same enzymes resulting in slower rate of parent drug metabolism. Administration of different doses of the drug produces different amounts of the metabolites that inhibit the metabolism of the parent drug to different degrees. Also, the metabolite concentration after administration of the parent drug is always changing, which makes the rate of drug metabolism change all the time. So the drug pharmacokinetics will be nonlinear.

Time-dependent pharmacokinetics is also considered a type of nonlinear pharmacokinetics. This is observed when the drug pharmacokinetic behavior changes with time. Some drugs like carbamazepine can induce their own metabolism in a phenomenon known as autoinduction [8]. After initiation of carbamazepine therapy in epileptic patients, the drug accumulates in the body until steady state is achieved. The drug clearance increases gradually during the first 4–5 weeks of the initiation of therapy and remains steady thereafter. If the dosing rate of the drug is kept constant, an initial steady state is approached followed by gradual decline in the drug concentration until a lower steady-state concentration is achieved. The new steady state depends on the dosing rate and the higher drug clearance reached after induction. For this reason, carbamazepine therapy should be initiated with only a fraction of the recommended dose and then the dose is increased gradually every 2–3 weeks depending on the response and adverse effects.

16.3 PHARMACOKINETICS OF DRUGS ELIMINATED BY DOSE-DEPENDENT METABOLISM: MICHAELIS–MENTEN PHARMACOKINETICS

Drugs that follow nonlinear pharmacokinetics due to saturable metabolism have to be used with caution since small change in dose can cause more than proportional increase in the steady-state drug concentration. Dose-dependent metabolism, also known as capacity-limited metabolism, is the main cause of nonlinearity in most drugs that show evidence of nonlinearity in the range of doses used clinically.

16.3.1 MICHAELIS–MENTEN ENZYME KINETICS

Enzymatic reaction involves an interaction between the enzyme (E) and the substrate (D, the drug) to form an enzyme-substrate complex (ED), which can then dissociate to give the product of the reaction (M, the metabolite) and the enzyme as in Equation 16.4:

$$E + D \leftrightarrow ED \rightarrow E + M \tag{16.4}$$

The enzyme can then go back to react with the drug to form another molecule of the metabolite and so on. According to the Michaelis-Menten enzyme kinetic principles, a quantitative relationship between the enzymatic reaction rate (V) and the substrate concentration (S) can be expressed as

$$V = \frac{V_{max}S}{K_m + S} \tag{16.5}$$

where
  V_{max} is the maximum rate of the enzymatic reaction
  K_m is the Michaelis-Menten constant (M-M constant) that is a measure of the affinity of the substrate to the enzyme [9,10]

The M-M constant, K_m, is the substrate concentration when the reaction rate is $\frac{1}{2}V_{max}$. Assuming that a drug is metabolized via a single metabolic pathway, a similar relationship between the drug metabolic rate and the plasma drug concentration (Cp) can be written:

$$Rate = \frac{V_{max}Cp}{K_m + Cp} \tag{16.6}$$

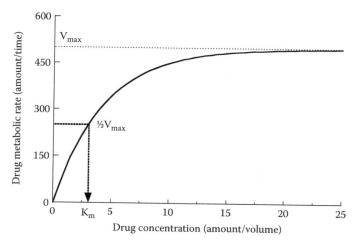

FIGURE 16.3 Relationship between the drug metabolic rate and the drug concentration. V_{max} is the maximum rate of drug metabolism, and K_m is the M-M constant and it is the drug concentration when the reaction rate is $\frac{1}{2}V_{max}$.

Graphically, this relationship can be presented as in Figure 16.3. This hyperbolic relationship indicates that as the drug concentration increases, the rate of drug metabolism increases until it reaches a plateau at very high drug concentration. At this plateau, the drug metabolizing enzymes are saturated and the metabolic rate is at its maximum value. Theoretically, all metabolic pathways can be saturated at very high drug concentration. However, saturable drug metabolism is of clinical significance when saturation occurs after administration of therapeutic doses of the drug.

The change in the drug metabolic rate as a function of the drug concentration is different at different drug concentrations as illustrated in Figure 16.3. At very low drug concentration (i.e., $K_m \gg Cp$), the drug metabolic rate is proportional to the drug concentration and the metabolic process follows first-order kinetic. Equation 16.6 can be approximated by

$$\text{Rate} \cong \left(\frac{V_{max}}{K_m} \right) Cp \tag{16.7}$$

On the contrary, at very high drug concentration (i.e., $K_m \ll Cp$), the metabolizing enzymes are saturated. The drug metabolic rate is constant and independent of the drug concentration and the metabolic process follows zero-order kinetic. Equation 16.6 can be approximated by

$$\text{Rate} \cong \left(\frac{V_{max} Cp}{Cp} \right) \cong V_{max} \tag{16.8}$$

16.3.2 Pharmacokinetic Parameters

The V_{max} of a metabolic pathway is the maximum rate of drug metabolism through this particular metabolic pathway. It has units of rate, that is, amount/time.

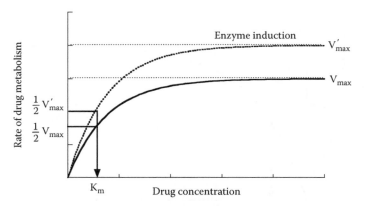

FIGURE 16.4 Enzyme induction causes an increase in V_{max} without affecting K_m.

Each metabolic pathway has its own V_{max} that depends on the amount of enzymes involved in the metabolic process. Enzyme induction increases the amount of the metabolizing enzymes that leads to the increase in V_{max}. The amount of enzyme increases without affecting the affinity of the enzyme to react with drugs. This means that enzyme induction does not affect K_m of the enzymatic process as in Figure 16.4.

The M-M constant, K_m, is a qualitative characteristic of how an enzyme interacts with the drug, and it is independent of the enzyme concentration. This constant is equal to the substrate concentration when the metabolic rate is half its maximum value, so it has units of concentration. In the presence of a competitive inhibitor for the metabolizing enzyme, the drug metabolic rate at any given drug concentration is slower than the rate in the absence of the inhibitor. However, as the drug concentration increases relative to the inhibitor concentration, the maximum metabolic rate is achieved. This means that in the presence of a competitive inhibitor, K_m increases without affecting V_{max} as illustrated in Figure 16.5.

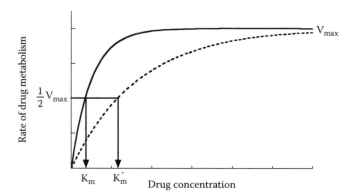

FIGURE 16.5 Competitive inhibition of the metabolizing enzyme increases K_m without affecting V_{max}.

16.3.3 DRUG CONCENTRATION–TIME PROFILE AFTER ADMINISTRATION OF A DRUG THAT IS ELIMINATED BY A SINGLE METABOLIC PATHWAY THAT FOLLOWS MICHAELIS–MENTEN KINETICS

16.3.3.1 After Single IV Bolus Administration

The model that describes the drug pharmacokinetic behavior after a single IV dose when the drug is eliminated via a single metabolic pathway that follows Michaelis-Menten kinetics is presented in Figure 16.6. The initial drug concentration is dependent on the dose and the drug Vd as in Equation 16.9. This means that administration of increasing doses produces initial drug concentrations (Cp_o) that are proportional to the administered dose:

$$Cp_o = \frac{\text{Dose}}{\text{Vd}} \tag{16.9}$$

The rate of decline in the amount of the drug in the body (A) is equal to the rate of drug metabolism. The differential equation that describes the rate of change of the amount of the drug in the body can be written as follows:

$$\frac{-dA}{dt} = \frac{V_{max}Cp}{K_m + Cp} \tag{16.10}$$

Integrating Equation 16.10 and dividing by the volume of distribution gives

$$Cp = Cp_o + K_m \ln\left(\frac{Cp_o}{Cp}\right) - \frac{V_{max}t}{Vd} \tag{16.11}$$

Equation 16.11 is not an explicit expression for the plasma concentration versus time relationship. This means that the equation cannot be used to calculate the plasma concentration at any time by substituting different values of time, because the term for the drug concentration is present in both sides of the equation and cannot be separated [9]. Numerical integration methods can be used to calculate the plasma drug concentration at different time points after drug administration. The plasma concentration–time profile after a single IV bolus dose of a drug that is eliminated by a single metabolic pathway that follows Michaelis-Menten kinetics is presented in Figure 16.7.

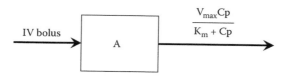

FIGURE 16.6 Schematic presentation of the pharmacokinetic model for a single IV bolus dose of a drug that is eliminated by a single metabolic pathway that follows Michaelis-Menten kinetics.

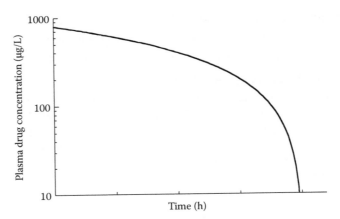

FIGURE 16.7 Plasma concentration–time profile after a single IV bolus dose of a drug that is eliminated by a single metabolic pathway that follows Michaelis-Menten kinetics.

16.3.3.2   During Multiple Drug Administration

Studying the pharmacokinetic behavior of the drugs that are eliminated by a process that follows Michaelis-Menten kinetics during multiple drug administration before reaching the steady state is not an easy task. However, at steady state the rate of drug administration is equal to the rate of drug elimination. When the drug is eliminated by a single metabolic pathway that follows Michaelis-Menten kinetics, the relationship between the dosing rate (FD/τ) and steady-state plasma drug concentration can be described by the following equation [10]:

$$\frac{FD}{\tau} = \frac{V_{max}Cp_{ss}}{K_m + Cp_{ss}} \qquad (16.12)$$

This equation can be rearranged to obtain an expression for the steady-state plasma drug concentration:

$$Cp_{ss} = \frac{(FD/\tau)K_m}{V_{max} - (FD/\tau)} \qquad (16.13)$$

This expression indicates that administration of increasing doses of the drug results in more than proportional increase in the steady-state plasma drug concentration as presented in Figure 16.8. When the dosing rate is close to the V_{max} of the drug, small change in the dose causes several-fold increase in the steady-state drug concentration. Also, if the dosing rate (FD/τ) exceeds V_{max}, the expected steady-state drug concentration will be a negative value according to Equation 16.11. The steady-state plasma drug concentration cannot be a negative value. From its definition, V_{max} is the maximum rate of drug elimination. So if the dosing rate exceeds V_{max}, steady state will never be achieved and continuous accumulation of the drug in the body will occur.

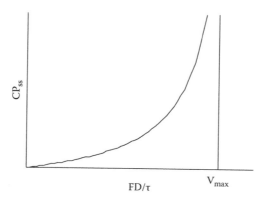

FIGURE 16.8 Relationship between the steady-state drug concentration and the dosing rate during multiple administration of a drug when the drug elimination process follows Michaelis-Menten kinetics.

16.3.4 DETERMINATION OF THE PHARMACOKINETIC PARAMETERS FOR DRUGS WITH ELIMINATION PROCESS THAT FOLLOWS MICHAELIS–MENTEN KINETICS

The pharmacokinetic behavior of the drug that is eliminated by a process that follows Michaelis-Menten kinetics depends on the pharmacokinetic parameters of the drug. Vd determines the relationship between the dose and the initial drug concentration after single drug administration, while the total body clearance determines the relationship between the dosing rate and the steady-state concentration during multiple drug administration, and the half-life determines the rate of decline in the drug concentration with time. So determination of the drug pharmacokinetic parameters is important to predict the pharmacokinetic behavior of the drug.

16.3.4.1 Volume of Distribution

Drug distribution is similar whether the drug elimination follows first-order or Michaelis-Menten kinetics. Vd can be calculated from the dose of the drug and the initial drug concentration achieved after a single IV dose of the drug. The relationship between dose, Cp_0, and Vd has been described in Equation 16.9.

16.3.4.2 Total Body Clearance

The total body clearance can be determined by dividing the drug metabolic rate by drug concentration:

$$CL_T = \frac{V_{max}}{K_m + Cp} \qquad (16.14)$$

Equation 16.14 indicates that the CL_T of the drug that is eliminated by a process that follows Michaelis-Menten kinetics is dependent on the drug concentration. As the drug concentration increases, CL_T decreases.

16.3.4.3 Half-Life

Half-life is the time required to decrease the plasma drug concentration by 50%. It can be calculated from the drug CL_T and Vd as follows:

$$t_{1/2} = \frac{0.693 \, \text{Vd}}{V_{max}} (K_m + Cp) \qquad (16.15)$$

Equation 16.15 indicates that the half-life of the drug that is eliminated by a process that follows Michaelis-Menten kinetics is dependent on the drug concentration. The half-life is longer when the drug concentration is higher. This is important because when a patient takes an overdose of a drug, toxic plasma drug concentration is achieved. In this case, it takes long time for the drug concentration to decrease to the therapeutic drug concentrations because the half-life is longer at high drug concentration.

CL_T and $t_{1/2}$ are different at different drug concentrations. So these parameters have to be calculated at a specific drug concentration. After a single drug administration, the drug concentration, and hence CL_T, and $t_{1/2}$, would change with time. The CL_T calculated from the dose and AUC similar to the drugs eliminated by the first-order process (CL_T = Dose/AUC) is an average value for the CL_T. At steady state, the plasma drug concentration will be fluctuating around an average steady-state concentration and CL_T and $t_{1/2}$ can be estimated at this average steady-state concentration.

16.4 ORAL ADMINISTRATION OF DRUGS THAT ARE ELIMINATED BY MICHAELIS–MENTEN PROCESS

The rate of drug absorption significantly affects the plasma concentration–time profile after a single oral dose when drug elimination is dose dependent. After oral administration of the same dose of a drug, rapidly absorbed formulations usually produce larger AUC compared to slowly absorbed formulations. This is because rapidly absorbed formulations achieve higher maximum drug concentration. At higher drug concentration, the total body clearance is lower and the half-life is longer when drug elimination is dose dependent. During multiple drug administration, the steady-state plasma drug concentration is dependent on the dose, V_{max} and K_m. The rate of drug absorption does not significantly affect the average steady-state plasma concentration. However, faster drug absorption may result in larger fluctuations in drug concentration at steady state.

The pharmacological effect of some drugs may be different after a single oral administration due to the difference in the rate of drug absorption. For example, alcohol is eliminated from the body by a saturable metabolic process. Consumption of the same amount of alcohol may produce different plasma concentration–time profiles depending on the rate of its absorption. The blood alcohol concentration–time profile after consumption of a certain amount of alcohol over a short period of time (rapid absorption) is much higher than that achieved after consumption of the same amount of alcohol over a longer period of time (slow absorption). Also, alcohol intake on an empty stomach results in faster absorption and higher alcohol blood concentration when compared to alcohol intake on a full stomach, which leads to slower alcohol absorption. The rapid absorption of alcohol may increase the bioavailability of alcohol due to saturable first-pass effect. The high alcohol blood concentrations achieved as a result of the rapid absorption and the higher bioavailability decreases alcohol clearance and prolongs its half-life, which leads to the higher alcohol concentration–time profile and the more intense pharmacological effect.

16.5 DETERMINATION OF THE MICHAELIS–MENTEN PARAMETERS AND CALCULATION OF THE APPROPRIATE DOSAGE REGIMENS

Dosage recommendation for drugs that are eliminated by the dose-dependent elimination process should be done with great caution especially for the drugs with narrow therapeutic window. This is because small change in dose can lead to significant change in the steady-state drug concentration. Also, the interpatient variability makes individualization of dosage regimen for these drugs difficult based on the patient's demographic information only. This demonstrates the importance of determination of the patient's specific Michaelis-Menten parameters for calculating the proper dosage requirements for each patient. All the methods used to calculate the Michaelis-Menten parameter, V_{max} and K_m, have several assumptions that can be summarized as follows [11,12]:

1. The drug is eliminated from the body by a single elimination pathway that follows Michaelis-Menten kinetics.
2. The drug is administered repeatedly in a fixed dose and dosing interval until steady state is achieved.
3. Information about two different dosing regimens and the steady-state drug concentration achieved while administration of each regimen is available.

16.5.1 MATHEMATICAL METHOD

The relationship between the dosing rate and the steady-state plasma drug concentration is described by Equation 16.12. When information is available about two different dosing rates and their corresponding steady-state drug concentrations, two different equations in the same form as Equation 16.10 can be constructed:

$$\frac{FD_1}{\tau} = \frac{V_{max}Cp_{ss1}}{K_m + Cp_{ss1}} \quad \text{and} \quad \frac{FD_2}{\tau} = \frac{V_{max}Cp_{ss2}}{K_m + Cp_{ss2}}$$

These two equations contain two different unknowns that are the two Michaelis-Menten kinetic parameters, V_{max} and K_m. The values for the dosing rates and the corresponding steady-state concentrations are substituted in the equations and the two equations can be solved simultaneously to determine V_{max} and K_m.

16.5.2 DIRECT LINEAR PLOT

Direct linear plot is a linear transformation method that is used to estimate V_{max} and K_m. This method requires knowledge of two different dosing rates and their corresponding steady-state plasma drug concentrations. The plot is constructed by plotting the dosing rate in the y-axis and the steady-state drug concentration on the left side of the x-axis. A line is drawn between each dosing rate and its corresponding steady-state concentration. The two lines for the two dosing rates are extrapolated until they intersect. The x-coordinate of the point of intersection corresponds to K_m, while the y-coordinate of the point of intersection corresponds to V_{max}/F as presented in Figure 16.9.

The direct linear plot can be used to estimate the steady-state plasma drug concentration achieved after administration of a specific dosing rate by drawing a line between the point of intersection and the dosing rate. Extrapolation of the line meets the x-axis at a point corresponding to the expected steady state that should be achieved after administration of this dosing rate. Also, the direct linear plot can be used to determine the dosing rate required to achieve a certain steady-state drug concentration by drawing a line between the point of intersection and the desired steady-state concentration. The line crosses the y-axis at a point corresponding to the dosing rate required to achieve the desired steady-state drug concentration.

Example

A 32-year-old, 75 kg female has been taking 200 mg of phenytoin daily. Because her average phenytoin plasma concentration was only 6 mg/L, her phenytoin dose was increased to 350 mg/day. The steady-state average phenytoin concentration was 21 mg/L (Vd of phenytoin is 0.75 L/kg and F = 1).

    a. Using the direct linear plot, calculate the phenytoin V_{max} and K_m in this patient.
    b. Calculate the dose required to achieve an average steady-state phenytoin plasma concentration around 15 mg/L.

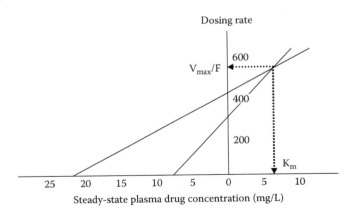

FIGURE 16.9 Direct linear plot.

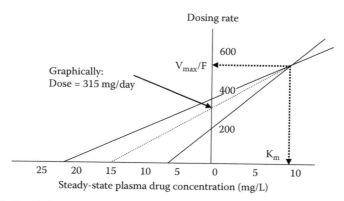

FIGURE 16.10 Estimation of the V_{max}, K_m, and the dose from the direct linear plot.

c. Calculate phenytoin half-life at steady state while the patient was taking 350 mg/day.
d. Because of poor seizure control, phenobarbitone was added to the patient's medications. After several weeks, phenytoin plasma concentration was 14 mg/L while taking 360 mg/day phenytoin. Comment on the decrease in phenytoin plasma concentration.

Answer

a. From the direct linear plot in Figure 16.10:
V_{max} = 500 mg/day
K_m = 9 mg/L
b. The dose required to achieve a steady-state concentration of 15 mg/L can be determined graphically and mathematically.
Graphically from Figure 16.10, the dose is approximately 315 mg/day.
Mathematically,

$$\frac{FD}{\tau} = \frac{V_{max}Cp_{ss}}{K_m + Cp_{ss}}$$

$$\frac{FD}{\tau} = \frac{500\,mg/day}{9 + 15\,mg/L} \cdot 15\,mg/L = 312.5\,mg/day$$

c. Steady state when the dose was 350 mg/day = 21 mg/L.

$$t_{1/2} = \frac{0.693Vd}{V_{max}}(K_m + Cp)$$

$$t_{1/2} = \frac{0.693(0.7\,L/kg \times 75\,kg)}{500\,mg/day}(9 + 21\ mg/L) = 2.18\,days$$

d. Phenobarbitone is an enzyme inducer that can increase the rate of phenytoin metabolism (increase V_{max}) and decrease its steady-state concentration.

16.5.3 LINEAR TRANSFORMATION METHOD

This method is based on a linear transformation of Equation 16.12 that relates the dosing rate and the achieved steady-state drug concentration and includes the Michaelis-Menten parameters, V_{max} and K_m:

$$\frac{FD}{\tau} = \frac{V_{max}Cp_{ss}}{K_m + Cp_{ss}}.$$

The principle of the linear transformation methods is to mathematically manipulate the aforementioned nonlinear equation to obtain an equation in the same form as the straight-line equation [13]:

$$\frac{FD}{\tau}K_m + \frac{FD}{\tau}Cp_{ss} = V_{max}Cp_{ss} \qquad (16.16)$$

Rearranging and dividing by FCp_{ss},

$$\frac{D}{\tau} = -K_m\frac{D/\tau}{Cp_{ss}} + \frac{V_{max}}{F} \qquad (16.17)$$

Equation 16.17 is a straight-line equation. A plot of the dosing rate (D/τ) versus the dosing rate divided by the average steady-state concentration yields a straight line with a slope equal to $-K_m$ and y-intercept equal to V_{max}/F as shown in Figure 16.11. The parameters V_{max} and K_m estimated from the slope and the y-intercept of the plot can be used to calculate the dosing rate required to achieve a certain Cp_{ss} or, conversely, to calculate the expected Cp_{ss} from administration of a given dosing rate.

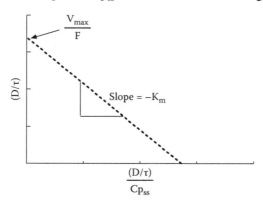

FIGURE 16.11 Plot of the dosing rate versus the dosing divided by the steady-state drug concentration. The slope is equal to $-K_m$, and the y-intercept is $\dfrac{V_{max}}{F}$.

16.6 MULTIPLE ELIMINATION PATHWAYS

In the previous discussion, it was assumed that the drug is eliminated by a single saturable elimination pathway that follows Michaelis-Menten kinetics. Many drugs are eliminated by more than one elimination pathways. If the drug is eliminated by two saturable elimination pathways that follow Michaelis-Menten kinetics, each pathway will have its own V_{max} and K_m as in Figure 16.12A. The rate of drug metabolism will be the sum of the rates for the two different pathways as in Equation 16.18:

$$\text{Rate} = \frac{V_{max1}Cp}{K_{m1}+Cp} + \frac{V_{max2}Cp}{K_{m2}+Cp} \tag{16.18}$$

As the drug concentration increases, one of the pathways is saturated first and then the second pathway is saturated at a different drug concentration. The fraction of dose that is eliminated by each of the pathways is dependent on the relative magnitude of the average clearances associated with each pathway. Since the clearances for the two pathways are dependent on the drug concentration, the fraction of dose eliminated by each pathway is different after administration of different doses. The drug will always follow nonlinear pharmacokinetics.

Some drugs are eliminated by two elimination pathways: one of them is saturable and the other follows first-order kinetics, Figure 16.12B. The rate of drug elimination in this case is the sum of the rates of the two pathways:

$$\text{Rate} = \frac{V_{max}Cp}{K_m+Cp} + kVdCp \tag{16.19}$$

Administration of increasing doses of the drug causes reduction of the clearance of the saturable elimination pathways while the clearance of the pathway that follows first-order kinetics remains constant. This makes larger fractions of the administered doses eliminated via the first-order pathway. At very high drug concentration, the contribution of the saturable pathway to the CL_T becomes very small. So the drug is still eliminated via the saturable pathway, but the majority of the drug is eliminated by the first-order pathway.

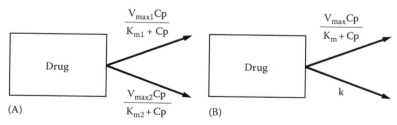

FIGURE 16.12 Schematic presentation of (A) the pharmacokinetic model for a drug eliminated by two parallel saturable elimination pathways that follow Michaelis-Menten kinetics and (B) the model for a drug eliminated by two elimination pathways: one saturable pathway follows Michaelis-Menten kinetics and the other follows first-order kinetics.

16.7 EFFECT OF CHANGING THE PHARMACOKINETIC PARAMETERS ON THE DRUG CONCENTRATION–TIME PROFILE

After a single IV dose of a drug that is eliminated by a single elimination pathway that follows Michaelis-Menten kinetics, the drug declines initially at slow rate and then the rate of decline increases as the drug concentration decreases. This is because the drug half-life is dependent on the drug concentration, while during multiple drug administration, the steady-state concentration is dependent on the dose and the drug CL_T, which is also dependent on the drug concentration.

16.7.1 PHARMACOKINETIC SIMULATION EXERCISE

Pharmacokinetic simulations can be used to examine how the change in the pharmacokinetic parameters affects the plasma drug concentration–time profile. The drug concentration–time profiles after a single IV administration and during multiple drug administrations can be simulated using average values for the pharmacokinetic parameters. Then, the pharmacokinetic parameters are changed one parameter at a time while keeping all the other parameters constant, and the simulation is repeated. The resulting profiles are examined to see how the change affects the rate of decline of the drug concentration after single IV administration and the drug steady-state concentration during multiple administrations. The plotting exercise of the nonlinear pharmacokinetics module in the basic pharmacokinetic concept section and the pharmacokinetic simulation section of the companion CD to this textbook can be used to run these simulations.

16.7.1.1 Dose

Administration of increasing IV bolus doses achieves higher initial plasma drug concentrations since Vd is constant. The drug CL_T is lower and the half-life is longer at higher drug concentration. So the rate of decline in the plasma drug concentration is slower at higher drug concentration and faster at lower drug concentration. However, at any given concentration the rate of decline of the drug concentration is similar since K_m and V_{max} are constant. Increasing the dose results in more than proportional increase in the steady-state concentration during multiple drug administration. It takes longer time to achieve steady state following administration of larger doses because the half-life is longer.

16.7.1.2 V_{max}

The drug CL_T is higher, and the half-life is shorter when V_{max} is higher. So after a single IV dose, the rate of decline in the drug concentration is faster and the AUC is smaller when V_{max} is high. During multiple administration of the same dose, the steady-state concentration is lower when V_{max} is higher and the time to achieve steady state is shorter because the half-life is shorter.

16.7.1.3 K_m

The drug CL_T is lower, and the half-life is longer when K_m is higher. So after a single IV dose of the drug, the rate of decline in the drug concentration is slower and the

AUC is larger when K_m is high. During multiple administration of the same dose, the steady-state concentration is higher when K_m is higher and the time to achieve steady state is longer because the half-life is longer.

PRACTICE PROBLEMS

16.1 A 78 kg, 28-year-old man is receiving phenytoin for the treatment of seizures. When this patient was taking a daily oral dose of 250 mg phenytoin, his steady-state plasma concentration was 7.2 mg/L. Because phenytoin plasma concentration was well below the therapeutic range, the patient's daily dose was increased to 450 mg phenytoin, which resulted in a steady-state plasma concentration of 30 mg/L. (Assume that the absolute bioavailability of oral phenytoin is 100%, and that the volume of distribution of phenytoin is 50 L.)
   a. Graphically calculate the patient's V_{max} and K_m.
   b. Calculate phenytoin half-life in this patient at steady state while taking 450 mg daily.
   c. What is the steady-state concentration that should be achieved if the dose was 300 mg daily?
   d. What is the daily phenytoin dose that should achieve a steady-state phenytoin plasma concentration of 20 mg/L in this patient?

16.2 A 65 kg male was started on 260 mg phenytoin daily at bed time to control his seizures. After 3 months of phenytoin therapy, his serum phenytoin concentration was found to be 5 mg/L. Because of the poor control of his seizures, his phenytoin dose was increased to 240 mg of phenytoin twice daily. One month after starting this new dosage regimen, the serum phenytoin concentration was found to be 24 mg/L. The volume of distribution of phenytoin is 0.7 L/kg.
   a. Calculate the V_{max} and K_m using a graphical method.
   b. Because the therapeutic range of phenytoin is 10–20 mg/L, recommend a dosage regimen to maintain steady-state serum phenytoin concentration around 15 mg/L.
   c. What will be the half-life of phenytoin at steady state if a dose of 200 mg every 12 h was given to this patient?
   d. If the phenytoin dose was changed and the steady-state serum phenytoin concentration was found to be exactly equal to the value of K_m that you have determined in part (a) in this problem, what will be the phenytoin elimination rate during this dosage regimen?

16.3 A 65 kg, 21-year-old woman is receiving phenytoin for the treatment of seizures. When she was taking a daily oral dose of 300 mg phenytoin, her steady-state plasma concentration was 5.1 mg/L. Because phenytoin plasma concentration was well below the therapeutic range, the patient's dose was increased to 500 mg phenytoin, which resulted in a steady-state plasma concentration of 20 mg/L. (Assume that the absolute bioavailability of oral phenytoin is 100%.)
   a. Graphically calculate the patient's V_{max} and K_m.
   b. Recommend a daily dose of phenytoin for this patient to achieve a phenytoin plasma concentration of 15 mg/L at steady state.

    c. Calculate the half-life and the total body clearance when the plasma concentration is 15 mg/L.

    d. What will be the steady-state concentration that should be achieved if the dose was 450 mg daily?

16.4 A 70 kg, 34-year-old man is receiving phenytoin for the treatment of seizures. When this patient was taking a daily oral dose of 350 mg phenytoin, his steady-state plasma concentration was 4.6 mg/L. Because phenytoin plasma concentration was well below the therapeutic range, the patient's dose was increased to 600 mg phenytoin, which resulted in a steady-state plasma concentration of 18 mg/L. (Assume that the absolute bioavailability of oral phenytoin is 100%.)

    a. Graphically calculate the patient's V_{max} and K_m.

    b. Although the patient's phenytoin plasma concentration is in the therapeutic range, the seizures were not controlled. Phenobarbitone, another drug used in the treatment of seizures that is known to be an enzyme inducer, was added to the patient's drug therapy. Four months later, while still taking 600 mg phenytoin/day in addition to the phenobarbitone, the patient's phenytoin plasma concentration was found to be 15 mg/L. Calculate the patient's new pharmacokinetic parameter responsible for this decrease in phenytoin plasma concentration (V_{max} and K_m).

    c. Recommend a daily dose of phenytoin at this induction state for this patient in order to achieve a steady-state plasma concentration of 20 mg/L.

16.5 A 25 kg, 14-year-old female was admitted to the hospital because of frequent episodes of seizures. She was diagnosed as having epileptic seizures and she was started on IV phenytoin. She received a loading dose of 5 mg/kg followed by 80 mg phenytoin IV given every 12 h. At steady state, the average plasma phenytoin concentration was found to be 8 mg/L. The phenytoin dose was increased to 100 mg phenytoin IV given every 12 h. At steady state, the plasma phenytoin concentration was 13.3 mg/L. Because the patient's condition was stable, the IV phenytoin was replaced with phenytoin oral suspension, which is known to have 100% bioavailability. The patient went home with a prescription for 225 mg phenytoin suspension at bed time every day. (The volume of distribution of phenytoin is 0.8 L/kg.)

    a. Graphically estimate phenytoin V_{max} and K_m in this patient.

    b. What is the expected average steady-state phenytoin concentration in this patient while taking the 225 mg phenytoin suspension at night?

    c. Calculate phenytoin CL_T and half-life in this patient while taking the phenytoin suspension (225 mg phenytoin at bed time) at steady state.

REFERENCES

1. Evans WE, Schentag JJ, and Jusco WJ (1992) *Applied Pharmacokinetics: Principles of Therapeutic Drug Monitoring*, 3rd edn., Lippincott Williams & Wilkins, Philadelphia, PA.
2. Ludden TM (1991) Nonlinear pharmacokinetics. Clinical applications. *Clin Pharmacokinet* 20:430–432.
3. Hsu F, Prueksritanont T, Lee MG, and Chiou WL (1987) The phenomenon and cause of the dose-dependent oral absorption of chlorothiazide in rats: Extrapolation to human data based on the body surface area concept. *J Pharmacokinet Biopharm* 15:369–386.

4. Yu HY, Shen YZ, Sugiyama Y, and Hanano M (1987) Dose-dependent pharmacokinetics of valproate in guinea pigs of different ages. *Epilepsia* 28:680–687.
5. Levy G (1979) Pharmacokinetics of salicylate in man. *Drug Metab Rev* 9:3–19.
6. Ludden TM, Hawkins DW, Allen JP, and Hoffman SF (1976) Optimum phenytoin dosage regimen. *Lancet* 1(7954):307–308.
7. Perrier D, Ashley JJ, and Levy G (1973) Effect of product inhibition in kinetics of drug elimination. *J Pharmacokinet Biopharm* 1:231–242.
8. Levy RH (1983) Time-dependent pharmacokinetics. *Pharmacol Ther* 17:383–392.
9. Wagner J (1973) Properties of the Michaelis-Menten equation and its integrated form which are useful in pharmacokinetics. *J Pharmacokinet Biopharm* 1:103–121.
10. Wagner JG, Szpunar GJ, and Ferry JJ (1985) Michaelis-Menten elimination kinetics: Areas under curves, steady-state concentrations, and clearances for compartment models with different types of input. *Biopharm Drug Dispos* 6:177–200.
11. Mullen PW (1978) Optimal phenytoin therapy: A new technique for individualizing dosage. *Clin Pharmacol Ther* 23:228–232.
12. Vozeh S, Muir KT, Sheiner LB, and Follath F (1981) Predicting individual phenytoin dosage. *J Pharmacokinet Biopharm* 9:131–146.
13. Mullen PW and Foster RW (1979) Comparative evaluation of six techniques for determining the Michaelis-Menten parameters relating phenytoin dose and steady-state serum concentrations. *J Pharm Pharmacol* 31:100–104.

17 Multicompartment Pharmacokinetic Models

OBJECTIVES

After completing this chapter you should be able to

- Describe the differences between the one-compartment and the two-compartment pharmacokinetic models
- Define all the parameters of the two-compartment pharmacokinetic model
- Describe the plasma concentration–time profile after a single IV and oral administration, during constant rate IV infusion, and multiple drug administration of drugs that follow two-compartment pharmacokinetic model
- Estimate all the pharmacokinetic parameters of the two-compartment pharmacokinetic model from plasma concentrations obtained after a single IV administration
- Analyze the effect of changing one or more of the pharmacokinetic parameters on the plasma concentration–time profile and the drug distribution between the central and the peripheral compartments after administration of drugs that follow the two-compartment pharmacokinetic model
- Describe the general steps for compartmental modeling and discuss the general approaches used to evaluate the goodness of model fit

17.1 INTRODUCTION

In the previous discussions, it was assumed that the drug is rapidly distributed to all parts of the body once it enters the systemic circulation. An immediate equilibrium is established between the drug in the systemic circulation and the drug in all parts of the body. The drug concentration in different parts of the body is different because of the differences in drug affinity to the different tissues. However, any change in the plasma drug concentration due to drug absorption or drug elimination is accompanied by a proportional change in the drug concentration in the different tissues. So the drug concentration–time profiles in the different parts of the body are parallel to each other. The rapid distribution equilibrium achieved between the different tissues makes the body act as one homogenous compartment.

The process of drug distribution to the different parts of the body can be demonstrated by a beaker that has a coating material covering its inner wall and is filled with a liquid as in Figure 17.1. In this example, the liquid in the center of the beaker represents the systemic circulation and the beaker wall coating materials represents the tissues. If a drop of dye is added to the liquid, the dye is distributed in the liquid

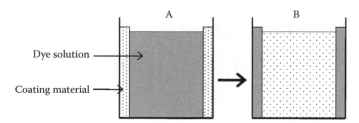

FIGURE 17.1 Diagrammatic presentation of the distribution of the dye from the solution in the center of the beaker to the beaker wall coating material. The distribution process causes decrease in the dye concentration in solution and increase in the dye concentration in the coating material. When the dye distribution to the beaker wall coating material (A → B) is fast, the beaker behaves as a single compartment, while when the dye distribution to the beaker wall coating material (A → B) is slow, the beaker behaves as if it consists of two different compartments.

in the center of the beaker first and then to the coating material of the beaker wall. If the dye is rapidly distributed from the liquid to the coating material, the dye distribution equilibrium is achieved rapidly. The dye concentration in the liquid in the center of the beaker becomes constant immediately after addition of the dye. In this case, the beaker behaves as a single compartment despite the difference in dye concentration in the liquid and in the beaker wall covering. For drugs that are rapidly distributed from the systemic circulation to the tissues, rapid distribution equilibrium between the drug in the systemic circulation and tissues is achieved. When the drug is eliminated, the drug concentrations in the systemic circulation and in all tissues decline at the same rate because of the rapid distribution equilibrium. Drugs that follow this behavior follow the one-compartment pharmacokinetic model. When these drugs are administered by a rapid IV bolus dose, the plasma drug concentration declines monoexponentially and the plasma drug concentration–time profile is linear on the semilog scale.

For some drugs, the distribution from the systemic circulation to the different tissues is slow. The beaker example mentioned earlier can be used to explain this condition. After addition of the dye to the beaker, it distributes in the liquid in the center of the beaker initially. Then the dye starts to distribute slowly to the beaker wall coating material. The distribution of the dye from the liquid in the center of the beaker to the beaker wall coating material causes gradual decrease in the dye concentration in the liquid and gradual increase in the dye concentration in the beaker coating material as illustrated in Figure 17.1. The dye concentration in the liquid reaches a constant value when equilibrium is achieved between the dye in the liquid and the beaker wall coating material as illustrated in Figure 17.2.

After IV administration of a drug that is slowly distributed to the tissues, the drug is immediately distributed in the systemic circulation and other highly perfused tissues. The drug concentration in the systemic circulation decreases initially at a fast rate due to drug distribution to the tissues and also due to drug elimination from the body. When equilibrium is established between the drug in the systemic circulation and all tissues, the drug concentration in the systemic circulation and tissues declines at a rate dependent on the rate of elimination, which is slower than

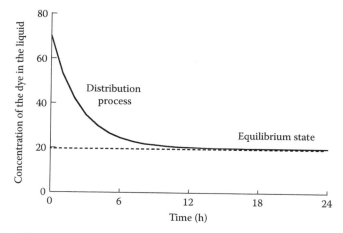

FIGURE 17.2 Dye concentration–time profile in the liquid with the decrease in the dye concentration representing the distribution of the dye from the liquid in the central of the beaker to the beaker wall coating material.

the initial rate of decline. After IV bolus administration of the drugs that follow this behavior, the plasma drug concentration–time profile is curvilinear on the semilog scale. These drugs follow the two-compartment, three-compartment, or any other multi-compartment pharmacokinetic model. This model consists of a central compartment that includes the vascular space and highly perfused tissues and one or more peripheral compartments that include the other organs of the body.

17.2 COMPARTMENTAL PHARMACOKINETIC MODELS

Pharmacokinetic modeling in general involves the development of a model that can quantitatively describe the pharmacokinetic behavior of the drug in the body. In compartmental modeling, the body is described by one or more interconnected compartments depending on the rate of drug distribution to the different parts of the body. The number of compartments in the model depends on the rate of drug distribution to the different parts of the body. Each of the compartments has its own volume of distribution and the intercompartmental clearances that govern the drug distribution and transfer between these compartments. The model includes an input function that describes the drug entry to the systemic circulation. The order of the elimination process and the compartment where the elimination process takes place are included in the model [1].

Compartmental pharmacokinetic models differ in the number of compartments, the compartment(s) where drug elimination occurs, and the arrangement of these compartments. The number of compartments in the model depends on the rate of drug distribution to the different parts of the body. If the drug in the systemic circulation is distributed rapidly to all parts of the body, the body behaves as a single compartment and the drug pharmacokinetic behavior can be described by one-compartment pharmacokinetic model, while if the drug is distributed rapidly to some tissues and organs and slowly to other tissues and organs, the two-compartment pharmacokinetic

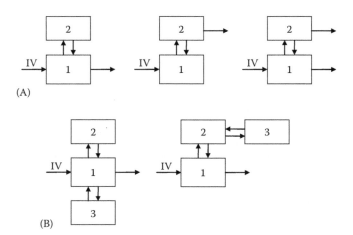

FIGURE 17.3 Diagram represents different compartmental pharmacokinetic models. (A) Examples of two-compartment pharmacokinetic models with elimination from compartment 1, compartment 2, or both compartments. (B) Examples of the many possible three-compartment pharmacokinetic models that differ in the arrangement of the compartments and in the compartment(s) where drug elimination takes place.

model can be used to describe the pharmacokinetic behavior of the drug in this case. On the contrary, when the drug is distributed to the different parts of the body at three distinguished rates, for example, rapid, slow, and very slow, the three-compartment pharmacokinetic model can be used to describe this pharmacokinetic behavior. The pharmacokinetic behavior of most drugs can be described by one-, two-, or three-compartment pharmacokinetic models; however, models with more compartments can be used if the obtained data can support these complicated models.

Pharmacokinetic models that have the same number of compartments can be different when drug elimination occurs from different compartments [2]. The different two-compartment pharmacokinetic models presented in Figure 17.3A differ in the compartment where drug elimination takes place. One of the models has drug elimination from compartment 1, the second model has drug elimination from compartment 2, and the third model has drug elimination from both compartments. For the three-compartment pharmacokinetic model, there are seven different possibilities for the compartment(s) where drug elimination takes place. Also, pharmacokinetic compartment models can differ in the way the compartments are arranged. For example, the models presented in Figure 17.3B are examples of the three-compartment pharmacokinetic models.

17.3 TWO-COMPARTMENT PHARMACOKINETIC MODEL

The two-compartment pharmacokinetic model with elimination from the central compartment is the most common model used to describe the pharmacokinetic behavior of drugs that follow two-compartment model. So this model will be used in the following discussion. After IV bolus dose, the drug is distributed rapidly to the body spaces and tissues that represent the central compartment. Then the drug is distributed by a first-order process from the central compartment to the other body spaces and tissues that represent the peripheral compartment. Because the blood is usually part of the central compartment, the drug can be delivered to the eliminating organ(s) once the drug is in the central compartment. So distribution and elimination occur simultaneously after drug administration, which causes rapid decline in the drug concentration in the central compartment. After the distribution process is completed and equilibrium is established between the drug in the central compartment and the drug in the peripheral compartment, the drug concentration in the central compartment declines at a rate dependent on drug elimination. The rate of decline in the drug concentration in the central compartment due to drug elimination is slower than the initial rate of decline due to distribution and elimination. So the plasma drug concentration–time profile that represents the drug profile in the central compartment consists of two phases on the semilog scale. An initial distribution phase characterized by rapid decline in drug concentration, followed by a terminal elimination phase with slower rate of decline in drug concentration. The drug concentration–time profile during the terminal elimination phase is linear on the semilog scale since it declines depending on the rate of drug elimination [3]. A typical plasma concentration–time profile after IV bolus administration of drugs that follow two-compartment pharmacokinetic model is presented in Figure 17.4.

The two-compartment pharmacokinetic model assumes that at time zero there is no drug in the tissues representing the peripheral compartment. After an IV dose, the drug is rapidly distributed in the central compartment. The amount of drug in the central compartment declines rapidly due to the transfer of drug out of the central compartment to the peripheral compartment and also due to drug elimination that occurs simultaneously. The drug in the central compartment is transferred to the peripheral compartment by a first-order process, and can return back to the central compartment also by a first-order process. Initially the amount of the drug in the central compartment is larger than the amount of the drug in the peripheral compartment, so the net drug transfer is from the central compartment to the peripheral

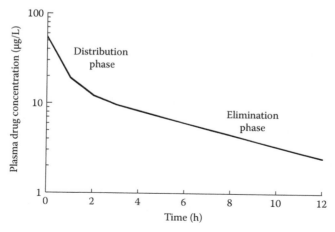

FIGURE 17.4   Plasma concentration–time profile of a drug that follows the two-compartment pharmacokinetic model after single IV bolus dose.

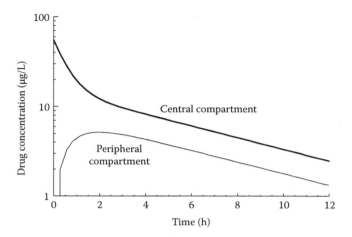

FIGURE 17.5 Drug concentration–time profile in the central and peripheral compartments after administration of a single IV bolus dose of a drug that follows two-compartment pharmacokinetic model.

compartment. This means that initially the amount of drug in the peripheral compartment increases with time.

As the amount of drug in the peripheral compartment increases, the rate of drug transfer from the peripheral to the central compartment approaches that from the central to the peripheral compartment. When these two rates become equal, the amount of drug in the peripheral compartment reaches a maximum value. Because the drug is continually eliminated from the central compartment, the amount of drug in the central compartment decreases and the rate of drug transfer from the peripheral to the central compartment becomes larger than that from the central to peripheral compartment. The net drug transfer is from the peripheral to the central compartment, and the amount of drug in the peripheral compartment starts to decline parallel to the decline in the amount of the drug in the central compartment. Figure 17.5 shows the drug concentration–time profile in the central and peripheral compartments after administration of a single IV bolus dose. The concentration of drug in the central compartment is determined by dividing the amount of drug in the central compartment by the volume of the central compartment. Likewise, the concentration of drug in the peripheral compartment is determined by dividing the amount of drug in the peripheral compartment by the volume of the peripheral compartment. So, the drug concentration in the peripheral compartment can be higher or lower than the drug concentration in the central compartment depending on the drug affinity to the tissues.

17.4 PARAMETERS OF THE TWO-COMPARTMENT PHARMACOKINETIC MODEL

The two-compartment pharmacokinetic model presented by the block diagram in Figure 17.6 assumes that the drug transport between the central and peripheral compartments follows first-order kinetics and that the drug is eliminated from the central compartment by a first-order process.

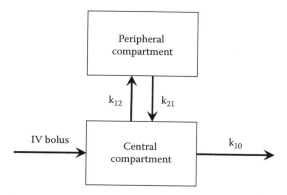

FIGURE 17.6   Block diagram that represents the two-compartment pharmacokinetic model with first-order transport between the central and peripheral compartments and first-order drug elimination from the central compartment.

17.4.1   DEFINITION OF THE PHARMACOKINETIC PARAMETERS

The following are the definitions of the pharmacokinetic parameters used in deriving the equations for the two-compartment pharmacokinetic model:

X is the amount of drug in the central compartment and has units of mass.

Y is the amount of drug in the peripheral compartment and has units of mass.

k_{12} is the first-order transfer rate constant from the central compartment to the peripheral compartment and has units of time^{-1}.

k_{21} is the first-order transfer rate constant from the peripheral compartment to the central compartment and has units of time^{-1}.

k_{10} is the first-order elimination rate constant from the central compartment and has units of time^{-1}.

A and B   are the hybrid coefficients and have units of concentrations.

α is the hybrid first-order rate constant for the distribution process and has units of time^{-1}.

β is the hybrid first-order rate constant for the elimination process and has units of time^{-1}.

$t_{1/2\alpha}$ is the half-life for the distribution phase and has units of time.

$t_{1/2\beta}$ is the half-life for the elimination phase and has units of time.

V_c is the volume of the central compartment and has units of volume. This term relates the administered dose to the initial plasma drug concentration (central compartment concentration) after administration of a single IV dose:

$$Cp_o = \frac{Dose}{V_c} \tag{17.1}$$

Vd_{ss} is the volume of distribution of the drug at steady state and has units of volume. This term relates the amount of the drug in the body and the plasma drug concentration at steady state:

Amount of the drug in the body at steady state $= Vd_{ss}Cp_{ss}$ (17.2)

Vd_β or Vd_{area} is the volume of distribution during the elimination phase and has units of volume. This term relates the amount of the drug in the body and the plasma drug concentration during the elimination phase (β-phase):

Amount of the drug in the body during the elimination phase $= Vd_\beta Cp_{\beta\text{-phase}}$ (17.3)

17.4.2 MATHEMATICAL EQUATION THAT DESCRIBES THE PLASMA CONCENTRATION–TIME PROFILE

The rate of change of the amount of the drug in any compartment is equal to the sum of the rates of drug transfer into the compartment minus the sum of the rates of drug transfer out of the compartment. After a single IV bolus dose and based on the pharmacokinetic model in Figure 17.6, the rate of change of the amount of the drug in the central compartment (X) at any time is equal to the rate of drug transfer from the peripheral compartment to the central compartment minus the rate of drug transfer from the central compartment to the peripheral compartment, minus the rate of drug elimination. Similarly, the rate of change of the amount of drug in the peripheral compartment (Y) is equal to the rate of drug transfer from the central compartment to the peripheral compartment minus the rate of drug transfer from the peripheral compartment to the central compartment. The differential equations that describe these two rates are

$$\frac{dX}{dt} = k_{21}Y - k_{12}X - k_{10}X \tag{17.4}$$

and

$$\frac{dY}{dt} = k_{12}X - k_{21}Y \tag{17.5}$$

Integrating the first differential equation yields the integrated equation for the amount of drug in the central compartment (X) as a function of time after a single IV bolus dose (D):

$$X = \frac{D(\alpha - k_{21})}{(\alpha - \beta)} e^{-\alpha t} + \frac{D(k_{21} - \beta)}{(\alpha - \beta)} e^{-\beta t} \tag{17.6}$$

This equation contains two exponents, one exponent describes the distribution process and the other describes the elimination process. These exponents contain the hybrid rate constants for the distribution and elimination processes, α and β. As a result of the integration process to get the integrated equation for the amount of the drug in the central compartment, the following two relationships were obtained:

$$\alpha + \beta = k_{12} + k_{21} + k_{10} \tag{17.7}$$

$$\alpha\beta = k_{21}k_{10} \tag{17.8}$$

where

$$\alpha = \frac{1}{2}\left[(k_{12} + k_{21} + k_{10}) + \sqrt{(k_{12} + k_{21} + k_{10})^2 - 4k_{21}k_{10}}\right] \qquad (17.9)$$

$$\beta = \frac{1}{2}\left[(k_{12} + k_{21} + k_{10}) - \sqrt{(k_{12} + k_{21} + k_{10})^2 - 4k_{21}k_{10}}\right] \qquad (17.10)$$

Since the distribution process is usually faster than the elimination process, the larger hybrid rate constant α is the rate constant for the distribution process and the smaller hybrid rate constant β is the rate constant for the elimination process as in Equations 17.9 and 17.10. During the distribution phase, the drug distribution rate does not depend only on k_{12}, the transfer rate constant from the central to peripheral compartment. This is because while the drug is distributing from the central to the peripheral compartment, there is drug returning back to the central compartment at a rate dependent on the rate constant k_{21}, and also there is elimination from the peripheral compartment affected by the rate constant k_{10}. So the observed rate of the distribution process is described by the hybrid rate constant α, which is dependent on the three rate constants k_{12}, k_{21}, and k_{10} as in Equation 17.9. Similarly, the drug elimination rate does not depend only on k_{10}, the elimination rate constant from the central compartment. This is because during the elimination of the drug from the central compartment, there is drug transfer from the central to the peripheral compartment at a rate dependent on the rate constant k_{12}, and drug returning back to the central compartment at a rate dependent on the rate constant k_{21}. So the observed rate for the elimination process is described by the hybrid rate constant β, which is dependent on the three rate constants k_{12}, k_{21}, and k_{10} as in Equation 17.10. The first-order rate constants k_{12}, k_{21}, and k_{10} are usually termed the micro rate constants, while α and β are termed the macro rate constants.

Dividing Equation 17.6 by the volume of the central compartment, V_c, gives the equation for the drug concentration in the central compartment, and hence the plasma drug concentration, at any time after a single IV bolus dose:

$$Cp = \frac{D(\alpha - k_{21})}{V_c(\alpha - \beta)}e^{-\alpha t} + \frac{D(k_{21} - \beta)}{V_c(\alpha - \beta)}e^{-\beta t} \qquad (17.11)$$

which can be simplified to

$$Cp = Ae^{-\alpha t} + Be^{-\beta t} \qquad (17.12)$$

where

$$A = \frac{D(\alpha - k_{21})}{V_c(\alpha - \beta)} \qquad (17.13)$$

and

$$B = \frac{D(k_{21} - \beta)}{V_c(\alpha - \beta)} \qquad (17.14)$$

Equation 17.11 and its simplified form Equation 17.12 are the equations that describe the plasma drug concentration at any time after a single IV bolus dose of a drug that follows the two-compartment pharmacokinetic model [4]. These equations include two exponents: one describes the distribution process and includes the larger hybrid rate constant, α, and the other describes the elimination process and includes the smaller hybrid rate constant, β. As time elapses after IV drug administration, the exponential term that has the distribution (larger) hybrid rate constant approaches zero and the plasma concentration declines at a rate dependent on the hybrid elimination rate constant, β. So the plasma drug concentration–time profile after a single IV bolus dose on the semilog scale has a rapidly declining distribution phase and a linear terminal elimination phase.

17.5   DETERMINATION OF THE TWO-COMPARTMENT PHARMACOKINETIC MODEL PARAMETERS

The pharmacokinetic parameters k_{21}, V_c, α, and β, in Equation 17.11, or the parameters A, B, α, and β, in Equation 17.12, can be estimated from the plasma drug concentrations obtained after a single IV dose (D) of the drug by nonlinear regression analysis utilizing specialized statistical programs. The estimated parameters in both equations can be used to calculate all the other parameters of the model. The pharmacokinetic parameters allow prediction of the drug steady-state plasma concentration during repeated drug administration and determination of the dose required to achieve certain drug concentration at steady state. The pharmacokinetic parameters in Equation 17.12, A, B, α, and β, can be estimated graphically utilizing the method of residuals.

17.5.1   METHOD OF RESIDUALS

The method of residuals is a graphical method used to estimate the two-compartment pharmacokinetic model parameters after a single IV dose. The basic principle of the method of residuals is to separate the two exponential terms in Equation 17.12 as illustrated in Figure 17.7. The method of residuals can be summarized by the following steps:

- The experimentally obtained plasma concentrations are plotted against their corresponding time values on the semilog scale.
- The plasma drug concentrations that decline linearly during the elimination phase are identified. The best line that passes through these points is drawn and the line is back extrapolated to meet the y-axis.
- This line is corresponding to the $(Be^{-\beta t})$ term in the biexponential equation. The y-intercept of the extrapolated line is equal to the coefficient B in the equation. The hybrid rate constant β can be determined from the slope of the line (slope = $-\beta/2.303$). Also, the $t_{1/2\beta}$ can be determined directly from the line by calculating the time required for any concentration on the line to decrease by 50%. Then β is calculated as

$$\beta = \frac{0.693}{t_{1/2\beta}}$$

(17.15)

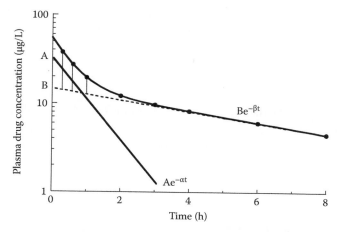

FIGURE 17.7 Method of residuals applied to separate the two exponential terms of the equation that describes the plasma concentration–time profile of drugs that follow the two-compartment pharmacokinetic model after a single IV dose.

- The residuals are calculated from the difference between the observed plasma concentration–time data and the corresponding values on the extrapolated line representing the elimination phase. The residuals are plotted versus their corresponding time values.
- The residual versus time plot is linear on the semilog scale and this line is corresponding to the $(Ae^{-\alpha t})$ term in the biexponential equation. The y-intercept of this line is equal to the coefficient A in the equation. The hybrid rate constant α can be determined from the slope of the line (slope $= -\alpha/2.303$). Also, the $t_{1/2\alpha}$ can be determined directly from the line by calculating the time required for any point on the line representing the α-phase to decrease by 50%. Then the hybrid rate constant α is calculated as

$$\alpha = \frac{0.693}{t_{1/2\alpha}} \tag{17.16}$$

- A is always the y-intercept of the faster process (the process with shorter $t_{1/2}$, the distribution process), and B is always the intercept of the slower process (the process with longer $t_{1/2}$, the elimination process).

17.5.2 DETERMINATION OF THE MODEL PARAMETERS

Once the parameters A, B, α, and β are determined from the method of residuals, the other model parameters can be calculated [1].

17.5.2.1 Volume of the Central Compartment, V_c

After IV bolus administration, the drug is distributed initially in the central compartment. So the volume of the central compartment can be determined from the dose and the initial drug concentration in the central compartment, which is same as the initial plasma drug concentration. The plasma concentration at time zero is determined from Equation 17.12 by substituting the time by zero, and it is equal to (A + B):

$$V_c = \frac{\text{Dose}}{\text{Cp}_o} = \frac{\text{Dose}}{A + B} \tag{17.17}$$

17.5.2.2 Area under the Plasma Concentration–Time Curve, AUC

The area under the plasma concentration–time curve is determined by integrating Equation 17.12, which describes the plasma concentration–time profile from time 0 to ∞:

$$\left.\text{AUC}\right|_{t=0}^{t=\infty} = \frac{A}{\alpha} + \frac{B}{\beta} \tag{17.18}$$

17.5.2.3 Total Body Clearance, CL_T

The CL_T is determined from the dose and the AUC similar to the one-compartment pharmacokinetic model:

$$CL_T = \frac{\text{Dose}}{\left.\text{AUC}\right|_{t=0}^{t=\infty}} \tag{17.19}$$

17.5.2.4 First-Order Elimination Rate Constant from the Central Compartment, k_{10}

The CL_T is the product of the first-order elimination rate constant k_{10} and V_c. When V_c and CL_T are known, k_{10} can be calculated:

$$CL_T = k_{10}V_c \tag{17.20}$$

$$k_{10} = \frac{CL_T}{V_c} \tag{17.21}$$

17.5.2.5 First-Order Transfer Rate Constant from the Peripheral Compartment to the Central Compartment, k_{21}

As a result of integrating the differential equation to obtain the integrated equation for the amount of the drug in the central compartment, the relationship in Equation 17.8 has been obtained ($\alpha\beta = k_{21}k_{10}$). Based on this relationship, k_{21} can be calculated:

$$k_{21} = \frac{\alpha\beta}{k_{10}} \tag{17.22}$$

17.5.2.6 First-Order Transfer Rate Constant from the Central Compartment to the Peripheral Compartment, k_{12}

Also, while integrating the differential equation to obtain the integrated equation for the amount of the drug in the central compartment, the relationship in

Equation 17.7 has been obtained $(\alpha + \beta = k_{12} + k_{21} + k_{10})$. Based on this relationship, k_{12} can be calculated:

$$k_{12} = (\alpha + \beta) - (k_{21} + k_{10}) \qquad (17.23)$$

17.5.3 DETERMINATION OF THE VOLUMES OF DISTRIBUTION FOR THE TWO-COMPARTMENT PHARMACOKINETIC MODEL

In the one-compartment pharmacokinetic model the drug is distributed rapidly to all parts of the body and the distribution equilibrium is established immediately after drug administration. So the drugs that follow one-compartment pharmacokinetic model are distributed in the same tissues once they enter the systemic circulation and they have only one volume of distribution. However, in the two-compartment pharmacokinetic model there is more than one volume of distribution. Initially, after IV drug administration the drug is distributed in the central compartment only. Then the drug distributes from the central compartment to the peripheral compartments. During the elimination phase the drug volume of distribution is equal to Vd_β and during steady state the drug volume of distribution is equal to Vd_{ss}. The volume of the central compartment is the smallest, while Vd_β is the largest of the three volumes in the two-compartment pharmacokinetic model. Vd_{ss} is larger than V_c and smaller than Vd_β. V_c can be calculated from the dose of the initial drug concentration as in Equation 17.17.

17.5.3.1 Volume of Distribution at Steady State, Vd_{ss}

Vd_{ss} is the factor that relates the amount of the drug in the body and the plasma drug concentration during steady state when the drug is administered by constant rate IV infusion and the drug concentration in the body is constant. When the drug concentration is constant, the rate of drug transfer from the central to the peripheral compartment is equal to the rate of drug transfer from the peripheral to the central compartment. Also, a transient steady state is achieved for brief moment after a single IV administration when the drug concentration in the peripheral compartment reaches its maximum value, and the net rate of drug transfer between the central and peripheral compartments is equal to zero. The rate of drug transfer can be expressed by the drug transfer rate constant and the amount of the drug in each compartment. At steady state,

$$k_{12}X = k_{21}Y \qquad (17.24)$$

$$Y = \frac{Xk_{12}}{k_{21}} = \frac{Cp_{ss}V_c k_{12}}{k_{21}} \qquad (17.25)$$

Since the amount of the drug in the central compartment is the product of the plasma drug concentration and V_c. At steady state, Vd_{ss} relates the amount of the drug in the body to the drug concentration in plasma:

$$Vd_{ss} = \frac{X + Y}{Cp_{ss}} = \frac{Cp_{ss}V_c + Cp_{ss}V_c(k_{12}/k_{21})}{Cp_{ss}} \qquad (17.26)$$

$$Vd_{ss} = V_c + V_c \frac{k_{12}}{k_{21}} \tag{17.27}$$

$$Vd_{ss} = V_c \left(1 + \frac{k_{12}}{k_{21}} \right) \tag{17.28}$$

17.5.3.2   Volume of Distribution in the Elimination Phase, Vd_β

During the elimination phase, distribution equilibrium is established between the drug in the central and peripheral compartments, which makes the drug concentration in the central and peripheral compartments decline at the same rate. However, there is more drug transfer from the peripheral compartment to the central compartment to compensate for the drug elimination that occurs from the central compartment. The volume of distribution during the elimination phase can be calculated from the CL_T and the first-order hybrid elimination rate constant:

$$Vd_\beta = \frac{CL_T}{\beta} = \frac{V_c k_{10}}{\beta} \tag{17.29}$$

Example

After a single IV bolus dose of 1000 mg of an antiarrhythmic drug, the following concentrations were obtained:

Time (h)	Concentration (mg/L)
0.2	120
0.5	84
1.0	53
2.0	29
4.0	18
6.0	15
8.0	12.5
12.0	8.8

    a. Using the method of residuals, calculate the following parameters:
       $t_{1/2\alpha}$, $t_{1/2\beta}$, k_{12}, k_{21}, k_{10}, V_c, Vd_β, Vd_{ss}, AUC, and CL_T
    b. What will be the amount of drug remaining in the body after 15 h?

Answer

a. The method of residuals used to solve the problem and presented in Figure 17.8 can be performed by the following steps:

- Plot the concentration versus time on a semilog scale.
- Identify the best line that represents the drug elimination process.

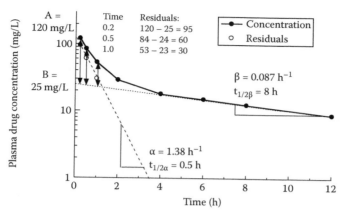

FIGURE 17.8 Application of the method of residuals in solving the example.

- The y-intercept is equal to B. The hybrid elimination rate constant (β) and β-half-life can be determined from the line.
- Calculate the residuals from the difference between the plasma drug concentration and the values on the extrapolated line during the distribution phase.
- Plot the residuals versus time, and draw the best line that goes through the points.
- The y-intercept of this line is equal to A. The hybrid distribution rate constant α and α-half-life can be determined from this line.

A 120 mg/L
B 25 mg/L

$$\alpha = 1.38\,h^{-1} \quad t_{1/2\alpha} = 0.5\,h$$

$$\beta = 0.087\,h^{-1} \quad t_{1/2\beta} = 8\,h$$

$$V_c = \frac{Dose}{A + B} = \frac{1000}{120 + 25\,mg/L} = 6.9\,L$$

$$AUC = \frac{A}{\alpha} + \frac{B}{\beta} = \frac{120\,mg/L}{1.38\,h^{-1}} + \frac{25\,mg/L}{0.087\,h^{-1}} = 374.4\,mg\,h/L$$

$$CL_T = \frac{Dose}{AUC} = \frac{1000\,mg}{374.4\,mg\,h/L} = 2.67\,L/h$$

$$k_{10} = \frac{CL_T}{V_c} = \frac{2.67\,L/h}{6.9\,L} = 0.387\,h^{-1}$$

$$k_{21} = \frac{\alpha\beta}{k_{10}} = \frac{1.38\,h^{-1} \times 0.087\,h^{-1}}{0.387\,h^{-1}} = 0.310\,h^{-1}$$

$$k_{12} = (\alpha + \beta) - (k_{21} + k_{10}) = (1.38 + 0.087\,h^{-1}) - (0.310 + 0.387\,h^{-1}) = 0.77\,h^{-1}$$

$$Vd_\beta = \frac{CL_T}{\beta} = \frac{2.67\,L/h}{0.087\,h^{-1}} = 30.7\,L$$

$$Vd_{ss} = V_c\left(1 + \frac{k_{21}}{k_{21}}\right) = 6.7\,L\left(1 + \frac{0.77\,h^{-1}}{0.310\,h^{-1}}\right) = 23.3\,L$$

b. $Cp = Ae^{-\alpha t} + Be^{-\beta t}$

$$Cp_{15h} = 120\,mg/L\ e^{-1.38h^{-1}15h} + 25\,mg/L\ e^{-0.087h^{-1}15h} = 6.78\,mg/L$$

Amount of the drug in the body during the elimination phase $= Cp \times Vd_\beta$
$Amount_{15h} = Cp_{15h} \times Vd_\beta = 6.78\,mg/L \times 30.7\,L = 208\,mg$

17.6 ORAL ADMINISTRATION OF DRUGS THAT FOLLOW THE TWO-COMPARTMENT PHARMACOKINETIC MODEL

After oral administration of a drug that follows two-compartment pharmacokinetic model, the drug is absorbed to the systemic circulation, which is part of the central compartment. Once in the central compartment, the drug can be eliminated from the body or distributed to the peripheral compartment. If the drug is rapidly absorbed, the decline in the plasma concentration–time profile after the end of the absorption phase will be biexponential, reflecting the distribution and the elimination phases. The biexponential decline in the drug plasma concentration after drug absorption will be clear only if the absorption, distribution, and elimination processes proceed at three distinctive rates. However, if the drug absorption is slow, the biexponential decline in the plasma concentration after the end of drug absorption may not be evident. Figure 17.9 represents the plasma concentration–time profile after a single oral dose of a drug that follows the two-compartment pharmacokinetic model. The decline of the drug concentration in the post-absorption phase is biexponential. The plasma drug concentration–time profile after oral administration of drugs that follow two-compartment pharmacokinetic model can be described by a triexponential equation that represents the absorption, distribution, and elimination processes as in Equation 17.30 [2]. The plasma drug concentrations obtained after single oral administration of drugs that follow two-compartment pharmacokinetic model can be fitted to Equation 17.30 to estimate the model parameters. Specialized computer programs are usually utilized in this fitting process.

$$Cp = \left(\frac{k_a FD}{V_c}\right)\left[\frac{(k_{21} - \alpha)e^{-\alpha t}}{(\beta - \alpha)(k_a - \alpha)} + \frac{(k_{21} - \beta)e^{-\beta t}}{(k_a - \beta)(\alpha - \beta)} + \frac{(k_{21} - k_a)e^{-k_a t}}{(\alpha - k_a)(\beta - k_a)}\right] \quad (17.30)$$

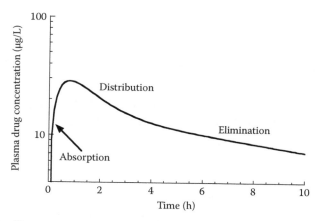

FIGURE 17.9 Plasma concentration–time profile for a drug that follows two-compartment pharmacokinetic model after administration of a single oral dose.

17.6.1 LOO–RIEGELMAN METHOD FOR DETERMINATION OF k_a AFTER ORAL ADMINISTRATION OF DRUGS THAT FOLLOW THE TWO-COMPARTMENT PHARMACOKINETIC MODEL

This method is similar in principle to the Wagner–Nelson method that is used for the determination of the absorption rate constant as discussed in Chapter 9. The Loo–Riegelman method can be applied to determine the absorption rate constant for drugs that follow linear kinetics, with zero-order or first-order absorption, and follow two-compartment pharmacokinetic model [5]. The method depends on calculation of the fraction of the dose remaining to be absorbed at different time points [1-(fraction of dose absorbed)] to determine the order of drug absorption process and to calculate the absorption rate constant. The amount of the drug absorbed up to any time is the sum of the amount of the drug in the body and the amount of the drug excreted, while the total amount of the drug absorbed is equal to the total amount of the drug excreted. The fraction of the dose absorbed at any time is the ratio of the amount of drug absorbed up to this time to the total amount of the drug absorbed. If the absorption process is first order, a plot of the fraction remaining to be absorbed versus time should give a straight line on the semilog scale. The slope of this line is equal to $-k_a/2.303$. On the contrary, if the absorption process is zero order, a plot of the fraction remaining to be absorbed versus time should give a straight line on the Cartesian scale. The slope of this line is equal to $-k_a$.

The only difference is that for the drugs that follow the two-compartment pharmacokinetic model, the amount of the drug in the body is the sum of the amount of the drug in the central compartment and the amount of the drug in the peripheral compartment. The drug amounts in the two compartments have to be calculated separately from the concentration and volume of each compartment because the drug in the two compartments is not at equilibrium all the time after a single drug administration. Calculation of the amount of the drug in each compartment requires the pharmacokinetic parameters for the two-compartment model that can only be obtained after IV administration of the drug. So IV administration of the drug is necessary to obtain these parameters before the absorption rate constant can be determined after oral administration. This limits the application of this method to drugs that can be administered intravenously.

17.7 CONSTANT RATE IV ADMINISTRATION OF DRUGS THAT FOLLOW THE TWO-COMPARTMENT PHARMACOKINETIC MODEL

The plasma concentration–time profile of drugs that follow two-compartment pharmacokinetic model during constant rate IV infusion increases gradually until it reaches the steady state. At steady state, the rate of drug administration is equal to the rate of drug elimination. The steady-state plasma concentration is dependent on the rate of the IV infusion and the CL_T of the drug as in Equation 17.31. This is similar to the drugs that follow one-compartment pharmacokinetic model.

$$Cp_{ss} = \frac{\text{Infusion rate}}{CL_T} = \frac{K_o}{CL_T} \qquad (17.31)$$

The time to reach steady state during constant rate IV infusion of drugs that follow two-compartment pharmacokinetic model is dependent on the drug elimination half-life ($t_{1/2\beta}$). It takes five to six times the elimination half-life of continuous IV infusion to reach the steady state. Termination of the IV infusion results in biexponential decline in the drug plasma concentration, a rapid distribution phase and a slow elimination phase.

Administration of a loading dose may be necessary to achieve faster approach to steady state especially in emergency situations. In this case, simultaneous administration of an IV loading dose and the constant rate IV infusion is necessary. Calculation of the loading dose based on V_c and the desired steady-state concentration ($Cp_{ss} \times V_c$) should achieve the desired concentration initially. However, due to drug distribution to the peripheral compartment the drug concentration declines transiently, possibly to subtherapeutic concentration, and then increases gradually to the desired steady-state concentration. Calculation of the loading dose based on Vd_β and the desired steady-state concentration ($Cp_{ss} \times Vd_\beta$) can avoid this transient decline in plasma drug concentration. However, this loading dose should produce very high drug concentration initially, which may be toxic for drugs with narrow therapeutic range. The loading dose should be calculated based on an average value for V_c and Vd_β. Another approach that can be used is to give a loading dose calculated based on V_c initially followed by smaller IV doses to compensate for the transient decline in drug concentration after the loading dose.

17.8 MULTIPLE DRUG ADMINISTRATION

Drugs that follow two-compartment pharmacokinetic model accumulate during repeated administration until steady state is achieved. At steady state, the plasma concentration will be changing during each dosing interval; however, the maximum and minimum plasma concentrations will be similar if the drug is administered as a fixed dose at equally spaced intervals. The average steady-state concentration is directly proportional to the dosing rate and inversely proportional to the CL_T:

$$Cp_{\text{average ss}} = \frac{F\,Dose}{CL_T \tau} \tag{17.32}$$

where
   τ is the dosing interval
   F is the bioavailability

This relationship is similar for one- and two-compartment pharmacokinetic models. It takes five to six elimination half-lives ($t_{1/2\beta}$) to reach the steady state during multiple administration of drugs that follow two-compartment pharmacokinetic model. Administration of a loading dose may be necessary to achieve faster approach to steady state.

17.9   RENAL EXCRETION OF DRUGS THAT FOLLOW THE TWO-COMPARTMENT PHARMACOKINETIC MODEL

For a drug that follows two-compartment pharmacokinetic model, the amount of the drug in the central compartment declines biexponentially. So the renal excretion rate (dA_e/dt) versus time profile will also decline biexponentially:

$$\frac{dA_e}{dt} = A'e^{-\alpha t} + B'e^{-\beta t} \tag{17.33}$$

where A' and B' are the hybrid coefficients and have units of amount/time. The renal clearance can be determined from the renal excretion rate and the average plasma concentration during the urine collection interval. This is similar to the drugs that follow one-compartment pharmacokinetic model.

$$CL_R = \frac{\Delta A_e / \Delta t}{Cp_{\text{t-mid}}} \tag{17.34}$$

The renal clearance can also be determined from the total amount of the drug excreted in urine and the drug AUC. This is similar to the drugs that follow one-compartment pharmacokinetic model.

$$CL_R = \frac{A_{e\infty}}{AUC|_{t=0}^{t=\infty}} \tag{17.35}$$

The fraction of the drug dose excreted in urine is determined from the ratio of the renal clearance to the total body clearance.

17.10 EFFECT OF CHANGING THE PHARMACOKINETIC PARAMETERSONTHEDRUGCONCENTRATION–TIMEPROFILE FOR DRUGS THAT FOLLOW THE TWO-COMPARTMENT PHARMACOKINETIC MODEL

After a single IV dose, the rate of drug distribution depends on the hybrid distribution rate constant, while the rate of elimination depends on the hybrid elimination rate constant. During multiple drug administration, the steady state is directly proportional to the administration rate and inversely proportional to the CL_T, and the time to reach the steady state is dependent on the hybrid elimination rate constant [6].

17.10.1 Pharmacokinetic Simulation Exercise

Pharmacokinetic simulations can be used to examine how the pharmacokinetic parameters affect the plasma concentration–time profile and the steady state drug concentration achieved after single and multiple drug administration. The drug plasma concentration–time profile is simulated using an average value of each of the pharmacokinetic parameters. The pharmacokinetic parameters are changed one parameter at a time, while keeping all the other parameters constant, and simulation of the drug concentration–time profile is repeated. The resulting profiles are examined to see how the changes affect the drug concentration–time profile. The plotting exercise of the two multicompartment pharmacokinetics modules in the basic pharmacokinetic concept section and the pharmacokinetic simulations section of the companion CD to this textbook can be used to run these simulations.

17.10.1.1 Dose

Administration of increasing doses results in proportional increase in the plasma concentrations. The plasma concentration–time profiles after administration of increasing doses will be parallel, while during multiple drug administration the average steady-state concentration is directly proportional to the administered dose, if the CL_T is constant.

17.10.1.2 Total Body Clearance

The change in CL_T will result in different elimination rate of the drug if the volume is kept constant. If the same dose is administered and the volume of distribution is kept constant, the decrease in clearance produces larger AUC and longer elimination half-life. During multiple drug administration of the same dose, the decrease in drug clearance will result in higher steady-state concentration and longer time to achieve the steady state, if the volume fd distribution is constant.

17.10.1.3 Volume of the Central Compartment

The change in the volume of the central compartment is accompanied by a proportional change in Vd_{ss} and Vd_β. Larger volume of distribution results in lower initial drug plasma concentration after administration of the same dose and similar AUC if the CL_T does not change. When the volume of distribution changes while CL_T remains constant, the elimination rate constant will be different. Multiple administration of the same dose should achieve the same average steady-state concentration if the clearance is similar, but the time to achieve steady state will be different if the volume is different because the elimination half-life will be different.

17.10.1.4 Hybrid Distribution Rate Constant

Larger hybrid distribution rate constant results in faster completion of the distribution process without affecting the rate of drug elimination. This is assuming that the three micro rate constants k_{12}, k_{21}, and k_{10} change in a way that will change the rate of the distribution process without affecting the elimination process.

17.10.1.5 Hybrid Elimination Rate Constant

Larger hybrid elimination rate constant results in faster drug elimination without affecting the rate of drug distribution. This is assuming that the three micro rate constants k_{12}, k_{21}, and k_{10} change in a way that will change the rate of the elimination process without affecting the distribution process.

17.11 EFFECT OF CHANGING THE PHARMACOKINETIC PARAMETERS ON THE DRUG DISTRIBUTION BETWEEN THE CENTRAL AND PERIPHERAL COMPARTMENTS

Drugs that follow the two-compartment pharmacokinetic model have different concentration–time profiles in the central and peripheral compartments after a single IV administration. During the elimination phase, distribution equilibrium is established and the ratio of the drug concentration in the central and peripheral compartments is dependent on the transfer rate constants.

17.11.1 Dose

The change in dose results in proportional change in the amount and concentration of the drug in the central and peripheral compartments. However, the distribution ratio between the central and peripheral compartments does not change. Changing the dose does not affect the ratio of the amount of the drug in the peripheral compartment to the amount of the drug in the central compartment when the distribution equilibrium is established.

17.11.2 First-Order Transfer Rate Constant from the Central to the Peripheral Compartment

The change in k_{12} affects the drug distribution rate, elimination rate, and the tissue distribution. Larger k_{12} results in higher amount of the drug distributing to the peripheral compartment, faster distribution rate, and slower elimination rate. The ratio of the amount of the drug in the peripheral compartment to the amount of the drug in the central compartment at steady state increases due to the increase in k_{12}/k_{21} ratio.

17.11.3 First-Order Transfer Rate Constant from the Peripheral to the Central Compartment

The change in k_{21} affects the drug distribution rate, elimination rate, and the tissue distribution. Larger k_{21} results in lower amount of the drug distributing to the peripheral compartment, faster distribution rate, and faster elimination rate. The ratio of the amount of the drug in the peripheral compartment to the amount of the drug in the central compartment at steady state decreases due to the decrease in k_{12}/k_{21} ratio.

17.11.4 First-Order Elimination Rate Constant from the Central Compartment

The change in k_{10} affects the drug distribution rate and elimination rate. Larger k_{10} results in faster distribution rate and faster elimination rate. However, the drug distribution ratio between the central and the peripheral compartments does not change. The ratio of the amount of the drug in the peripheral compartment to the amount of the drug in the central compartment at steady state does not change due to the change in k_{10} because the ratio k_{12}/k_{21} does not change.

17.12 THREE-COMPARTMENT PHARMACOKINETIC MODEL

With the development of accurate sampling methods and sensitive analytical techniques it has been shown that some drugs follow three-compartment pharmacokinetic model. After drug administration into the central compartment, the drug is distributed slowly to the tissues. However, the distribution of the drug to some tissues is much slower than its distribution to other tissues. This results in two distinct rates of distribution and a biexponential distribution phase followed by a terminal elimination phase. Figure 17.10 is an example of the plasma concentration–time profile for a drug that follows three-compartment pharmacokinetic model. The diagram presented in Figure 17.11 is an example of a three-compartment pharmacokinetic model in which the elimination of the drug is from the central compartment, and the two peripheral compartments are connected to the central compartment.

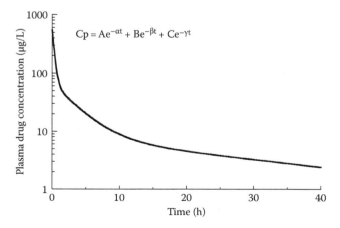

FIGURE 17.10 Plasma concentration–time profile for a drug that follows three-compartment pharmacokinetic model after administration of a single IV bolus dose.

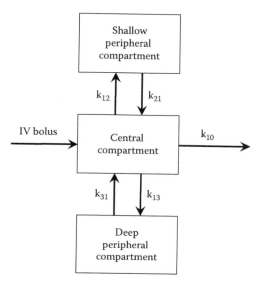

FIGURE 17.11 Block diagram representing the three-compartment pharmacokinetic model with the two peripheral compartments connected to the central compartment and drug elimination from the central compartment.

The equation that describes the plasma concentration–time profile after a single IV bolus dose is triexponential with the three exponential terms describing the rapid and slow distribution processes and the elimination process. Equation 17.36 is the mathematical expression that describes the plasma concentration–time profile for a drug that follows three-compartment pharmacokinetic model after administration of a single IV bolus dose [2]:

$$Cp = \left(\frac{D}{V_c}\right)\left[\frac{(k_{21}-\alpha)(k_{31}-\alpha)}{(\beta-\alpha)(\gamma-\alpha)}e^{-\alpha t} + \frac{(k_{21}-\beta)(k_{31}-\beta)}{(\alpha-\beta)(\gamma-\beta)}e^{-\beta t} + \frac{(k_{21}-\gamma)(k_{31}-\gamma)}{(\alpha-\gamma)(\beta-\gamma)}e^{-\gamma t}\right]$$

(17.36)

This equation can be simplified to

$$Cp = Ae^{-\alpha t} + Be^{-\beta t} + Ce^{-\gamma t}$$

(17.37)

The pharmacokinetic parameters for three-compartment pharmacokinetic models are usually obtained by nonlinear regression analysis utilizing specialized data analysis software.

17.13   COMPARTMENTAL PHARMACOKINETIC DATA ANALYSIS

The first step in compartmental pharmacokinetic data analysis is to construct the model that can describe the pharmacokinetic behavior of the drug. The choice of the compartmental pharmacokinetic model is usually based on the observed drug concentrations after drug administration. So compartmental modeling is considered data-based modeling. For example, when the plasma drug concentrations observed after a single IV bolus dose of the drug decline as a straight line on the semilog scale, this suggests that the one-compartment model is the appropriate model to describe the drug pharmacokinetic behavior, while if the decline in the drug concentrations is curvilinear on the semilog scale, the two-compartment pharmacokinetic model will be appropriate in this case. On the contrary, if the drug concentrations after a single IV bolus dose on the semilog scale decline at three distinct rates, this pharmacokinetic behavior may be described by the three-compartment pharmacokinetic model.

In addition to the number of the compartments, other model components such as the input function that depends on the route of drug administration and the output function that describes the drug elimination process should be included. Drug input into the systemic circulation, which is usually part of the central compartment, can be instantaneous such as in the case of IV bolus administration, first order as in oral administration, or zero order as in constant rate IV infusion and drugs absorbed by zero-order process, while drug elimination can follow first-order process, Michaelis-Menten process, or a combination of the two. The compartment where drug elimination occurs is usually the central compartment because most of the eliminating organs are highly perfused organs, unless there are evidences that drug elimination takes place in organs that are part of the peripheral compartments. Once all the model components are included, the model is defined mathematically.

17.13.1 MATHEMATICAL DESCRIPTION OF THE MODEL AND ESTIMATION OF THE MODEL PARAMETERS

Based on the constructed compartmental model, a set of differential equations are usually utilized to describe the rate of change of the dependent variable that is usually the drug amount or concentration with respect to time, which is the independent variable. These equations usually include the pharmacokinetic parameters that control the drug pharmacokinetic behavior in addition to constants like the administered dose. For each compartment, the rate of change of the dependent variable is the difference between the rate of drug entering the compartment and the rate of drug leaving the compartment. The differential equations describe the rate of change of the dependent variable with time at a finite period of time. Integration of these differential equations gives the integrated equations which can be used to calculate the dependent variable at any time. The integrated equations contain the pharmacokinetic model parameters that have to be estimated to allow prediction of the drug concentration at any time. The pharmacokinetic parameters are estimated from the drug concentration data obtained from pharmacokinetic studies. Since most pharmacokinetic studies involve determination of the plasma drug concentrations, the observed plasma drug concentrations and their corresponding time values are fitted to the integrated equation that describes the drug concentration–time profile in the central compartment to estimate the pharmacokinetic model parameters.

17.13.2 FITTING THE EXPERIMENTAL DATA TO THE MODEL EQUATION

Fitting of the experimentally observed data to the model equation to estimate the pharmacokinetic parameters utilizes nonlinear regression analysis, which is usually performed with the aid of specialized statistical software. The basic principle for estimation of the pharmacokinetic parameters involves selecting the best values for the pharmacokinetic parameters, which will minimize the sum of the squared differences between the experimentally observed drug concentrations and the model predicted drug concentrations [7]. The model predicted concentrations are determined by substituting the estimated pharmacokinetic parameters to the model equation and calculating the drug concentration at different time points. The process is not simple because the data analysis program has to check all possible combinations of the parameter values to find the combination of the parameter values that will minimize the sum of the squared error for all data points. So most programs require the input of an initial estimate for each parameter to be used as the starting point for the parameter estimation process. Different programs utilize different algorithms to search for the best estimates for the pharmacokinetic parameters.

For example, the pharmacokinetic parameters in the equation for the two-compartment pharmacokinetic model for drugs administered by IV bolus dose are A, B, α, and β, Equation 17.12. The dose and the experimentally determined drug concentrations at different time points are used to estimate the pharmacokinetic parameters. The best estimates for these parameters are the values that should minimize the sum of the squared differences between all the observed and predicted concentrations, whereas the pharmacokinetic parameters in the equation for the three-compartment pharmacokinetic model for drugs administered by a single IV bolus dose are A, B, C, α, β, and γ, Equation 17.37. These parameters are estimated by selecting the best values for the six parameters that when used together minimizes the sum of the squared differences between all the observed and predicted concentrations. When the pharmacokinetic experiment is repeated several times, the data for each individual experiment are fitted to the model equation to estimate the parameters for that particular experiment. The fitting is repeated for each data set and the parameters for the different experiments can be summarized using descriptive statistics.

Estimation of the pharmacokinetic parameters depends primarily on the drug concentrations in the experimentally obtained samples. So the quality of the obtained data is important in improving the accuracy in pharmacokinetic parameter estimation. The quality of data is dependent on the number of samples, the period of time over which the samples were obtained, and the accuracy of the analytical method used for determination of the drug concentration in the samples. Accurate estimation of the three-compartment pharmacokinetic parameters cannot be obtained if only few samples were obtained after a single IV drug administration. In general, complicated models have more parameters that require larger number of samples for their accurate estimation. Also, samples obtained over a short period of time cannot be used to accurately estimate the parameters of a drug that follows two-compartment pharmacokinetic model with long elimination half-life even if large number of samples were obtained after drug administration. Enough samples should be obtained during each phase of the plasma drug concentration–time profile to obtain accurate estimation of all model parameters. There is no strict rule for the number and the timing of samples that should be obtained in pharmacokinetic experiments because frequent sampling can be obtained in some experimental settings, while samples can be very limited in other settings. However, the minimum number of samples required to obtain reasonable estimates for the pharmacokinetic parameters should not be less than three samples for each phase of the drug profile, and samples should be spread over the entire drug concentration–time profile. In addition to the number and the timing of the obtained samples, the analytical procedures used for the determination of the drug concentration in the obtained samples have to be accurate and precise to minimize the error in the experimental data. So, fewer number of samples obtained at the proper time and analyzed using accurate analytical method can be used to obtain estimates for the pharmacokinetic parameters that are better than the parameter estimates obtained from larger number of samples obtained at inappropriate time schedule and analyzed using inaccurate method.

After drug administration, the drug concentration declines exponentially and usually there is big difference in the concentrations measured shortly after drug administration and during the terminal elimination phase specially after IV bolus doses. Since the objective of the fitting procedures is to obtain the parameter estimates that will minimize the sum of the squared errors, the samples with the high concentrations usually have larger influence in the estimation of the parameters. This is because absolute error of 1 mg/L represents 2% relative error if the drug concentration is 50 mg/L and represents 200% relative error if the drug concentration is 0.5 mg/L. So the fitting program will usually fit the high concentration values better than the low concentration values when all the data points are treated equally, that is, weighted equally. In this case, fitting of the measured concentrations to the model equation during the distribution phase will be much better compared to fitting the concentrations during the elimination phase.

Weighting of the pharmacokinetic data is used during the fitting procedures to give the different data points different weights to compensate for the difference in their magnitude [7]. Different weighting schemes can be used for weighting the pharmacokinetic data. The reciprocal of the variance at each data point has been used as a weighting function to make all the data points have approximately the same influence while estimating the pharmacokinetic parameters. So if the pharmacokinetic experiment is repeated several times, the drug concentrations measured at specific time point in all of these experiments are used to calculate the variance for the concentrations obtained at this time. The value for 1/variance is used as the weight for the drug concentrations at this particular time. The same is done for each time point to determine the weight for each data point. When the variance for each data point cannot be determined, other weighting functions can be used such as 1/(predicted concentration)^2, 1/(observed concentration)^2, or 1/(observed concentration), that is, $1/\hat{y}^2$, $1/y^2$, or $1/y$, respectively. These weighting functions give less weight to the high drug concentration and higher weight to the lower drug concentrations, which compensate for the difference in the absolute values of the concentrations. So when the appropriate weighting function is used, all the drug concentrations should have similar influence in the estimation of the pharmacokinetic parameters.

17.13.3   Evaluation of the Pharmacokinetic Model

The primary goal of modeling in pharmacokinetics is to choose the best model that can describe the drug pharmacokinetic behavior in the body and to estimate the model parameters with acceptable accuracy. For example, in the previous discussion of the two-compartment pharmacokinetic model, it was mentioned that after IV bolus administration the drug is distributed rapidly to the tissues of the central compartment and slowly to the tissues of the peripheral compartment. This does not mean that the drug distribution to the different tissues is either rapid or slow. In reality, the drug may be distributed to the different tissues at different rates but the drug distribution can be approximated by two rates and the two-compartment model can approximate the overall behavior of the drug in the body. So the observed plasma drug concentrations should fit with reasonable accuracy to the equation for the two-compartment pharmacokinetic model. Using the three-compartment pharmacokinetic model may improve fitting the observed data to the model equation and usually decreases the sum of the squared deviations between the observed and the predicted concentrations. However, the use of more complicated models is not necessarily better because increasing the number of compartments increases the number of pharmacokinetic parameters as in Equations 17.12 and 17.32. When the same number of data points is used to estimate larger number of pharmacokinetic parameters, the accuracy of the parameter estimates is compromised. So it is necessary to evaluate the goodness of fit of the experimental data to the pharmacokinetic model.

There is no single diagnostic procedure or statistical test that can be used to determine the validity of the model to describe the observed data. However, there are several statistical and graphical methods that are generally used to evaluate how well the model fits the data set [7]. Most data analysis programs provide information regarding the variability for each of the estimated parameters such as the standard error or the coefficient of variation. Coefficient of variation >20% for any parameter indicates uncertainty of this parameter estimate, which usually results from overparameterization of the model or insufficient data. Also, the Akaike information criteria are used to determine if going to more complex model improves the fit without compromising the accuracy in model parameter estimation.

Several graphical methods can be used to evaluate the goodness of fit including a scattered plot of the observed concentrations around the model predicted drug concentration–time curve to determine how well the model fit the data. Small differences between the observed and model predicted values and random distribution of the observed values around the predicted values indicate good fit, as in Figure 17.12A. The existence of trend in the data points that is presented by a series of consecutive data points above or below the predicted profile is an indication of inappropriate fit as in Figure 17.12B. Also, the observed versus the model predicted drug concentration values is a very useful diagnostic plot to evaluate the goodness of fit. A good model fit can be concluded when the values are gathered uniformly and closely around the line with slope equal to one as in Figure 17.12C, while the presence of trend in the data points is an indication of inappropriate fit as in Figure 17.12D. Also, several residuals plots can be utilized in the model evaluation. The residuals are the difference between the observed drug concentration and the model predicted drug concentration, which

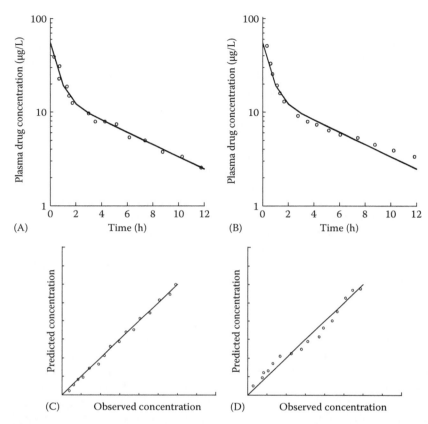

FIGURE 17.12 Examples of the diagnostic graphs for compartmental pharmacokinetic data analysis. The scattered plot of the observed concentration and the model predicted drug plasma profile. Random distribution of the data around the predicted profile indicates good data fitting (A), while the presence of a trend that appears as series of observations above or below the model predicted values indicates inappropriate data fitting (B). The observed versus predicted plasma drug concentration. Uniform and random distribution of data around the line with slope of 1 indicates good data fitting (C), while the presence of trend indicates unacceptable data fitting (D).

is a measure of the error at each data point. For example, the residual versus predicted concentration plot to examine the error value at different drug concentrations and determine if the model fit one end of the curve better than the other. Also, the residual versus time plot to evaluate if the model accurately accounts for all the different phases in the drug concentration–time profile. Furthermore, the plot of the weighed residuals versus predicted values and weighed residuals versus time are useful to evaluate the model fit as in Figure 17.13A–D. When the model fits the observed data properly, the magnitude of the weighted residuals in the weighted residuals versus predicted value plot and the weighted residuals versus time plot, should be small with approximately uniform magnitude, and randomly distributed around the zero residual line, as in Figure 17.13A and C. While the existence of trend or inconsistent weighted residual magnitude indicates improper fit, as in Figure 17.12B and D.

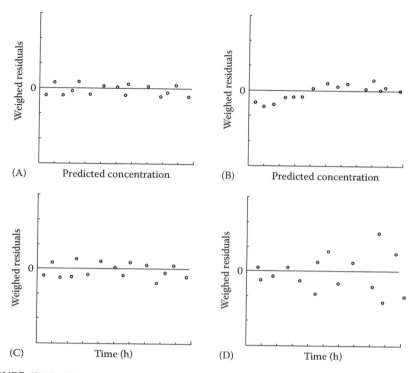

FIGURE 17.13 Examples of the residual plot used as a diagnostic test for evaluating curve fitting. (A and B) is the weighted residuals versus predicted concentrations, and (C and D) is the weighted residuals versus time. Small, uniform, and randomly distributed weighted residuals indicate good fitting of data (A and C), while the presence of trend or unequal weighed residuals suggest improper data fitting (B and D).

PRACTICE PROBLEMS

17.1 A drug that follows a two-compartment pharmacokinetic model is given to a patient by rapid IV injection. Would the drug concentration in each tissue be the same after the drug equilibrates between the plasma and all the tissues in the body? Explain.

17.2 A drug follows two-compartment pharmacokinetic model. If a single IV bolus dose is given, what is the cause of the initial rapid decline in the plasma concentration (α-phase)? What is the cause of the slower decline in the plasma concentration (β-phase)?

17.3 A drug that follows two-compartment pharmacokinetic model was given as a single IV bolus dose of 5.6 mg/kg. The equation that describes the plasma concentration–time data is

$$CP\ (mg/L) = 18e^{-2.8t} + 6e^{-0.11t}$$

a. Calculate the plasma concentration after 0.5, 3, and 12 h of drug administration.
b. What will be the equation that describes the plasma concentration–time profile if the dose given was 11.2 mg/kg?

17.4 After administration of a single IV bolus dose of 75 mg of a drug to a healthy volunteer, the pharmacokinetics of this drug followed the two-compartment model. The following parameters were obtained:

$$A = 4.62\,\text{mg/L} \quad B = 0.64\,\text{mg/L}$$

$$\alpha = 8.94\,\text{h}^{-1} \quad \beta = 0.19\,\text{h}^{-1}$$

a. Calculate the following parameters:
    $t_{1/2\alpha}$, $t_{1/2\beta}$, k_{12}, k_{21}, k_{10}, V_c, Vd_β, Vd_{ss}, AUC, and CL_T.
b. What will be the amount of drug remaining in the body after 8 h?

17.5 A single dose of 500 mg of a drug was administered by a rapid IV injection into a 70 kg patient. Plasma samples were obtained over a 7 h period and assayed for the drug. The results are tabulated as follows:

Time (h)	Concentration (mg/L)
0.00	70.0
0.25	53.8
0.5	43.3
0.75	35.0
1.0	29.1
1.5	21.2
2.0	17.0
2.5	14.3
3.0	12.6
4.0	10.5
5.0	9.0
6.0	8.0
7.0	7.0

a. Calculate the following parameters:
    $t_{1/2\alpha}$, $t_{1/2\beta}$, k_{12}, k_{21}, k_{10}, V_c, Vd_β, Vd_{ss}, AUC, and CL_T.
b. What will be the plasma concentration 12 h after drug administration?
c. What will be the initial plasma concentration if a dose of 1500 mg is administered as an IV bolus?
d. Which of the aforementioned pharmacokinetic parameters will change with the increase in the dose to 1500 mg?
e. Calculate the new values for these parameters.
f. What will be the IV infusion rate required to achieve a steady-state plasma concentration of 10 mg/L?

17.6 The plasma concentration time data following a 50 mg IV bolus dose of lidocaine is tabulated as follows:

Time (min)	Concentration (mg/L)
2.0	1.51
4.0	1.20
10	0.796
15	0.639
20	0.462
40	0.329
60	0.271
90	0.242
120	0.179
180	0.112
240	0.081

a. Using the method of residuals, calculate the following parameters: $t_{1/2\alpha}$, $t_{1/2\beta}$, k_{12}, k_{21}, k_{10}, V_c, Vd_β, Vd_{ss}, AUC, and CL_T

b. Calculate the plasma concentration at the time of each sample from the equation that describes the plasma concentration–time profile, and comment on the differences between the measured and the calculated concentrations.

c. What will be the amount of lidocaine remaining in the body after 240 min?

d. What will be the plasma concentration when 90% of the administered dose is eliminated?

REFERENCES

1. Gibaldi M and Perrier D (1982) *Pharmacokinetics*, 2nd edn., Marcel Dekker, New York.
2. Wagner JG (1993) *Pharmacokinetics for the Pharmaceutical Scientist*, Technomic Publishing Co., Lancaster, PA.
3. Loughnan PM, Sitar DS, Ogilvie RI, and Neims AH (1976) The two-compartment open-system kinetic model: A review of its clinical implications and applications. *J Pediatr* 88:869–873.
4. Mayersohn M and Gibaldi M (1971) Mathematical methods in pharmacokinetics II: Solution of the two-compartment open model. *Am J Pharm Ed* 35:19–28.
5. Loo JCK and Riegelman S (1968) New method for calculating the intrinsic absorption rate of drugs. *J Pharm Sci* 57:918–928.
6. Jusko WJ and Gibaldi M (1972) Effects of change in elimination on various parameters of the two-compartment open model. *J Pharm Sci* 61:1270–1273.
7. Bourne DWA (1995) *Mathematical Modeling of Pharmacokinetic Data,* Technomic Publishing Co., Lancaster, PA.

18 Drug Pharmacokinetics Following Administration by Intermittent Intravenous Infusion

OBJECTIVES

After completing this chapter you should be able to

- Describe the drug concentration–time profile after the first dose, before steady state and at steady state for drugs administered by intermittent IV infusion
- Analyze the effect of changing the pharmacokinetic parameters on the maximum and minimum steady-state drug concentration
- Calculate the steady-state maximum and minimum drug concentration during intermittent IV infusion
- Predict aminoglycoside half-life based on the patient's kidney function
- Describe the method for estimating the patient's specific aminoglycoside pharmacokinetic parameters
- Recommend the appropriate aminoglycoside dosing regimen based on the patient's specific pharmacokinetic parameters

18.1 INTRODUCTION

Drug administration by intermittent IV infusion involves administration of short IV infusion repeatedly every fixed dosing interval. Following repeated administration of these short IV infusions, the drug accumulates in the body until steady state is achieved. At steady state, the maximum and minimum plasma drug concentrations will be constant if the dose, infusion duration, and dosing interval are kept constant. This route of administration is usually used when bolus IV drug administration produces high plasma drug conchration that can produce serious adverse effects. Examples of drugs administered by this route of administration are vancomycin and aminoglycosides.

Vancomycin and aminoglycosides are drugs with pharmacokinetic behavior that can be described by multicompartment pharmacokinetic models. Rapid IV administration of these drugs produces high plasma drug concentration in the central compartment because of the slow distribution to the peripheral compartment. Administration of vancomycin doses over a period of less than 30 min has been associated with erythematous reactions, intense flushing known as the "red-neck" syndrome, tachycardia, and hypotension. These adverse effects have been well correlated with the rate of drug administration. Vancomycin is usually administered as a constant rate IV infusion over a period of 1 h. This slow rate of administration allows distribution of the drug to all parts of the body during administration to avoid the high plasma drug concentration achieved after rapid drug administration. Similarly, rapid IV administration of aminoglycoside can produce high plasma drug concentration at the end of drug administration, which can increase the risk of aminoglycoside ototoxicity. Aminoglycosides are usually administered by IV infusion over a period of 0.5–1.0 h. Although it is well documented that vancomycin and aminoglycosides follow multicompartment pharmacokinetic models, most of the methods used for individualization of therapy for these drugs based on pharmacokinetic calculations assume that they follow one-compartment pharmacokinetic model. This is because during the clinical use of these drugs, the obtained samples after administration are not enough to characterize their multicompartment pharmacokinetic behavior. Also, the use of the one-compartment model does not introduce significant error.

During intermittent IV infusion, the drug is administered over a period of t' and the dose is repeated every τ. The time between the maximum and the minimum drug concentration is $\tau - t'$ as illustrated in Figure 18.1. If the infusion time is neglected and it is assumed that the drug is administered by IV bolus administration, the calculation will miss significant amount of the drug eliminated during the infusion time. This miscalculation can be significant for drugs with short half-lives, which can influence the calculation of the pharmacokinetic parameters for these drugs.

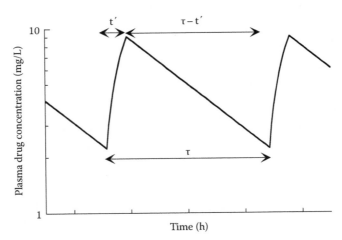

FIGURE 18.1 Plasma drug concentration–time profile during repeated administration of intermittent IV infusion. The dosing interval (τ) is the sum of the duration of the infusion (t') and the post-infusion time ($\tau - t'$).

18.2   DRUG CONCENTRATION–TIME PROFILE DURING INTERMITTENT IV INFUSION

Studying the drug pharmacokinetic behavior when the drug is administered by intermittent IV infusion requires the development of the equations that describe this profile during and after drug administration. There are three different situations that have to be considered. These are when the drug is administered for the first time, when the drug is administered repeatedly before reaching steady state, and when the drug is administered repeatedly at steady state. The following discussion assumes that the drug is eliminated by first-order process and that the drug follows the one-compartment pharmacokinetic model [1,2].

18.2.1   AFTER THE FIRST DOSE

The rate of change of the amount of drug in the body during the constant rate IV infusion is equal to the difference between the rate of drug administration and the rate of drug elimination as in Equation 18.1:

$$\frac{dA}{dt} = K_o - kA \tag{18.1}$$

where

   K_o is the rate of the IV infusion that is equal to dose/infusion time and has units of mass/time
   k is the first-order elimination rate constant
   A is the amount of drug in the body

Integrating Equation 18.1 gives the equation that describes the change in the amount of drug in the body during a constant rate IV infusion:

$$A = \frac{K_o}{k}(1 - e^{-kt}) \tag{18.2}$$

Dividing Equation 18.2 by Vd gives the expression for the plasma concentration at any time during constant rate IV infusion:

$$Cp = \frac{K_o}{kVd}(1 - e^{-kt}) \tag{18.3}$$

If the drug infusion continues for a long period of time (t is large), Equation 18.3 is reduced to Equation 18.4, which describes the steady-state plasma concentration during constant rate infusion:

$$Cp_{ss} = \frac{K_o}{kVd} \tag{18.4}$$

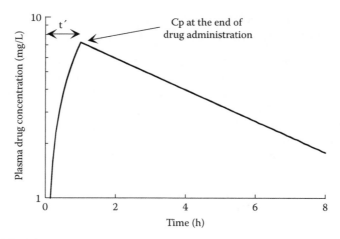

FIGURE 18.2 Plasma drug concentration–time profile during and after administration of the first dose of a drug on the semilog scale. The drug is administered as a constant rate IV infusion over a period of t'.

For drugs that are administered as IV infusion over a short period, the plasma concentration at the end of the infusion administered over a period of t' is described by the following equation:

$$Cp = \frac{K_o}{kVd}(1 - e^{-kt'}) \tag{18.5}$$

If the drug IV infusion is terminated after time, t', the drug concentration declines monoexponentially as shown in Figure 18.2. The equation that describes the drug concentration during and after the drug infusion is as follows:

$$Cp = \left[\frac{K_o}{kVd}(1 - e^{-kt'})\right]e^{-k(t-t')} \tag{18.6}$$

where
    t is the time from starting drug administration
    t' is the infusion time

This is the general equation that describes the drug concentration during and after a constant rate IV infusion. During the IV infusion, t is equal to t' and Equation 18.6 is reduced to Equation 18.5. After termination of the IV infusion, t becomes larger than t' and Equation 18.6 describes the drug concentration at any time after termination of the drug infusion.

18.2.2 AFTER REPEATED ADMINISTRATION BEFORE REACHING STEADY STATE

During repeated intermittent IV infusion, the drug concentration during the IV infusion is the sum of the drug concentration resulting from drug infusion plus the drug

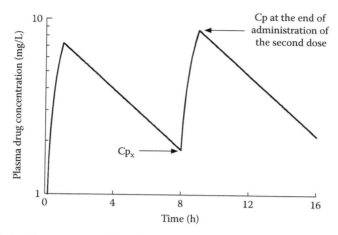

FIGURE 18.3 Plasma concentration–time profile during repeated administration of intermittent IV infusion before reaching steady state.

concentration remaining in the body from previous doses. If we assume that the drug concentration just before drug administration is equal to Cp_x as illustrated in Figure 18.3, the drug concentration at the end of the infusion can be described by the following equation:

$$Cp = \frac{K_o}{kVd}(1 - e^{-kt'}) + Cp_x e^{-kt'} \tag{18.7}$$

When the IV infusion is terminated after time equal to t', the drug concentration declines monoexponentially as shown in Figure 18.3. The drug concentration after termination of the IV infusion can be described by the following equation:

$$Cp = \left[\frac{K_o}{kVd}(1 - e^{-kt'}) + Cp_x e^{-kt'}\right] e^{-k(t-t')} \tag{18.8}$$

Equation 18.8 is the general equation for drug administration as short constant rate IV infusion. During the infusion, t is equal to t' and Equation 18.8 is reduced to Equation 18.7, while after the end of infusion, t becomes bigger than t' and the equation can be used to calculate the drug concentration at any time after termination of the infusion. On the contrary, if the drug is administered for the first time, Cp_x is equal to zero and the equation is reduced to Equation 18.5 or 18.6.

18.2.3 At Steady State

Repeated drug administration by intermittent IV infusion leads to drug accumulation in the body until steady state is achieved. At steady state the drug concentration right after the end of drug administration is equal to $Cp_{max\ ss}$ and the drug concentration just before drug administration is equal to $Cp_{min\ ss}$, providing that the same dose is administered at a fixed dosing interval as shown in Figure 18.4. An expression similar

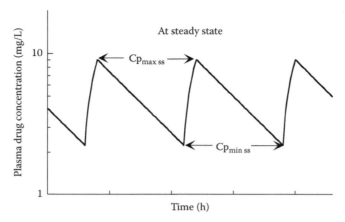

FIGURE 18.4 Plasma concentration–time profile during repeated administration of intermittent IV infusion at steady state.

to Equation 18.7 can be written to describe the drug concentration after the end of the short IV infusion at steady state. However, at steady state, Cp_x, which is the drug concentration just before drug administration, is equal to $Cp_{min\,ss}$ as in Equation 18.9:

$$Cp_{max\,ss} = \frac{K_o}{kVd}(1 - e^{-kt'}) + Cp_{min\,ss}e^{-kt'} \qquad (18.9)$$

Since $Cp_{min\,ss}$ is equal to the concentration remaining from $Cp_{max\,ss}$ after the post infusion period $(\tau - t')$, $Cp_{min\,ss}$ can be expressed as

$$Cp_{min\,ss} = Cp_{max\,ss}e^{-k(\tau-t')} \qquad (18.10)$$

By substituting the value of $Cp_{min\,ss}$ in Equation 18.9 and solving for $Cp_{max\,ss}$, the following relationship can be obtained for $Cp_{max\,ss}$:

$$Cp_{max\,ss} = \frac{K_o(1 - e^{-kt'})}{kVd(1 - e^{-k\tau})} \qquad (18.11)$$

18.3 EFFECT OF CHANGING THE PHARMACOKINETIC PARAMETERS ON THE STEADY-STATE PLASMA CONCENTRATION DURING REPEATED INTERMITTENT IV INFUSION

The steady-state drug concentration achieved during multiple intermittent IV infusion is directly proportional to the administered dose and inversely proportional to the CL_T. It takes five to six elimination half-lives to achieve the steady state. Administration of a loading dose leads to faster approach to steady state without affecting the steady-state concentration.

18.3.1 Pharmacokinetic Simulation Exercise

Pharmacokinetic simulations can be used to examine how the pharmacokinetic parameters affect the steady-state drug concentration achieved during multiple intermittent IV infusion. The drug plasma concentration–time profile is simulated using an average value for each of the pharmacokinetic parameters and the steady-state concentration and the time to achieve steady state are observed. Then the pharmacokinetic parameters are changed one parameter at a time, while keeping all the other parameters constant, and the simulation is repeated. The resulting profile is examined to see how the change affects the drug steady-state concentration and the time to achieve steady-state concentration. The plotting exercise of the intermittent IV infusion module in the basic pharmacokinetic concept section and the pharmacokinetic simulations section of the companion CD to this textbook can be used to run these simulations.

18.3.1.1 Dose

The steady-state plasma concentration is directly proportional to the administered dose. Increasing the dose leads to proportional increase in the steady-state maximum and minimum plasma concentrations if the CL_T of the drug remains constant. The AUC during each dosing interval at steady state increases with the increase in dose. Although increasing the dosing rate increases the average steady-state concentration, the time to achieve steady state should be the same if CL_T and Vd are constant.

18.3.1.2 Infusion Time

Administration of the same dose of the drug over longer duration of time results in lower maximum drug concentration and higher minimum drug concentration at steady state, that is, smaller fluctuations in the drug concentrations at steady state. This is because larger amount of the drug is eliminated during drug administration when the infusion time is longer.

18.3.1.3 Total Body Clearance

The steady-state plasma concentration is inversely proportional to CL_T. Lower CL_T results in higher maximum and minimum steady-state concentrations when the dose is kept constant. Administration of the same dose of a drug to patients with different CL_T achieves higher steady-state drug concentration in the patients with lower CL_T. Assuming that the Vd is constant, patients with lower CL_T should achieve steady state slower than those with higher clearance. This is because lower CL_T means smaller k and longer $t_{1/2}$ when Vd is constant.

18.3.1.4 Volume of Distribution

The Vd does not affect the steady-state concentration if the CL_T and the dose are constant. When Vd is different in patients with similar CL_T, the $t_{1/2}$ and k (the dependent parameters) will be different. In these patients, the steady state will be the same (same CL_T and K_o); however, the approach to steady state will be faster in the individuals with larger CL_T/Vd ratios (larger k and shorter half-life).

18.4 APPLICATION OF THE PHARMACOKINETIC PRINCIPLES FOR INTERMITTENT IV INFUSION TO THE THERAPEUTIC USE OF AMINOGLYCOSIDE

The classical example of drugs that are administered by intermittent IV infusion and are frequently monitored in patients is the aminoglycosides. Aminoglycosides such as gentamicin, tobramycin, amikacin, and netilmicin are antibacterial agents that have bactericidal activity against gram-negative aerobic bacteria.

18.4.1 PHARMACOKINETIC CHARACTERISTICS OF AMINOGLYCOSIDES

Aminoglycosides are not absorbed after oral administration. However, some aminoglycoside antibiotics such as neomycin and streptomycin are administered orally for their local gastrointestinal effect. After intramuscular administration, the maximum aminoglycoside plasma concentration is achieved after 30–60 min in patients with normal kidney function and after 2–5 h in patients with reduced kidney function, depending on the severity of the kidney dysfunction. Aminoglycosides are distributed primarily in the extracellular fluid because of their poor lipid solubility. Their average Vd is 0.2–0.25 L/kg. After parenteral administration, aminoglycosides are completely eliminated unchanged in urine [3].

18.4.2 GUIDELINES FOR AMINOGLYCOSIDE PLASMA CONCENTRATION

The most common adverse effects of aminoglycosides are nephrotoxicity, ototoxicity, and neuromuscular blockade. The goal of conventional aminoglycoside dosing adjustment strategies is to maintain the steady-state maximum and minimum plasma concentration within a certain range to ensure optimal efficacy with minimal toxicity. Table 18.1 lists the general guidelines for the desired maximum and minimum aminoglycoside plasma concentrations at steady state using the conventional dosing.

TABLE 18.1
Guidelines for the Steady-State Aminoglycoside Concentrations while Using the Conventional Dosing Regimen

	Drug	
	Gentamicin Tobramycin Netilmicin	Amikacin
Maximum (peak) concentration (mg/L)		
Serious infections	6–8	20–25
Life-threatening infections	8–10	25–30
Minimum (trough) concentration (mg/L)		
Serious infections	0.5–1	1–4
Life-threatening infections	1–2	4–8

18.4.3 EXTENDED-INTERVAL AMINOGLYCOSIDE DOSING REGIMEN

The total daily dose of aminoglycosides administered once a day has been utilized effectively to treat systemic infections. Aminoglycosides have concentration-dependent bactericidal effect and concentration dependent postantibiotic effect. This means that higher concentration produces faster rate of bacterial killing and the duration of the bactericidal effect of aminoglycosides extends for a period of time after their plasma concentrations fall below the minimum inhibitory concentration. Also, administration of larger doses while extending the dosing intervals does not significantly increase the aminoglycoside toxicity. These factors provide the basis for the rationale of once daily aminoglycoside dosing. The effectiveness of once daily aminoglycoside dosing in all patients to treat all infections is yet to be determined. There are no known optimal maximum and minimum plasma drug concentrations when aminoglycosides are administered once daily [4,5]. The guidelines in Table 18.1 do not apply to the once-daily dosing method. The following discussion covers the conventional aminoglycoside dosing adjustment method only.

18.5 INDIVIDUALIZATION OF AMINOGLYCOSIDE THERAPY

Individualization of drug therapy in general is the process of selecting the dosing regimen for each patient based on his/her own specific pharmacokinetic characteristics. The process starts by estimating the pharmacokinetic parameters of the drug in the patients and then using these parameters to calculate the appropriate dosing regimen for the patient. An important component in the individualization of drug therapy is to select the target steady-state drug concentration and the pharmacokinetic model that describes the drug pharmacokinetic behavior. The guidelines for the maximum and minimum steady-state aminoglycoside concentrations presented in Table 18.1 are usually used as the target concentration when selecting the dosing regimen. The Sawchuk-Zaske method for adjusting the aminoglycoside doses will be used as the basis of the following discussion. It is one of the first methods developed to calculate the patient's specific pharmacokinetic parameters from few blood concentrations and utilizes these drug concentrations in calculating the proper dosing regimen for specific patients. The assumption that aminoglycosides follow one-compartment pharmacokinetic model makes this method relatively simple without significantly compromising its accuracy [2,6,7]. This method is widely used for the individualization of aminoglycoside therapy.

18.5.1 ESTIMATION OF THE PATIENT'S PHARMACOKINETIC PARAMETERS

The proper dosing regimen is calculated based on the aminoglycoside pharmacokinetic parameters. Before the start of aminoglycoside therapy it is not possible to determine the patient's specific pharmacokinetic parameters. The initial dosing regimen is usually calculated using the aminoglycoside parameters estimated based on the patient demographic information. However, with the start of drug therapy, it becomes possible to estimate the patient's specific pharmacokinetic parameters. The estimated patient's specific pharmacokinetic parameters are used to modify the dosing regimen if necessary.

18.5.1.1 Estimation of the Patient's Pharmacokinetic Parameters Based on the Patient Information

The patient demographic information is used to estimate the patient's pharmacokinetic parameters based on the reported parameters for the different patient populations. The factors that affect the pharmacokinetic parameters of aminoglycosides are evaluated in the patient. Then aminoglycoside pharmacokinetic parameters in a population similar to that of the patient are used as the initial parameter estimate for the patient.

18.5.1.1.1 Half-Life

Aminoglycosides are completely eliminated by the kidney. This makes their elimination half-lives highly correlated with the patient's kidney function. The patient's kidney function can be determined from the creatinine clearance (CrCL). The CrCL is either determined directly or estimated from the serum creatinine and some patient's information. Direct CrCL determination requires 24 h urine collection and determination of serum creatinine as discussed in Chapter 14, while the method of Cockroft and Gault, for example, can provide a reasonable estimate for the CrCL in mL/min from the age, weight, serum creatinine, and gender. According to this method, the CrCL can be estimated in men from Equation 18.12 and in women from Equation 18.13. The estimated CrCL can be used to estimate the half-life or the elimination rate constant of aminoglycosides:

$$CrCL = \frac{(140 - age)(Wt \text{ in } kg)}{72(s.Cr. \text{ in } mg/dL)} \qquad (18.12)$$

$$CrCL = 0.85\left(\frac{(140 - age)(Wt \text{ in } kg)}{72(s.Cr. \text{ in } mg/dL)}\right) \qquad (18.13)$$

Since aminoglycosides are eliminated completely by the kidney, the kidney function measured as the CrCL is directly proportional with aminoglycoside elimination rate constant and inversely proportional with the half-life. The half-life of aminoglycoside can be estimated empirically from the average aminoglycoside half-life and the patient's kidney function. The patient's kidney function (KF) is determined by comparing the patient's CrCL with the normal CrCL, which is usually in the range of 120 mL/min:

$$Patient \text{ } KF = \frac{Patient \text{ } Cr \text{ } CL}{120 \text{ } mL/min} \qquad (18.14)$$

The aminoglycoside half-life can be estimated, assuming that the average half-life of aminoglycoside is 2.5 h, as follows:

$$Estimated \text{ } t_{1/2} = \frac{Average \text{ normal } t_{1/2}(2.5 \text{ } h)}{Patient \text{ } KF} \qquad (18.15)$$

When the estimated creatinine clearance is more than 120 mL/min, the patient's kidney function is considered equal to unity and the half-life in this case can be estimated as the average half-life of aminoglycosides. Studying the elimination rate of aminoglycosides in large number of patients with different kidney functions resulted in the development of Equation 18.16 that relates the elimination rate constant of aminoglycosides to the CrCL. So the patient's CrCL can be substituted in this equation to estimate the elimination rate constant of aminoglycoside [3]:

$$k(\text{for aminoglycosides in h}^{-1}) = 0.00293(\text{CrCL in mL/min}) + 0.014 \qquad (18.16)$$

18.5.1.1.2   Volume of Distribution
Aminoglycosides are very polar drugs so they are distributed mainly in the extracellular space. Their average Vd is 0.25 L/kg based on the ideal body weight since adipose tissues have lower extracellular fluid contents. Conditions like ascites and overhydration can increase the Vd of aminoglycosides. The estimated aminoglycoside elimination rate constant and Vd are used to calculate the initial aminoglycoside dosing regimen.

18.5.1.2   Estimation of the Patient's Specific Pharmacokinetic Parameters from Aminoglycoside Blood Concentrations
After starting aminoglycoside therapy, the patient's specific parameters should be determined by designing an appropriate sampling schedule that allows pharmacokinetic parameter determination. The assumption is that aminoglycosides are administered by intermittent IV infusion over a period of t', and drug administration is repeated every τ, and that aminoglycosides follow one-compartment pharmacokinetic model. Although aminoglycosides follow multicompartment pharmacokinetic model, the use of one-compartment pharmacokinetic model can generally provide clinically acceptable estimates for drug disposition.

18.5.1.2.1   If the Patient Is to Receive the First Aminoglycoside Dose
After administration of the first dose of the drug as a constant rate IV infusion over a period of t' and at a rate equal to K_o (this is equal to dose/t'), the plasma drug concentration at the end of the drug administration can be determined from Equation 18.3:

$$Cp = \frac{K_o}{kVd}(1 - e^{-kt'})$$

To estimate the pharmacokinetic parameters, three samples are obtained over a period of time equivalent approximately to the estimated aminoglycoside half-life. For example, for a patient with normal kidney functions, samples should be drawn over a 2.5 h period (e.g., at 0.5, 1.5, and 3 h) after the end of drug administration. Patients with reduced kidney functions may require obtaining the samples over a longer period of time according to their estimated aminoglycoside half-lives. The samples are analyzed for aminoglycoside, and the measured drug concentrations are plotted on a semilog graph paper as in Figure 18.5.

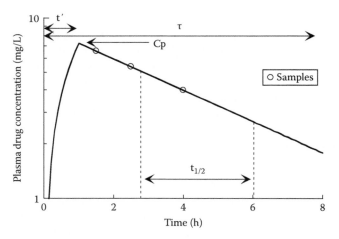

FIGURE 18.5   Graphical determination of aminoglycoside half-life and the concentration at the end of drug administration from the plasma concentration–time profile after administration of the first dose as a short IV infusion of duration t′.

The best line that fits the three points is drawn and back extrapolated to the time when the infusion was terminated to determine the drug concentration at the end of the drug administration (Cp). Figure 18.5 represents the entire aminoglycoside plasma concentration time profile during and after the end of drug administration. However, for the determination of the drug half-life and the drug concentration right at the end of drug administration, a plot of the drug concentration versus time after the end of drug administration is sufficient. In this plot, the y-intercept will be equal to the drug plasma concentration at the end of drug administration. The elimination rate constant can be determined from the slope of the line, where the slope of the resulting line on the semilog scale is equal to −k/2.303. The half-life can be calculated from k or determined graphically by finding the time required for the drug concentration to decrease by 50% as in Figure 18.6. Knowing either the elimination rate constant or the half-life, the other parameter can be calculated ($k = 0.693/t_{1/2}$). The drug elimination rate constant can also be determined mathematically by using any two plasma drug concentrations on the fitted line from Equation 18.17:

$$Cp_{t2} = Cp_{t1}e^{-kt} \tag{18.17}$$

where

Cp_{t1} and Cp_{t2} are two different plasma concentrations after the end of drug administration, Cp_{t1} is the sample obtained at earlier time and Cp_{t2} is the sample obtained at later time

k is the first-order elimination rate constant

t is the time difference between the two samples

After determination of Cp and the elimination rate constant, aminoglycoside Vd can be determined by substitution in Equation 18.3.

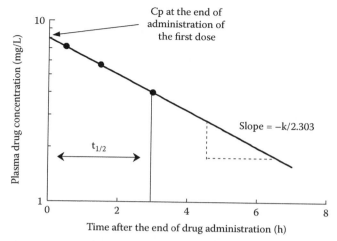

FIGURE 18.6 Graphical determination of aminoglycoside half-life and concentration at the end of drug administration from the drug concentrations versus time plot after the end of drug administration.

18.5.1.2.2   If the Patient Received Aminoglycosides before but the Steady State Was Not Achieved

The plasma concentration after the end of administration of the second dose of the drug by constant rate IV infusion (or repeated administration before steady state is achieved) is the sum of the drug concentration resulting from the administered drug and the drug remaining from previous drug administration. In this case the drug concentration at the end of drug administration can be expressed by Equation 18.7 as described previously:

$$Cp = \frac{K_o}{kVd}(1 - e^{-kt'}) + Cp_x e^{-kt'}$$

To determine aminoglycoside k, $t_{1/2}$ and Vd, one plasma sample should be obtained just before drug administration and two or three samples after the end of drug administration as shown in Figure 18.7. The drug plasma concentration obtained just before drug administration is equal to Cp_x in Equation 18.7. The samples obtained after the end of drug administration should be obtained over a period of time equivalent approximately to the estimated aminoglycoside $t_{1/2}$ in the patient. Aminoglycoside $t_{1/2}$ or k can be determined as mentioned earlier from the plasma concentrations obtained after the end of drug administration. The plasma concentration at the end of drug administration is determined graphically by back extrapolation to the time of termination of the infusion. By substituting Cp, Cp_x, and k in Equation 18.7, aminoglycoside Vd can be estimated.

18.5.1.2.3   If the Patient Received Aminoglycosides and Steady State Was Achieved

At steady state, $Cp_{max\ ss}$ and $Cp_{min\ ss}$ are constant in consecutive dosing intervals. So the drug concentration in the sample obtained just before drug administration should be equal to the drug concentration at the end of the following dosing interval. So two

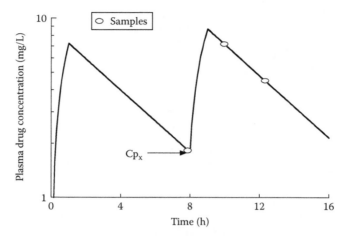

FIGURE 18.7 Plasma samples obtained for the determination of the pharmacokinetic parameters during repeated intermittent IV infusion before reaching steady state.

plasma samples are obtained, one sample just before drug administration and the other at 1 h after the end of drug administration as shown in Figure 18.8. The $Cp_{max\,ss}$ is expressed by Equation 18.11:

$$Cp_{max\,ss} = \frac{K_o(1-e^{-kt'})}{kVd(1-e^{-k\tau})}$$

where
 K_o is the infusion rate (dose/t′)
 k is the first-order elimination rate constant
 Vd is the volume of distribution
 τ is the dosing interval

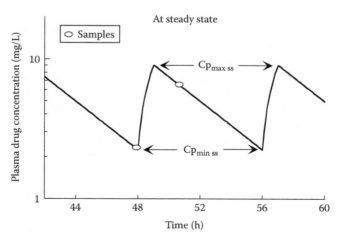

FIGURE 18.8 Plasma samples obtained for the determination of the pharmacokinetic parameters during repeated intermittent IV infusion at steady state.

Drug concentrations determined before and after the drug administration can be used to calculate k. The two different concentrations are known and the time difference between the two concentrations is known, so k can be calculated. Also, the drug concentration right after the end of drug administration can be determined graphically or mathematically. By substituting k and the $Cp_{max\ ss}$ in Equation 18.11, Vd can be estimated.

18.5.2 DETERMINATION OF THE DOSING REGIMEN BASED ON THE PATIENT'S SPECIFIC PARAMETERS

The estimated aminoglycoside k and Vd are used to determine the dose (D) and the dosing interval (τ) that should achieve a specific $Cp_{max\ ss}$ (peak) and $Cp_{min\ ss}$ (trough).

18.5.2.1 Selection of the Dosing Interval (τ)

After selecting the drug infusion time (t') and the target $Cp_{max\ ss}$ and $Cp_{min\ ss}$, τ can be calculated from Equation 18.10. The calculated τ should be approximated to the nearest practical dosing interval, that is, 4, 6, 8, 12, 24, 48, or 72 h.

18.5.2.2 Selection of Dose

The approximated value of τ, the infusion time t', the target $Cp_{max\ ss}$, and the calculated pharmacokinetic parameters are used to calculate aminoglycoside dose from Equation 18.11. The calculated dose should be approximated to the nearest practical dose (approximate to the nearest 5 mg for aminoglycosides).

18.5.2.3 Selection of the Loading Dose

When administration of a loading dose is necessary, the loading dose should be selected to achieve plasma concentration equal to $Cp_{max\ ss}$ after the loading dose. The loading dose is calculated from Equation 18.3 after substation for t', k, Vd, and the Cp.

The actual values of the $Cp_{max\ ss}$ (peak) and $Cp_{min\ ss}$ (trough) that should be achieved by using the approximated values of the dose and the dosing interval can be calculated from Equations 18.10 and 18.11. The patient should be monitored for the therapeutic and adverse effects of aminoglycoside therapy and the dosing regimen is modified if necessary. Reassessment of aminoglycoside regimen is necessary when the patient's condition changes in a way that can alter aminoglycoside pharmacokinetics.

Example

A 43-year-old, 68 kg male was admitted to the hospital to treat lung infection with gentamicin. He received his first dose of 140 mg administered by constant rate IV infusion over a period of 1 h. Three plasma samples were drawn after the end of drug administration, and the concentrations were as follows:

Time after end of administration	2 h	4 h	8 h
Gentamicin concentration (mg/L)	8.4	5.85	2.84

a. Estimate the $t_{1/2}$ and Vd of gentamicin in this patient.
b. Recommend a dosing regimen (dose and dosing interval) that should achieve maximum and minimum steady-state plasma gentamicin concentration of 8 and 1 mg/L, respectively. Gentamicin is administered by constant rate IV infusion over 1 h.

Answer

a. The $t_{1/2}$ and the plasma concentration achieved at the end of drug administration can be determined graphically as in Figure 18.9:
The half-life = 3.85 h
Plasma concentration at the end of drug administration = 12 mg/L

$$Cp = \frac{K_o}{kVd}(1 - e^{-kt'})$$

$$12\,mg/L = \frac{140\,mg/h}{0.18h^{-1}\,Vd}(1 - e^{-0.18h^{-1}1\,h})$$

$$Vd = 10.68\,L$$

b. Dosing regimen:

$$Cp_{min\,ss} = Cp_{max\,ss}\,e^{-k(\tau-t')}$$

$$1\,mg/L = 8\,mg/L\,e^{-0.18h^{-1}(\tau-1\,h)}$$

$$(\tau - t') = 11.55h$$

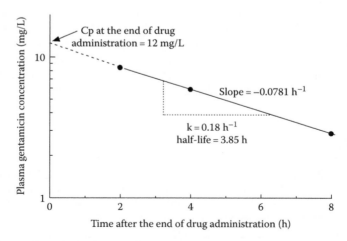

FIGURE 18.9 Graphical determination of the drug half-life and drug concentration at the end of drug administration from a plot of the drug concentrations versus time after the end of drug administration.

An appropriate dosing interval = 12 h

$$Cp_{maxss} = \frac{K_o(1-e^{-kt'})}{kVd(1-e^{-k\tau})}$$

$$8\,mg/L = \frac{K_o(1-e^{-0.18h^{-1}1h})}{0.18h^{-1}\,10.68L(1-e^{-0.18h^{-1}12h})}$$

K_o = 82.6 mg administered over 1 h

Recommendation: 85 mg of gentamicin administered as a constant rate IV infusion over 1 h and repeated every 12 h.

Example

A 38-year-old, 68 kg male was admitted to the hospital because of acute pneumonia and he is to receive tobramycin. His serum creatinine was found to be 1.6 mg/dL upon admission to the hospital.

a. Estimate the $t_{1/2}$ of tobramycin in this patient based on his kidney function.
b. A loading dose of 2 mg/kg tobramycin given as a constant rate infusion of 1 h duration followed by 150 mg tobramycin every 8 h given as a constant rate infusion of 1 h duration were prescribed. The patient received his first dose of tobramycin and before administration of the second dose you were asked to determine the pharmacokinetic parameters of tobramycin in this patient. Recommend a sampling schedule around the second dose that can allow the determination of gentamicin pharmacokinetic parameters in this patient (please give the exact number and time of samples).
c. Despite the pharmacokinetic consultation, the patient continued to receive 150 mg tobramycin every 8 h given as a constant rate infusion of 1 h duration. At steady state, the maximum and the minimum plasma concentrations of tobramycin (measured immediately after the end of drug administration and just before drug administration at steady state) were 11.3 and 3.85 mg/L, respectively. Calculate the $t_{1/2}$ and the Vd of tobramycin in this patient.
d. Recommend a dosing regimen (a dose and dosing interval) that will achieve steady-state maximum and minimum plasma concentrations of 6 and 1 mg/L, respectively.

Answer

a.
$$CrCL = \frac{(140-age)(Wt\ in\ kg)}{72(s.Cr.\ in\ mg/dL)}$$

$$CrCL = \frac{(140-38\,year)(68\,kg)}{72(1.6\,mg/dL)} = 60\,mL/min$$

$$Fraction\ of\ KF = \frac{Patient\ CrCL}{120\ mL/min} = \frac{60\ mL/min}{120\ mL/min} = 0.5$$

$$\text{Estimated tobramicin } t_{1/2} = \frac{\text{Normal } t_{1/2}(2.5\,h)}{\text{Fraction of KF}} = \frac{2.5\,h}{0.5} = 5h$$

Also, using Equation 18.16, the elimination rate constant can be estimated:

$$k \text{ (for aminoglycosides in } h^{-1}) = 0.00293 \text{ (CrCL in mL/min)} + 0.014$$

$$k\,(h^{-1}) = 0.00293\,(60) + 0.014 = 0.1898\,h^{-1}$$

$$\text{Half-life} = 3.7\,h$$

b. The blood samples will be obtained around the second sample (before reaching steady state). So one sample should be obtained before administration of the second dose and two to three samples should be obtained after the end of drug administration over a period of time equivalent approximately to the estimated tobramycin half-life (5 h).

First sample	Just before drug administration
Second sample	0.5 h after the end of drug administration
Third sample	2 h after the end of drug administration
Fourth sample	5 h after the end of drug administration

c. $Cp_{min\ ss} = Cp_{max\ ss}e^{-k(\tau - t')}$

$$3.85\,mg/L = 11.3\,mg/L\ e^{-k(8-1\,h)}$$

$$k = 0.154\,h^{-1} \quad t_{1/2} = 4.5h$$

$$Cp_{maxss} = \frac{K_o(1 - e^{-kt'})}{kVd(1 - e^{-k\tau})}$$

$$11.3\,mg/L = \frac{150\,mg/h(1 - e^{-0.154h^{-1}1\,h})}{0.154h^{-1}Vd(1 - e^{-0.154h^{-1}8\,h})}$$

$$Vd = 17.4\,L$$

d. Dosing regimen:

$$Cp_{minss} = Cp_{max\ ss}e^{-k(\tau - t')}$$

$$1\,mg/L = 6\,mg/L\ e^{-0.154h^{-1}(\tau - 1\,h)}$$

$$(\tau - t') = 11.6h$$

An appropriate dosing interval $= 12\,h$

$$Cp_{max\ ss} = \frac{K_o(1-e^{-kt'})}{kVd(1-e^{-k\tau})}$$

$$6\,mg/L = \frac{K_o(1-e^{-0.154h^{-1}1h})}{0.154h^{-1}7.4L(1-e^{-0.154h^{-1}12\,h})}$$

$K_o = 95\,mg$ administered over $1\,h$

Recommendation: 95 mg of gentamicin administered as a constant rate IV infusion over 1 h and repeated every 12 h.

PRACTICE PROBLEMS

18.1 A 60 kg patient received a 1 h infusion of gentamicin, and the pharmacokinetic study showed that the half-life is 2.7 h and the volume of distribution is 0.21 L/kg. The desired maximum and minimum steady-state concentrations for this patient are 6 and 1 mg/L, respectively.
   a. Calculate the dosing regimen to achieve steady-state concentrations around these desired concentrations.
   b. Calculate the actual steady-state maximum and minimum plasma concentrations for the regimen you recommended.

18.2 A patient is receiving 75 mg gentamicin every 4 h as an infusion of 1 h duration. The maximum and minimum plasma gentamicin concentrations achieved at steady state are 6 and 2.35 mg/L, respectively.
   a. Calculate gentamicin half-life in this patient.
   b. Calculate gentamicin volume of distribution in this patient.
   c. Recommend a dosing regimen to achieve steady-state maximum and minimum plasma gentamicin concentrations around 8 and 1 mg/L, respectively.
   d. Calculate the actual steady-state maximum and minimum plasma concentrations that should be achieved with the regimen you recommended in (c).

18.3 A patient is receiving 50 mg every 6 h of tobramycin as intermittent IV infusion of 1 h duration. At steady state, three plasma samples were obtained and tobramycin concentrations were as follows:

Time	Before the dose	0.5 h after the infusion	2 h after the infusion
Conc (mg/L)	1.26	3.56	2.52

   a. Calculate tobramycin half-life in this patient.
   b. Calculate tobramycin volume of distribution in this patient.

    c. Recommend a dosing regimen to achieve steady-state maximum and minimum plasma tobramycin concentrations around 10 and 1.5 mg/L, respectively.

    d. Calculate the actual steady-state maximum and minimum plasma concentrations that should be achieved with the regimen you recommended in (c).

18.4 A 60-year-old, 60 kg male was admitted to the hospital because of acute pneumonia. Gentamicin 75 mg every 12 h given as a short infusion of 1 h was prescribed. Because his serum creatinine was found to be 2.5 mg/dL, the pharmacokinetic service was consulted to adjust gentamicin dosing regimen.

    a. Estimate the creatinine clearance in this patient.

    b. What is the percentage renal function remaining in this patient?

    c. What is the estimated half-life of gentamicin in this patient?

    Four plasma samples were drawn around the second dose, just before giving the second dose and 1, 4, and 10 h after the second dose. Samples were analyzed for gentamicin and the results came back as follows:

Time	Just before	1 h post	4 h post	10 h post
Conc (mg/L)	2.1	6.5	5.11	3.13

    d. Calculate the half-life and the volume of distribution of gentamicin in this patient.

    e. What was the maximum plasma concentration after the first dose?

    f. What would be the steady-state maximum and the minimum plasma concentrations if the 75 mg every 12 h was continued?

    g. Comment on the difference between the maximum plasma concentration after the first dose and the maximum plasma concentration at steady state (during the 75 mg every 12 h regimen).

    h. Recommend a dosing regimen (dose and dosing interval) to achieve steady-state maximum and minimum plasma concentrations of 7 and 1 mg/L, respectively.

18.5 A patient is receiving tobramycin as 100 mg every 8 h as a short infusion over half an hour. His serum creatinine was 1 mg/dL. At steady state, two plasma samples were obtained 0.5 h before the administration of the dose and 1 h after the end of the infusion, and the tobramycin plasma concentrations were 2.18 and 8.73 mg/L in the two samples, respectively.

    a. Calculate the half-life and volume of distribution of tobramycin in this patient.

    b. Recommend a dosing regimen to achieve steady-state maximum and minimum plasma concentrations of 9 and 1 mg/L, respectively.

    c. Calculate the actual maximum and minimum plasma concentrations achieved at steady state with the regimen you recommended in (b).

    d. The patient came back to the hospital 6 months later and the serum creatinine was 2 mg/dL. What is the estimated new half-life of tobramycin in this patient?

18.6 An 84-year-old, 50 kg male is admitted to the hospital and he is to receive gentamicin. His serum creatinine was 1.2 mg/dL. Gentamicin 65 mg/12 h given as short infusion of 1 h duration was prescribed.

    a. Estimate the half-life of gentamicin in this patient.

    b. Recommend a sampling schedule around the second dose that will allow the determination of the pharmacokinetic parameters in this patient.

       Samples were obtained and a dose of 75 mg every 24 h as short infusion (1 h duration) was recommended. At steady state, two samples were obtained, 1 and 8 h after the end of the dose, and the gentamicin plasma concentrations were 9.25 and 5.4 mg/L, respectively.

    c. Calculate the half-life and volume of distribution of gentamicin in this patient.

    d. Recommend a dosing regimen to achieve steady-state maximum and minimum plasma concentrations of 9 and 1 mg/L, respectively.

    e. Calculate the actual maximum and minimum plasma concentrations achieved at steady state with the regimen you recommended in (d).

REFERENCES

1. Murphy JE and Winter ME (1996) Clinical pharmacokinetic pearls: Bolus versus infusion equations. *Pharmacotherapy* 16:698–700.
2. Sawchuk RJ, Zaske DE, Cippolle JR, Wargin WA, and Strate RG (1977) Kinetic model for gentamicin dosing with the use of individual patient parameter. *Clin Pharmacol Ther* 21:362–365.
3. Bauer LA (2008) *Applied Clinical Pharmacokinetics*, 2nd edn., McGraw-Hill Companies, Inc., New York.
4. Nicolau DP, Freeman CD, Belliveau PP, Nightingale CH, Ross JW, and Quintiliani R (1995) Experience with a once-daily aminoglycoside program administered to 2184 adult patients. *Antimicrob Agents Chemother* 39:650–655.
5. Barclay ML, Begg EJ, and Hickling KG (1994) What is the evidence for once-daily aminoglycoside therapy? *Clin Pharmacokinet* 27:32–48.
6. Zaske DE, Sawchuk RJ, Gerding DN, and Strate RG (1976) Increased dosage requirements of gentamicin in burn patients. *J Trauma* 16:824–828.
7. Zaski DE, Sawchuk RJ, and Strate RG (1978) The necessity of increased doses of amikacin in burn patients. *Surgery* 84:603–608.

19 Pharmacokinetic–Pharmacodynamic Modeling

OBJECTIVES

After completing this chapter you should be able to

- Describe the different components of the pharmacokinetic/pharmacodynamic models
- Discuss the approaches used to measure the drug effect and differentiate between biomarkers, surrogate endpoints, and clinical endpoints
- Describe the different pharmacodynamic models that can relate the drug concentration at the site of action and the drug pharmacological effect
- Discuss the differences between the direct and indirect response models, the direct and indirect link models, and time variant and invariant response models
- Describe the pharmacokinetic/pharmacodynamic modeling approaches for the different models
- Analyze the effect of changing the pharmacokinetic or pharmacodynamic parameters on the plasma concentration–time profile and the drug effect-time profile after single and multiple drug administration

19.1 INTRODUCTION

Pharmacokinetics involves studying the kinetics of drug absorption, distribution, and elimination processes. These are the processes that define the quantitative relationship between the administered dose of the drug and the drug concentration–time profile in different body fluids and tissues, while pharmacodynamics involves studying the quantitative relationship between the drug concentration at the site of action and the resulting therapeutic and/or toxic effects. It is obvious that these two disciplines are related because the drug concentration–time profile in the body fluids is related to the drug profile at the site of action, which in turn determines the intensity and the time course of the drug effect, as illustrated in Figure 19.1.

The pharmacokinetic information obtained from the pharmacokinetic investigations will only be important when there is a relationship between the plasma drug concentration and the drug therapeutic and adverse effects. Also, pharmacodynamic studies that involve monitoring the drug effects will be useful only when these effects

Pharmacokinetics   Pharmacodynamics

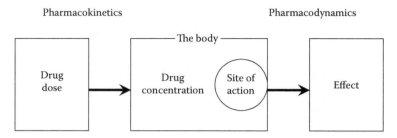

FIGURE 19.1   Schematic presentation of the relationship between pharmacokinetics and pharmacodynamics.

are linked to the drug dose and concentration in plasma or at the site of action. So the interest in linking the pharmacokinetic and the pharmacodynamic information for the drug is usually directed to quantify the relationship between the administered dose, the resulting drug concentration–time profile in the body, and the subsequent time course of the drug effects. This relationship can be useful for determining the dose required to produce the desired effect, predicting the effect produced by a certain dose, and identifying the temporal pattern of drug effect. Pharmacokinetic/pharmacodynamic (PK/PD) modeling is the process of constructing a mathematical model that can link the administered drug dose, the drug concentration–time profile in the body, and the drug effect-time profile. This concept has numerous applications in drug development and clinical drug use.

19.2   COMPONENTS OF THE PK/PD MODELS

The PK/PD model usually includes a pharmacokinetic model and a pharmacodynamic model that are combined together. The way these two models are combined or linked together depends on the available pharmacokinetic and pharmacodynamic information, the mechanism of drug effect, the site of action of the drug, and if the concentration-effect relationship changes with time [1–3].

19.2.1   Pharmacokinetic Model

The pharmacokinetic model is used to describe the drug concentration–time profile in the systemic circulation after administration of a certain dose. The time course of the drug concentration in the body usually serves as a measure for the exposure of the site of effect to the drug. Both compartmental and noncompartmental approaches for pharmacokinetic data analysis can be used. The choice usually depends on the study design and the nature of the drug exposure-effect relationship. When the drug effect varies substantially due to the change in drug concentration within the dosing interval, the maximum information can be gained from relating multiple effect values to their corresponding drug concentrations. In this case, compartmental pharmacokinetic models can be useful to fully characterize the drug concentration–time profile that can be used to characterize the concentration-effect relationship over a period of time, while if the drug effect can only be obtained once on a given sampling day, this effect can be related to the drug AUC that represents the average drug concentration over the dosing intervals. Other measures of drug exposure that can be used include C_{max}, C_{min}, or sparse drug concentration obtained during the dosing interval. In this case, noncompartmental analysis of the pharmacokinetic data will be appropriate since the drug concentration–time profile does not need to be fully characterized.

When the drug is the only active moiety responsible for the drug effect and the drug binding to plasma and tissue proteins is constant, the total drug concentration in the plasma can be used to characterize the drug concentration-effect relationship. However, free drug concentration should be used when the drug binding in plasma or tissues is concentration dependent or in case of diseases that can significantly affect the drug protein binding. This is because the free drug molecules are usually responsible for producing the drug effect. Also, if the drug is metabolized to a pharmacologically active metabolite, both the parent drug and the active metabolite concentrations should be included in the process of characterizing the concentration-effect relationship. In this case, the difference in potency between the parent drug and the metabolite should be considered. Furthermore, when a chiral drug is used as the racemate, the difference in the pharmacokinetic and pharmacodynamic properties of individual enantiomers should be considered when characterizing the concentration-effect relationship for this drug. Moreover, in some complex mixture of drugs derived from animal or plant origin, all the individual components cannot be identified. In this case, one or more of the active moieties can be used in characterizing the concentration-effect relationship.

19.2.2 Measuring the Response

The therapeutic and adverse effects of the drug can be quantified using a variety of efficacy measures. These efficacy measures have to be predictive for the long-term outcome of the drug to increase the predictive power of the PK/PD model. These efficacy measures are classified as biomarkers, surrogate markers, and clinical outcome [4].

19.2.2.1 Biomarkers

Biomarkers are defined as quantifiable physiological, pathological, biochemical, or anatomical measurements that are affected by the drug. These measurements should be related to the progression of the disease, the susceptibility to the disease, the mechanism of action of the drug, or the actual clinical response to the treatment. Biomarkers may or may not be relevant for monitoring the clinical outcome of the drug treatment. When a biomarker is shown to function as a valid indicator of clinical benefit, it is considered an acceptable surrogate marker or a surrogate endpoint. Biomarkers are very useful in the drug discovery and development processes even if their validity for predicting the clinical outcome is not established. Changes in the biomarkers follow a time course that is directly related to the time course of the plasma drug concentration, with possible delay in some instances. For these reasons, concentration-effect studies based on biomarkers can help in linking the preclinical and early clinical concentration-response relationship and can help in selecting the dose range in clinical trials. Examples of biomarkers that reflect the drug action but are not indicative of the clinical outcome include ACE inhibition in response to ACE inhibitor therapy and inhibition of ADP-dependent platelet aggregation as the effect of antiplatelet therapy.

19.2.2.2 Surrogate Endpoint

Surrogate endpoints are biomarkers that are used in clinical trials as a substitute for clinical endpoints that are expected to predict the effect of therapy. The usefulness of these surrogate endpoints in predicting the drug efficacy and clinical endpoint has to be validated by examining the correlation between the change in these measurements and the change in the disease state and therapeutic outcome. A validated surrogate endpoint should predict the clinical endpoint of drug treatment with acceptable reproducibility, repeatability, and sensitivity. Examples of surrogate markers are blood pressure measurement to assess the effect of antihypertensive drugs, cholesterol level to determine the effect of cholesterol lowing drugs, viral load to assess the efficacy of anti-HIV drugs, and tumor marker as a measure for the response to anticancer drug therapy.

19.2.2.3 Clinical Endpoint

Clinical endpoints are characteristics or variables that reflect how the patients feel or function, such as cure or decreased morbidity. They usually reflect the desired effect of the treatment and they are the most credible response measurements. However, the assessment of these clinical endpoints is usually difficult to perform, so they are often predicted from surrogate endpoints.

19.2.3 INTEGRATING THE PHARMACOKINETIC AND PHARMACODYNAMIC INFORMATION

The common strategies used to combine the pharmacokinetic and pharmacodynamic information will be discussed in detail later in this chapter. Briefly, the following four model characteristics have to be considered while selecting the appropriate strategy to integrate the pharmacokinetic and pharmacodynamic data [5].

19.2.3.1 Direct Response versus Indirect Response Models

For the direct response models, the observed drug effect results from the drug concentration at the site of action without any time delay. Any change in the drug concentration at the site of action is immediately reflected in the observed drug effect, with no drug effect observed once the drug disappears from the site of action. An example of drugs that produce direct response is the general anesthetics, which usually produce their anesthetic effect as long as the drug is present in the body in sufficient quantities. Once the general anesthetic agents are eliminated from the body, their effect disappears and the patients start to gain conscious.

For the indirect response models, the drug produces its effect by inhibiting or stimulating a receptor, mediator, enzyme, precursor, or cofactor that leads to the production of the drug effect, which appears at a later time. In this case, the drug effect may be observed after the drug disappears from the body. So there is no direct relationship between the drug concentration and the observed effect. Despite the temporal dissociation between the drug concentration–time profile and the effect-time profile, higher drug concentrations usually lead to more intense drug effect. An example of drugs that produce their effect by indirect response is the oral anticoagulants that inhibit vitamin K reductase, leading to interference with synthesis of vitamin K-dependent coagulating factors. The effect of oral anticoagulants is usually observed after few days when the already existing clotting factors disappear.

19.2.3.2 Direct Link versus Indirect Link Models

In the direct response models where there is a direct relationship between the drug at the site of action and the drug effect, the plasma drug concentration can be directly or indirectly linked to the drug concentration at the site of action. In the direct link models, rapid equilibrium is achieved between the drug concentration in plasma and the drug concentration at the site of action, indicating that the plasma drug concentration is always proportional to the drug concentration at the site of action. Any change in the plasma drug concentration produces proportional change in the drug concentration at the site of action, so the plasma concentration is considered to be directly linked to the effect site concentration. In this case, the plasma drug concentration can be used to characterize the drug concentration-effect relationship.

The indirect link models are used when there is a delay between the plasma concentration–time profile and the drug effect-time profile. This time delay is usually caused by the delay in drug distribution from the plasma to the site of action. The simplest example to demonstrate this distributional delay is when the site of drug action is in the peripheral compartment of a multicompartment pharmacokinetic model. The delay in the distribution of the drug from the central compartment to the peripheral compartment will be responsible for the delay in observing the drug effect. In this case, the drug effect will be related to the drug concentration in the peripheral compartment rather than the drug concentration in the central compartment. It is important to point out that the indirect link model is a type of the direct response models, but the delay between the drug concentration and drug effect profiles is due to distributional delay and not due to the mechanism of action of the drug.

19.2.3.3 Soft Link versus Hard Link Models

In the soft link models, both drug concentration and drug effect data are used to define the characteristics of the link between the pharmacokinetic and pharmacodynamic models. The link can then serve as a buffer to account for misspecification of the PK/PD relationship. On the contrary, in the hard link models only the pharmacokinetic data in addition to some in vitro parameters are used to predict the pharmacodynamic data. These in vitro parameters may include drug binding affinity to the receptors or enzymes, the minimum inhibitory concentration for antibiotics or parameters related to the drug mechanism of action. So the hard link models are mechanism-based models that utilize the drug concentration–time data with in vitro measurements to predict the time course of the drug effect.

19.2.3.4   Time-Variant versus Time-Invariant Models

Most PK/PD models assume time invariant, meaning that the drug concentration-effect relationship does not change with time. However, there are instances where the drug concentration-effect relationship changes with time. In this case, the same drug concentration may produce lower or higher effects during repeated drug administration. Tolerance is the decrease in the drug effect over time, while sensitization is the increase in drug effect over time, when the drug concentration at the site of action is kept constant. This means that in these cases, the pharmacodynamic parameters and the drug concentration-effect relationship change with time. The time variant models should be designed to account for the time dependent change in the pharmacodynamic parameters.

19.3   DIRECT LINK PK/PD MODELS

The direct link PK/PD models are models with rapid equilibrium achieved between the drug in plasma and the drug at the site of action, and the drug effect is related to the drug concentration at the site of action. These are also known as the steady-state models because at steady state the drug in plasma is at equilibrium with the drug at the site of action. The time course of the drug effect including the onset, intensity, and duration of effect is dependent on the drug concentration–time profile at the site of action. In general, the onset of drug effect is observed once the drug reaches the site of action in adequate concentration. Achievement of higher drug concentration at the site of action usually produces higher intensity of drug effect. Also, the duration of effect is related to the length of time the drug concentration is maintained above certain concentration at the site of action.

For the direct link models, the drug concentration–time profile and the drug effect-time profile are correlated with the maximum drug effect observed at the same time of the maximum plasma drug concentration. However, the change in the drug effect due to the change in the plasma drug concentration depends on the nature of the concentration-effect relationship. Different drugs usually have different concentration-effect relationships. The pharmacodynamic models describe the relationship between the drug concentration at the site of action and the drug effect. It is usually very difficult and in many cases impossible to determine the drug concentration at the site of action. However, this concentration can be determined from the pharmacokinetic model that describes the drug pharmacokinetic behavior in the body. In case of the direct link models, the plasma drug concentration is proportional to the drug concentration at the site of action, so it can be used as the input function in the pharmacodynamic models to characterize the drug concentration-effect relationship.

The pharmacodynamic model that describes the drug concentration-effect relationship for a certain drug is determined experimentally by measuring the drug effect resulting from different drug concentrations. Characterization of the drug concentration-effect relationship will be better when the drug effect is measured over a wide range of drug concentrations. Then the concentration-effect data are fitted to the different equations for the different pharmacodynamic models to determine the best model that can describe the concentration-effect relationship. The following are the different pharmacodynamic models that can describe the relationship between the drug concentration at the effect site and the observed drug effect [1,6–8]. These pharmacodynamic models describe the drug concentration-effect relationship for direct and indirect link models. In the direct link models, the plasma drug concentration is used as the input concentration for the pharmacodynamic models, while in indirect link models, other approaches are used to estimate the drug concentration at the site of action. The estimated drug concentrations at the site of action are used as the input concentration for the pharmacodynamic models.

19.3.1 FIXED EFFECT MODEL

It is also known as the quantal effect model. This is the simplest pharmacodynamic model that relates a certain drug concentration to a fixed effect that is either present or not, as, for example, cure or no cure, sleep or awake. In this model, there is only one parameter, which is the drug concentration at which the effect appears. This model has limited applications in PK/PD modeling because of the limited ability of the model to predict the effect at different time points.

19.3.2 LINEAR MODEL

This model assumes a linear relationship between the drug concentration at the site of action and the observed effect over a certain range of drug concentrations:

$$E = SC \qquad (19.1)$$

where
  E is the intensity of effect
  C is the drug concentration at the site of action
  S is the slope parameter that determines the rate of change of the intensity of
     effect with the change in drug concentration

The slope of this linear relationship reflects the potency of the drug.

The linear model expressed by Equation 19.1 and presented in Figure 19.2 assumes that there is no effect in absence of the drug (at drug concentration = 0). If the measured effect has some value in absence of the drug (e.g., blood pressure), the model can be expressed as

$$E = E_o + SC \qquad (19.2)$$

where E_o is the effect in the absence of the drug or the baseline effect. In this case, the concentration-effect relationship can be presented as in Figure 19.3.

If a linear relationship exists between the drug concentration and the observed effect, linear regression can be performed between the measured drug effect at different concentrations to estimate the model parameter(s): the slope (S) and baseline effect (E_o). The linear relationship between the drug concentration and effect usually exist only over a certain range of drug concentrations, and outside this range this

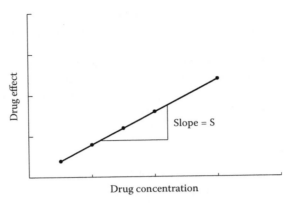

FIGURE 19.2 Drug concentration-effect relationship for a drug that follows the linear pharmacodynamic model.

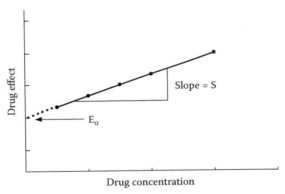

FIGURE 19.3 Drug concentration-effect relationship for a drug that follows the linear pharmacodynamic model in presence of a baseline effect.

linear relationship is not certain. In this case, it has to be specified that the model should be used only over this range of concentrations, and extrapolation outside this range is not appropriate.

19.3.3 LOG-LINEAR MODEL

This model assumes a linear relationship between the drug effect and the logarithm of the drug concentration at the site of action over a certain range of drug concentrations:

$$E = S \log C + I \tag{19.3}$$

where
    E is the drug effect
    S is the slope of the line
    C is the drug concentration at the effect site
    I is a constant

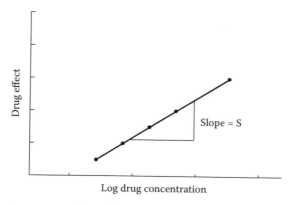

FIGURE 19.4 Drug concentration-effect relationship for a drug that follows the log-linear pharmacodynamic model.

The slope of the line reflects the potency of the drug. As mentioned under the linear pharmacodynamic model, it is important to specify the range of drug concentration over which the log-linear relationship between the drug concentration and effect exists as presented in Figure 19.4. This log-linear relationship may not exist outside this range of concentration and extrapolation outside this range is not appropriate.

The measured drug effect should be in the range of 20%–80% of the maximum response to obtain the log-linear relationship. However, the log-linear model does not allow prediction of the maximum drug effect that should be observed if the drug concentration is allowed to increase indefinitely. This makes it difficult to ensure that all the effect measurements are in this range. The log-linear model has been applied extensively to the description of in vitro pharmacodynamic studies. When the concentration-effect relationship can be described by the log-linear model, linear regression is performed between log drug concentrations and the measured drug effect at each concentration to determine the slope of this log-linear relationship. The estimated slopes for different drugs can be used to compare the relative potencies of these drugs and also to determine the combined effect of drugs.

19.3.4 E_max Model

This model assumes that the effect of the drug increases as the drug concentration increases until it reaches a plateau or a maximum effect at very high drug concentration as presented in Figure 19.5. The concentration-effect relationship can be described mathematically by a hyperbolic function:

$$E = \frac{E_{max}C}{EC_{50} + C} \qquad (19.4)$$

where
E_{max} is the maximum effect resulting from the drug that actually represents the intrinsic activity of the drug
EC_{50} is the drug concentration when the effect is 50% of the maximum effect which is a measure of the drug potency

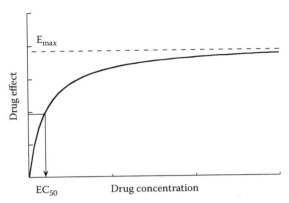

FIGURE 19.5 Drug concentration-effect relationship for a drug that follows the E_{max} pharmacodynamic model.

This model can be used to describe the concentration-effect relationship when a baseline effect is observed in the absence of the drug. In this case, Equation 19.4 can be modified to account for the baseline effect, E_o, as in Equation 19.5:

$$E = E_o + \frac{E_{max}C}{EC_{50} + C} \tag{19.5}$$

The model can also be used to describe the concentration-effect relationship when the drug causes reduction in the value of the measured effect, such as lowering the blood pressure by antihypertensive drugs as in Equation 19.6:

$$E = E_o - \frac{E_{max}C}{EC_{50} + C} \tag{19.6}$$

In this case, the maximum effect E_{max} (maximum reduction in blood pressure) can be calculated from the difference between the baseline blood pressure (blood pressure before using the drug) and the lowest blood pressure observed while using increasing doses of the drug. When the drug concentration-effect relationship follows the E_{max} model, the drug concentrations and the measured drug effect at each concentration are fitted to the model equation with nonlinear regression to estimate the model parameters, E_{max} and EC_{50}.

19.3.5 SIGMOID E_{max} MODEL

When the concentration-effect relationship does not follow the typical hyperbolic function, the sigmoid E_{max} model can be used to describe the concentration-effect relationship. If the drug concentration-effect curve is S-shaped or if the response

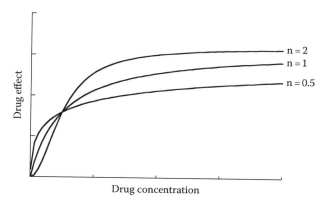

FIGURE 19.6 Drug concentration-effect relationship for a drug that follows the sigmoid E_{max} pharmacodynamic model.

approaches E_{max} very slowly, then deviation from the simple hyperbola can be described by

$$E = \frac{E_{max}C^n}{EC_{50}^n + C^n} \tag{19.7}$$

where n is the parameter affecting the shape of the curve. If n is greater than 1, then the curve will be S-shaped and if it is less than 1, then the initial portion of the curve has slope greater than the simple hyperbola and beyond EC_{50} the slope is less than the simple hyperbola as shown in Figure 19.6:

The sigmoid E_{max} model is applied when the interaction between a drug molecule with the receptor affects the interaction between the other drug molecules and the receptors [6,8]. For example, the interaction of one drug molecule with the receptor can make the other receptors more sensitive for interaction with the other drug molecules. In this case, n is >1 in the model equation. On the other hand, the drug receptor interaction may decrease the sensitivity of the other receptors for interaction with the other drug molecules. In this case, n is <1 in the model equation. If the interaction of one drug molecule with the receptor does not affect the interaction of the other drug molecules with the receptor, n is equal to 1 and Equation 19.7 is reduced to the equation for the E_{max} model. The sigmoid E_{max} model should not be used if the maximum effect is not clearly defined. When the drug concentration-effect relationship follows the sigmoid E_{max} model, the drug effect measurements and their corresponding drug concentrations are fitted to the model equation with nonlinear regression to estimate the model parameters, E_{max}, EC_{50}, and n.

19.4 INDIRECT LINK PK/PD MODELS

Under some instances, the drug effect may lag behind the plasma drug concentration. The delay in observing the drug effect results from delay in the drug distribution to its site of action. The lag between the plasma drug concentration and response becomes

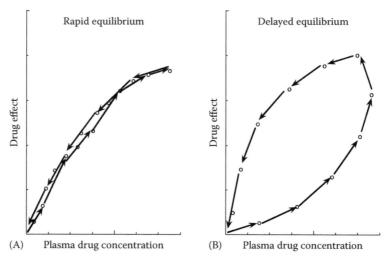

FIGURE 19.7 Plot of the plasma drug concentration versus the observed drug effect with the arrows representing the chronological order of the data points. In (A) rapid equilibrium exists between the drug in plasma and the drug at the site of action as in the direct link models, while in (B) the equilibrium between the drug in plasma and the drug at the site of action is delayed as in the indirect link models.

evident by examining the plot of the drug concentration–time and drug effect-time profiles. Also, plotting the plasma drug concentration-effect data and connecting the points in chronological order will give the characteristic counterclockwise hysteresis. This hysteresis is not observed when rapid equilibrium is achieved between the drug in plasma and the drug at the site of action as in Figure 19.7. The delayed equilibrium leads to the counterclockwise hysteresis; however, there are other conditions that can lead to this hysteresis too.

The simplest example to demonstrate the equilibrium delay is when the drug follows multicompartment pharmacokinetic model, and the drug site of action is in a tissue or an organ, which is part of the peripheral compartment. The drug concentration in the plasma, which is part of the central compartment, is not in rapid equilibrium with the drug in the peripheral compartment all the time. In this case, the use of the estimated drug concentration in the peripheral compartment as the input concentration for the pharmacodynamic model can avoid the distributional delay and can characterize the drug concentration-effect relationship better. This approach has been successfully used to describe the concentration-effect relationship for some drugs [9,10]. However, there is no reason to believe that the drug effect site concentration must have the same time course of the drug concentration in any of the compartments in the pharmacokinetic model. A more general approach that involves the introduction of an effect compartment to the PK/PD model has been used to describe the drug concentration-effect relationship in the presence of equilibrium delay.

19.4.1 Effect Compartment Approach

This modeling approach involves introduction of a hypothetical effect compartment that links the pharmacokinetic model and the pharmacodynamic model [11,12]. This approach assumes that the drug transfer to the effect compartment is negligible, so it does not affect the pharmacokinetic behavior of the drug. It also assumes that the drug transfer into and out of the effect compartment follows first-order processes, and that the drug effect is determined by the drug concentration in the effect compartment. In this case, the PK/PD model consists of three different components: the pharmacokinetic model that describes the plasma drug concentration–time profile, the pharmacodynamic model that relates the drug concentration in the effect compartment to the drug effect, and the effect compartment that provides the link between the pharmacokinetic and the pharmacodynamic model. The basic idea of this approach is to use the plasma concentrations-time data to estimate the drug pharmacokinetic parameters. Then the estimated pharmacokinetic model parameters and the drug effect-time data are used to estimate the drug concentration–time profile in the effect compartment, characterize the drug concentration-effect relationship, and estimate the pharmacodynamic model parameters.

The model in Figure 19.8 represents the one-compartment pharmacokinetic model that is linked to an effect compartment. The plasma drug concentration at any time after a single IV bolus dose can be described by Equation 19.8:

$$Cp = \frac{D}{Vd} e^{-kt} \qquad (19.8)$$

Writing the differential equation that describes the rate of change in the amount of the drug in the effect compartment and integrating this equation and dividing by the

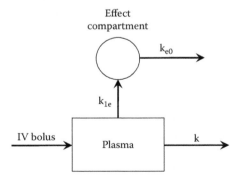

FIGURE 19.8 One-compartment pharmacokinetic model linked to an effect compartment. The parameters: k is the first-order elimination rate constant; k_{1e} and k_{e0} are the first-order transfer rate constant into and out of the effect compartment, respectively.

volume of the effect compartment yields the equation for the drug concentration in the effect compartment as follows:

$$C_e = \frac{Dk_{1e}}{V_e(k_{e0} - k)}(e^{-kt} - e^{-k_{e0}t})$$ (19.9)

where
  C_e is the drug concentration in the effect compartment
  D is the dose
  k is the first-order elimination rate constant
  k_{1e} is the first-order transfer rate constant from the plasma to the effect compartment
  k_{e0} is the first-order exit rate constant from the effect compartment
  V_e is the volume of the effect compartment

By assuming that the rate of appearance and removal of drug from the effect compartment are governed by the same process, it follows that the clearances into and out of the effect compartment are equal, that is,

$$Vdk_{1e} = V_e k_{e0}$$ (19.10)

where Vd is the drug volume of distribution.

By rearrangement and substituting for k_{1e} by $V_e k_{e0}/Vd$, the following expression for the drug concentration in the effect compartment can be obtained:

$$C_e = \frac{Dk_{e0}}{Vd(k_{e0} - k)}(e^{-kt} - e^{-k_{e0}t})$$ (19.11)

If we assume that the drug concentration-effect relationship follows the sigmoid E_{max} pharmacodynamic model, the relationship between the drug concentration in the effect compartment, C_e, and the drug effect will be described by the following equation [6–8]:

$$E = \frac{E_{max}C_e^n}{EC_{50}^n + C_e^n}$$ (19.12)

The plasma concentration–time data and the drug effect-time data are used to determine the pharmacokinetic and pharmacodynamic model parameters. The entire PK/PD model can be described mathematically by three different equations: The equation that describes the plasma concentration–time profile, which includes the pharmacokinetic parameters of the drug (e.g., Equation 19.8); also, the equation that describes the drug concentration–time profile in the effect compartment and includes the drug pharmacokinetic parameters and also k_{e0}, which is considered one of the pharmacodynamic parameters since it influences the rate of disappearance of the drug effect (e.g., Equation 19.11); in addition to the equation that describes the drug concentration-effect relationship, which includes the other pharmacodynamic parameters (e.g., Equation 19.12). Estimation of the PK/PD model parameters usually starts with fitting the drug concentration–time data to Equation 19.8 to estimate the pharmacokinetic parameters Vd and k. Then the estimated pharmacokinetic parameters and the drug effect-time data are fitted to Equations 19.11 and 19.12 to estimate the pharmacodynamic model parameters, E_{max}, EC_{50}, n, and k_{e0}. It is also possible to fit both the plasma drug concentration–time and effect-time data to the equations for the plasma drug concentration, the effect compartment drug concentration, and the drug concentration-effect relationship simultaneously. In this case, the pharmacokinetic model parameters and the pharmacodynamic model parameters are estimated simultaneously.

Similar approach can be used if the drug follows the two-compartment pharmacokinetic model where the effect compartment can be linked to the central or the peripheral compartment as shown in Figure 19.9. The plasma drug concentrations and the drug effect data are used to estimate the pharmacokinetic parameters and the drug concentration in the effect compartment at different time points, which is then substituted in the equation for the pharmacodynamic model to estimate the pharmacodynamic parameters. When the effect compartment is linked to the peripheral compartment in a multicompartment pharmacokinetic model, accurate characterization of the concentration-effect relationship and precise estimation of the pharmacodynamic parameters can only be achieved when information about the drug concentration in the peripheral compartment is available.

The aforementioned approach requires the assumption of a pharmacokinetic model to estimate the effect compartment drug concentration that can be related to the observed effect by the pharmacokinetic model. Another nonparametric approach has been used to analyze the pharmacokinetic and pharmacodynamic data when distributional delay exists leading to the counterclockwise hysteresis in the plasma concentration-effect relationship as in Figure 19.7B. This nonparametric approach does not require any assumption about the pharmacokinetic model. With fewer assumptions for the structure of the pharmacokinetic and the pharmacodynamic model, this approach can describe the delay between the concentration–time and

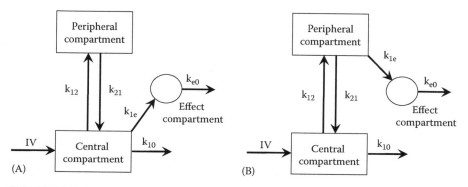

FIGURE 19.9 Two-compartment pharmacokinetic model linked to an effect compartment. (A) The effect compartment is linked to the central compartment and (B) the effect compartment is linked to the peripheral compartment.

effect-time profiles. It estimates the rate constant for the linking model as the value that causes the plasma concentration-effect hysteresis curve to collapse to a single curve, which describes the relationship between the drug concentration at the effect site and drug effect [13,14].

19.5   INDIRECT RESPONSE MODELS

The lag between the time course of the drug concentration and the observed drug response is not always due to delayed equilibrium. This delay can result from indirect response mechanism, which can also lead to counterclockwise hysteresis when the drug concentration-effect data are plotted in chronological order. When the drug mechanism of action involves synthesis or degradation of endogenous substances or when the drug effect is the result of inhibition or stimulation of an intermediary factor, the lag between the drug profile and the drug effect is observed. The indirect response models have been used to describe the pharmacodynamic effect of oral anticoagulants as mentioned previously. The maximum plasma concentration of the oral anticoagulants is usually achieved few hours after administration; however, their effect may be observed few days later after depletion of the already existing clotting factors. Despite this temporal dissociation between drug concentration and effect, higher drug concentrations usually result in more intense drug effect. The indirect response models are usually used to characterize the drug concentration-effect relationship for these drugs.

Four basic models have been proposed to relate the time course of the drug concentration and the drug effect for drugs with indirect pharmacodynamic response [15–18]. These general models assume that the rate of change of the response is controlled by a zero-order process for the production of the drug response and a first-order process for the loss of the response. So the differential equation that describes the change in drug response in the absence of the drug can be written as

$$\frac{dR}{dt} = k_{in} - k_{out}R_{Baseline} \qquad (19.13)$$

where
   k_{in} is the zero-order rate constant for the production of response R
   k_{out} is the first-order rate constant for the loss of response
   $R_{Baseline}$ is the value of the response in the absence of the drug

The drug response can be affected by either stimulation or inhibition of the production or loss of effect. The degree of this stimulation or inhibition is related to the drug concentration at the effect site via the sigmoid E_{max} pharmacodynamic model. So depending on the mechanism of action of the drug one can determine if the observed response results from inhibition or stimulation of the production or loss of the response. Then the model appropriate to the mechanism of action for the drug can be chosen to describe the drug concentration-effect relationship. For this reason, the indirect response models are also known as the mechanism-based models. For example, oral anticoagulants produce their effect by inhibition of the clotting factor synthesis. So the indirect response model for the inhibition of the production of effect can be selected to describe the concentration-effect relationship of these drugs based on their mechanism of action.

The differential equations that describe the rate of change in the response with time for the four different models can be written as follows:

- For inhibition of the production of response model:

$$\frac{dR}{dt} = k_{in} \left(1 - \frac{I_{max} C^n}{IC_{50}^n + C^n} \right) - k_{out} R \qquad (19.14)$$

- For inhibition of the loss of response model:

$$\frac{dR}{dt} = k_{in} - k_{out} \left(1 - \frac{I_{max} C}{IC_{50}^n + C} \right) R \qquad (19.15)$$

- For stimulation of the production of response model:

$$\frac{dR}{dt} = k_{in} \left(1 + \frac{S_{max} C^n}{SC_{50}^n + C^n} \right) - k_{out} R \qquad (19.16)$$

- For simulation of the loss of response model:

$$\frac{dR}{dt} = k_{in} - k_{out} \left(1 + \frac{S_{max} C^n}{SC_{50}^n + C^n} \right) R \qquad (19.17)$$

where
k_{in} is the zero-order rate constant for the production of response R
k_{out} is the first-order rate constant for the loss of response
n is the parameter affecting the shape of the concentration-effect curve known as the sigmoidicity factor
C is the drug concentration at the site of action
I_{max} is the maximum inhibition that can be produced by the drug
IC_{50} is the drug concentration when the inhibition is 50% of I_{max}
S_{max} is the maximum stimulation that can be produced by the drug
SC_{50} is the drug concentration when the stimulation is 50% of S_{max}

Figure 19.10 represents a schematic presentation of the four basic indirect response models.

The indirect response models become a good choice for describing the drug concentration-effect relationship when there are evidences that the lag between the drug concentration–time and effect-time profiles is not due to distributional delay.

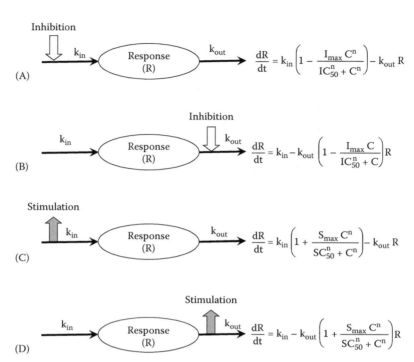

FIGURE 19.10 Schematic representation of the four basic indirect response models and the differential equations that describe the rate of change in the drug response with respect to time for each model. The four models are (A) inhibition of production of response model, (B) inhibition of loss of response model, (C) stimulation of production of response model, and (D) stimulation of the loss of response model.

The process starts with the selection of the appropriate indirect response model based on the drug pharmacological activity and mechanism of action. Also, an appropriate pharmacokinetic model is used to describe the pharmacokinetic behavior of the drug. The drug concentration–time data are fitted to the equation that describes the drug pharmacokinetic behavior to estimate the drug pharmacokinetic parameters and to characterize the drug concentration–time profile at the site that is most probably associated with the drug effect. This can be the plasma concentration, the concentration in the peripheral compartment of a multicompartment model or even in a hypothetical effect compartment. Then the drug effect-time data and the drug concentrations estimated from the pharmacokinetic model are fitted to the equation of the selected indirect response model to estimate the pharmacodynamic model parameters, k_{in}, k_{out}, the parameter for the maximum effect I_{max} or S_{max}, the parameter for the drug concentration at half maximum effect IC_{50} or SC_{50}, and n. It is also possible to fit both drug concentration–time and effect-time data to the pharmacokinetic and pharmacodynamic equations simultaneously to estimate all the parameters for the PK/PD model.

19.6   TIME-VARIANT PHARMACODYNAMIC MODELS

Time-variant models are also known as the time-dependent pharmacodynamic models. Drugs that follow these models have their concentration-effect relationships change with time, meaning that the same drug concentration produces higher or lower response during continuous exposure to the drug. When the drug effect decreases with time it is called tolerance, while the increase in drug effect with time is called sensitization. So in these models, the pharmacodynamic parameters, for example, E_{max} and EC_{50} in the E_{max} model, change with time. The rate of change of these parameters depends on the mechanism by which tolerance or sensitization occurs. The change in the pharmacodynamic parameters can be rapid, so the same drug concentration during the absorption and the elimination phases after oral drug administration produces different intensities of drug effect, in the absence of any distributional delay, while in other situations tolerance or sensitization can be developed over days or weeks.

Tolerance is defined as the decrease in drug pharmacological response after prolonged exposure to the drug. Plotting the drug concentration-effect data in chronological order will show a clockwise hysteresis due to the development of tolerance. Tolerance has been documented in many drugs such as glyceryl nitrate, morphine, cocaine, nicotine, and benzodiazepines. The mechanism of developing tolerance to drug response vary for different drugs and can be due to receptor downregulation, decrease in affinity between the drug and receptor, decrease in the receptor generated response, or other reasons. Pharmacodynamic models that describe the drug concentration-effect relationship for drugs that develop tolerance over time should account for the change in the pharmacodynamic parameters over time.

Several modifications in the pharmacodynamic models have been suggested to account for the change in the pharmacodynamic parameters with time. For example, the inclusion of a time-dependent exponential term to decrease the value of E_{max} as time increases (e.g., $E_{max}e^{-St}$) to describe receptor downregulation can be used. Also, the exponential term can be used to increase the value of EC_{50} with time (e.g., $EC_{50}e^{St}$) to describe the decrease in receptor affinity. The constant S in the exponential terms controls the rate of change in the parameter. This modification suggests that the parameters change continuously with time, which may not be correct. Another approach is to have a lower boundary for E_{max} and higher boundary for EC_{50}. These two approaches assume that the development of tolerance depends only on time. However, it has been well documented that tolerance development depends on the intensity of drug exposure, which is a function of drug concentration and time. A more general approach has been developed that suggests the formation of a hypothetical drug metabolite that noncompetitively antagonizes the effect of the drug. The rate of formation of this hypothetical metabolite depends on the drug concentration and also a rate constant that control the rate of appearance and disappearance of tolerance. This model has been used to describe the development of acute tolerance to the effect of nicotine on heart rate [19].

Sensitization is defined as the increase in drug pharmacological response after prolonged exposure to the drug. Plotting the drug concentration-effect data in chronological order will show an anticlockwise hysteresis when the development of sensitization is rapid.

Sensitization can occur due to upregulation of receptors. Example of the development of sensitization is the hypersensitivity to catecholamines after sudden withdrawal of β-blockers. Pharmacodynamic models have been modified to account for the change in the pharmacodynamic parameters due to sensitization.

19.7 OTHER PHARMACODYNAMIC MODELS

The models described earlier are the general PK/PD models that have been utilized to analyze the drug concentration-effect relationship for many drugs. However, there are drugs with special response characteristics that necessitate modification of these general models or development of new modeling approaches to suit this special response features.

19.7.1 IRREVERSIBLE EFFECT MODELS

When the drug effect on the target site is irreversible, the time course of the drug effect is dependent on the turnover rate of the target rather than the pharmacokinetics of the drug. For example, the covalent acetylation of the platelet membrane cyclooxygenase by aspirin leads to irreversible effect on platelet aggregation because the platelet cannot synthesize new protein. So the effect will last for the life span of the platelet. Other drugs that produce irreversible effects include omeprazole, which irreversibly inhibits the proton pump (H^+, K^+-ATPase) in the parietal cells causing inhibition of gastric acid secretion that lasts for more than 24 h despite the short half-life of the drug [20]. Pharmacodynamic models used to describe the time course of the effect of these drugs should include the turnover rate of the affected target, including the rate of formation and degradation of this target in addition to the drug concentration-effect relationship.

19.7.2 TRANSDUCTION PROCESS MODELING

The pharmacodynamic effect of the drug may be produced as a result of a cascade of events initiated by the interaction of the drug with its receptor. Advances in the field of molecular pharmacology helped in understanding the signal transduction pathways that occur between the time of drug-receptor interaction until the generation of the pharmacological effect. These transduction pathways may involve gene transcription, protein phosphorylation, activation of ionic channel, second messenger, and other processes that usually take time and cause the delay in the observation of the drug response. The concept of the transit compartments has been used to account for the delay in the drug pharmacological effect [21]. One or more hypothetical transit compartments, depending on the number of distinctive steps involved in the generation of effect, are connected in series to the compartment representing the systemic circulation in the pharmacokinetic model. Each transit compartment represents an intermediary or a second messenger that is formed or degraded at a rate dependent on the transit time, which represents the time delay resulting from this transit compartment. Since the transit compartments are connected in series, the time delay for the generation of the drug response is dependent on the transit time for all the transit compartments. These models are very useful in reflecting the mechanism of drug action when information is available about the time dependent signal transduction or actual measurements of secondary messenger or intermediates can be obtained.

19.7.3 PHARMACOKINETIC MODELS WITHOUT DRUG CONCENTRATIONS

The time course of the pharmacodynamic effect of the drug can provide useful information about the drug at the site of action and the drug response in the absence of drug concentration data. The dose-effect-time relationship can be investigated utilizing the time course of the drug response after administration of different doses of the drug. For example, the effect of calcium receptor agonist on the parathyroid hormone concentration was described by an indirect response model with inhibition of the production of effect. The dose-response relationships are related by the E_{max} model, as in Equation 19.18, which is a slight modification of Equation 19.14. This is because the response, which is the parathyroid hormone plasma concentration, is dependent on the rate of formation (k_{in}) and the rate of elimination (k_{out}) and, the calcium receptor agonist is expected to inhibit the secretion of the hormone.

$$\frac{dR}{dt} = k_{in}\left(1 - \frac{I_{max}A}{IA_{50} + A}\right) - k_{out}R \tag{19.18}$$

where
    A is the dose of the drug
    IA_{50} is the dose of the drug that produces 50% of the maximum effect [22]

This approach can be useful in characterizing the dose-effect-time relationship in the absence of pharmacokinetic data; however, extensive pharmacodynamic data are usually required to accurately estimate the model parameters. This approach can be used to study the different factors that can affect the time course of the drug response.

19.7.4 DISEASE PROGRESSION MODELS

Conventional PK/PD models assumes that the baseline condition of the biological system before administration of the drug stay constant during the treatment period. However, in progressive and chronic diseases, the status of the biological system may deteriorate over the course of the drug treatment and the concentration-effect relationship may change over time [23]. In such cases, the effect of the drug treatment on the disease progression should be incorporated in the model especially if the drug treatment is intended to modify the disease progression. The indirect response models assume that the drug effect results from inhibition or stimulation of the production of response (k_{in}) or the rate of loss of the response (k_{out}). In the previous discussion k_{in} and k_{out} were assumed to be constants. Modeling of the disease progression can be achieved by changing the value of k_{in} or k_{out}, as a function of time depending on the natural disease progression rate. This is appropriate when the drug effect results from relieving the symptoms without affecting the process of disease progression. However, when the drug effect occurs due to modification of the process underlying the disease, resulting in change in the time course of disease progression, the rate of change in the k_{in} or k_{out} can be changed to account for the effect of the drug on the rate of disease progression.

19.8   PK/PD MODELING PROCESS

The PK/PD modeling usually goes through several iterative steps that start usually with proposing a tentative model based on the available information about the drug and its response. The experimental data are fitted to the proposed model and the model is evaluated and modified. The process is repeated to refine the model until an appropriate model is developed. An appropriate model is the simplest model with reasonable goodness of fit and has good predictability. The following is a summary of the steps that are followed in the modeling process [5].

19.8.1   STATING THE OBJECTIVES, PROPOSING A TENTATIVE MODEL, AND DESIGNING THE STUDY

The objectives of performing the modeling have to be stated clearly because the PK/PD study design including the measured surrogate measured has to be selected to fulfill these objectives. All the available pharmacokinetic and pharmacodynamic information about the drug under investigation have to be used to propose a preliminary model to describe the drug concentration-effect relationship. This information includes the drug pharmacokinetic behavior, the factors that affect the drug pharmacokinetics and/or the pharmacodynamics of the drug, formation of pharmacologically active metabolite, mechanism of action for the drug, the surrogate markers for drug response, existence of time delay between the time course of drug concentration and effect, and development of tolerance or sensitization. Based on this information the PK/PD study is designed and executed to obtain the necessary pharmacokinetic and pharmacodynamic data. Study design factors such as the number of subjects included in the study, number of samples obtained, and the distribution of the samples over all phases of the study have great influence on the validity of the constructed models.

19.8.2   INITIAL DATA EXPLORATION AND DATA TRANSFORMATION

This step is very important in exploring how the experimentally generated data agree with the proposed PK/PD model. Data exploration usually includes plotting drug concentration–time curve, response-time curve, and concentration-response curve. In these plots, the linear and log-transformed data can be used. Also, the response can be expressed as the actual measured values, the change in base line effect, the absolute change in baseline effect, or the percentage change in baseline effects.

The drug concentration–time curve is usually important in characterizing the pharmacokinetic behavior of the drug and to determine if the drug follows one- or multicompartment pharmacokinetic model, while the drug effect-time curve can be used together with the drug concentration–time curve to determine if there is delay between the drug concentration–time and the drug response-time profiles. Also, the existence of counterclockwise hysteresis in the plot of the drug concentration versus response when the data points are plotted in chronological sequence suggests delay between the time courses of the drug concentration and drug effect. It is also possible to determine if the delay results from distributional delay or due to the mechanism of action of the drug. Furthermore, the drug concentration-effect plot can help in determining if the linear, log-linear, E_{max}, or sigmoid E_{max} pharmacodynamic model can describe the concentration-effect relationship. Based on this initial exploration of data the initial assumptions for the concentration-effect relationship are revised and the preliminary model is modified to concur with the observed results.

19.8.3 Refining and Evaluation of the PK/PD Model

The obtained experimental data are fitted to the mathematical expressions that describe the PK/PD model using specialized data analysis software, and the model parameters are estimated. The ability of the model to describe the obtained results is determined from how well the data are fitted to the model or the goodness of fit. Most of the available PK/PD data analysis softwares have some diagnostic statistics that can be used to examine the model goodness of fit. This include, but not limited to, the standard error of the parameter estimates, 95% confidence interval, and the coefficient of variation for the parameter estimates, which are measures of the variability in the parameter estimates. Large values in these statistical measures usually indicate uncertainty of this parameter estimate and poor description of the obtained data by the model. Also, graphical methods can be used to evaluate the goodness of fit including a scattered plot of the observed concentrations around the model predicted concentration–time and effect-time profiles to determine how well the model fits the data. A plot of the observed versus model predicted concentrations or effect can be useful to examine how well the model describes the data. Furthermore, several residuals plots can be utilized in model evaluation. The residuals are the difference between the observed drug concentration and the model predicted concentration or the observed effect and the model predicted effect. A plot of the residuals versus predicted concentration and the residual versus time can be used to examine if the model fit all parts of the profiles equally. When the model fits the observed data properly, the residuals plotted versus time or versus predicted values should be small, with approximately uniform relative magnitude, and randomly distributed around the zero residual line. Based on this evaluation, the PK/PD model may be refined and the process is repeated again until a model that can properly describe the data is obtained. If the model seems to appropriately describe the data, further validation of the model is usually necessary to determine the other situations where the model can be applied.

19.8.4 Validation of the PK/PD Model

The ability of the PK/PD model to describe the pharmacokinetic and pharmaco-dynamic behavior of the drug is usually evaluated by the diagnostic statistics for the model goodness of fit as described earlier. However, the real model validity is determined from its ability to predict the drug pharmacokinetic and pharmacody-namic behavior in situations that were not used to develop or refine the model. The predictability of the PK/PD models is important especially when it provides evi-dences of safety and efficacy and supports new doses and dosage regimen in the target population or subpopulations. One of the common methods used to test the predictive power of the model is to split the data into two parts. One set of data is used to construct and refine the model and the other set of data is used to test the model predictive power. The developed model is used to simulate the drug pharma-cokinetic and pharmacodynamic behavior under the conditions of the second data set. The agreement between the experimentally obtained data set and the predicted data is tested to evaluate the predictive power of the model. The predictability of the model can also be evaluated by performing a separate validation study and compar-ing the obtained data with the predicted data using model simulations. PK/PD model simulations can also be used to explore the effect of factors like model assumptions, design constrains, parameter sensitivity, and dosage regimen on the performance of the model. All the validation techniques are important in defining the situations within which the model can be applied.

19.9 APPLICATIONS OF THE PK/PD MODELING IN DRUG DEVELOPMENT AND CLINICAL USE OF DRUGS

PK/PD modeling and simulation are very useful tools for enhancing the effective utilization of resources in all stages of drug development. During the preclinical phase of drug development, studies that relate the pharmacokinetic information of the candidate drug with its pharmacodynamic properties usually provide important information that is necessary for subsequent development activities. During this early phase of drug development, biomarkers can be tested and evaluated for their potential use as surrogate marker for the drug clinical efficacy and toxicity. The development of mechanism-based PK/PD models to describe the dose-concentration-effect rela-tionship in different animal species allows the prediction of the concentration-effect relationship in humans, which is very important in selecting the appropriate drug doses in early phase I clinical studies. Also, the PK/PD models allow the compari-son of the potencies and intrinsic activities of different drugs and prediction of drug potency in humans from the animal PK/PD data. Furthermore, the different physi-ological and pathological factors and the potential drug interactions that can alter the drug pharmacokinetic and pharmacodynamic properties can be investigated. Characterization of the drug concentration-effect relationship allows the selection and optimization of the dosage form and dosage regimen that can achieve the drug concentration–time profile required to produce the desired effect.

During the different phases of clinical drug development, integration of the phar-macokinetic and pharmacodynamic information provide beneficial information to determine the range of doses that can be tolerated and to learn how to use the drug in the target patient population. The dose escalation studies provide the opportunity to examine the dose-concentration-effect relationship for therapeutic and adverse effects over a wide range of doses. Correlation of the drug concentration and drug effect profiles can be used to determine the impact of the route of administration and the rate of drug absorption on the drug effect, which is useful in deciding if a controlled-release formulation can be clinically beneficial. Population PK/PD modeling is frequently applied to examine the dose-concentration-effect relationship in patients and also to identify the different factors that can contribute to the interindividual variability in response. Factors such as age, gender, disease, other drugs, and tolerance development are usually investigated in population PK/PD studies, and the dosage requirements in the different patient subpopulations are usually determined. Also, the PK/PD information can be used to examine the effect of ethnic and genetic factors on the dose-concentration-effect relationship, which can provide the necessary information for global drug development.

19.10   PK/PD SIMULATIONS

The companion CD to this book includes a section for PK/PD simulations. This section allows simultaneous simulation of the plasma drug concentration–time profile and the drug effect-time profile after single and multiple drug administrations. These simulations include direct link models, indirect link models using the effect compartment approach, and the indirect response models. The sigmoid E_{max} pharmacodynamic model is used in these simulations to describe drug concentration-effect relationship. The following discussions cover few examples of the important factors that significantly affect the drug concentration-effect relationship for the different PK/PD models. The PK/PD simulations can be used to visualize drug concentration-effect relationship under different situations.

19.10.1   Direct Link Models

The relationship between EC_{50} and the plasma drug concentrations: The range of drug concentrations achieved during the therapeutic use of the drug usually depends on the therapeutic range of the drug. So the relationship between this range of drug concentrations and the drug EC_{50} can have significant effect on the observed drug effect. When the plasma drug concentrations achieved are much lower than the EC_{50}, the relationship between the drug concentration and drug effect profiles can be approximated by a linear relationship. So the drug concentration-effect relationship will be linearly related. On the contrary, when the drug concentration is in the range of EC_{50}, a small change in the drug concentration will produce significant change in the drug effect. In this case, fluctuation in drug concentration during multiple drug administration produces significant fluctuations in the drug effect. Whereas if the drug concentrations achieved is much higher than the EC_{50}, even large change in the drug concentration produces small fluctuation in the drug effect.

The sigmoidicity factor n: When n is larger than 1, the change in the drug effect due to the change in the drug concentration will be faster especially when the drug concentration is in the range of the EC_{50}. Values of n less than 1 result in smaller change in effect with the change in concentration over a wide range of concentrations.

19.10.2   INDIRECT LINK MODEL USING EFFECT COMPARTMENT

The drug effect is related to the drug concentration in the effect compartment. The relationship between the drug concentration achieved in the effect compartment and the EC_{50} and how this influences the change in drug effect as a result of the change in drug concentration can also be applied for the effect compartment models.

The rate constant k_{e0}: The smaller the value of k_{e0} the slower is the equilibration between the drug in the systemic circulation and the effect compartment and the slower is the emergence of the effect. So the time to achieve the maximum effect is dependent on k_{e0} with longer delay in effect observed when k_{e0} is smaller. Changing the dose will change the intensity of effect but it does not affect the time to achieve the maximum effect. Smaller values of k_{e0} delay the time for maximum effect but also prolong and increase the exposure of the effect compartment to the drug. The higher exposure of the effect compartment to the drug is reflected by the larger AUC in the effect compartment, and also the increase in drug effect is reflected by the larger area under the effect-time curve. When k_{e0} is very small, the drug effect may be observed after the disappearance of the drug from the plasma.

19.10.3   INDIRECT RESPONSE MODELS

The different basic indirect response models have some similar properties. The models for inhibition of the production of effect and the stimulation of the loss of response usually have a decrease and then increase in the measured response, while the models for the inhibition of the loss of response and the stimulation of production of response have increase and then decrease in response. All four models have maximum effect achieved after the maximum drug concentration is achieved. The increase in dose results in delay in the observation of the maximum effect when both rate constants for the production and loss of response were kept constant [18].

REFERENCES

1. Holford NHG and Sheiner LB (1981) Pharmacokinetic and pharmacodynamic modeling in vivo. *CRC Crit Rev Bioeng* 5:273–322.
2. Meibohm B and Derendorf H (1997) Basic concepts of pharmacokinetic/pharmacodynamic (PK/PD) modeling. *Int J Clin Pharmacol Ther* 35:401–413.
3. Derendorf H and Meibohm B (1999) Modeling of pharmacokinetic/pharmacodynamic (PK/PD) relationships: Concepts and perspectives. *Pharm Res* 16:176–185.
4. Center for Drug Evaluation and Research, U.S. Food and Drug Administration (2002) Guidance for industry: Exposure-response relationships: Study design, data analysis, and regulatory applications.

5. Rohatagi S, Martin NE, and Barrett JS (2004) Pharmacokinetic/pharmacodynamic modeling in drug development, in Krishna R (Ed.) *Applications of Pharmacokinetic Principles in Drug Development*, Kluwer Academic/Plenum Publisher, New York.
6. Wagner JG (1968) Kinetics of pharmacologic response. *J Theor Biol* 20:173–201.
7. Holford NHG and Shiner LB (1981) Understanding the dose-effect relationship: Clinical application of pharmacokinetic-pharmacodynamic models. *Clin Pharmacokinet* 6:429–453.
8. Holford NHG and Shiner LB (1982) Kinetics of pharmacologic response. *Pharmacol Ther* 16:141–166.
9. Wagner JG, Aghajanian GK, and Bing OH (1968) Correlation of performance test scores with tissue concentration of lysergic acid diethylamide in human subjects. *Clin Pharmacol Ther* 9:635–638.
10. Kramer WG, Kolibash AJ, Lewis RP, Bathala MS, Visconti JA, and Reuning RH (1979) Pharmacokinetics of digoxin: Relationship between response intensity and predicted compartmental drug levels in man. *J Pharmacokinet Biopharm* 7:47–61.
11. Segre G (1968) Kinetics of interaction between drugs and biological systems II. *Farmaco* 23:906–918.
12. Sheiner LB, Stanski DR, Vozeh S, Miiller RD, and Ham J (1979) Simultaneous modeling of pharmacokinetics and pharmacodynamics: Application to d-tubocurarine. *Clin Pharmacol Ther* 25:358–371.
13. Fuseau E and Sheiner LB (1984) Simultaneous modeling of pharmacokinetics and pharmacodynamics with a nonparametric pharmacodynamic model. *Clin Pharmacol Ther* 35:733–741.
14. Unadkat JD, Bartha F, and Sheiner LB (1984) Simultaneous modeling of pharmacokinetics and pharmacodynamics with a nonparametric kinetic and dynamic models. *Clin Pharmacol Ther* 40:86–93.
15. Daneyka NL, Garg V, and Jusko WJ (1993) Comparison of four basic models of indirect pharmacologic response. *J Pharmacokinet Biopharm* 21:457–478.
16. Jusko WJ and Ko HC (1994) Physiologic indirect response models characterize diverse type of pharmacodynamic effects. *Clin Pharmacol Ther* 56:406–419.
17. Levy G (1994) Mechanism-based pharmacodynamic modeling. *Clin Pharmacol Ther* 56:356–358.
18. Sharma A and Jusko WJ (1996) Characterization of four basic models of indirect pharmacodynamic responses. *J Pharmacokinet Biopharm* 24:611–635.
19. Porchet HC, Benowitz NL, and Shiner LB (1988) Pharmacodynamic modeling of tolerance: Application to nicotine. *J Pharmacol Exp Ther* 244:231–236.
20. Äbelö A, Erikson UG, Karlsson MO, Larsson H, and Gabrielsson J (2000) A turnover model for the irreversible inhibition of gastric acid secretion by omeprazole in the dog. *J Pharmacol Exp Ther* 295:662–629.
21. Mager DE and Jusco WJ (2001) Pharmacodynamic modeling of time-dependent transduction systems. *Clin Pharmacol Ther* 70:210–216.
22. Lalonde RL, Gaudreault J, Karhu DA, and Marriott TB (1999) Mixed-effects modeling of the pharmacodynamic responses to the calcimimetic agent R-568. *Clin Pharmacol Ther* 65:40–49.
23. Chan PL and Holforrd NH (2001) Drug treatment effect on disease progression. *Annu Rev Pharmacol Toxicol* 41:625–659.

20 Noncompartmental Approach in Pharmacokinetic Data Analysis

OBJECTIVES

After completing this chapter you should be able to

- Discuss the situations when the noncompartmental data analysis approach is appropriate
- Define the mean residence time
- Calculate the AUC, the AUMC, and the MRT from the plasma concentration–time data
- Analyze the drug absorption characteristics after extravascular administration using the noncompartmental approach
- Determine the pharmacokinetic parameters using the noncompartmental approach and describe how they are related to their estimates from the compartmental approach

20.1 INTRODUCTION

In the previous discussions, the compartmental approach was used to describe the pharmacokinetic behavior of the drug in the body. The compartmental approach for data analysis requires model specification and setting the assumptions to identify the space within which the model can be applied. This approach of data analysis is usually performed utilizing special computer software, which requires special skills and knowledge of pharmacokinetics and statistics to ensure proper model specification and suitability for the obtained results. Also, complex compartmental pharmacokinetic models in most cases describe the drug profile in the body better than the simpler models. However, complex pharmacokinetic models usually have more parameters and the accuracy of parameter estimation is usually compromised in the presence of limited data. So it is important to statistically test if going to complex pharmacokinetic models significantly improves the description of the drug concentration–time profile in the body without compromising the accuracy of the model parameter estimates. When all these issues are considered, the compartmental approach can be a very valuable tool for the analysis of pharmacokinetic data.

The noncompartmental approach for pharmacokinetic data analysis provides an alternative data analysis method that can be used when the required pharmacokinetic information can be obtained without the need to assume a specific compartmental model. The comparison between the compartmental and noncompartmental methods is not to determine which one is superior to the other, but to determine the situations when each method can be applied and the information that can be obtained when using each approach. When deciding which approach to use in the pharmacokinetic data analysis, the choice usually depends on the objectives of the data analysis and the suitability of each approach to achieve these objectives. The classical example of important pharmacokinetic studies, which are usually analyzed using the noncompartmental approach, is the bioequivalent studies. The main objective of the bioequivalent study is to compare the rate and extent of drug absorption after administration of test and reference products for the same active drug. The rate and extent of drug absorption after administration of the two products can be evaluated by comparing the t_{max}, C_{max}, and AUC for the two products. The parameters t_{max}, C_{max}, and AUC can be calculated without the need to assume a specific compartmental model, which makes the noncompartmental data analysis approach appropriate for these studies.

20.2   NONCOMPARTMENTAL APPROACH IN DATA ANALYSIS

The only assumption for the noncompartmental approach in pharmacokinetic data analysis is that the drug elimination is first order. The noncompartmental approach is based on the statistical moment theory, which has been utilized in chemical engineering. This theory views the drug molecules in the body as randomly distributed and each molecule has a certain probability to be eliminated at a certain time (t). So according to this theory the time course for the drug concentration in plasma can be regarded as a probability density function. This probability density function multiplied by time raised to a certain power (0, 1, or 2) and integrated over time yields the area under the moment curve. For example, the area under the zero moment curve can be determined from Equation 20.1, which is equal to the AUC. Also, the area under the first moment curve (AUMC) can be determined as in Equation 20.2. Only the area under the zero and first moments are utilized in pharmacokinetics since higher moments are subjected to large computational errors.

$$\text{Area under the zero moment curve} = \int_{t=0}^{t=\infty} t^0 Cp\,dt = \int_{t=0}^{t=\infty} Cp\,dt = AUC \qquad (20.1)$$

$$\text{Area under the first moment curve} = \int_{t=0}^{t=\infty} t^1 Cp\,dt = \int_{t=0}^{t=\infty} tCp\,dt = AUMC \qquad (20.2)$$

The principle of moment analysis has been utilized to estimate the pharmacokinetic parameters such as the mean residence time (MRT), drug clearance (CL_T), and also the volume of distribution at steady state (Vd_{ss}) [1,2].

20.3 MEAN RESIDENCE TIME AFTER IV BOLUS ADMINISTRATION

Drug molecules are distributed throughout the body after IV administration. Some drug molecules are eliminated from the body faster than other molecules despite the fact that all the molecules are similar. The difference in the residence time of different molecules in the body occurs by chance according to the statistical moment theory. The MRT is defined as the average time for the residence of all the drug molecules in the body [3]. In other words, the MRT can be calculated from the total residence time for all drug molecules (by adding the residence time for all molecules) and dividing this by the number of drug molecules as in Equation 20.3:

$$MRT = \frac{\text{Total residence time for all drug molecules}}{\text{Number of drug molecules}} \tag{20.3}$$

Equation 20.3 helps in explaining the meaning of the MRT; however, practically it cannot be used in the calculation. The MRT can be calculated from the area under the zero and first moment curves according to Equation 20.4:

$$MRT = \frac{AUMC}{AUC} \tag{20.4}$$

where

AUMC is the area under the first moment–time curve
AUC is the area under the zero moment–time curve or the area under the plasma concentration–time curve

The MRT has units of time.

20.3.1 Calculation of the AUC and AUMC

20.3.1.1 Area under the Plasma Concentration–Time Curve

The AUC can be calculated utilizing the trapezoidal rule as described in detail in Chapter 10. The plasma concentration–time profile is divided into trapezoids and the area of each trapezoid is calculated according to Equation 20.5:

$$\text{Area of a trapezoid} = \left(\frac{C_n + C_{n+1}}{2} \right) \cdot (t_{n+1} - t_n) \tag{20.5}$$

The AUC_{0-t} is calculated by adding the area of all the trapezoids, while the $AUC_{t-\infty}$ is calculated by extrapolation to time ∞ as in Equation 20.6:

$$AUC_{t-\infty} = \frac{C_{last}}{\lambda} \tag{20.6}$$

where

C_{last} is the last measured plasma drug concentration
λ is the rate constant for the terminal decline phase in the plasma drug concentration

The total $AUC_{0-\infty}$ is calculated by adding the two areas as in Equation 20.7:

$$AUC_{0-\infty} = AUC_{0-t} + AUC_{t-\infty} \tag{20.7}$$

20.3.1.2 Area under the First Moment–Time Curve

The AUMC can also be calculated utilizing the trapezoidal rule after dividing the curve to trapezoids. The area of each trapezoid is calculated according to Equation 20.8:

$$\text{Area of a trapezoid} = \left(\frac{t_n C_n + t_{n+1} C_{n+1}}{2} \right) \cdot (t_{n+1} - t_n) \tag{20.8}$$

The $AUMC_{0-t}$ is calculated by adding the area of all the trapezoids. The $AUMC_{t-\infty}$ is calculated as in Equation 20.9:

$$AUMC_{t-\infty} = \frac{t_{last} Cp_{last}}{\lambda} + \frac{C_{last}}{\lambda^2} \tag{20.9}$$

where
  C_{last} is the last measured plasma drug concentration
  λ is the rate constant for the terminal elimination phase in the plasma drug concentration

The total $AUMC_{0-\infty}$ is calculated by adding both areas as in Equation 20.10:

$$AUMC_{0-\infty} = AUMC_{0-t} + AUMC_{t-\infty} \tag{20.10}$$

Example

After a single IV bolus administration of 50 mg of a drug, the following plasma concentrations were obtained:

Time (h)	Concentrations (μg/L)
0	250
1	225
3	185
6	135
9	105
12	77
18	40
24	22

The terminal rate constant for the decline in the drug concentration = 0.1 h^{-1}.
  Calculate the MRT.

Answer

The MRT is calculated from the AUC and AUMC.

- Calculation of the AUC by the trapezoidal rule:

$$\text{Area of trapezoid 1} = \left(\frac{250 + 225}{2}\right) \cdot (1 - 0) = 237.5\,\mu g\,h/L$$

$$\text{Area of trapezoid 2} = \left(\frac{225 + 185}{2}\right) \cdot (3 - 1) = 410\,\mu g\,h/L$$

$$\text{Area of trapezoid 3} = \left(\frac{185 + 135}{2}\right) \cdot (6 - 3) = 480\,\mu g\,h/L$$

$$\text{Area of trapezoid 4} = \left(\frac{135 + 105}{2}\right) \cdot (9 - 6) = 360\,\mu g\,h/L$$

$$\text{Area of trapezoid 5} = \left(\frac{105 + 77}{2}\right) \cdot (12 - 9) = 273\,\mu g\,h/L$$

$$\text{Area of trapezoid 6} = \left(\frac{77 + 40}{2}\right) \cdot (18 - 12) = 351\,\mu g\,h/L$$

$$\text{Area of trapezoid 7} = \left(\frac{40 + 22}{2}\right) \cdot (24 - 18) = 186\,\mu g\,h/L$$

$$AUC_{t-\infty} = \frac{22}{0.1} = 220\,\mu g\,h/L$$

$$AUC_{0-\infty} = 237.5 + 410 + 480 + 360 + 273 + 351 + 186 + 220 = 2517.5\,\mu g\,h/L$$

- Calculation of the AUMC
  To calculate the AUMC it is easier to add a column to the available data that includes the product of the time and the plasma concentration as follows:

Time (h)	Concentrations (µg/L)	Time × Concentration (µg h/L)
0	250	0
1	225	225
3	185	555
6	135	810
9	105	945
12	77	924
18	40	720
24	22	528

$$\text{Area of trapezoid } 1 = \left(\frac{0+225}{2}\right) \cdot (1-0) = 112.5 \,\mu g\,h^2/L$$

$$\text{Area of trapezoid } 2 = \left(\frac{225+555}{2}\right) \cdot (3-1) = 780 \,\mu g\,h^2/L$$

$$\text{Area of trapezoid } 3 = \left(\frac{555+810}{2}\right) \cdot (6-3) = 2047.5 \,\mu g\,h^2/L$$

$$\text{Area of trapezoid } 4 = \left(\frac{810+945}{2}\right) \cdot (9-6) = 2632.5 \,\mu g\,h^2/L$$

$$\text{Area of trapezoid } 5 = \left(\frac{945+924}{2}\right) \cdot (12-9) = 2803.5 \,\mu g\,h^2/L$$

$$\text{Area of trapezoid } 6 = \left(\frac{924+720}{2}\right) \cdot (18-12) = 4932 \,\mu g\,h^2/L$$

$$\text{Area of trapezoid } 7 = \left(\frac{720+528}{2}\right) \cdot (24-18) = 3744 \,\mu g\,h^2/L$$

$$AUMC_{t-\infty} = \frac{t_{last}Cp_{last}}{\lambda} + \frac{Cp_{last}}{\lambda^2} = \frac{528}{0.1} + \frac{22}{(0.1)^2} = 7480 \,\mu g\,h^2/L$$

$$AUC_{0-\infty} = 112.5 + 780 + 2047.5 + 2632.5 + 2803.5 + 4932 + 3744 + 7480$$

$$= 24532 \,\mu g\,h^2/L$$

$$MRT = \frac{AUMC}{AUC} = \frac{24532 \,\mu g\,h^2/L}{2517.5 \,\mu g\,h/L} = 9.74 \,h$$

Note that when calculating the MRT there was no assumption of any compart-mental model. The only needed information is the rate constant for the terminal elimination phase.

20.3.2 MRT AFTER DIFFERENT ROUTES OF ADMINISTRATION

20.3.2.1 MRT after Extravascular Administration

The mean residence time for a specific drug in a given patient should be constant after a single IV bolus administration when the drug follows linear pharmacokinet-ics. However, after oral (or any extravascular route) administration, the drug molecules spend additional time at the site of administration. In this case, the observed MRT_{oral} is equal to the sum of the MRT in the body after reaching the systemic circulation (similar to the MRT observed after a single IV dose) and the mean absorption time (MAT), which is the average time the drug molecules spend at the site of absorption [2,4]:

$$MRT_{oral} = MRT_{IV} + MAT \tag{20.11}$$

This means that the noncompartmental data analysis can be used to compare the rate of drug absorption after administration of different products for the same active drug. This is because if the products contain the same active drug, the MRT_{IV} in the body should be similar in a given patient. The difference in the observed MRT_{oral} for the different products results from the difference in the MAT. Longer MRT_{oral} indicates slower absorption. The MRT is calculated after oral administration from the plasma concentration–time data after calculating the AUC and AUMC as described previously.

This approach allows comparison of the rate of absorption of different drug products without the need to assume specific compartmental model or knowledge of the order of drug absorption. If the objective of the study is to compare the rate of absorption of two different oral products for the same active drug, the MRT is calculated for the two products and the difference will be the difference in the MAT for the two products. However, if the objective of the study is to calculate the MAT, in this case the drug has to be administered by IV and by oral administration in two different occasions and the MAT is calculated from the difference in the MRT_{oral} and MRT_{IV} as in Equation 20.11.

Example

In an experiment to investigate the drug absorption from two different oral products of the same active drug, a normal volunteer received a single IV bolus dose of 100 mg, a single oral dose of 100 mg of formulation A, and a single oral dose of 100 mg of formulation B in three different occasions. The following data were obtained:

Formulation	AUC (μg h/L)	AUMC (μg h^2/L)
IV bolus (100 mg)	352	1232
Formulation A (100 mg)	264	1056
Formulation B (100 mg)	299	1495

- How would you interpret these data?

Answer

The available information can be used to compare the rate and the extent of drug absorption from the two oral formulations:

- The rate of absorption:

$$MRT_{IV} = \frac{AUMC_{IV}}{AUC_{IV}} = \frac{1232\,\mu g\,h^2/L}{352\,\mu g\,h/L} = 3.5\,h$$

$$MRT_{\text{Formulation A}} = \frac{AUMC_{\text{Formulation A}}}{AUC_{\text{Formulation A}}} = \frac{1056\,\mu g\,h^2/L}{264\,\mu g\,h/L} = 4.0\,h$$

$$MRT_{\text{Formulation B}} = \frac{AUMC_{\text{Formulation B}}}{AUC_{\text{Formulation B}}} = \frac{1495\,\mu g\,h^2/L}{299\,\mu g\,h/L} = 5.0\,h$$

The MAT can be calculated for the two oral formulations to compare their rate of absorption:

$$MAT_{\text{Formulation A}} = MRT_{\text{Formulation A}} - MRT_{\text{IV}} = 4.0 - 3.5\,h = 0.5\,h$$

$$MAT_{\text{Formulation B}} = MRT_{\text{Formulation B}} - MRT_{\text{IV}} = 5.0 - 3.5\,h = 1.5\,h$$

This means that formulation A is absorbed faster than formulation B
• The extent of absorption (bioavailability):

$$F_{\text{Formulation A}} = \frac{AUC_{\text{Formulation A}}}{AUC_{\text{IV}}} = \frac{264\,\mu g\,h/L}{352\,\mu g\,h/L} = 0.75$$

$$F_{\text{Formulation B}} = \frac{AUC_{\text{Formulation B}}}{AUC_{\text{IV}}} = \frac{299\,\mu g\,h/L}{352\,\mu g\,h/L} = 0.85$$

The absolute bioavailability of the drug from formulation A is 75% and the absolute bioavailability of the drug from formulation B is 85%.

20.3.2.2 MRT after Constant Rate IV Infusion

When the drug is administered by constant rate IV infusion for a certain duration of time equal to (T), the MRT is usually longer than the MRT after IV bolus administration because the drug stays in the syringe for a period of time. So the MRT after constant rate IV infusion can be determined as in Equation 20.12:

$$MRT_{\text{IV infusion}} = MRT_{\text{IV}} + \frac{T}{2} \qquad (20.12)$$

where T is the duration of the IV infusion.

20.4 OTHER PHARMACOKINETIC PARAMETERS THAT CAN BE DETERMINED USING THE NONCOMPARTMENTAL APPROACH

The noncompartmental approach can also be used to calculate other pharmacokinetic parameters such as the bioavailability, CL_T, and Vd_{ss}. Estimation of the bioavailability and clearance has been discussed previously without stating that the methods were independent of any compartmental assumptions. The absolute bioavailability is determined from the ratio of the AUC after oral and IV administration as in Equation 20.13, and the relative bioavailability of two oral products is determined from the ratio of the AUC for the two different oral products as in Equation 20.14:

$$F_{Absolute} = \frac{AUC_{oral}}{AUC_{IV}} \tag{20.13}$$

$$F_{Relative} = \frac{AUC_{Product\ A}}{AUC_{Product\ B}} \tag{20.14}$$

The drug clearance can be determined after IV administration from the dose and the AUC as in Equation 20.15 and after oral administration as in Equation 20.16:

$$CL_T = \frac{Dose_{IV}}{AUC_{IV}} \tag{20.15}$$

$$\frac{CL_T}{F} = \frac{Dose_{oral}}{AUC_{oral}} \tag{20.16}$$

Vd_{ss} represents the proportionality constant that relates the amount of the drug in the body at steady state during continuous IV infusion and the resulting steady state plasma drug concentration. Also, Vd_{ss} relates the average amount of the drug in the body at steady state during multiple drug administration and the resulting average steady state plasma drug concentration. At steady state the drug is in a state of equilibrium in all parts of the body regardless of the number of compartments. Estimation of Vd_{ss} does not require drug administration to reach steady state, because according to the statistical moment theory Vd_{ss} is the product of the clearance and MRT [3]. So after a single IV bolus administration, Vd_{ss} can be estimated as follows:

$$Vd_{ss} = CL_T \times MRT_{IV} \tag{20.17}$$

$$Vd_{ss} = \frac{Dose_{IV}}{AUC} \times \frac{AUMC}{AUC} = \frac{Dose_{IV}AUMC}{AUC^2} \tag{20.18}$$

Vd_{ss} can also be determined after constant rate IV infusion as follows:

$$Vd_{ss} = CL_T \times MRT_{infusion} = CL_T\left(MRT_{IV} - \frac{T}{2}\right) \tag{20.19}$$

which can be rearranged to

$$Vd_{ss} = \frac{\text{Infused dose (AUMC)}}{(AUC)^2} - \frac{\text{Infused dose (T)}}{2(AUC)} \qquad (20.20)$$

where T is the duration of the IV infusion, and the infused dose is the total amount of drug administered during the IV infusion and can be calculated from the product of the infusion rate and the infusion duration. Vd_{ss} after oral drug administration cannot be determined this way unless we make some assumptions regarding the bioavailability and the mean absorption time.

20.5 DETERMINATION OF THE MRT FOR COMPARTMENTAL MODELS

The previous discussion dealt with the determination of the MRT using a noncompartmental approach. However, when the pharmacokinetic model is known, it is possible to use the equations that describe the pharmacokinetic model to calculate the MRT. The following are the MRT for selected compartmental models:

- For a single IV bolus dose when the drug follows one-compartment pharmacokinetic model:

$$MRT_{IV} = \frac{1}{k} \qquad (20.21)$$

  where k is the first-order elimination rare constant
- For a single oral dose when the drug follows one-compartment pharmacokinetic model:

$$MRT_{oral} = \frac{1}{k} + \frac{1}{k_a} \qquad (20.22)$$

and

$$MAT = \frac{1}{k_a} \qquad (20.23)$$

where
   k is the first-order elimination rate constant
   k_a is the first-order absorption rate constant

- For drugs administration by constant rate infusion when the drug follows one-compartment pharmacokinetic model:

$$MRT_{infusion} = \frac{1}{k} + \frac{T}{2} \qquad (20.24)$$

where
   k is the first-order elimination rate constant
   T is the duration of the IV infusion

- For a single IV bolus dose when the drug follows two-compartment pharmacokinetic model:

$$MRT_{IV\,2\,comp} = \frac{1}{\alpha} + \frac{1}{\beta} - \frac{1}{k_{21}} \qquad (20.25)$$

where

α and β are the first-order hybrid rare constant for the distribution and elimination, respectively

k_{21} is the first-order transfer rate constant from the peripheral compartment to the central compartment

- For a single oral dose when the drug follows two-compartment pharmacokinetic model:

$$MRT_{oral\,2\,comp} = \frac{1}{k_a} + \frac{1}{\alpha} + \frac{1}{\beta} - \frac{1}{k_{21}} \qquad (20.26)$$

PRACTICE PROBLEMS

20.1 After administration of a single IV bolus dose of 1 mg, the following plasma concentrations were obtained:

Time (h)	Concentration (µg/L)
0	50
1	39
3	24
6	12
9	6.8
12	4.1
18	1.8
24	0.94

If the terminal rate for decline of the plasma drug concentration is $0.1\,h^{-1}$, calculate for this drug the

a. MRT

b. Clearance

c. Vd_{ss}

20.2 In a study to compare the absorption characteristics of three different oral formulations for the same active drug, a group of volunteers received a single dose of the 25 mg as IV solution and the three oral formulations in four different occasions. The following data were obtained:

Formulation	AUC (µg h/L)	AUMC (µg h²/L)
IV solution	6,250	40,625
Formulation A	3,750	31,875
Formulation B	2,500	17,500
Formulation C	4,375	39,375

a. Arrange formulations A, B, and C according to the extent of drug absorption.
b. Arrange formulations A, B, and C according to the rate of drug absorption.

20.3 A volunteers received a single dose of 20 mg of IV solution, capsule, and tablet for the same active drug on three different occasions. The following plasma concentrations were obtained:

Time (h)	IV Solution Concentration (µg/L)	Oral Capsule Concentration (µg/L)	Oral Tablet Concentration (µg/L)
0	400	0	0
0.5	371	32	56
1	344	58	97
2	296	92	149
3	255	111	172
4	220	119	178
6	162	116	162
8	120	101	133
10	89	83	105
12	66	66	80
18	27	30	34
24	11	13	14

a. Calculate the MRT for this drug after IV administration.
b. Calculate the MRT after the two oral formulations.
c. Calculate the MAT for the two oral formulations.
d. Calculate the clearance and the Vd_{ss} for this drug.

REFERENCES

1. Yamaoka K, Nakagawa T, and Uno T (1978) Statistical moment in pharmacokinetics. *J Pharmacokinet Biopharm* 6:547–558.
2. Cutler DJ (1978) Theory of the mean absorption time, and adjunct to conventional bioavailability studies. *J Pharm Pharmacol* 30:476–478.
3. Benet LZ and Galeazzi RL (1979) Noncompartmental determination of the steady-state volume of distribution. *J Pharm Sci* 6:1071–1074.
4. Riegelman S and Collier P (1980) The application of the statistical moment theory to the evaluation of in vivo dissolution time and absorption time. *J Pharmacokinet Biopharm* 8:509–534.

21 Physiological Approach to Hepatic Clearance

OBJECTIVES

After completing this chapter you should be able to

- Describe the physiological meaning of the organ clearance in terms of organ blood flow, intrinsic clearance, and extraction ratio
- Describe the effect of changing the hepatic intrinsic clearance and blood flow on the efficiency of the liver to eliminate the drug (extraction ratio)
- Analyze the effect of changing the intrinsic clearance on the plasma concentration–time profile of high and low extraction ratio drugs after IV and oral administration
- Analyze the effect of changing the liver blood flow on the plasma concentration–time profile of high and low extraction ratio drugs after IV and oral administration
- Discuss the drug characteristics that will make the drug elimination rate sensitive to changes in the protein binding
- Predict the potential for clinically significant drug interactions that involve enzyme induction or inhibition, modification of the hepatic blood flow, and change in protein binding based on the characteristics of the interacting drugs

21.1 INTRODUCTION

The physiological approach to organ clearance is a simple approach that uses the organ's ability to eliminate the drug, organ blood flow, and protein binding to describe the rate of drug elimination by the organ and the drug profile in the body. This approach allows prediction of the change in drug disposition that occurs due to changes in organ blood flow, enzymatic activity, and drug protein binding. For example, the hepatic clearance of a drug is dependent on the liver intrinsic ability to metabolize the drug, which is dependent on the enzyme activity, and the rate of delivery of the drug to the liver, which is dependent on the liver blood flow. Enzyme induction and enzyme inhibition can alter the liver ability to metabolize the drug and can lead to changes in hepatic clearance. Also, diseases such as congestive heart failure and drugs such as beta-blockers can decrease the cardiac output and decrease the liver blood flow, which may change the hepatic clearance of the drug.

21.2 ORGAN CLEARANCE

Organ clearance is defined as the volume of blood completely cleared of the drug per unit time by that particular organ. This is a measure of the efficiency of the organ in eliminating the drug from the blood reaching the organ. Based on the aforementioned definition, the clearance can be estimated from the organ blood flow and the difference in the arterial and venous drug concentration across the organ. Equation 21.1 describes the general relationship between the drug clearance, excretion rate, and concentration, which can be modified to describe the drug clearance by a particular organ as in Equation 21.2:

$$CL = \frac{\text{Drug excretion rate}}{\text{Drug concentration}} \tag{21.1}$$

$$CL_{organ} = \frac{\text{Amount of drug entering the organ} - \text{Amount of drug leaving the organ}}{\text{Concentration of drug entering the organ}}$$

$$\tag{21.2}$$

The amount of drug entering the organ is equal to the product of drug concentration in the arterial side and the organ blood flow, while the amount of drug leaving the organ is equal to the product of drug concentration in the venous side and the organ blood flow [1]. Based on this definition, hepatic clearance, CL_H, can be expressed as follows:

$$CL_H = \frac{QCp_a - QCp_v}{Cp_a} \tag{21.3}$$

where

Q is the hepatic blood flow

Cp_a is the drug concentration in the arterial side of the liver (portal and arterial)

Cp_v is the drug concentration in the venous side of the liver

$$CL_H = Q\left[\frac{Cp_a - Cp_v}{Cp_a}\right] \tag{21.4}$$

$$CL_H = QE \tag{21.5}$$

where E is the extraction ratio, which is a measure of the efficiency of the organ in eliminating the drug during a single pass through the organ.

21.3 HEPATIC EXTRACTION RATIO

The hepatic extraction ratio is the fraction of the amount of drug presented to the liver that is eliminated during a single pass through the liver. When the drug that reaches the liver is completely eliminated, that is, Cp_v is equal to zero, the hepatic extraction ratio becomes equal to unity. On the other hand, when no drug is eliminated while going through the liver, that is, $Cp_v = Cp_a$, the extraction ratio is equal to zero. The extraction ratio can take values from zero to unity (0–1), and can be expressed as percentage from 0% to 100%. It is important to note that the hepatic extraction ratio is a measure of the liver elimination efficiency during a single pass for the drug through the liver.

This is different from the fraction of dose metabolized, which is a fraction of the administered dose that will be eliminated from the body through the metabolic pathway. There are examples of drugs that are completely metabolized but have low hepatic extraction ratio and drugs that have high hepatic extraction ratio and are not completely metabolized. The hepatic extraction ratio is a function of the intrinsic ability of the liver to eliminate the drug (intrinsic clearance, CL_{int}) and the hepatic blood flow [2]:

$$E = \frac{CL_{int}}{Q + CL_{int}} \tag{21.6}$$

Drugs are classified as low extraction ratio drugs if their hepatic extraction ratio is less than 0.3 (e.g., diazepam, warfarin, salicylic acid, phenytoin, and procainamide) or high extraction ratio drugs if their hepatic extraction ratio is larger than 0.7 (e.g., lidocaine, propranolol, morphine, verapamil, and propoxyphene). If the hepatic extraction ratio is between 0.3 and 0.7, then the drugs are considered intermediate extraction ratio drugs. Drugs in the same class based on their hepatic extraction ratio usually share some common characteristics of how the change in the physiological parameters affects the overall elimination of the drug. So the effect of some physiological and pathological changes on the elimination of a particular drug can be predicted based on the extraction ratio of the drug. Drugs eliminated by the kidney can also be classified according to their renal extraction ratio. Atenolol, digoxin, and methotrexate are examples of low extraction ratio drugs because their extraction ratio by the kidney is <0.3, while metformin and p-aminohippuric acid are examples of high extraction ratio drugs because their extraction ratio by the kidney is >0.7.

21.4   INTRINSIC CLEARANCE

CL_{int} is the maximum ability of the organ to eliminate the drug in the absence of any flow limitation. In the liver, for example, CL_{int} is the inherent ability of the hepatic enzymes to metabolize drugs, and it reflects the maximum capacity of the liver to metabolize the drug [3]. On the other hand, the actual observed CL_H depends on the probability of the drug molecules to get in contact with the metabolizing enzymes. This depends on the amount of enzymes available, which is reflected by CL_{int}, and the ability of the drug to diffuse to the organ to get in contact with the enzymes that are dependent on the organ blood flow. The expression that relates CL_H to Q and CL_{int} is as follows:

$$CL_H = QE = Q \left[\frac{CL_{int}}{Q + CL_{int}} \right] \tag{21.7}$$

By rearrangement, an expression for CL_{int} can be obtained:

$$CL_{int} = \frac{QE}{1 - E} \tag{21.8}$$

This relationship indicates that CL_{int} for high extraction ratio drugs is much higher than CL_H, while for low extraction ratio drugs the value of CL_{int} is close to that of the CL_H.

21.5   SYSTEMIC BIOAVAILABILITY

When the orally administered drug is absorbed completely to the portal circulation, the only cause for incomplete bioavailability will be the hepatic metabolism during the first-pass through the liver. In this case, the bioavailability (F) will be dependent on the hepatic extraction ratio [4]:

$$F = 1 - E \qquad (21.9)$$

This means that F of drugs with high hepatic extraction ratio is much lower than F of drugs with low hepatic extraction ratio when drugs are absorbed completely to the portal circulation. Factors that can alter the hepatic extraction ratio such as the change in Q and/or CL_{int} can affect F of orally administered drugs. The F of drugs that is not absorbed completely from the gastrointestinal tract (GIT) to the portal circulation is determined from the fraction of dose absorbed to the portal circulation and the fraction of dose that escapes the first-pass hepatic metabolism.

21.6   EFFECT OF CHANGING INTRINSIC CLEARANCE AND HEPATIC BLOOD FLOW ON THE HEPATIC CLEARANCE, SYSTEMIC AVAILABILITY, AND DRUG CONCENTRATION–TIME PROFILE

The CL_{int} and Q may change due to some physiological and pathological conditions or as a result of using some drugs. Liver diseases such as liver cirrhosis can significantly decrease the CL_{int} of many drugs, while diseases like congestive heart failure usually decrease the hepatic blood flow. Drugs like beta-blockers decrease the cardiac output and the hepatic blood flow, and many drugs are known to induce or inhibit the hepatic metabolizing enzymes that can significantly affect the CL_{int} of other drugs. In general, the effect of the change in CL_{int} or Q on the clearance, bioavailability, and elimination rate of low extraction ratio drugs and high extraction ratio drugs will be different. However, within each class of drugs the effect of change in CL_{int} or Q is approximately similar [1]. This is important because based on the drug extraction ratio it is possible to expect the changes in the drug pharmacokinetic behavior in some physiological and pathological conditions and to predict the outcome of some drug–drug interactions.

The CL_H of any drug is dependent on the drug CL_{int} and Q as presented in Equation 21.7. For drugs that have $CL_{int} \ll Q$, Equation 21.7 can be reduced to

$$CL_H = Q \frac{CL_{int}}{Q} = CL_{int} \qquad (21.10)$$

Equation 21.10 indicates that the CL_H for drugs that have $CL_{int} \ll Q$ (i.e., low extraction ratio drugs) is about equal to the drug CL_{int}. Any change in the enzyme activity by induction or inhibition that affects the CL_{int} will affect the CL_H of these low extraction ratio drugs. Changes in Q will not have a significant effect on the CL_H of low extraction ratio drugs. On the other hand when $CL_{int} \gg Q$, Equation 21.7 can be reduced to

$$CL_H = Q \qquad (21.11)$$

Equation 21.11 indicates that the CL_H for drugs with $CL_{int} \gg Q$ (i.e., high extraction ratio) is about equal to Q. Any change in Q will affect the CL_H of high extraction ratio drugs. Changes in the drug CL_{int} will not have significant effect on the CL_H of high extraction ratio drugs.

The previous discussion indicates that drugs within the same class based on their extraction ratio (low, high, or intermediate) are affected similarly by the change in CL_{int} and Q. The following numerical examples demonstrate how the change in CL_{int} and Q affects the CL_H, F, and overall plasma drug concentration–time profile in low and high extraction ratio drugs.

21.6.1 Low Extraction Ratio Drugs

Assume that we have a low extraction ratio drug that is completely metabolized meaning that the CL_H is equal to CL_T. After oral administration, the drug is completely absorbed to the portal circulation indicating that the hepatic metabolism during the first-pass through the liver is the cause of its incomplete bioavailability. The drug extraction ratio is equal to 0.05, and Q is 1.5 L/min. The CL_{int} of this drug can be calculated from Equation 21.8:

$$CL_{int} = \frac{QE}{1-E} = \frac{1.5\,\text{L/min}\ 0.05}{1-0.05} = 0.079\,\text{L/min}$$

CL_H can be calculated from Equation 21.5:

$$CL_H = QE = 1.5\,\text{L/min} \times 0.05 = 0.075\,\text{L/min}$$

F can be calculated from Equation 21.9:

$$F = 1 - E = 1 - 0.05 = 0.95$$

- If the CL_{int} increases to double its original value due to enzyme induction and Q stays the same, the new CL_{int} after induction can be calculated as follows:

$$CL_{int} = 0.079\,\text{L/min} \times 2 = 0.158\,\text{L/min}$$

The extraction ratio after induction

$$E = \frac{CL_{int}}{Q + CL_{int}} = \frac{0.158\,\text{L/min}}{1.5 + 0.158\,\text{L/min}} = 0.095$$

CL_H after induction

$$CL_H = QE = 1.5\,\text{L/min} \times 0.095 = 0.143\,\text{L/min}$$

F after induction

$$F = 1 - E = 1 - 0.095 = 0.905$$

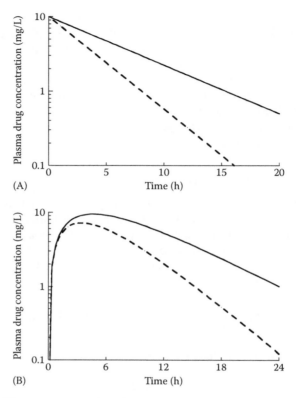

FIGURE 21.1 Plasma concentration–time profile for a low extraction ratio drug after administration of (A) a single IV bolus dose and (B) a single oral dose, before (—) and after (---) enzyme induction.

Based on these calculations, enzyme induction causes an increase in the extraction ratio from 0.05 to 0.095. This small change represents about 90% increase in the extraction ratio, which results in a significant increase in the CL_H from 0.075 to 0.143 L/min (about 90% increase). The change in extraction ratio also causes a change in F from 0.95 to 0.905 (about 5% decrease). So enzyme induction significantly increases the CL_H (and CL_T in this example) of low extraction ratio drugs after IV and oral administration, which significantly increases the rate of decline in the drug concentration–time profile after IV and oral administration, assuming that Vd does not change. However, enzyme induction does not significantly affect F of low extraction ratio drugs as illustrated in Figure 21.1.

Pharmacokinetic Parameters	Before Induction	After Induction
Q	1.5 L/min	1.5 L/min
E	0.05	0.095
CL_{int}	0.079 L/min	0.158 L/min
CL_H and CL_T	0.075 L/min	0.143 L/min
F	0.95	0.905

- If Q decreases by 50% (i.e., new Q = 0.75 L/min) without affecting CL_{int}, the new extraction ratio after the reduction in Q can be calculated as follows:

$$E = \frac{CL_{int}}{Q + CL_{int}} = \frac{0.079\,L/min}{0.75 + 0.079\,L/min} = 0.095$$

CL_H after the decrease in Q

$$CL_H = QE = 0.75\,L/min \times 0.095 = 0.0712\,L/min$$

Pharmacokinetic Parameters	Normal Hepatic Blood Flow	Low Hepatic Blood Flow
Q	1.5 L/min	0.75 L/min
E	0.05	0.079
CL_{int}	0.079 L/min	0.079 L/min
CL_H and CL_T	0.075 L/min	0.0712 L/min
F	0.95	0.905

F after the decrease in Q

$$F = 1 - E = 1 - 0.095 = 0.905$$

Based on these calculations, the decrease in Q results in an increase in the extraction ratio from 0.05 to 0.095, which represents about 90% increase in the extraction ratio. The CL_H decreases from 0.075 to 0.0712 L/min (about 5% decrease), and F decreases from 0.95 to 0.905 (about 5% decrease). So the change in Q does not significantly affect the CL_H (and CL_T in this example) and F of low extraction ratio drugs, which should not affect the plasma concentration–time profile of the drug after IV and oral administration as illustrated in Figure 21.2.

21.6.2 HIGH EXTRACTION RATIO DRUGS

Assume that we have a high extraction ratio drug that is completely metabolized meaning that the CL_H is equal to CL_T. After oral administration, the drug is completely absorbed to the portal circulation, which means that the hepatic metabolism during the first-pass through the liver is the cause of its incomplete bioavailability. The drug extraction ratio, E, is equal to 0.95, and Q is 1.5 L/min. The CL_{int} of this drug can be calculated from Equation 21.8:

$$CL_{int} = \frac{QE}{1 - E} = \frac{1.5\,L/min\;0.95}{1 - 0.95} = 28.5\,L/min$$

CL_H can be calculated from Equation 21.5:

$$CL_H = QE = 1.5\,L/min \times 0.95 = 1.425\,L/min$$

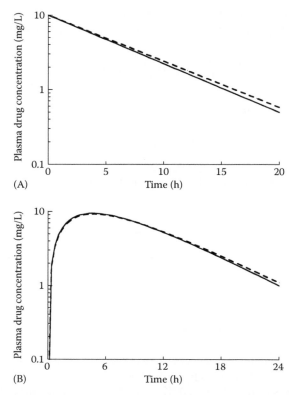

FIGURE 21.2 Plasma concentration–time profile for a low extraction ratio drug after administration of (A) a single IV bolus dose and (B) a single oral dose, when the hepatic blood flow is 1.5 L/min (—) and after the reduction of the hepatic blood flow to 0.75 L/min (---).

F can be calculated from Equation 21.9:

$$F = 1 - E = 1 - 0.95 = 0.05$$

- If the drug CL_{int} increases to double its original value due to enzyme induction and Q stays the same, the new CL_{int} will be

$$CL_{int} = 28.5 \, L/min \times 2 = 57.0 \, L/min$$

The extraction ratio after induction

$$E = \frac{CL_{int}}{Q + CL_{int}} = \frac{57 \, L/min}{1.5 + 57 \, L/min} = 0.974$$

CL_H after induction

$$CL_H = QE = 1.5 \, L/min \times 0.974 = 1.461 \, L/min$$

F after induction

$$F = 1 - E = 1 - 0.974 = 0.026$$

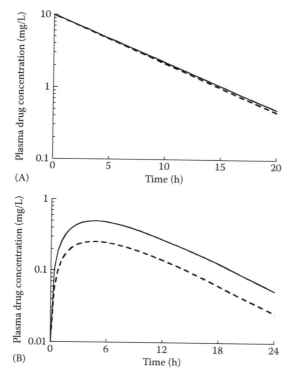

FIGURE 21.3 Plasma concentration–time profile for a high extraction ratio drug after administration of (A) a single IV bolus dose and (B) a single oral dose, before (—) and after (---) enzyme induction.

Based on these calculations, enzyme induction results in the increase in the extraction ratio from 0.95 to 0.974 (about 2.5% increase), which results in a very small increase in CL_H from 1.425 to 1.461 L/min (about 2.5% increase) and a significant decrease in F from 0.05 to 0.026 (about 50% decrease). So enzyme induction does not significantly affect the CL_H (and CL_T in this example) of high extraction ratio drugs and will not significantly affect the rate of decline in the plasma concentration–time profile after a single IV and oral drug administration. However, enzyme induction decreases F of high extraction ratio drugs, which results in a significant decrease in the drug AUC as illustrated in Figure 21.3.

Pharmacokinetic Parameters	Before Induction	After Induction
Q	1.5 L/min	1.5 L/min
E	0.95	0.974
CL_{int}	28.5 L/min	57.0 L/min
CL_H and CL_T	1.425 L/min	1.461 L/min
F	0.05	0.026

- If Q decreases by 50% (new Q = 0.75 L/min) without affecting CL_{int}, the extraction ratio after the reduction in Q will be

$$E = \frac{CL_{int}}{Q + CL_{int}} = \frac{28.5\,L/min}{0.75 + 28.5\,L/min} = 0.974$$

CL_H after the decrease in Q

$$CL_H = QE = 0.75\,L/min \times 0.974 = 0.7305\,L/min$$

F after the decrease in Q

$$F = 1 - E = 1 - 0.974 = 0.026$$

Based on these calculations, the decrease in Q results in the increase in the extraction ratio from 0.95 to 0.974 (about 2.5% increase), which results in a significant decrease in CL_H from 1.425 to 0.7305 L/min (about 50% decrease), and significant decrease in F from 0.05 to 0.026 (about 50% decrease). So the decrease in Q significantly decreases the CL_H (and CL_T in this example) of high extraction ratio drugs after IV and after oral administration, which is reflected by the slower rate of decline in the drug concentration–time profile. After oral administration, the decrease in clearance of the high extraction ratio drugs as a result of the reduction in Q increases the drug AUC. However, the decrease in Q also causes a reduction in F of this high extraction ratio drug that decreases the AUC. So the increase in AUC due to the reduction in drug clearance is compensated by the decrease in AUC due to the reduction in F and the drug AUC does not change significantly as illustrated in Figure 21.4.

The effect of altered Q and CL_{int} on the pharmacokinetics of drugs depends on whether the drug is classified as a low or high extraction ratio drug. The clearance of low extraction ratio drugs is affected mainly by changes in CL_{int} and is not affected by changes in Q, while the clearance of high extraction ratio drugs is affected mainly by the change in Q and is not affected by changes in CL_{int}. After oral administration, F of low extraction ratio drugs is high and changes in the extraction ratio due to changes in CL_{int} or Q does not cause significant change in F. On the other hand, changes in CL_{int} and Q cause small changes in the extraction ratio and F of high extraction ratio drugs after oral administration. However, since F of high extraction ratio drugs is usually very low, small changes in F cause a significant change in the bioavailable amount of the drug. For intermediate extraction ratio drugs, the clearance and the half-life are partially dependent on liver blood flow to an extent that is only estimated by knowing the extraction ratio.

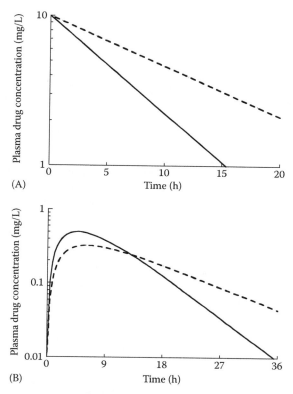

FIGURE 21.4 Plasma concentration–time profile for a high extraction ratio drug after administration of (A) a single IV bolus dose and (B) a single oral dose, when the hepatic blood flow is 1.5 L/min (——) and after the reduction of the hepatic blood flow to 0.75 L/min (---).

Pharmacokinetic Parameters	Normal Hepatic Blood Flow	Low Hepatic Blood Flow
Q	1.5 L/min	0.75 L/min
E	0.95	0.974
CL_{int}	28.5 L/min	28.5 L/min
CL_H and CL_T	1.425 L/min	0.7305 L/min
F	0.05	0.026

Example

An experimental antiarrhythmic drug (MMH-98) is completely metabolized by the liver to inactive metabolites. In clinical trials, this drug was found to have a hepatic extraction ratio of 0.89 in a congestive heart failure patient who has a hepatic blood flow of 1.22 L/min. This drug is 96% bound to plasma protein. Although the oral bioavailability of this drug is less than 100%, when it is administered orally all the dose is absorbed from the GIT and reaches the portal circulation.

a. Calculate the CL_T of this drug in this patient.
b. Calculate the CL_{int} of this drug in this patient.
c. What is the AUC produced after administration of a single dose of 300 mg orally?
d. In addition to the antiarrhythmic drug, the patient started taking an inotropic drug that increases the cardiac output with no effect on any other organs. Due to this increase in cardiac output, the liver blood flow increased to 1.62 L/min.

How does the increase in the hepatic blood flow affect the value of each of the following parameters?

Hepatic intrinsic clearance	Increase	Decrease	No change
Hepatic extraction ratio	Increase	Decrease	No change
Total body clearance	Increase	Decrease	No change
Oral bioavailability	Increase	Decrease	No change

Answer

a. Since the drug is completely metabolized, CL_H is equal to CL_T:

$$CL_T = CL_H = QE = 1.22 \text{L/min} \times 0.89 = 1.086 \text{L/min}$$

b. $$CL_{int} = \frac{QE}{1-E} = \frac{1.22 \text{L/min} \times 0.89}{1-0.89} = 9.87 \text{L/min}$$

c. $$AUC = \frac{F \, Dose}{CL_T} = \frac{(1-E) \, Dose}{CL_T} = \frac{0.11 \times 300 \text{mg}}{1.086 \text{L/min}} = 30.4 \text{mg min/L}$$

d. The hepatic intrinsic clearance is dependent on the intrinsic ability of the liver to metabolize the drug and is independent of the hepatic blood flow. So the hepatic intrinsic clearance will not change due to the increase in hepatic blood flow.
   - Hepatic extraction ratio

$$E = \frac{CL_{int}}{Q+CL_{int}} = \frac{9.87 \text{L/min}}{1.62+9.87 \text{L/min}} = 0.859$$

The increase in hepatic blood flow decreases the extraction ratio.
   - Total body clearance

$$CL_T = CL_H = QE = 1.62 \text{L/min} \times 0.859 = 1.392 \text{L/min}$$

The CL_T that is equal to CL_H for this drug increases with the increase in the hepatic blood flow.
   - Oral bioavailability

$$Bioavailability \ (F) = 1-E = 1-0.859 = 0.141$$

The oral bioavailability increases because the hepatic extraction ratio decreases due to the increase in hepatic blood flow.

21.7 PROTEIN BINDING AND HEPATIC EXTRACTION

The previous discussion has been concerned with the total drug concentration in the blood. However, it is known that almost all drugs are bound to blood constituents to some extent. So it is important to consider the effect of drug protein binding on drug clearance and half-life. It is usually assumed that only the free (unbound) drug is available for elimination. However, many examples exist in which the hepatic extraction is sufficiently high that the drug can be removed (stripped) from its binding sites during passage through the liver. Two different extraction processes are usually observed. One restricted or limited to the free drug and one that is nonrestricted in which both free and bound drugs can be removed by the liver [5]. When the free drug concentration is considered, the following relationship can be obtained:

$$CL_H = QE = Q\left[\frac{f_u CL'_{int}}{Q + f_u CL'_{int}}\right] \qquad (21.12)$$

where
f_u is the free unbound fraction of the drug in the blood
CL'_{int} is the intrinsic clearance of the unbound free drug

The effect of protein binding on the hepatic clearance of drugs is different depending on the drug characteristics. The clearance of high extraction ratio drugs is considered flow dependent and so changes in the protein binding of these drugs do not affect their hepatic clearance. This is because during drug passage through the liver, both free and bound drug molecules are extracted and eliminated by the liver.

The hepatic clearance of drugs that have low extraction ratio and are not bound to a large extent (<75% protein bound) does not change significantly by the change in their protein binding. However, the hepatic clearance of drugs that have low extraction ratio and are highly bound to plasma protein is very sensitive to small change in protein binding. This is because small displacement in the protein binding of these drugs will cause large increase in the free drug concentration and will increase the liver ability to eliminate the drug (due to increase in f_u).

21.8 PHARMACOKINETIC SIMULATION EXERCISE

The physiological approach to clearance module of the companion CD to this book includes a plotting exercise that allows the selection of CL_{int} and Q values and simulates the plasma drug concentration–time profile. The idea is to select values for CL_{int} and Q that correspond to E in the low extraction ratio range or the high extraction ratio range, and then the plasma concentration–time profile is simulated after IV or oral drug administration. The values for CL_{int} and Q can be changed one at a time and the simulation is repeated. Examination of the plasma concentration–time profiles for the different simulations allows visualization of the effect of change in CL_{int} and Q on the plasma concentration–time profile for low and high extraction ratio drugs after IV and oral administration.

PRACTICE PROBLEMS

21.1 Why does a drug with high extraction ratio (e.g., propranolol) demonstrate greater difference between individuals after oral administration than after IV administration?

21.2 Why does a drug with low hepatic extraction ratio (e.g., theophylline) demonstrate greater differences between individuals after hepatic enzyme induction than a drug with high extraction ratio?

21.3 A drug has intrinsic clearance of 40 mL/min in a normal adult patient whose hepatic blood flow is 1.5 L/min.
   a. Calculate the hepatic clearance of this drug.
   b. If the patient develops congestive heart failure that reduces hepatic blood flow to 1.0 L/min without affecting the intrinsic clearance, calculate the hepatic clearance of the drug in this patient.
   c. If the patient was receiving medication such as phenobarbital that increased the intrinsic clearance to 90 mL/min but did not alter the hepatic blood flow (1.5 L/min), calculate the hepatic clearance of the drug in this patient.

21.4 A drug has intrinsic clearance of 12 L/min in a normal adult patient whose hepatic blood flow is 1.5 L/min.
   a. Calculate the hepatic clearance of this drug.
   b. If this patient develops congestive heart failure that reduces his hepatic blood flow to 1.0 L/min without affecting the intrinsic clearance, calculate the hepatic clearance of the drug in this patient.
   c. Calculate the extraction ratio for the liver in this patient before and after congestive heart failure develops.
   d. From the aforementioned information, estimate the drug bioavailability, assuming that when the drug is given orally, all the drug is absorbed to the portal vein.

21.5 The following drugs have the following characteristics:

Drug	A	B	C	D	E	F	G	H
Fraction metabolized	0.98	0.1	0.94	0.5	0.1	0.9	0.5	0.95
Protein binding	0.94	0.6	0.94	0.93	0.96	0.6	0.6	0.5
Extraction ratio	0.1	0.1	0.92	0.11	0.1	0.1	0.11	0.93

What are the expected changes in the total body clearance, the biological half-life, and the systemic bioavailability for each of these drugs in the following cases?
   a. Administration of an enzyme inducer that increases the activity of the metabolizing enzymes.
   b. Administration of an enzyme inhibitor that decreases the activity of the metabolizing enzymes.
   c. Administration of a highly protein-bound drug that can displace the aforementioned drugs from their binding protein and increases their free fraction.
   d. Decrease in the hepatic blood flow due to congestive heart failure.

REFERENCES

1. Wilkinsin GR and Shand DG (1975) A physiological approach to hepatic drug clearance. *Clin Pharmacol Ther* 18:377–390.
2. Rane A, Wilkinson GR, and Shand DG (1977) Prediction of hepatic extraction ratio from in vitro measurements of intrinsic clearance. *J Pharmacol Exp Ther* 200:420–424.
3. Gibaldi P and Perrier D (1982) *Pharmacokinetics*, 2nd edn., Marcel Dekker Inc., New York.
4. Rowland M, Benet LZ, and Graham GG (1973) Clearance concepts in pharmacokinetics. *J Pharmacokinet Biopharm* 1:123–136.
5. Blaschke TF (1977) Protein binding and kinetics of drugs in liver diseases. *Clin Pharmacokinet* 1:32–44.

22 Physiologically Based Pharmacokinetic Models

OBJECTIVES

After completing this chapter you should be able to

- Discuss the information that can be obtained from using the PBPK models
- Discuss the general features of the PBPK models
- Describe the general principles of drug distribution to different tissues
- State the basic steps for developing a PBPK model
- Show how the absorption, distribution, and elimination processes in the PBPK models can be described by mathematical expressions
- Describe how the different PBPK model parameters can be obtained
- Demonstrate how the PBPK models can be used in inter-dose, inter-route, inter-tissue, and interspecies extrapolation
- Discuss some applications of the PBPK models in drug development and clinical practice

22.1 INTRODUCTION

Characterization of the pharmacokinetic behavior of drugs in the body is important in determining the drug concentration–time profile and predicting the therapeutic and toxic effects after administration of different dosing regimens by different routes of administrations. The pharmacokinetic behavior of drugs in the body depends on a variety of factors including the drug physicochemical properties, blood flow to different organs, the ability of the drug to cross the biological membranes, the affinity of the drug to different tissues, and the ability of some organs to eliminate the drug. The compartmental pharmacokinetic models have been used to describe the pharmacokinetic behavior in the body by dividing the body into a number of interconnected compartments without identifying the organs and tissues that make up each compartment. This approach utilizes the observed drug concentration in the systemic circulation and other biological fluids to select the best compartmental model that can describe the drug pharmacokinetics. The estimated pharmacokinetic parameters for the compartmental model can be used to describe the drug concentration–time profiles in the central and peripheral compartments that can be linked to the observed drug effects after drug administration. On the contrary, the noncompartmental approach, which can be used when the drug elimination follows first-order kinetics, describes the general drug pharmacokinetic behavior without the exact characterization of the drug concentration–time profile. This approach can be useful when comparing the in vivo performance of different dosage forms, the rate and extent of drug absorption from different routes of administration, and the pharmacokinetic behavior in different patient populations. It is also useful for bioequivalence testing, studying drug–drug interactions, and other pharmacokinetic investigations that do not require determination of the time course of the drug concentration in the body. Both the compartmental and noncompartmental modeling approaches provide important and useful information about the drug pharmacokinetics in the body.

A third modeling approach known as the physiologically based pharmacokinetic modeling (PBPK) has been used to describe the drug pharmacokinetics in the systemic circulation and various organs and tissues simultaneously [1]. The PBPK smodels consist of a series of compartments with each compartment representing one or more organ, tissue, or body space. So the general structure of the PBPK models is physiologically realistic because it is derived from the anatomical and physiological properties of the body and it is independent of the drug under investigation. The PBPK models utilize the blood flow to the different organs, the size of each organ, and the affinity of the drug to the different organs to determine the amount of drug delivered to each organ and describe the drug distribution to different organs. Inclusion of information about the elimination efficiency of the eliminating organs allows characterization of the time course of the drug concentration in the blood and different organs and estimation of the exposure of different organs to the drug. So the information needed to construct the PBPK models include anatomical and physiological parameters that are readily available for humans and different animal species and are independent of the drug under investigation. This is in addition to drug-specific information that affects the drug distribution and elimination and can be determined experimentally.

22.2 PHYSIOLOGIC PHARMACOKINETIC MODELS

The PBPK models can be constructed to represent the entire body, isolated body systems, or a single organ. Our focus in the following discussion will be the whole body PBPK models, which usually consist of a series of connected compartments representing the different organs and tissues of the body. The blood circulation represents the link between these compartments that are arranged and connected in a physiologically relevant manner [2].

22.2.1 GENERAL MODEL STRUCTURE

The model presented in Figure 22.1 consists of nine different compartments representing the heart, lung, brain, muscles, skin, intestine, liver, kidney, and the last compartment represents all the other remaining organs of the body. The venous blood that returns from all organs to the heart is pumped entirely to the lung for oxygenation. The oxygenated blood returns to the heart, where it is pumped to all the organs with each organ receiving a relatively constant blood flow rate. The blood flow into the organ is equal to the blood flow out of the organ. The model in Figure 22.1 assumes that the drug is eliminated by the liver and the kidney. The blood flow to the liver as presented in the model comes partially from the arterial

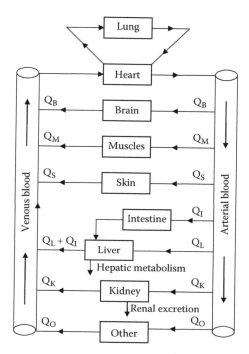

FIGURE 22.1 Representative example of the whole body PBPK models consists of nine different compartments. Each of the first eight compartments represents one organ with the ninth compartment representing all the remaining organs and tissues. The term Q represents the blood flow, with the subscript indicating a specific organ. The blood flow entering the organ is equal to the blood flow leaving the organ. The arrows coming out of the liver and the kidney indicate drug elimination by these organs, while the arrows in the closed circulation loop indicate the direction of blood flow (From Nestorov, I., *Clin. Pharmacokinet.*, 42,883, 2003.)

blood and partially from the blood leaving the small intestine. So the general structure of the model is based on the real anatomical and physiological information.

22.2.2 GENERAL PRINCIPLES OF TISSUE DISTRIBUTION

The drug is distributed to all organs of the body with the systemic circulation, where a fraction of the drug delivered to each organ distributes to the tissues of the organ and the remaining drug leaves the organ and returns to the heart with the venous circulation. The concentration of the drug in each organ depends on the blood drug concentration, the organ blood flow, and the affinity of the drug to the different tissue constituents of that particular organ. Generally, there are three distinct anatomical regions in the organ: the vascular space, the interstitial space, and the intracellular space. The drug delivered to the organ in the vascular space can cross the capillary membrane and distribute into the interstitial fluid. In the interstitial fluid, the drug can cross the cellular membrane and distribute intracellularly where it can bind to different cell constituents as in Figure 22.2. In eliminating organs, the drug can also be metabolized or excreted unchanged from the body by the organ.

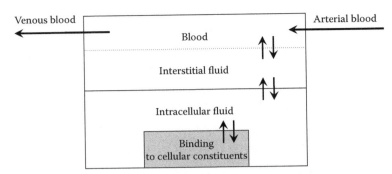

FIGURE 22.2 Diagram representing the three different subcompartments included in noneliminating organ structure. The double arrows indicate that the drug can distribute in both directions in the three different subcompartments.

In general, the drug distribution to the different tissues can either follow blood-flow-limited or membrane-limited models. The blood-flow-limited model assumes that the organ blood flow is the rate limiting step to the drug uptake into the tissues. According to the model, the drug delivered to the organ with the arterial blood is distributed rapidly to all parts of the organ and the blood capillary membrane does not present any resistance to the drug permeation. Since some of the drug delivered to the organ is distributed to the tissues, the venous drug concentration is lower than the arterial drug concentration in each organ. Rapid distribution equilibrium is established between the drug in the organ and the drug in the venous blood leaving the organ. The ratio of the drug concentration in the organ to the drug concentration in the venous blood is constant and depends on the affinity of the drug to the organ constituents. This concentration ratio is known as the tissue-to-blood partition coefficient, and it is different for different tissues. The distribution of low molecular weight, lipophilic, weakly ionized drugs to organs with low blood flow usually follows the flow-rate-limited models [3,4].

If the capillary membrane and/or the cell membrane act as barriers for the drug distribution into the organ, the rate determining step for the drug distribution into the organ will be the diffusion across these membranes. In this case, the drug distribution to the organ follows the membrane-limited model [5–7]. When the blood flow is faster than the membrane permeation, a concentration gradient is established between the drug in the organ and the drug in blood, which becomes the driving force for the drug diffusion accross the membrane. The distribution of hydrophilic drugs to highly perfused organs usually follows the membrane-limited model. If both the capillary membrane and the cell membrane act as barriers to slow the drug distribution to all parts of the organ, the organ behaves as if it consists of three distinctly different subcompartments as shown in Figure 22.2. Expressing the change in the drug concentration within the organ will have to consider the drug distribution between the three subcompartments [8]. On the contrary, when the capillary membrane represents the only barrier to drug distribution into the organ, the drug that reaches the interstitial space can be distributed rapidly across the cell membrane. In this case, the organ behaves as if it consists of two subcompartments: the first includes the vascular space and the second includes both the interstitial and intracellular spaces together.

Describing the change in the drug concentration in the organ will have to consider the diffusion of the drug from the vascular subcompartment to the rest of the organ. Similarly, the organ behaves as if it consists of two subcompartments if the cellular membrane is the only barrier to the drug distribution to the organ. The first consists of the vascular and interstitial spaces and the second is the intracellular space. It is possible that for the same drug, some organs or tissues follow the flow-rate-limited model and other organs or tissues follow the membrane-limited model.

22.3 PHYSIOLOGICALLY BASED PHARMACOKINETIC MODEL DEVELOPMENT

The development of a PBPK model usually goes through a series of steps, which starts with construction of the components of the model. This includes the general structure of the models as well as the mathematical expressions that describe the change in drug concentrations in all parts of the model. The next step is model parameterization, which involves the inclusion of the values of all the model parameters including anatomical and physiological parameters and also parameters related to drug properties. The model is then used to simulate the drug concentration–time profile in all components of the model and the simulated data are compared with the experimentally obtained information. Modification of the model may be necessary until the simulated drug concentration–time profiles in the different model components agree with the experimental data.

22.3.1 MODEL PRESENTATION

The objectives of the PBPK model development have to be well defined because this will determine the information that needs to be included when presenting the model. The model presentation includes identification of the model components and also a mathematical description of the drug behavior in all model components.

22.3.1.1 Model Components

As mentioned previously the model usually consists of a number of compartments each representing an organ, part of an organ, tissue, or body space. The general rule is to include all the relevant organs and body spaces while keeping the number of organs as little as possible. The included organs and body spaces are determined from the objective of the modeling process and also the drug behavior in the body. All organs and tissues where the drug can exert its pharmacological and adverse effects should be included in the model. This is because the calculated tissue exposure from these models can be correlated with the drug effects. Also, the eliminating organs and organs where drug absorption takes place should be included in the model because the rate of absorption and elimination is important in determining the time course of the drug in the body. Furthermore, inclusion of organs and tissues that receive a large amount of the drug will make it easier to account for the total amount of the drug in the body. Moreover, it is important to include easily sampled body spaces because the experimentally determined drug concentrations are usually compared with the model predicted concentrations to evaluate and validate the developed model [2].

For example, models developed for gaseous anesthetic agents should include the lung, which is the main site for inhalation and excretion of these drugs as in Figure 22.3A. Adipose tissues should be included in the models for highly lipophilic drugs or chemicals because these drugs are extensively distributed in fatty tissues. PBPK models for drugs that undergo enterohepatic recycling should account for this process as presented in Figure 22.3B because this recycling process affects the drug behavior in the body [9]. Orally administered drugs should include the intestine as part of the model while transdermally applied drugs should include the skin in their model. The kidney should be included in the models for renally excreted drugs, and the liver for drugs that are eliminated by hepatic metabolism as in Figure 22.3C [10]. So although the whole body PBPK models deal with the same body structure, each model emphasizes and deemphasizes certain structures depending on the drug properties and the objectives of the model development.

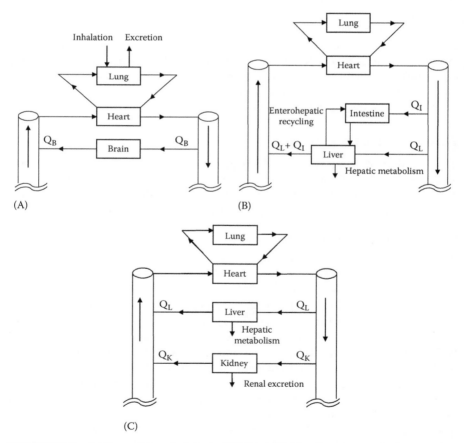

FIGURE 22.3 Sections of the whole body PBPK models that demonstrate the presentation of (A) lung inhalation and excretion of drugs, (B) enterohepatic recycling, and (C) renal and hepatic drug elimination.

22.3.1.2   Mathematical Presentation of the Model

Once the model general structure is defined, all the relevant pharmacokinetic processes that affect the pharmacokinetic behavior of the drug in all parts of the body are expressed by mathematical equations. This should include a set of equations that describe the rate of change of the amount of drug in each organ or tissue included in the model. Differential equations that describe the mass balance for the drug reaching the organ and the drug leaving the organ are used. Mathematical expressions that describe drug absorption, protein binding, drug transport, drug metabolism, renal excretion, and all other relevant pharmacokinetic processes should be included in the model description [2,11,12].

22.3.1.2.1   Mathematical Presentation of the Drug Distribution to Tissues

The rate of change of the drug amount in the organ is the difference between the amount of drug reaching the organ and the amount of drug leaving the organ to the venous circulation in noneliminating organs, while for the eliminating organs, the rate of change of the amount of the drug in the organ is the difference between the amount of drug reaching the organ and the sum of the amount of drug leaving the organ to the venous circulation and the amount of the drug eliminated by the organ. The amount of the drug reaching the organ can be expressed by the product of the organ blood flow and the arterial drug concentration, while the amount of the drug leaving the organ can be expressed by the product of the organ blood flow and the venous drug concentration. Equation 22.1 describes the rate of change in the amount of drug in a noneliminating organ:

$$\frac{dA_T}{dt} = Q_T C_a - Q_T C_{v,T} \tag{22.1}$$

where
   A_T is the amount of the drug in the tissue
   Q_T is the blood flow rate to the tissue
   C_a and $C_{v,T}$ are drug concentrations in the arterial blood and the venous blood for the tissue, respectively

Similarly the differential equation for the rate of change in the drug concentration in the tissue can be expressed as in Equation 22.2:

$$V_T \frac{dC_T}{dt} = Q_T C_a - Q_T C_{v,T} \tag{22.2}$$

where
   C_T is the concentration of the drug in the tissue
   V_T is the volume of the tissue

One differential equation can be written for each noneliminating organ. For the eliminating organ, the differential equation will include an additional term for the rate of drug elimination as in Equation 22.3:

$$V_T \frac{dC_T}{dt} = Q_T C_a - Q_T C_{v,T} - \text{Rate of drug elimination} \tag{22.3}$$

Writing the differential equations for the rate of change of the drug concentration in each organ is dependent on whether the drug distribution to the organ follows the flow-rate-limited model or the membrane-limited model, and also whether the drug is eliminated by that particular organ or not.

22.3.1.2.1.1 Mathematical Presentation of the Drug Distribution to Tissues That Follow the Flow-Rate-Limited Model Equation 22.2 that describes the rate of change in the drug concentration in a noneliminating organ uses the drug concentration in the arterial and venous blood for each organ. The drug concentration in the arterial blood for all organs is similar because each organ receives a fraction of the cardiac output. However, the drug concentration in the venous blood of different organs is not similar because it depends on the affinity of the drug to the organ constituents. Determination of the venous blood drug concentration is not possible for each organ because it has to be determined in the organ venous drainage before it is mixed with the venous blood coming from other organs. As mentioned previously, when the drug distribution to the organ follows the flow-rate-limited model, the tissue to blood distribution coefficient (Kp) is the ratio of the drug concentration in the tissue to that in the venous blood leaving the tissue as in Equation 22.4:

$$Kp = \frac{C_T}{C_{v,T}} \tag{22.4}$$

So the venous blood drug concentration leaving the tissue in Equation 22.2 can be expressed in terms of the tissue drug concentration and Kp as follows:

$$V_T \frac{dC_T}{dt} = Q_T C_a - Q_T \frac{C_T}{Kp} \tag{22.5}$$

For example, the differential equation that describes the rate of change of the drug concentration in the muscles can be written as follows:

$$V_M \frac{dC_M}{dt} = Q_M C_B - Q_M \frac{C_M}{Kp_M} \tag{22.6}$$

where
  V_M is the volume of the muscles
  C_M is the muscle drug concentration
  Q_M is the muscle blood flow
  C_B is the arterial blood drug concentration
  Kp_M is the muscle to blood distribution coefficient

The equation for an eliminating organ like the kidney can be written as follows:

$$V_K \frac{dC_K}{dt} = Q_K C_B - Q_K \frac{C_K}{Kp_K} - CL_R C_K \tag{22.7}$$

where
- V_K is the volume of the kidney
- C_K is the kidney drug concentration
- Q_K is the kidney blood flow
- C_B is the arterial blood drug concentration
- Kp_K is the kidney to blood distribution coefficient
- CL_R is the renal clearance

In this equation, the two kidneys are considered as one organ, so the volume and blood flow for both kidneys should be used.

22.3.1.2.1.2   Mathematical Presentation of the Drug Distribution to Tissues That Follow the Membrane-Limited Model   The mass balance expression when the tissue distribution of the drug follows a membrane-limited model is more complicated. Assume the situation when the drug distribution across the capillary membrane is the rate limiting step, and once the drug reaches the extracellular space it is rapidly distributed to the intracellular components. In this case, the organ is divided into two different subcompartments and the drug distribution to the organ will have to be described in each subcompartment separately. Consider the example in Figure 22.4 where the organ is divided into the vascular space and the cellular space, which include the extracellular and intracellular spaces. The rate of change of the amount of drug in the cellular space is the net flux of the drug between the two subcompartments in noneliminating organs. So it is the difference between the rate of drug diffusion from the vascular to the cellular space and the rate of drug

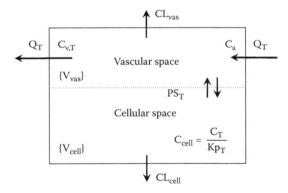

FIGURE 22.4   Diagram representing a membrane-limited organ, where drug diffusion across the capillary membrane is the rate determining step, and the drug that reaches the extracellular space is distributed rapidly to the intracellular space. V_{cell} and V_{vas} are the volume of the cellular and vascular spaces in the tissue, C_{cell} is the drug concentration in the cellular space, C_a is the arterial drug concentration, $C_{v,T}$ is the drug concentration in the venous blood leaving the tissue, C_T is the tissue drug concentration, Q_T is the blood flow to the tissue, Kp_T is the tissue to blood concentration ratio or the partition coefficient of the drug between tissue and blood, PS_T is the mass transfer coefficient and is the permeability surface area product for the tissue, CL_{cell} is the drug clearance from the cellular space, and CL_{vas} is the drug clearance from the vascular space.

back diffusion from the cellular to the vascular space as in Equation 22.8. Also, the rate of drug elimination should be considered when the drug is eliminated from the cellular space of the tissue as in Equation 22.9:

$$V_{cell}\frac{dC_{cell}}{dt} = PS_T(C_{v,T} - C_{cell}) = PS_T\left(C_{v,T} - \frac{C_T}{Kp_T}\right) \tag{22.8}$$

$$V_{cell}\frac{dC_{cell}}{dt} = PS_T\left(C_{v,T} - \frac{C_T}{Kp_T}\right) - CL_{cell} \cdot \frac{C_T}{Kp_T} \tag{22.9}$$

where

V_{cell} is the volume of the cellular space in the tissue

C_{cell} is the drug concentration in the cellular space

PS_T is the mass transfer coefficient and it is the permeability surface area product for the tissue

$C_{v,T}$ is the drug concentration in the venous blood leaving the tissue

C_T is the tissue drug concentration

Kp_T is the tissue to blood concentration ratio or the partition coefficient of the drug between tissue and blood

CL_{cell} is the drug clearance from the cellular space

On the other hand, the rate of change in the amount of drug in the vascular space in the tissue is equal to the difference between the amount of drug entering and leaving the tissue and the net flux between the vascular and cellular spaces as in Equation 22.10 when no drug is eliminated from the vascular space. However, the rate of drug elimination should be considered when the drug is eliminated from the vascular space of the tissue as in Equation 22.11:

$$V_{vas}\frac{dC_{v,T}}{dt} = Q_T(C_a - C_{v,T}) + PS_T\left(\frac{C_T}{Kp_T} - C_{v,T}\right) \tag{22.10}$$

$$V_{vas}\frac{dC_{v,T}}{dt} = Q_T(C_a - C_{v,T}) + PS_T\left(\frac{C_T}{Kp_T} - C_{v,T}\right) - CL_{vas} \cdot C_{v,T} \tag{22.11}$$

where

V_{vas} is the volume of the vascular space in the tissue

$C_{v,T}$ is the drug concentration in the venous blood leaving the organ

Q_T is the blood flow to the tissue

C_a is the arterial drug concentration

CL_{vas} is the drug clearance from the vascular space, and the other terms as defined previously

Example

Figure 22.5 represents part of a whole body PBPK model for a drug that includes the liver, intestine, adipose tissues, and blood. The drug is eliminated from the liver. The distribution of the drug to the adipose tissues, liver, and intestine follows the flow-rate-limited model. Write the differential equations that describe the rate of change of the drug concentration in the adipose tissues, liver, and blood.

Answer

According to Figure 22.5, the adipose tissues are noneliminating tissues while the liver can eliminate the drug, and the blood flow that leaves the liver is the sum of the blood flow to the liver and intestine.

- For the adipose tissues:

$$V_F \frac{dC_F}{dt} = Q_F C_B - Q_F \frac{C_F}{Kp_F}$$

where
    V_F is the volume of the adipose tissues
    C_F is the adipose tissues drug concentration
    Q_F is the adipose tissues blood flow
    C_B is the arterial blood drug concentration
    Kp_F is the adipose tissues to blood distribution coefficient

- For the liver:

$$V_L \frac{dC_L}{dt} = Q_L C_B + Q_I \frac{C_I}{Kp_I} - (Q_L + Q_I) \frac{C_L}{Kp_L} - CL_L C_L$$

where
    V_L is the volume of the liver
    C_L is the liver drug concentration
    Q_L is the liver blood flow
    Q_I is the intestine blood flow
    C_B is the blood drug concentration
    Kp_I is the intestine to blood distribution coefficient
    Kp_L is the liver to blood distribution coefficient
    CL_L is the liver drug clearance

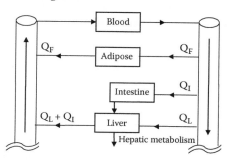

FIGURE 22.5   Part of a whole body PBPK model for the drug described in the solved example.

- For the blood:

$$V_B \frac{dC_B}{dt} = Q_F \frac{C_F}{Kp_F} + Q_L \frac{C_L}{Kp_L} - Q_B C_B$$

The equation for the blood includes the terms for the adipose tissues and liver only; however, when all the components of the model are known, the terms for the venous return for all organs have to be included.

22.3.1.2.2 Mathematical Presentation of the Administration/ Absorption Processes

IV bolus drug administration involves direct introduction of the entire dose to the venous blood, so the initial venous drug concentration in the model is determined by dividing the dose by the volume of the blood as in Equation 12.12, while for constant rate IV infusion, the drug concentration in the venous blood will be determined from the infusion rate and the drug concentration in the venous blood from different organs. So the rate of change in the drug concentration in the blood (C_B) can be expressed by Equation 22.13:

$$C_{Binitial} = \frac{Dose}{V_B} \tag{22.12}$$

$$V_B \frac{dC_B}{dt} = K_o + \sum Q_T C_{v,T} - Q_B C_B \tag{22.13}$$

where
  K_o is the rate of drug infusion
  $\sum Q_T C_{v,T}$ is the sum of the products of the blood flow and the venous drug concentration for all organs

After oral drug administration, the rate of change of the amount of drug in the gastrointestinal tract (GIT) at the absorption site is equal to the rate of drug absorption, assuming that the entire dose is absorbed. The expression for the rate of drug absorption can be included in the mass balance expression for the intestine. The rate of drug absorption can be generally described as in Equation 22.14:

$$\frac{dA_G}{dt} = k_a F D e^{-k_a t} \tag{22.14}$$

where
  A_G is the amount of the drug in the GIT at the absorption site
  k_a is the absorption rate constant if the absorption is first order
  F is the fraction of dose absorbed to account for incomplete absorption
  D is the dose

The mass balance equation for the intestine can be expressed as in Equation 22.15:

$$V_I \frac{dC_I}{dt} = Q_I C_B + k_a F D e^{-k_a t} - Q_I \frac{C_I}{Kp_I}$$ (22.15)

where
   V_I is the volume of the intestine
   C_I is the drug concentration in the intestine
   C_B is the arterial blood drug concentration
   Q_I is the blood flow to the intestine
   Kp_I is the intestine to blood distribution coefficient

Transdermal drug absorption can also be included in the mass balance equation that describes the rate of change of the amount of drug in the skin as in Equation 22.16:

$$\frac{dA_S}{dt} = PS\left(C_{surface} - \frac{C_S}{Kp_S}\right) + Q_S\left(C_B - \frac{C_S}{Kp_S}\right)$$ (22.16)

where
   A_S is the amount of the drug in the skin
   PS is the product of the permeability constant and the surface area exposed to the drug
   $C_{surface}$ is the drug concentration at the surface of the skin
   C_S is the skin drug concentration
   Kp_S is the skin to blood distribution coefficient
   Q_S is the skin blood flow
   C_B is the arterial blood drug concentration

22.3.1.2.3 Mathematical Presentation of the Distribution Process

The blood or plasma drug concentration can be expressed as the free or the total drug concentration. However, the free drug concentration is better correlated with the therapeutic and adverse effects of the drug. This is because the free drug is the moiety that can cross the biological membranes and distribute into different tissues to interact with the receptors. When the drug plasma protein binding is linear, the free drug concentration is always proportional to the total plasma drug concentration. However, the plasma protein binding of drugs can be nonlinear, which necessitates the expression of the drug concentration as the free drug concentration. Equation 22.17 expresses the relationship between the free and total drug concentrations when the plasma protein binding is linear:

$$C_{free} = f_u C_{total}$$ (22.17)

where
   C_{free} is the free unbound drug concentration
   f_u is the free fraction of the drug
   C_{total} is the total drug concentration

On the contrary, for nonlinear plasma protein binding, the relationship between the bound and free drug concentration can be expressed as in Equation 22.18:

$$C_{bound} = \frac{N_{tot}C_{free}}{K_D + C_{free}} \qquad (22.18)$$

where

C_{bound} is the bound drug concentration

C_{free} is the free drug concentration

K_D is the equilibrium dissociation constant for the drug-protein complex

N_{tot} is the total binding capacity or the capacity constant that is the product of the number of binding sites per mole of protein times the molar concentration of the protein, assuming that there is one type of binding and the sites are independent, that is, binding of drug to one site does not affect the binding of other drug molecules to another site

The relationships in Equations 22.17 and 22.18 can be used to express the plasma drug concentration as the free drug concentration in the mathematical equations for the PBPK model.

The drug tissue distribution may occur by passive diffusion or by carrier-mediated transport. In the case of passive diffusion across a membrane, the drug tissue distribution is dependent on the permeability area product and the concentration gradient across the membrane as described previously, while when the drug distribution involves a carrier-mediated transport, the mathematical expression that describes the kinetics of drug transport should be included in the model. Assuming that the carrier transport system can transfer the drug in both directions of the membrane and that the transport characteristics for the inward and outward directions are different, the net flux of the drug across the membrane can be expressed by Equation 22.19:

$$Flux = \frac{T_{max1}V_1C_1}{K_{T1} + C_1} - \frac{T_{max2}V_2C_2}{K_{T2} + C_2} \qquad (22.19)$$

where

T_{max1} and T_{max2} are the maximum rate of inward and outward transport

K_{T1} and K_{T2} are the association rate constants between the drug and the carrier protein on both directions of the membrane

V_1 and V_2 are the volume of the spaces on the two sides of the membrane

C_1 and C_2 are the drug concentrations on both sides of the membrane

In case of nonlinear protein binding in one or both of the tissue spaces separated by the membrane, the free drug concentration should be used. This expression can be modified if the carrier protein transfers the drug in only one direction across the membrane, or if the drug can be transported by passive as well as carrier-mediated transport across the membrane.

22.3.1.2.4 Mathematical Presentation of the Elimination Process

Drug elimination by organs should also be included in the mathematical presentation of the PBPK model. Drug metabolism can follow first-order kinetics or Michaelis-Menten (M-M) kinetics. In the case of first-order metabolism, the rate of drug metabolism is equal to the rate of metabolite formation dA_{met}/dt and it is determined from the first-order metabolic rate constant, k_m, and the amount of the drug available to be metabolized, A_T, as in Equation 22.20:

$$\frac{dA_{met}}{dt} = k_m A_T \tag{22.20}$$

On the contrary, in the case of saturable drug metabolism, the rate of metabolite formation can be expressed by the M-M-type equation as in Equation 22.21:

$$\frac{dA_{met}}{dt} = \frac{V_{max1} C_{v,T}}{K_m + C_{v,T}} \tag{22.21}$$

where
  V_{max} is the maximum rate of metabolism
  K_m is the M-M constant
  $C_{v,T}$ is the drug concentration in the venous blood of the eliminating organ

Also, the renal excretion of drugs should be included in the model. For first-order renal excretion, the renal excretion rate, dA_e/dt, is determined from the first-order renal excretion rate constant, k_e, and the amount of the drug available to be excreted in the kidney, A_k, as in Equation 22.22:

$$\frac{dA_e}{dt} = k_e A_k \tag{22.22}$$

When the renal excretion process does not follow first-order kinetics, the renal excretion rate can be expressed in terms of the three processes involved in the renal excretion of drugs: the glomerular filtration, tubular secretion, and tubular reabsorption.

22.3.2 Model Parameterization

The first step involved construction of the model structure and writing the differential equations that describe the rate of change of the amount of drug in all parts of the model. Using these differential equations, the drug concentration–time profile in all model components can be computed using numerical integration or simulation programs. However, before the start of the simulation process, estimates for the model parameters should be included in the model equations. These parameters include anatomical, physiological, physicochemical, and biochemical parameters.

Anatomical and physiological parameters include tissue and organ volumes, and blood flow rate, cardiac output, and breathing rate can also be included.

This type of information has been compiled for humans and different species and is available in the literature [13–15].

Physicochemical parameters such as the tissue partition coefficient can be determined experimentally using in vitro or in vivo techniques. Experiments that involve equilibration of the drug with tissue homogenates and then using appropriate techniques like equilibrium dialysis or ultrafiltration can be performed to estimate the drug partitioning to tissue components. Also, incubation of tissue slices with drug solutions has been used to estimate the tissue partition coefficient for some drugs. Furthermore, drug administration by IV infusion until steady state is achieved and then measuring the drug concentration in the blood and tissues can be used to estimate the tissue to blood distribution ratio. Estimates for drug permeability and diffusion parameters can be obtained using in vitro techniques. Biochemical model parameters such as the metabolic activity can also be estimated experimentally. The drug metabolic rate can be determined in vitro using hepatocytes or microsomal preparations by monitoring the rate of drug disappearance or the rate of metabolite formation. The M-M parameters (V_{max} and K_m) calculated in vitro can be scaled to predict the full metabolic activity of the liver and estimate the in vivo intrinsic clearance. The hepatic clearance can be predicted from the estimated in vivo intrinsic clearance and information as the hepatic blood flow and the drug-binding characteristics in the blood [16,17]. Other biochemical model parameters include drug-protein binding, and blood to plasma distribution ratio, which can be determined experimentally. Parameters that can describe drug absorption after extravascular administration derived from in vitro techniques such as the Caco-2 cells or from sophisticated simulation software are also incorporated in the model.

The parameters used in the model have to be suitable for the population being modeled. In models developed for special populations such as obese individuals, children, pregnant women, or elderly, the parameters used have to be appropriate for this population. Also, the parameters included in the model should be modified in the presence of factors that can modify these physiological parameters. For example, drugs such as beta adrenergic blockers can significantly alter the cardiac output that will affect blood flow to the different organs. Other factors such as diseases, physical activity, food, stress, or posture can affect the physiological parameters.

22.3.3 MODEL SIMULATION AND PARAMETER ESTIMATION

The PBPK models can be used for simulation of the time course of the drug concentration in all tissues and organs included in the model or for estimation of model parameters. When the PBPK model is used for simulation, all the model parameters obtained from the literature or estimated experimentally should be included in the model equations. These equations are used to simulate the time course of the drug concentration in all parts of the model using numerical integration methods utilizing specialized software [12]. The simulations can be used for model evaluation by comparing the simulated concentration–time profiles and the experimentally determined concentration–time profiles. Once the model presentation is optimized, the simulations can be used to simulate the drug pharmacokinetic behavior under different conditions that are difficult to duplicate experimentally, for example, when the experimental subjects are exposed to the risk of toxicity, when long-term exposure to the drug is investigated, or when the cost of performing the experiment is very high.

PBPK models can also be used for parameter estimation. In this case, it is required to experimentally determine the drug concentration–time profile in a number of organs and tissues that are included in the model. The experimental drug concentration–time data are fitted to the equations of the PBPK model. Specialized software is used to estimate the model parameter values that minimize the sum of the squared deviations between the experimentally obtained and the model predicted concentrations [18,19].

22.3.4 MODEL VALIDATION

The PBPK model validation involves evaluation of the adequacy of model construction and presentation. This is important to ensure that all the determinants and processes that affect the pharmacokinetic behavior of the drug have been accounted for. Experimental data such as plasma drug concentrations, tissue drug concentrations, and urinary excretion rate data obtained at different time points after drug administration are compared with the model predicted concentrations. Agreement between the model predicted values and experimental data indicates adequacy of the model and increases confidence in the model for extrapolation and prediction. The appropriate diagnostic and statistical tests should be used in this comparison. Also, the estimated model parameters are examined to determine the precision of the parameter estimates, and the expected variability in the model parameters in a particular population. It is important to determine sensitivity of the parameter, which is the extent of change in the model predictions as a result of change in the value of a particular parameter.

The existence of significant deviations between the experimentally obtained data and the model predicted data is an indication of model inadequacy. This may result from incorrect presentation of the model, failure to include key processes in the model, or using inaccurate estimates for model parameters. In this case, the model can be refined by revising the model structure and presentation. Also, examination of the parameter sensitivity can identify important processes and parameters that require careful modeling and additional experiments for better characterization. The process is repeated using the revised model until accurate and precise estimates for the model parameters are obtained and the model predicted drug pharmacokinetic behavior agrees with the experimentally obtained data.

22.3.5 MODEL IMPLEMENTATION

The whole body PBPK models are usually developed and utilized for descriptive and predictive purposes. These models can be used to describe general or specific aspects of the drug pharmacokinetic behavior under conditions within which the model was developed. However, the more important utility of these models is to predict the drug pharmacokinetic behavior in conditions other than those under which the model was developed. The most important of those is to predict the drug pharmacokinetic behavior in different animal species and in humans, an issue that is discussed later in this chapter. The other includes inter-dose, inter-route, inter-tissue extrapolation, and inter-drug extrapolation.

22.3.5.1   Inter-Dose Extrapolation

The PBPK models that describe the drug pharmacokinetic behavior after administration of a low dose of the drug can be used to predict the behavior after administration of a high dose of the drug under the same conditions. This can be achieved usually by accounting for all the possible nonlinear pharmacokinetic behavior that can happen when a high dose is administered. This includes accounting for nonlinear protein binding, nonlinear metabolism, nonlinear transport, and other processes that can be affected by the high dose. So the model developed for a certain dose of the drug can be used to predict the drug tissue distribution and disposition after administration of different doses.

22.3.5.2   Inter-Route Extrapolation

The PBPK model developed following a certain route of administration can be used to predict the drug pharmacokinetic behavior after a different route of administration. Most PBPK models are developed for IV bolus or constant rate IV administration. Introduction of the appropriate expression that represents drug absorption after different extravascular administration can allow the prediction of the drug pharmacokinetic behavior after different routes of administration. The pharmacokinetic behavior of drugs after oral, subcutaneous, or topical administration can be predicted from a model developed for IV administration. Most of the models used to investigate the long-term exposure to environmental pollutants by inhalation are extrapolated from models developed after IV administration.

22.3.5.3   Inter-Tissue and Inter-Drug Extrapolation

Drug concentration–time profiles in tissues and organs included in the PBPK models can be utilized to predict the drug profile in other tissues and organs. This is important because this extrapolation allows prediction of drug concentration in less accessible tissues. This can be achieved by examining the available information about the tissue to plasma partition coefficient, the drug characteristics, and the tissue composition for all the organs and tissues included in the model. Then, based on the available information about the composition of the tissue of interest, the tissue to plasma partition coefficient can be predicted [20]. Similarly, the pharmacokinetic behavior of a drug can be predicted from PBPK models developed for other related drugs [21].

22.4   INTERSPECIES SCALING

The objective of the interspecies scaling is to use the pharmacokinetic behavior of the drug characterized in one species to predict the drug pharmacokinetic behavior in different species. Most often, scientists try to predict the drug pharmacokinetic behavior in humans based on data obtained in experimental animals. The two main approaches for interspecies scaling are the PBPK modeling approach and the empirical allometric scaling approach.

22.4.1   PBPK Modeling Approach for Interspecies Scaling

The general principle of this scaling approach involves the development of the PBPK model for the drug in one species usually called the test species, and to use this model to predict the drug pharmacokinetic behavior in different species. In most cases, the interest is to use the drug pharmacokinetic properties in experimental animals to predict the drug pharmacokinetic behavior in humans. This usually involves replacing the physiological parameters for the test species in the PBPK model by the parameters for the species of interest [22,23]. For example, if the goal is to scale the drug pharmacokinetic behavior to humans, different organ volumes, blood flow, and cardiac output in humans are incorporated in the model. Also, drug-specific parameters related to drug absorption, metabolic rate, blood to plasma ratio, and protein binding in humans should be incorporated in the model. Scaling of the drug tissue distribution is done under the assumption that the tissue to blood partition coefficient is similar in the different species because of the similarities in the tissue composition in mammals.

Once the PBPK model is scaled to the species of interest, the model is used to simulate drug concentration–time profiles in the blood and tissues. At this point, the scaled PBPK model has to be validated. The most appropriate way to validate the scaled model is to obtain blood and tissue samples and then compare the model predicted concentrations with the experimentally determined concentrations. In the case of scaling to humans, it may be possible to use only the blood concentration for the model validation because it may not be possible to obtain tissue concentrations. Agreement between the predicted and experimentally determined blood drug concentration can be a good indication of successful model scaling. However, when the model validation is necessary it may be possible to scale the model to different animal species in addition to human scaling. The model is validated in the different animal species, and successful scaling to other animal species is a good indication of successful scaling to humans.

22.4.2   Allometric Approach for Interspecies Scaling

The allometric scaling is an empirical approach for interspecies scaling, which is still widely used to predict the human pharmacokinetic behavior from animal data. This is because it is simple and usually provides useful and reasonable predictions. This approach is based on the observation that a number of physiological parameters and processes in different species have been shown to vary with the body weight of these species according to a power function in the form presented in Equation 22.23:

$$y = a \cdot W^b \tag{22.23}$$

where
   y is the parameter of interest
   W is the body weight
   a is a coefficient
   b is the power

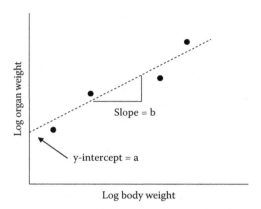

FIGURE 22.6 Hypothetical example of the relationship between log body weight and log organ size in different species.

Taking the logarithm of both sides of Equation 22.23 gives a straight-line equation as in Equation 22.24:

$$\log(y) = \log(a) + b \log(W) \tag{22.24}$$

This means that a linear relationship has been observed between log many of the physiological parameters in different species and log body weight of these species. For example, Figure 22.6 represents the relationship between log organ weight in different species and log body weight in these species. The y-intercept of the plot is equal to a, and the slope is equal to b. The values of a and b can be estimates and used in the power equation to predict the value of this parameter in an untested species [24].

Using the same principle, it has been proposed that the pharmacokinetic parameters (e.g., CL_T, Vd, $t_{1/2}$) of a drug in different species are related to the body weight of these species by the same power function. So the pharmacokinetic parameters for the drug of interest are determined in four or more animal species, and then the log parameter value is plotted versus the log weight of the corresponding animal species. Using linear regression, the y-intercept and the slope are estimated, which represent the coefficient and the exponent of the power equation, respectively. If the goal is to determine the pharmacokinetic parameter in humans, an average weight of 70 kg is substituted in the power equation to predict the value of the pharmacokinetic parameter in humans. Different pharmacokinetic parameters usually have different power equations, that is, different coefficients and exponents.

Another approach for interspecies scaling is based on the concept of "equivalent time" or the pharmacokinetic time in different species. This concept suggests that the biological time, which is the time necessary to complete a biological event, is different in different species. For example, the heart rate and the breathing rate are different in different species indicating that the time required for one heart beat or one breathing cycle is different in different species. So the rate of drug elimination in different species can be correlated if the chronological time in different species uses an intrinsic biological property (e.g., creatinine clearance, heart rate, breathing rate, blood circulation velocity) as the scaling time to determine the equivalent time. Biological rates in different species have been related to the species body weight by a power function as follows:

$$\text{Biological rate} = \text{Constant} \cdot W^{0.25} \qquad (22.25)$$

which indicates that the equivalent time can be obtained by dividing the chronological time by $W^{0.25}$. This principle suggests that plots of the plasma drug concentration–time profiles obtained in different species after administration of dose normalized for body weight and transforming the time scales by dividing by $W^{0.25}$ should be superimposable [25]. So this approach allows the prediction of the expected drug concentration–time profile in any species by transforming the time scale from the equivalent time to the chronological time for the species of interest by multiplying by $W^{0.25}$.

The allometric scaling approach is simple and usually provides reasonable and useful predictions. However, it should be used with caution because there are conditions when the use of the allometric scaling approach may not be appropriate. For example, when interspecies differences in drug metabolism and protein binding exist, the use of the allometric scaling may not be appropriate. In this case, the physiological method offers the flexibility for accommodating specific species information such as qualitative and quantitative differences in drug metabolism. Also, allometric scaling cannot be used to predict the drug behavior in specific human population. However, the physiological approach can be used to predict the modification in drug behavior due to physiological and pathological conditions by adjusting the model parameters. Furthermore, the physiological interspecies scaling procedures can be more appropriate for predicting the pharmacokinetic behavior of highly lipophilic drugs and chemicals. This is because different species have different body fat contents that result in large interspecies variation in the distribution and elimination of these compounds and increase the variability in the allometric scaling predictions.

22.5   APPLICATIONS OF THE PBPK MODELS

The PBPK modeling approach has been applied in numerous biomedical research areas such as drug development, therapeutic drug use, environmental toxicology, and risk assessment. In this section, we will only mention few examples for the application of PBPK models in drug development and therapeutic drug use.

22.5.1   ESTIMATING THE STARTING DOSE FOR ENTRY TO HUMANS

The first step in the clinical phases of development of any molecule involves the selection of the starting dose for entry to humans based on the information generated during the preclinical phase of drug development. The objective usually is to select the starting dose that should be administered as a single escalating dose to healthy volunteers to evaluate the tolerability of the new compound and to obtain some pharmacokinetic information if possible. There are four main methods that are commonly used to select the starting dose for noncytotoxic drugs [26].

The pharmacokinetically guided approach is the method of choice since it utilizes the systemic exposure instead of dose for extrapolation from animals to humans. The desired systemic exposure, usually measured as the AUC or C_{max}, in humans is defined as the systemic exposure corresponding to the no observable adverse effect level (NOAEL). When the AUC corresponding to the NOAEL is available for more than one species, the species with the lowest AUC is used. The clearance of the drug in humans is predicted using the physiological or the allometric approach. The starting dose can be calculated as follows:

$$\text{Starting Dose} = AUC_{preclinical} \cdot CL_{humans} \qquad (22.26)$$

where
   $AUC_{preclinical}$ is the AUC associated with NOAEL determined in animals
   CL_{humans} is the predicted drug clearance in humans using animal scale-up

There are few points that should be considered when utilizing the pharmacokinetically guided approach in calculating the starting dose in humans. This approach assumes that the concentration-effect relationship is similar in humans and other species, which may not be true for all drugs. When there is a large difference in the protein binding between species, it will be more appropriate to use the free drug concentration to describe drug exposure. Also, the approach described earlier assumes linear pharmacokinetics, and the parent drug is the only active moiety. The estimated dose should be corrected in case of evidence of nonlinearity or the presence of active metabolites. Also, the differences in rate and extent of drug absorption from the animal and human formulations should be considered when calculating the dose.

Other methods for estimating the starting doses in humans are empirical. These include the dose by a factor method that utilizes the animal dose associated with NOAEL multiplied by a safety factor. The other methods includes the similar drug approach that can be used when clinical data are available about another compound from the same pharmacological class as the drug under investigation, while the comparative approach utilizes two or more methods to estimate the starting dose for humans and then compares the results to come to the optimal starting dose.

22.5.2 Applications of PBPK Models in Therapeutic Drug Use

PBPK models have been developed to describe anticancer drug distribution to normal and cancerous tissues. The primary aim of these models is to quantify the normal and cancerous tissue exposure to the drugs and predict the therapeutic and adverse effects of the drug. This has been very useful for optimization of the anticancer drug therapy by developing new approaches for maximizing the cancerous tissue and minimizing the normal tissue drug exposure. Also, the drug distribution to the fetus from the mother through the placenta and to neonates through breast milk has been described by developing PBPK models for pregnant and lactating women. These models can quantify the fetal and neonatal drug exposure and characterize the time course of the drug concentration in different tissues and organs of the fetus and the neonate. It is very important to assess the possible pharmacological and toxicological effects that can result from the fetal and neonatal drug exposures. The PBPK models have been used to describe the tissue distribution of several antibiotics. This can be useful since the drug concentration in the infected tissue is the important determinant of the therapeutic effect of these drugs. The pharmacokinetic behavior of many other drugs such as anesthetics, sedatives, antibodies, and large molecular weight oligonucleotides has been described using PBPK models.

REFERENCES

1. Bischoff KB (1986) Physiological pharmacokinetics. *Bull Math Biol* 48:309–322.
2. Nestorov I (2003) Whole body pharmacokinetic models. *Clin Pharmacokinet* 42:883–908.
3. Blakey GE, Nestorov IA, Arundel PA, Aarons LJ, and Rowland M (1997) Quantitative structure-pharmacokinetics relationships: I. Development of a whole-body physiologically based model to characterize changes in pharmacokinetics across a homologous series of barbiturates in the rat. *J Pharmacokinet Biopharm* 25:277–312.
4. Bernareggi A and Rowland M (1991) Physiological modeling of cyclosporine kinetics in rat and man. *J Pharmacokinet Biopharm* 19:21–50.
5. Dedrick RL and Bischoff BK (1968) Pharmacokinetics in application of the artificial kidney. *Chem Eng Progr Symp Ser* 64:32–44.
6. Gerlovski LE and Jain RK (1983) Physiologically-based pharmacokinetic modeling: Principles and applications. *J Pharm Sci* 72:1103–1129.
7. Björkman S, Stanski DR, Harashima H, Dowrie R, Harapat SR, Wada DR, and Ebling WF (1993) Tissue distribution of fentanyl and alfentanil in the rat cannot be described by a blood flow limited model. *J Pharmacokinet Biopharm* 21:255–279.
8. Gallo JM, Hung CT, Gupta PK, and Perrier DG (1989) Physiological pharmacokinetic model of adriamycin delivered via magnetic albumin microspheres in the rats. *J Pharmacokinet Biopharm* 17:305–326.
9. Ploeger B, Mensinga T, Sips A, Meulenbelt J, and DeJongh, J (2000) A human physiologically based model for glycyrrhizic acid, a compound subject to presystemic metabolism and enterohepatic cycling. *Pharm Res* 17:1516–1525.
10. Clewell HJ, Gentry PR, Gearhart JM, Covington TR, Banton MI, and Andersen ME (2001) Development of a physiologically-based pharmacokinetic model of isopropanol and its metabolite acetone. *Toxicol Sci* 63:160–172.
11. Gallo JM (2002) Physiologically based pharmacokinetic models, in Schoenwald RD (Ed.) *Pharmacokinetics in Drug Discovery and Development.* CRC Press, Boca Raton, FL.
12. Espié P, Tytgat D, Sargentini-Maier ML, Poggesi I, and Watelet JB (2009) Physiologically based pharmacokinetics (PBPK). *Drug Metab Rev* 41:391–407.
13. Broun RP, Delp MD, Lindstedt SL, Rhomberg LR, and Beliles RP (1997) Physiological parameter values for physiologically-based pharmacokinetic models. *Toxicol Ind Health* 13:407–484.
14. Davies B and Morris T (1993) Physiological parameters in laboratory animals and humans. *Pharm Res* 10:1093–1095.
15. Leggert RW and Williams LR (1989) Suggested reference values for regional blood volumes in humans. *Health Phys* 60:139–154.
16. De Buck SS and Mackie CE (2007) Physiologically-based approaches towards the prediction of pharmacokinetics: In vitro–in vivo extrapolation. *Expert Opin Drug Metab Toxicol* 3:865–878.

17. Houston JB (1994) Utility of in vitro drug metabolizing data in predicting *in vivo* metabolic clearance. *Biochem Pharmacol* 47:1469–1479.
18. Ebling WF, Wada DR, and Stanski DR (1994) From piecewise to full pharmacokinetic modeling: Applied to thiopental disposition in the rat. *J Pharmacokinet Biopharm* 22:259–292.
19. Woodruff TJ, Bois FY, Auslander D, and Spear RC (1992) Structure and parameterization of pharmacokinetic models: Their impact on model predictions. *Risk Anal* 12:189–201.
20. Pelekis M, Poulin P, and Krishnan K (1995) An approach for incorporating tissue composition data into physiologically-based pharmacokinetic models. *Toxicol Ind Health* 11:511–522.
21. Nestorov I, Aarons L, and Rowland M (1998) Quantitative structure-pharmacokinetics relationships: II. Mechanistically based model for the relationship between the tissue distribution parameters and the lipophilicity of the compounds. *J Pharmacokinet Biopharm* 26:521–546.
22. Mordenti J (1986) Man versus beast: Pharmacokinetic scaling in mammals. *J Pharm Sci* 75:1028–1040.
23. Ings RMJ (1990) Interspecies scaling and comparisons in drug development and toxicokinetics. *Xenobiotica* 11:1201–1231.
24. Mahmood I (2007) Application of allometric principles for the prediction of pharmacokinetics in human and veterinary drug development. *Adv Drug Deliv Rev* 59:1177–1192.
25. Dedrick RL, Bischoff KB, and Zaharko DS (1970) Interspecies correlation of plasma concentration, history of methotrexate (NSC-740). *Cancer Chemother Rep* 54:95–101.
26. Reigner BG and Blesch KS (2002) Estimating the starting dose for entry into humans: Principles and practice. *Eur J Clin Pharmacol* 57:835–845.

23 Therapeutic Drug Monitoring

OBJECTIVES

After completing this chapter you should be able to

- Describe the importance of therapeutic drug monitoring in the initiation and management of drug therapy
- Compare the dose-response and concentration-response relationships
- Define the therapeutic range of drugs
- Discuss the characteristics that make drugs good candidates for therapeutic drug monitoring
- Describe the proper procedures that should be followed for obtaining and analyzing samples for therapeutic drug monitoring
- Recommend the general requirements and resources needed to establish a therapeutic drug monitoring service

23.1 INTRODUCTION

Therapeutic drug monitoring (TDM) is a concept that utilizes the drug concentration measurement in biological fluids as a tool for individualization of drug therapy and dosage adjustment. This concept is based on the strong correlation observed between the drug concentration in the systemic circulation and the therapeutic as well as toxic effects for many drugs. This strong correlation indicates that most drugs exert their desired therapeutic effects with minimal adverse effects in the majority of patients when their blood or plasma concentrations are maintained within a certain concentration range, which is known as the therapeutic range. The drug concentration achieved at steady state in a particular patient is dependent on the dosing rate of the drug and the drug total body clearance in this particular patient. When the same dose of a drug is administered to a group of patients, different drug concentrations are achieved in different patients due to many factors related to the drug product and the patient-specific characteristics. This explains why the correlation between the blood drug concentration and effect is stronger than the correlation between the drug dose and effect.

TDM is a multidisciplinary activity that utilizes pharmaceutical, pharmacokinetic, and pharmacodynamic knowledge for optimization of drug therapy in a variety of clinical situations [1]. The process starts with the selection of an initial dosing regimen based on the patient's specific characteristics. Then the blood drug concentrations measured while the patient is receiving the initial dosing regimen are used to estimate the patient-specific pharmacokinetic parameters for the drug. These pharmacokinetic parameters are used to determine the dosing regimen that should maintain the blood drug concentration within the desired range of drug concentrations. The desired blood concentrations are usually the concentrations that have been associated with the optimal therapeutic effects and minimal adverse effects. Periodic determination of the blood drug concentration may be necessary during long-term drug use to monitor the change in drug concentration that might happen due to changes in the patient's condition. The application of this concept became possible after the development of analytical procedures and techniques for rapid determination of the blood drug concentration with acceptable accuracy and precision. Also, this concept became attractive because several studies have proven the cost-effectiveness of its application in a variety of clinical settings.

23.2 GENERAL PRINCIPLES OF INITIATION AND MANAGEMENT OF DRUG THERAPY

The process of initiating drug therapy, which is simplified in the scheme in Figure 23.1, usually starts with the diagnosis of the patient's condition based on all the available subjective and objective patient information. Once the patient's condition is diagnosed, one or more drugs are usually prescribed to treat all the patient's medical problems, and the desired therapeutic outcomes for each of the patient's problems are determined. The dosing regimens of the drugs are selected based on the patient's demographic characteristics and a set of clinical monitoring parameters are selected

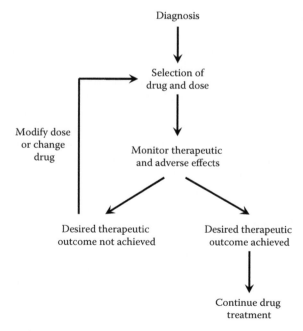

FIGURE 23.1   Basic steps in the process of initiation and management of drug therapy.

for the evaluation of the therapeutic and adverse effects for each drug. After initiation of drug therapy and allowing enough time for the drug to achieve the steady state, the patient is usually monitored to evaluate if the desired therapeutic outcomes are achieved. If the desired therapeutic outcomes are achieved, the selected drug and dosing regimen should continue as long as continuous drug use is required and the desired therapeutic goals are maintained. However, if the therapeutic outcomes are not achieved, the drug dosing regimen should be modified and the patient is monitored after allowing enough time to achieve the new steady-state drug concentration. The process is repeated until the desired therapeutic outcomes are achieved. If modification of the dosing regimen does not result in achieving the therapeutic goal, changing the drug or addition of another drug may be necessary and the process is repeated until the desired therapeutic outcomes are achieved [2,3].

For example, when oral hypoglycemic drugs are used by diabetes mellitus patients, the desired therapeutic outcome is usually to maintain the blood glucose level within the normal range without experiencing any adverse effects. After using the oral hypoglycemic drug for at least five elimination half-lives, the blood glucose level is evaluated. Adequate control of the blood glucose level without the appearance of any adverse drug reaction indicates that the desired therapeutic outcome of the drug is achieved and the drug use should be continued using the same dosing regimen, while inadequate reduction of the blood glucose level to the normal range may necessitate increasing the dose of the oral hypoglycemic drugs, and the appearance of adverse effects may call for holding or reduction of the oral hypoglycemic doses. After using the modified dosing regimen for enough time to achieve the new steady-state concentration, the drug effect is evaluated to determine if the desired therapeutic outcome is achieved and the process is repeated until the desired goal is achieved. When the blood glucose level cannot be maintained within the normal range using the selected oral hypoglycemic drug, the use of a different oral hypoglycemic drug or the addition of a second glucose-lowering drug may be necessary. The same process is repeated to evaluate if the new drug or drug combination can achieve the desired therapeutic goal. Different medical conditions usually have different desired therapeutic outcomes and different clinical monitoring parameters.

23.2.1 Use of Therapeutic Drug Monitoring in the Management of Drug Therapy

For many drugs, it is possible to utilize the approach described earlier for assessing the success or failure of therapy by monitoring the patient clinically. However, under certain medical conditions, completely relying on this approach may not be appropriate and can expose the patient to serious medical problems. Blood drug concentration measurements can be a valuable guiding tool for avoiding these serious problems and for achieving the desired therapeutic outcomes in a timely manner. Measuring the blood drug concentration in the early course of starting the drug therapy can help in the speedy selection of the appropriate dosing regimen for each patient. This practice usually cuts down the time required for making the necessary decisions to achieve the desired therapeutic outcomes.

Measuring the blood drug concentration can be very useful for differentiating between therapeutic failure, undertreatment, and noncompliance. When the drug is administered and the desired therapeutic effects of the drug are not observed, this may result from the use of the wrong drug, the wrong dose, or due to noncompliance. If the drug concentration is in the upper end of the therapeutic range, it indicates that a different drug should be used or an additional drug should be added to the first drug, while if the drug concentration is in the lower end or below the therapeutic range, it may be appropriate to increase the dose and make sure that the patient is taking the drug correctly before attempting to change the drug or to add a new drug. TDM is also very useful when the drug is used for prophylaxis because relying on the drug therapeutic effect may not be appropriate. Examples of the prophylaxis use of drugs includes the use of lithium in manic-depressive illness, the use of phenytoin to prevent the development of seizures after trauma or neurosurgical procedures, and the use of cyclosporine and tacrolimus to prevent organ rejection. In these cases, developing the symptoms that indicate insufficient drug doses can have serious consequences. Measuring the blood drug concentrations can help in making sure that the drug is present in the body in sufficient quantities to produce its desired effects and also to avoid the development of toxicity.

Measurement of the drug concentration can help in differentiating between drug toxicity and other medical conditions and also in making decisions regarding the drug therapy. For example, digoxin toxicity may result in the development of cardiac arrhythmias, which may mimic the symptoms of heart conditions that can develop in the patient population usually treated with digoxin. Also, the nephrotoxicity that is a common adverse effect of the immunosuppressive drug cyclosporine usually results in an increase in serum creatinine, which is similar to the common symptoms of graft rejection in renal transplant patients. Furthermore, the nephrotoxicity of the aminoglycoside antibiotics may be hard to differentiate from the decrease in kidney function caused by severe generalized infection. TDM can also be useful when monitoring the therapeutic effect of the drug is not readily accomplished such as in the case of antiepileptic drugs when the incidence of seizures is infrequent or in psychiatric conditions that are not easy to evaluate. Also, when the drug adverse effect is very serious or irreversible, it is not possible to use these adverse effects as monitoring parameters such as in the case of irreversible aminoglycoside ototoxicity. In these cases, the blood drug concentration provides additional information that can be utilized to achieve optimum patient care.

23.3   DRUG BLOOD CONCENTRATION VERSUS DRUG DOSE

Once the administered drug reaches the systemic circulation, the drug concentration–time profile will depend on the pharmacokinetic characteristics of the drug in each patient. This means that administration of the same dosing regimen of the same drug to different individuals usually produces different drug profiles due to the interindividual variability in the drug pharmacokinetic characteristics. The drug in the systemic circulation is distributed to all parts of the body to exert its therapeutic and adverse effects. The intensity of the therapeutic and the toxic effects for most drugs usually depends on their concentrations at the site of action, which is usually

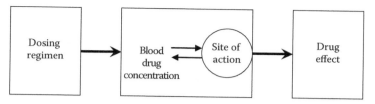

FIGURE 23.2   Schematic presentation for the relationship between the dosing regimen, the blood concentration, the concentration at the site of action, and the drug effect.

at equilibrium with the drug in blood as presented in Figure 23.2. Based on this discussion, the correlation between the blood drug concentrations and the therapeutic and adverse effects are much stronger than the correlation between the drug dosing regimen and the therapeutic and adverse effects [1,4].

The inter-patient variability in drug pharmacokinetics and response usually weakens the correlation between the drug dose and response. So drugs should not be administered to patients at fixed doses. The drug doses should be tailored according to the specific patient's characteristics. The variability in drug pharmacokinetics and response results from many factors such as genetic factors, age, weight, disease state, drug interactions, factors related to the drug formulations, nonlinear disposition, environmental factors, dietary factors, occupational exposure, stress, smoking, and seasonal variations. Some of these factors contribute significantly to the variation in drug disposition, and the effect of some other factors is minor. However, it is important to note that the overall variability in the drug disposition results from the additive effect of all these factors. Chapters 24 through 26 of this book cover some of the important factors that can contribute to the variability in drug disposition and response.

23.4   THERAPEUTIC RANGE

The correlation between the blood drug concentration and the drug therapeutic effect is well documented, with higher drug concentrations usually producing more intense effects for most drugs. This may indicate that a higher serum drug concentration may be more beneficial to obtain better therapeutic effects. However, the relationship between the drug blood concentration and the drug adverse effects is also well established, with higher drug concentrations increasing the probability of developing adverse effects. For example, as phenytoin concentration increases above 20 mg/L, patients develop nystagmus, then ataxia in the concentration range of 30–40 mg/L, while mental changes occur when phenytoin concentration exceeds 40 mg/L. The appearance of toxic effects usually requires holding or decreasing the drug dosage to decrease its serum concentration. So the blood drug concentration should be kept within the range of concentrations that produce the maximum therapeutic effect and the minimum adverse effects. This range of blood drug concentrations is known as the therapeutic range.

The therapeutic range is defined as the range of drug concentrations in the blood within which the probability of the desired therapeutic effect is relatively high and the probability of the unacceptable adverse effects is relatively low [1].

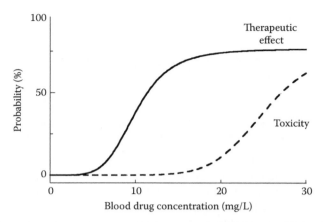

FIGURE 23.3   Therapeutic range is chosen to produce the highest probability of the therapeutic effect and the lowest probability of toxicity.

Figure 23.3 represents a hypothetical example, which shows that the probability of the desired therapeutic effect is very low when drug concentrations are low and also the probability of toxicity is very low. As the drug blood concentration increases, the probability of achieving the therapeutic effect increases then stays relatively constant. Over the same concentration range, the probability of developing toxicity increases more slowly. As the blood concentration increases, the probability of developing toxicity increases more rapidly. According to Figure 23.3, if one selects 10 mg/L as the lower end of the range, then the probability of the desired therapeutic effect would be about 40%, while if 20 mg/L was chosen as the upper end of the therapeutic range, then the probability of response would be about 80%. Over the same concentration range, the probability of unacceptable toxicity would remain less than about 10%. So the therapeutic range represents the range of drug blood concentration within which the majority of patients will have the desired therapeutic response with minimum incidence of adverse effects. It is important to note that few patients may have the desired therapeutic effect when the drug blood concentration is below the therapeutic range and few patients may not show any therapeutic effects even if the drug blood concentration is within the therapeutic range. Also, few patients may develop toxicity while their drug blood concentration is within the therapeutic range and some patients may not develop toxicity even if their blood drug concentration is slightly above the therapeutic range. So the decision regarding dosage adjustment should be guided by the blood drug concentration in conjunction with the clinical response of the patient.

The drug therapeutic and adverse effects are usually correlated with the drug concentration at the site of action. This means that the therapeutic range should be expressed in terms of the drug concentration at the site of action rather than the blood drug concentration. However, at steady state, when most drugs are monitored, equilibrium exists between the drug concentrations in all parts of the body. This does not mean that the drug concentration is similar in all parts of the body at steady state, but it means that the ratio of the blood drug concentration to the drug concentration in any particular organ is relatively constant at steady state. The decrease in blood drug concentration is usually accompanied by a proportional decrease in the drug concentration in all tissues including the site of action at steady state. So when the drug concentration in blood is in the therapeutic range, the drug concentration at the site of action is not known but this concentration should produce the optimal therapeutic effect with minimal toxicity.

23.5 DRUG CANDIDATES FOR THERAPEUTIC DRUG MONITORING

Application of the TDM is not recommended for all drugs. The use of blood drug concentration measurements for dosage optimization has been used for antibiotics such as aminoglycoside and vancomycin; antiepileptic drugs such as phenytoin, carbamazepine, valproic acid, phenobarbital, and ethosuximide; cardiovascular drugs such as digoxin, lidocaine, and procainamide; immunosuppressants such as cyclosporine, tacrolimus, and sirolimus; cytotoxic drugs such as methotrexate; bronchodilator such as theophylline; and psychiatric medications such as lithium, benzodiazepines, and tricyclic antidepressants in addition to many other drugs. All these drugs fall into one of the following drug categories that include the candidate drugs for TDM [5].

23.5.1 DRUGS WITH LOW THERAPEUTIC INDEX

Drugs with low therapeutic index, that is, the ratio of the minimum toxic concentration to the minimum effective concentration is low, require accurate determination of the drug dosing regimen to avoid drug toxicity or subtherapeutic effects. This is because the therapeutic ranges for these drugs are narrow and any small deviation from the appropriate dosing regimen can produce drug concentrations outside of the therapeutic range during the doing interval. TDM can serve as a tool for choosing the appropriate dosing regimen that can maintain the drug concentration within the therapeutic range all the time. On the other hand, drugs with high therapeutic index, that is, the ratio of the minimum toxic concentration and the minimum effective concentration is high, are considered safe drugs. This is because different dosing regimens from these drugs can achieve drug concentrations within the therapeutic range due to their wide therapeutic range. When these drugs are used clinically, an average dosage regimen is administered and the resulting drug concentrations usually fall within the therapeutic range all the time despite the inter-patient variability in the drug disposition. A wide range of dosing regimens should produce the desired therapeutic effect with minimal toxicity. So application of TDM may not be necessary for these high therapeutic index drugs.

23.5.2 DRUGS WITH LARGE VARIABILITY IN THEIR PHARMACOKINETIC PROPERTIES

Drugs with large variability in their pharmacokinetic behavior have a poor correlation between the blood drug concentrations and drug dose. Administration of the same dosing regimen of these drugs to a group of patients can produce a wide range of drug concentrations at steady state. This makes it very difficult to choose the drug dosing regimen that can maintain the blood drug concentration within the therapeutic range, based only on the patient's characteristics. For these drugs, TDM can serve as a guide to choose the appropriate dosing regimen required to achieve blood drug concentrations within the therapeutic range.

23.5.3 Drugs Commonly Used in High-Risk Patients or Patients with Multiple Medical Problems

Patients with multiple medical problems can face serious medical consequences if they develop drug toxicity or when there is delay in receiving therapeutic doses of the prescribed drugs. So careful selection of the appropriate dosing regimens for these patients is very important. However, this is not an easy task because these patients usually have other diseases that may affect the drug pharmacokinetic behavior, and they usually receive multiple medications that increase the probability of drug interactions. TDM can be very useful in the selection of the appropriate dosing regimens for these high-risk patients.

23.6 DETERMINATION OF THE DRUG CONCENTRATION IN BIOLOGICAL SAMPLES

Application of TDM involves the use of drug concentration in biological samples as a guide for selecting the appropriate dosing regimen for each individual patient. The right recommendation of dosing regimens cannot be made unless the measured drug concentration in biological fluid is reliable. The reliability of the drug concentration comes from the collection of the right biological fluid sample at the right time using the proper procedures. Also, the appropriate drug moiety should be determined in these samples utilizing accurate and precise analytical techniques.

23.6.1 Biological Samples

The biological samples used in TDM for the majority of drugs are whole blood, plasma, or serum. Some drugs can also be measured in urine and saliva samples; however, the measured concentrations in these cases have to be carefully interpreted. The drug properties and the technique used in the analysis usually determine the suitable sample matrix, the type of collection tubes, and the proper anticoagulant to be used when whole blood and plasma samples are needed [6]. Adherence to the sample collection instruction for each drug is necessary to obtain a reliable sample that can be used to determine the drug concentration accurately. Stability of the drug in the collected samples is an important issue that should be considered. Although most of the samples drawn for TDM in hospitals are analyzed shortly after collection, there are situations when this is not the case, such as when samples are drawn in the doctor's office and then sent to the clinical laboratory for analysis. In this case, the samples should be stored in a condition that will ensure the maximum stability of the drug in the sample.

23.6.2   Time of Sampling

The blood drug concentration is continually changing during the dosing interval when the drug is administered repeatedly. Large fluctuations in the blood drug concentration are usually observed when the drug is rapidly absorbed and rapidly eliminated. So the time of blood samples should be selected carefully to facilitate the interpretation of the measured drug concentration. There is usually optimal time for obtaining the blood samples for each drug. However, during multiple drug administration of the drug, the general role is that blood samples should be obtained after the steady-state concentration is achieved, that is, after receiving the drug for a period equivalent to at least five elimination half-lives for the drug [7]. The exception of this role is some cases where multiple samples are obtained before reaching a steady state to estimate the patient-specific pharmacokinetic parameters and to calculate the proper dosing regimen such as in the case of aminoglycoside antibiotics and vancomycin. When drug efficacy is the reason for blood concentration monitoring, the minimum drug concentration at steady state is usually determined by measuring the drug concentration just before drug administration, while if toxicity is the reason for monitoring, the maximum drug concentration at steady state is usually determined by measuring the drug concentration at the time when the highest drug concentration is expected [6]. When steady state is achieved while using aminoglycosides and vancomycin, the maximum and minimum blood concentrations are usually measured to make sure that the drug concentration is in the range that produces the optimal effect with minimum toxicity [8]. For drugs with long elimination half-lives and that follow multicompartment pharmacokinetic models such as lithium and digoxin, blood samples are usually obtained 6–8 h after drug administration to reflect the average drug concentration at steady state.

23.6.3   Measured Drug Moiety

The free drug is the drug moiety that is responsible for the drug therapeutic and adverse effects. This is because the free drug molecules can cross the biological membranes to become available at the site of drug action. However, measuring the free drug concentration is not simple and is not routinely performed in clinical laboratories. When the percentage of the drug bound to plasma protein is constant, the total drug concentration (free + bound) represents a simple alternative to measuring the free drug concentration. The measured total drug concentration in biological samples can be used for dosage adjustment keeping in mind that the free drug concentration is always a constant fraction of the total drug concentration. For example, the plasma protein binding for the antiepileptic drug phenytoin is 90%, and the therapeutic range for the free phenytoin concentration is 1–2 μg/mL. This means that when the total phenytoin concentration is measured, the therapeutic range for the total phenytoin concentration ranges from 10 to 20 μg/mL, as long as the phenytoin protein binding is relatively constant. So when the plasma protein binding for the drugs is relatively constant in the monitored patients, the total drug concentration can be measured and the therapeutic range for these drugs should be expressed in terms of the total drug concentration.

However, there are situations when the drug of interest is highly bound to plasma protein and the patient has conditions that can alter the drug protein binding. The conditions that can alter the drug plasma protein binding include hepatic diseases, renal failure, or concurrent administration of medications that can cause displacement of the drug protein binding. In these cases, the percentage of the drug bound to plasma protein is different from the average value and measuring the total drug concentration may not be appropriate. Under these conditions, measuring the free drug concentration is necessary [9,10]. Examples of these drugs are phenytoin, carbamazepine, valproic acid, antiretroviral drugs, digoxin, and immunosuppressant drugs in conditions that can alter the protein binding such as renal failure, liver disease, malnourishment, elderly, hyperbilirubinemia, and cystic fibrosis.

Measuring the free drug concentration involves an additional step to separate the free drug from the bound drug in the biological matrix. The equilibrium dialysis, ultrafiltration, and ultracentrifugation techniques can be used; however, the ultrafiltration technique is commonly used by the clinical laboratories because it is the simplest and quickest. Recently, a solid-phase microextraction technique has been developed that allows separation of the free drug from the bound drug in biological matrices. Once the free drug is separated, the same analytical technique is used for determination of the free drug concentration. The therapeutic range for the free drug concentration has to be considered when interpreting the measured free drug concentrations in patients.

Some drugs are metabolized to pharmacologically active metabolites that have therapeutic effects similar to that of the parent drug. The observed therapeutic effect usually results from the parent drug and the drug metabolite. In this case, TDM should involve measuring the parent drug and the metabolite concentration in the biological samples to account for all the drug moieties responsible for the observed therapeutic effect of the drug. Dosage adjustment recommendation should consider the contribution of both the parent drug and the metabolite to the therapeutic effect. The therapeutic range for these drugs should include recommendations for the parent drug and the active metabolite concentrations. Examples of such drugs include the antiarrhythmic drug procainamide and its active metabolite N-acetylprocainamide, which has antiarrhythmic effects similar to that of the parent drug. The therapeutic range for procainamide is 4–10 µg/mL and many laboratories recommend the range of 10–30 µg/mL for the sum of procainamide and N-acetylprocainamide concentrations [11].

Similarly when the drug is metabolized to a metabolite that can contribute significantly to the drug adverse effect, both the parent drug and the toxic metabolite should be measured, such as in the case of the antiepileptic drug carbamazepine that is metabolized to carbamazepine-10,11-epoxide. This metabolite contributes significantly to the therapeutic and toxic effects of carbamazepine. The therapeutic range for carbamazepine is 4–12 µg/mL, and it is recommended to keep the carbamazepine-10,11-epoxide concentration between 0.4 and 4 µg/mL [11].

23.6.4 ANALYTICAL TECHNIQUE

The application of TDM has been facilitated by the development of rapid, selective, sensitive, accurate, and precise analytical techniques that are suitable for quantifying the drug concentration in biological fluids. Currently, the majority of the drug assays performed in clinical settings utilize the commercially available immunoassays. This includes the fluorescence polarization immunoassay (FPIA), the enzyme immunoassay (EMIT), and the enzyme-linked immunoassay (ELISA). These methods are widely used because they are easily automated to ensure short turnaround time. The main disadvantage of these methods is their potential lack of selectivity due to cross-reactivity with compounds that are structurally related to the analyte of interest leading to overestimation or underestimation of the drug concentration. Also, these methods can only be applied for the analysis of drugs when the special reagents required for their analysis are commercially available. So the immunoassays cannot be readily applied for the analysis of newly developed drugs or the drugs that are not routinely monitored.

The other commonly used analytical techniques include the high-performance liquid chromatography (HPLC) and ultra-performance liquid chromatography (UPLC), which can be applied for a variety of drugs with minimal sample preparation procedures. Also, gas chromatography (GC) can be used for the analysis of volatile drugs or drugs that can be derivatized to form a volatile derivative. GC involves extensive sample preparation procedures, so it is usually used for the analysis of drugs that cannot be analyzed by the HPLC and UPLC techniques such as valproic acid. The coupling of the mass spectrometry (MS) with the HPLC and UPLC techniques led to the development of the LC-MS and LC-MS-MS techniques that revolutionized the analytical approach to TDM. The LC-MS-MS technique has the advantage of extreme sensitivity, the ability to analyze more than one drug simultaneously, and the ability to quantify the drug and its metabolite in the same run. The analytical assays developed utilizing the HPLC, UPLC, GC, and LC-MS-MS techniques are usually selective, sensitive, accurate, and precise. However, using these techniques requires extensive analytical skills and shifting from one analytical condition to the other takes time, which prolongs the turnaround time compared to the immunoassays. These techniques are usually used as the reference methods for the validation of the immunoassays [6].

The other analytical techniques used for the analysis of drug in biological samples include the radioimmunoassay (RIA). This technique is not commonly used for the routine analysis of samples in clinical settings because of the complexity associated with the handling of radioactive materials. Other techniques include the use of ion-selective electrodes in the analysis of lithium in biological fluids. All the analytical techniques used for the analysis of drugs in biological fluids to support the TDM should be fully validated. The analytical technique should be validated for accuracy, precision, selectivity, sensitivity, linearity, reproducibility, and robustness to ensure that the measured drug concentrations are reliable.

23.7 ESTABLISHING A THERAPEUTIC DRUG MONITORING (CLINICAL PHARMACOKINETIC) SERVICE

The TDM is a multidisciplinary activity that involves cooperation between the clinicians, pharmacists, nurses, and analysts. It is well documented that application of this service can facilitate the achievement of the desired therapeutic outcomes and decrease the incidence of adverse effects. So application of this service can be beneficial for the patients and can have pharmacoeconomic benefits.

23.7.1 Major Requirements

Establishing a TDM service in a healthcare institution requires the availability of trained healthcare professionals to run the service in addition to laboratory facility for drug analysis. The drug analysis facility to support the TDM service should have sensitive, accurate, specific, and rapid techniques for drug analysis in blood and other biological fluids. The pharmacy department that usually runs this service should have trained pharmacists who have the basic pharmacokinetic knowledge required to interpret the measured drug concentrations and examine the clinical data to recommend the appropriate dosing regimen for each patient. In addition to the clinical judgment, the pharmacists usually utilize computer software that can use the patient dosing history and the measured drug concentrations for estimating the patient-specific pharmacokinetic parameters and calculating the recommended dose for each patient. A wide variety of software are available ranging from simple software for handheld calculators to sophisticated software that stores the patient information every time it is used in a database and uses the stored database in subsequent recommendations.

23.7.2 Procedures

Optimization of drug therapy can be achieved empirically sometimes at considerable expense, time, and occasional toxicity. However, drug concentration in biological fluids can serve as a therapeutic endpoint to guide and assess drug therapy, and to guard against toxicity. Application of TDM usually goes through the following steps [11].

23.7.2.1 Determination of the Initial Dosing Regimen

The first step usually involves the selection of an initial dosing regimen for the patient to start the drug therapy. The patient's specific demographic information including age, sex, weight, organ function, nutritional status, and other medications are used to estimate the patient's pharmacokinetic parameters for the drug under consideration. The estimated drug pharmacokinetic parameters for the patient are used to calculate the initial dosage requirements for the patient. So the pharmacokinetic parameters used in the calculation of the initial dosing regimen for the patient are the pharmacokinetic parameters of the drug in a population similar to that of the patient being monitored.

23.7.2.2 Determination of the Patient's Specific Pharmacokinetic Parameters

After the start of drug therapy, the next step should be the determination of the patient's specific pharmacokinetic parameters for the drug. This is usually achieved by planning a sampling strategy that will allow calculation of the patient's specific drug pharmacokinetic parameters. The number of samples and the timing of these samples can be different depending on the drug being monitored as described previously. Knowledge of the clinical pharmacokinetics of the drug used by the patient can help in determining the number of samples required to estimate the patient's specific pharmacokinetic parameters and the time of these samples relative to the administered dose. The obtained sample(s) should be analyzed to determine the drug concentration using a validated analytical technique. The measured concentrations can be used to estimate the patient's specific pharmacokinetic parameters for the drug using the appropriate data analysis software.

23.7.2.3 Calculation of the Dosage Requirements Based on the Patient's Specific Pharmacokinetic Parameters of the Drug

The third step is to use the patient's estimated specific pharmacokinetic parameters to calculate the dosing regimen that should achieve a steady-state drug concentration within the therapeutic range. This calculated dosing regimen is specific for this particular patient because it is calculated based on the patient's specific pharmacokinetic parameters. Recommendations should be made to adjust the dosing regimen to achieve the desired therapeutic concentration. If the patient continues to receive the drug for a long time, such as in the treatment of chronic diseases as in epilepsy and cardiovascular diseases, it is important to periodically check the blood drug concentration to make sure that the drug concentrations continue to fall within the therapeutic range. Further dosage adjustment can be made based on the results of these follow-up samples.

23.7.3 PHARMACOECONOMICS OF THERAPEUTIC DRUG MONITORING

It has been well documented that the application of TDM service improves the patient response to many drugs and decreases the incidence of adverse drug reactions. Application of this service usually utilizes many resources such as equipment, space, analysis cost, software, training of the clinical and laboratory staff, and personnel effort in addition to other costs associated with applying this service. However, this cost is supposed to be counterbalanced by the positive patient outcomes such as decreased incidence of adverse drug reactions and decreased length of hospitalization. Pharmacoeconomic analysis of the impact of the TDM in adult patients with tonic-colonic epilepsy showed that application of TDM improved the seizure control, reduced the incidence of adverse reactions, increased the chance for remission, improved the patient earning capacity, and decreased the cost for patients due to lower hospitalization per seizures [12]. Also, a meta-analysis of TDM studies showed that TDM is beneficial for patients taking digoxin and theophylline. This study also showed that the TDM service run by clinical pharmacists had higher chances of achieving desirable drug concentrations and decreased the frequency of inappropriately collected samples [13]. Several studies also examined the role of TDM in optimization of aminoglycoside therapy by targeting the maximum and minimum blood concentrations associated with increased efficacy and reducing the incidence of aminoglycoside toxicity. These studies demonstrated high cost-effectiveness of dose individualization of aminoglycosides using TDM [14].

REFERENCES

1. Gross AS (2001) Best practice in therapeutic drug monitoring. *Br J Clin Pharmacol* 52(Suppl 1):5S–10S.
2. Rowland M and Tozer TN (2011) *Clinical Pharmacokinetics and Pharmacodynamics: Concepts and Applications*, 4th edn., Lippincott Williams & Wilkins, Philadelphia, PA.
3. Kang JS and Lee MH (2009) Overview of therapeutic drug monitoring. *Korean J Intern Med* 24:1–10.
4. Aronson JK and Hardman M (1992) ABC of monitoring drug therapy: Measuring plasma drug concentrations. *BMJ* 305:1078–1080.
5. Reynolds DJ and Aronson JK (1993) ABC of monitoring drug therapy: Making the most of plasma drug concentration measurements. *BMJ* 306:48–51.
6. Llorente Fernández E, Parés L, Ajuria I, Bandres F, Castanyer B, Campos F, Farré C, Pou L, Queraltó JM, and To-Figueras J (2010) State of the art in therapeutic drug monitoring. *Clin Chem Lab Med* 48:437–446.
7. Mann K, Hiemke C, Schmidt LG, and Bates DW (2006) Appropriateness of therapeutic drug monitoring for antidepressants in routine psychiatric inpatient care. *Ther Drug Monit* 28:83–88.
8. Hammett-Stabler CA and Johns T (1998) Laboratory guidelines for monitoring of antimicrobial drugs. National Academy of Clinical Biochemistry. *Clin Chem* 44:1129–1140.
9. Chan K and Beran RG (2008) Value of therapeutic drug level monitoring and unbound (free) levels. *Seizure* 17:572–575.
10. Sproule B, Nava-Ocampo AA, and Kapur B (2006) Measuring unbound versus total valproate concentrations for therapeutic drug monitoring. *Ther Drug Monit* 28:714–715.
11. Bauer LA (2008) *Applied Clinical Pharmacokinetics*, McGraw-Hill Companies Inc., New York.
12. Rane CT, Dalvi SS, Goptay NJ, and Shah PU (2001) A pharmacoeconomic analysis of the impact of therapeutic drug monitoring in adult patients with generalized tonic-clonic epilepsy. *Br J Clin Pharmacol* 52:193–195.
13. Ried LD, Horn JR, and McKenna DA (1990) Therapeutic drug monitoring reduces toxic drug reactions: A meta-analysis. *Ther Drug Monit* 12:72–78.
14. Streetman DS, Nafziger AN, Destache CJ, and Bertino AS Jr. (2001) Individualized pharmacokinetic monitoring results in less aminoglycoside-associated nephrotoxicity and fewer associated cost. *Pharmacotherapy* 21:443–451.

24 Pharmacokinetics in Special Patient Populations

OBJECTIVES

After completing this chapter you should be able to

- Discuss the regulatory requirements for pharmacokinetic studies in special populations
- List the factors that affect the change in drug pharmacokinetics in patients with renal dysfunction
- Analyze the effect of changing the kidney function and the liver function on the drug pharmacokinetics behavior after IV and oral administration
- Describe the general approaches for dosage recommendation in patients with kidney dysfunction and liver diseases
- Discuss the drug properties that increase the drug elimination during continuous renal replacement therapy
- Describe the effect of obesity on the pharmacokinetics of different drugs
- Discuss the age-related changes in the gastrointestinal secretion and motility, body composition, and eliminating organ function that can affect the drug pharmacokinetic behavior
- Describe the factors that can contribute to the change in drug pharmacokinetics during pregnancy
- List the drug properties that can increase its excretion in milk

24.1 INTRODUCTION

The drug pharmacokinetic behavior and response observed in different patients after administration of the same dose of the same drug can be variable. There are many factors that can contribute to this variability including genetic factors, diseases, body weight, age, drug interactions, gender, nutritional status, smoking, environmental factors, seasonal variation, and so on. Some of these factors can be quantitatively correlated with the variation in the drug pharmacokinetics and response, such as the eliminating organ dysfunction, while quantitative relationship cannot be established between the pharmacokinetic variability and other factors such as gender, nutritional status, environmental factors, and seasonal variation. Also, the effect of each of these factors on the pharmacokinetics behavior of different drugs is not the same. The effect of the reduction in kidney function on the rate of drug elimination is more significant on the renally eliminated drugs, and the effect of obesity on the pharmacokinetic behavior of hydrophilic and lipophilic drugs is different.

Classification of the entire patient population based on the factors that affect the drug pharmacokinetics and response such as age, weight, and eliminating organ function creates a group of subpopulations with relatively homogenous demographic characteristics. The differences in the drug response between the different subpopulations can be large; however, the variability between the individuals within each of these subpopulations is relatively small. The variability in drug response between the different patient subpopulations arises from differences in the drug pharmacokinetic behavior and the sensitivity of the individuals in different subpopulations to the therapeutic and toxic effects of the drug compared to the "normal" subjects. So it is important to identify the potential pharmacokinetic behavior modification in different patient populations to guide the proper dosing regimen recommendations for these populations. This is because achieving a specific therapeutically relevant systemic exposure measure can be considered an appropriate target to calculate the dose required for different patients. For example, the appropriate dose for patients of a special population should achieve AUC in these patients similar to the AUC achieved in the general patient population after administration of the average recommended drug dose for the general population. The assumption is that similar systemic exposure in different patients should produce similar therapeutic and adverse drug effects. Understanding the mechanisms by which the physiological and pathological changes in different populations affect different pharmacokinetic processes can help in predicting the pharmacokinetic behavior of drugs in these patient populations. This can be valuable for the design of pharmacokinetic studies in special patient populations to guide the recommendation of the appropriate dosing regimens of the drug in these special populations as required by the regulatory authorities.

24.2   REGULATORY ASPECTS OF PHARMACOKINETIC STUDIES IN SPECIAL POPULATIONS

All the drug regulatory authorities around the world recommend studying the drug pharmacokinetic behavior in special patient populations [1–3]. The primary objectives of these studies are to determine if any patient subpopulation requires special dosage recommendations to ensure optimal drug efficacy and safety and to guide these recommendations. The required pharmacokinetic studies in special populations differ from one drug to the other depending on several factors including the intended drug use, drug pharmacokinetic characteristics, and the therapeutic window of the drug. For example, drugs intended for use in fertile women do not require pharmacokinetic studies to investigate the gender effect on drug pharmacokinetics, and pharmacokinetic differences in children and elderly. Also, drugs that are eliminated mainly by renal excretion and are not highly bound to plasma protein require studies to investigate their elimination in patients with kidney dysfunction and do not require studies in patients with liver diseases. Furthermore, the pharmacokinetic studies in special populations become necessary only when the change in the drug pharmacokinetics in these populations results in change in the efficacy and safety of the drug.

Investigation of the pharmacokinetic behavior in special populations is usually carried out either by conventional pharmacokinetic studies where many samples are obtained from small number of subjects or by population pharmacokinetic studies where sparse samples are obtained from a large number of patients. Studying the factors that affect the drug pharmacokinetics should cover the widest range of factors because extrapolation of the results outside the range of the factors studied is not appropriate. For example, studies designed to investigate the effect of reduced renal function on drug pharmacokinetics should include patients with mild, moderate, severe, and end-stage renal failure. In this case, the conclusions and recommendations of the studies will cover all patients with varying degrees of kidney dysfunction. The drug concentration-effect relationship developed during phase II and phase III of clinical drug development is used to define a target exposure range for safe and effective treatments. The assumption is that the drug concentration-effect relationship in these special populations is similar to that of the general patient population. These target exposure measures can be achieved by maintaining the entire drug concentration–time profile within a certain concentration range. Also, summary variables that can reflect the drug exposure can be utilized by defining a range of AUC and minimum drug concentrations at steady state to assess drug efficacy and a range of the maximum drug concentration at steady state to assess drug toxicity.

If the results of the special population pharmacokinetic studies show that the drug exposure in any of the patient groups falls outside the accepted target exposure range for safety and efficacy, appropriate treatment recommendation should be developed for this specific patient population. The recommendation is made to ensure that the majority of patients in this special population get drug exposure within the range of the desired target exposure. When it is not possible to develop a suitable dosing recommendation for a special population for any reason, it is appropriate to include a warning in the drug label for possible compromised efficacy and/or safety when using the drug in this special population. It is also possible to include a recommendation for monitoring parameters that should be followed whenever the drug is used in this patient population. Exclusion of a special population from the drug indication is also possible when appropriate dosage recommendation in this special population is not possible and there is great potential for serious clinical consequences related to the efficacy and safety of the drug if used in this special population.

24.3 PATIENTS WITH RENAL DYSFUNCTION

The majority of hydrophilic drugs are excreted unchanged to a certain extent by the kidney. The nephron, which is the functional unit in the kidney, is responsible for the excretory function of the kidney. The free drug in the blood reaching the kidney is filtered through the glomerular membrane. The drug can be actively secreted by specific transport system mainly in the proximal tubules, and a fraction of the filtered and secreted drug can be reabsorbed from the renal tubules by passive and active mechanisms. The remaining drug in the renal tubules is collected in the collecting ducts and then in the urinary bladder until it is excreted with urine. The functional loss of the nephrons in renal diseases results in reduction in the renal excretion rate of drugs depending on the degree of kidney dysfunction. This usually causes alteration in the drug pharmacokinetics and hence pharmacodynamics depending on the contribution of the renal elimination pathway to the overall drug elimination process.

The main effect of renal dysfunction on the drug pharmacokinetics results from the reduction in the renal excretion of the drug and its metabolites. However, renal dysfunction can also affect the drug absorption, metabolism, protein binding, and distribution. These effects are more pronounced in patients with severe renal dysfunction and have been observed even when the renal elimination pathway is not the primary route for drug elimination. The reduction in hepatic metabolism in these patients has been attributed to the renal dysfunction-associated pathological and physiological alterations in every organ system in the body including the liver. Other evidences suggest that the accumulation of unspecified endogenous inhibitors known as uremic toxins in renal dysfunction patients can reduce the hepatic enzyme activity and expression [4]. In addition to their effect on the metabolizing enzymes, uremic toxins have been implicated in alteration of the transport system or transport activity in the kidney, liver, and intestine in normal and renal failure patients. This can contribute to the alteration in the distribution and nonrenal elimination of drugs in patients with renal dysfunction [5]. All the commonly used methods for calculating the dosing regimen requirements in renal dysfunction patients assume that the reduction in renal function only affects the renal elimination of the drugs.

24.3.1 DOSING REGIMENS IN RENAL DYSFUNCTION PATIENTS BASED ON CREATININE CLEARANCE

The initial dose estimation for renally eliminated drugs in renal dysfunction patients is usually based on the patient's creatinine clearance. This is because the decrease in kidney function, which is reflected by the decrease in creatinine clearance, results in the decrease in renal clearance of the drug. Determination and estimation of creatinine clearance as a measure of renal function has been discussed in Chapter 14. The creatinine clearance can be determined from the 24 h urine collection and calculation of the average creatinine excretion rate. The creatinine clearance is determined by dividing the average creatinine excretion rate by the serum creatinine concentration. Several empirical methods have been used to estimate the creatinine clearance from different parameters that can affect the creatinine clearance such as age, weight, and serum creatinine. The Cockoroft and Gault method mentioned in Chapter 14 can be used to estimate the creatinine clearance in adults from 18 years and older with stable serum creatinine. Other methods are available for estimating creatinine clearance in patients with unstable serum creatinine, in children, and other patient populations. The creatinine clearance can be used using the Cockoroft and Gault method as in Equations 24.1 and 24.2:

For men:

$$\text{CrCL} = \frac{(140 - \text{age})(\text{wt in kg})}{72(\text{S.Cr. in mg/dL})} \tag{24.1}$$

For women:

$$CrCL = 0.85 \left(\frac{(140 - age)(wt \text{ in kg})}{72(S.Cr. \text{ in mg/dL})} \right) \tag{24.2}$$

Dosage modification in patients with kidney dysfunction can be empirically based on kidney function and on the fraction of the drug dose excreted unchanged in urine. A modest reduction in drug dose is recommended when creatinine clearance decreases below 60 mL/min, moderate reduction in dose when creatinine clearance decreases below 30 mL/min, and significant reduction when creatinine clearance is lower than 15 mL/min. This empirical guidance is for selecting the initial dose, and further dose adjustment is usually based on the clinical drug response. The reduction in drug dose in renal failure patients can be achieved by reducing the dose or prolongation of the dosage intervals. In drugs like the aminoglycoside antibiotics where target concentrations are required for maximum and minimum plasma drug concentrations, modification of dose and dosing interval may be necessary to achieve these target concentrations.

It is also possible to use the patient's creatinine clearance to calculate the drug pharmacokinetic parameter based on prior data obtained in other renal dysfunction patients. The estimated pharmacokinetic parameters of the drug are used to calculate the dosage requirement in the patient. For example, digoxin CL_T can be calculated from creatinine clearance based on the following equation:

$$CL_{Digoxin} \text{ (mL/min)} = 1.303 \, CrCL \text{ (mL/min)} + CL_{NR} \tag{24.3}$$

where CL_{NR} is the nonrenal clearance of digoxin and it is equal to 40 mL/min in patients with mild heart failure and 20 mL/min in moderate to severe heart failure [6]. Also, digoxin Vd can be estimated based on the following equation:

$$Vd_{Digoxin}(L) = 226 + \frac{298 \, CrCL \text{ (mL/min)}}{29.1 + CrCL \text{ (mL/min)}} \tag{24.4}$$

The decrease in renal function manifested by a decrease in creatinine clearance results in smaller Vd for digoxin. This results from accumulation of the uremic toxins that cause displacement of digoxin from its tissue binding sites [7]. Another example is the estimation of the elimination rate constant (k) for the aminoglycoside antibiotics from the patient creatinine clearance as follows [8]:

$$k \, (h^{-1}) = 0.00293 \, CrCL \text{ (mL/min)} + 0.014 \tag{24.5}$$

The mathematical relationships as in Equations 24.3 through 24.5 are derived from the drug pharmacokinetic parameters and the creatinine clearance calculated in a large number of renal dysfunction patients. These relationships can only be applied for calculating the initial dosage regimen for the specific drugs that they were developed for. After initiation of the drug therapy, the patients should be monitored clinically or by measuring the plasma drug concentrations, and the dosage regimen should be modified as warranted.

24.3.2 GENERAL APPROACH FOR CALCULATION OF DOSING REGIMENS IN RENAL DYSFUNCTION PATIENTS

The magnitude of the change in the drug CL_T in renal dysfunction patients depends on the extent of drug excretion by the kidney and the degree of kidney dysfunction. Drugs that are mainly excreted by the kidney are affected more by the decrease in kidney function and require larger reduction in their doses to achieve therapeutic drug concentrations in this patient population. Also, patients with lower kidney function require larger reduction of their doses to achieve therapeutic drug concentrations.

The general method described by Giusti and Hayton and the Tozer approach for dose adjustment in renal dysfunction patients has the following assumptions [9]:

- The kidney dysfunction does not affect the concentration-effect relationship, that is, the therapeutic range does not change due to the change in kidney function.
- The decrease in kidney function results in a proportional decrease in the rate of renal drug elimination.
- The decrease in kidney function does not affect the nonrenal drug elimination.
- The decrease in kidney function does not affect drug absorption or distribution.

This approach requires knowledge of the average drug dose in patients with normal kidney function, the kidney function of the patient, and the fraction of the IV drug dose excreted unchanged in urine in patient with normal kidney function. This information can be used to calculate the dose required for patients with kidney dysfunction to achieve an average steady-state concentration similar to that achieved in patients with normal kidney function when they use the average dose of the drug. The kidney function (KF) is expressed as the fraction remaining of the normal kidney function and is determined from the ratio of creatinine clearance in the patient to normal creatinine clearance:

$$KF = \frac{CrCL_{failure}}{CrCL_{normal}} \qquad (24.6)$$

The fraction of the IV dose excreted unchanged in urine (f) can be determined from the ratio of the total amount of the drug excreted in urine and the IV dose or the bioavailable oral dose as in Equations 24.7 and 24.8:

$$Fraction~(f) = \frac{A_{e\infty}}{Dose_{IV}} \qquad (24.7)$$

$$Fraction~(f) = \frac{A_{e\infty}}{F~Dose_{oral}} \qquad (24.8)$$

Also, the fraction excreted unchanged in urine can be determined from the ratio of the renal excretion rate constant to the elimination rate constant or the ratio of the renal clearance to the total body clearance as follows:

$$\text{Fraction (f)} = \frac{k_e}{k} = \frac{CL_R}{CL_T} \qquad (24.9)$$

The fraction of the dose normally excreted unchanged in the urine, the kidney function, and the average dose used in patients with normal kidney function can be used to calculate the dose required in patients with renal dysfunction as follows:

$$\text{Dose}_{\text{failure}} = \text{Dose}_{\text{normal}}[f(KF-1)+1] \qquad (24.10)$$

Administration of the dose calculated using Equation 24.10 at the same dosing interval as the average dose should achieve average drug concentrations in renal dysfunction patients similar to that achieved in patients with normal kidney function when they receive the average dose of the drug. Also, the half-life in patients with renal dysfunction patients can be determined from the following relationship:

$$t_{1/2\,\text{failure}} = \frac{t_{1/2\,\text{normal}}}{[f(KF-1)+1]} \qquad (24.11)$$

Example

A patient admitted to the hospital because of acute myocardial infarction was started on oral antiarrhythmic medication. He received the average recommended dose for patients with normal kidney function, which is 600 mg every 12 h from an oral formulation that is known to be rapidly and completely absorbed. At steady state, the maximum and minimum plasma concentrations were 40 and 10 mg/mL, respectively.

a. Calculate mathematically the half-life and the volume of distribution of this drug in this patient.
b. The patient suddenly developed acute renal failure and the kidney function dropped to 30% of its normal value. If the renal clearance of this drug is 70% of the total body clearance, recommend an appropriate dose for this patient after developing the renal failure.
c. Calculate the maximum and minimum plasma concentration achieved at steady state from the regimen you recommended in part (b).

Answer

a.
$$Cp_{\text{max ss}} - Cp_{\text{min ss}} = \frac{\text{Dose}}{Vd}$$

$$40 - 10\,\text{mg/L} = \frac{600\,\text{mg}}{Vd}$$

$$Vd = \frac{600\,mg}{30\,mg/L} = 20 \text{ L}$$

$$Cp_{min\,ss} = Cp_{max\,ss}e^{-k\tau}$$

$$10\,mg/L = 40\,mg/L\ e^{-k\,12h}$$

$$\ln\frac{10\,mg/L}{40\,mg/L} = -k\,12\,h$$

$$-1.386 = -k\,12\,h$$

$$k = 0.1155\,h^{-1} \quad t_{1/2} = 6h$$

b.
$$f = \frac{CL_R}{CL_T} = \frac{70}{100} = 0.7$$

$$KF = 0.3$$

$$Dose_{failure} = Dose_{normal}[f(KF-1)+1]$$

$$Dose_{failure} = 600\,mg/12\,h[0.7(0.3-1)+1]$$

$$Dose_{failure} = 294\,mg/12\,h$$

c.
$$t_{1/2failure} = \frac{t_{1/2normal}}{[f(KF-1)+1]} = \frac{6h}{[0.7(0.3-1)+1]} = 12.24\,h$$

$$k_{failure} = \frac{0.693}{12.24} = 0.0566\,h^{-1}$$

$$Cp_{max\,ss} = \frac{D}{Vd(1-e^{-k\tau})}$$

$$Cp_{max\,ss} = \frac{294\,mg}{20L(1-e^{-0.0566\,h^{-1}\,12\,h})} = 29.8\,mg/L$$

$$Cp_{min\,ss} = Cp_{max\,ss}e^{-k\tau}$$

$$Cp_{min\,ss} = 29.8\ mg/L\ e^{-0.0566\,h^{-1}\,12\,h} = 15.1\ mg/L$$

24.4 PATIENTS RECEIVING RENAL REPLACEMENT THERAPY

Renal replacement therapy (RRT) is an approach used in acute and chronic renal failure patients for the removal of metabolic products accumulated in their systemic circulation due to impaired renal function as in intermittent hemodialysis (IHD). Continuous RRT (CRRT) such as hemofiltration and hemodiafiltration has been used in critically ill patients to remove the pro-inflammatory cytokines produced in response to infections that have been implicated for the development of multiple organ failure in these patients [10]. However, the use of these intermittent and continuous RRT leads to extracorporeal removal of drugs from the patients' circulation, which may significantly affect the pharmacokinetic behavior of drugs. This can have serious clinical consequences in cases such as antibiotic being significantly removed from the body during RRT in a critically ill patient with life-threatening infection. So the factors that affect the extracorporeal clearance of drugs and the measures that should be installed to compensate for this clearance should be considered.

24.4.1 PRINCIPLE OF HEMODIALYSIS AND HEMOFILTRATION

The removal of solutes from the blood through a semipermeable membrane during RRT occurs by diffusion or convection. In hemodialysis, the blood and the dialysis fluid are separated by a semipermeable membrane, and the drug removal from the blood occurs by passive diffusion according to the concentration gradient. The blood flows in the opposite direction of the flow of the dialysis fluid to maintain the highest concentration gradient and increase the efficiency of solute removal as in Figure 24.1. The cutoff for modern dialyser membranes allows removal of almost all small molecular weight drugs from the blood during the dialysis process. Only protein molecules and drug molecules that are bound to plasma proteins cannot be cleared during the hemodialysis process. However, in hemofiltration, a positive pressure is applied to the blood, which produces pressure gradient that forces the removal of substances by convection through a membrane that acts as a hemofilter as in Figure 24.2. The hemofilter has molecular weight cutoff that allows filtration of all small molecular weight drug molecules that are not bound to plasma protein

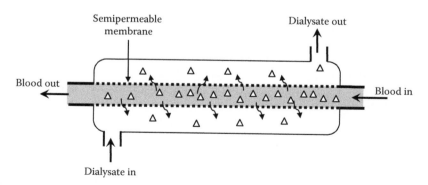

FIGURE 24.1   Schematic presentation of the principle of hemodialysis. Δ, free drug molecules.

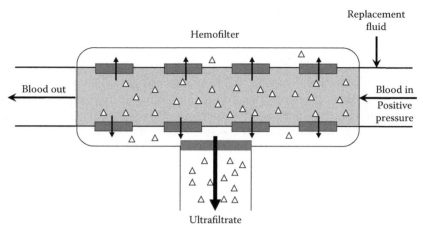

FIGURE 24.2 Schematic presentation of the principle of hemofiltration. Δ, free drug molecules.

and prevent passage of protein molecules. The fluid lost from the blood with the ultrafiltrate during the process is usually replaced either before or after the blood filtration process.

24.4.2 FACTORS AFFECTING DRUG CLEARANCE DURING RRT

The efficiency of RRT in clearing drugs from the blood depends on several factors related to the drug, the device, and the patient. In general, RRT and CRRT are used to replace the impaired renal function in clearing the blood from all the metabolic waste products that are normally excreted by the kidney. During these processes, drug molecules can also be removed from the blood. In general, hydrophilic drugs with relatively small Vd that are not highly bound to plasma protein are significantly cleared from the blood during RRT. Hydrophilic drugs are usually excreted unchanged by the kidney and do not have significant nonrenal clearance. So the excretion of hydrophilic drugs during RRT has significant contribution to their overall elimination. When the drug has small Vd, the amount of the drug cleared from the blood during RRT represents significant portion of the total amount of the drug in the body. So the blood concentration of drugs that have small Vd declines during RRT faster than that for drugs with high Vd. Because of the cutoff limit for the clearance of compounds across the semipermeable membrane in the RRT devices, only free drug molecules can be cleared from the blood. So drugs that are not significantly bound to plasma protein are cleared from the blood during the RRT better than highly bound drugs. The drug protein binding may be reduced in patients with lower plasma protein concentration, which may increase the drug clearance during RRT due to the increased drug-free fraction.

IHD is usually performed in patients for a period of 3–4 h and is repeated two to three times a week. When the drug is cleared from the blood during hemodialysis, this clearance will only occur during the hemodialysis period, while CRRT causes continuous clearance of the drug from the blood and may cause rapid decline in blood drug concentration. Other factors that can affect the clearance of drugs during RRT are the characteristics of the device used including the surface area and the dialyser membrane molecular weight cutoff limit. Devices with higher surface area usually clear the drug more efficiently from the blood. Although the clearance of drug molecules across the dialyser membrane depends on the molecular size, most new devices include high-flux dialyser membranes that have molecular weight cutoff limit that allows clearance of all nonprotein drugs.

24.4.3 Dose Adjustment during RRT

In general, patients undergoing IHD may have significant amount of the drug removed during the dialysis period. In this case, supplemental doses of the drugs can be administered after the end of the hemodialysis period to compensate for the amount of the drug cleared by the dialyser. The dose of the drug administered after hemodialysis is dependent on the extent of drug removal during the hemodialysis process. For example, the aminoglycosides antibiotics are hydrophilic drugs with relatively small Vd and very limited plasma protein binding, which make large fractions of the amount of these drugs in the body to get eliminated during hemodialysis. So it is recommended that patients receiving the aminoglycosides antibiotic to treat life-threatening infections should get additional doses of aminoglycosides after the end of hemodialysis to compensate for the amount of aminoglycosides cleared during hemodialysis.

On the other hand, CRRT represents a continuous mean of clearance of endogenous compounds as well as exogenous compounds including drugs. Drugs that are significantly cleared from the body during CRRT usually need significant increase in dose to compensate for the increased drug clearance. The important parameter that reflects the efficiency of drug clearance during CRRT is the extracorporeal clearance. The estimated drug clearance during CRRT is compared with the normal renal clearance of each drug to determine the role of CRRT in drug elimination. Drugs that have low clearance during CRRT may not require any modification in their doses. However, drugs that are significantly cleared during CRRT may require significant increase in dose compared to the doses used in renal failure or during IHD. This is usually achieved either by the increase in dose or administration of the same dose more frequently. The choice usually depends on the dosing regimen that can maintain the plasma drug concentration within the target range all the time. Increasing the dose while keeping the dosing regimen fixed results in higher $Cp_{max\ ss}$ and lower $Cp_{min\ ss}$, while administration of the same dose at shorter dosing interval usually achieves lower $Cp_{max\ ss}$ and higher $Cp_{min\ ss}$. A compiled list of recommendations is available for the doses of many antimicrobial drugs when used during CRRT [11].

24.5 PATIENTS WITH HEPATIC INSUFFICIENCY

The liver plays a central role in the pharmacokinetic behavior of most drugs. The decrease in the liver function results in reduction in the rate of hepatic drug metabolism and biliary excretion. Hepatic dysfunction can also affect the plasma protein binding, which can affect the drug distribution and elimination. The presystemic metabolism of orally administered drugs can also be affected in patients with impaired liver function leading to increase in bioavailability especially for high extraction ratio drugs. Liver dysfunction is usually associated with nonuniform reduction in the hepatic metabolizing enzymes with different cytochrome P450 (CYP450) enzymes affected to different degrees. The glucuronidation metabolic pathway is usually affected to lesser extent compared to CYP450 enzymes. Patients with advanced liver cirrhosis often have impaired renal function and the rate of renally eliminated drugs is also affected.

The two major types of hepatic diseases are hepatitis and cirrhosis. Hepatitis is characterized by inflammation of the liver and as a result the hepatocyte function may be compromised. In acute hepatitis, minor dosage modification may be required, while in chronic hepatitis the hepatocyte damage can be widespread and dosage adjustment may be required at some point. Hepatic cirrhosis is characterized by fibrosis and reduction of the number and activity of the hepatocytes and a reduction of the hepatic blood flow. These changes lead to the development of clinical manifestations such as esophageal varices, edema, ascites, and hepatic encephalopathy, which contribute to the pharmacokinetic and pharmacodynamic changes observed in liver dysfunction. Also, there is reduction in albumen synthesis leading to change in the drug protein binding in these patients, which can have pharmacokinetic and pharmacodynamic consequences. Furthermore, the function of other organs such as the intestine, lung, and kidney can be affected by liver cirrhosis and may develop into hepatorenal syndrome, which leads to severe renal impairment.

24.5.1 PHARMACOKINETIC AND PHARMACODYNAMIC CHANGES IN HEPATIC DYSFUNCTION

The absorption, distribution, metabolism, and elimination of many drugs can be affected by hepatic dysfunction. The extent of drug absorption of intermediate and high extraction ratio drugs is significantly increased in patients with hepatic dysfunction due to the reduction in their presystemic metabolism. These drugs normally undergo extensive first-pass effect and their systemic bioavailability is usually low. Even a small change in the fraction of the administered dose that escapes the presystemic elimination due to hepatic dysfunction results in significant increase in drug bioavailability. There are evidences that both hepatic and intestinal metabolism are diminished in patients with hepatic dysfunction. Low extraction ratio drugs do not undergo significant presystemic metabolism, so their bioavailability is not significantly affected in patients with hepatic dysfunction.

The drug distribution is dependent on the drug binding to plasma proteins, blood cells, and tissue proteins. Drugs that are highly bound to plasma proteins such as albumin or α_1-acid glycoprotein have significantly higher free fraction in patients with hepatic dysfunction. The reduction in the drug plasma protein binding in hepatic diseases can be due to the decrease in albumin and α_1-acid glycoprotein synthesis, the accumulation of endogenous compounds such as bilirubin that can compete with the drug for the binding sites, and the qualitative changes in the plasma proteins that can affect the drug binding [12,13]. The increase in drug-free fraction increases the Vd of drugs. Also, water-soluble drugs usually have larger Vd in patients with ascites. The change in drug protein binding can also affect the clearance of drugs especially the low extraction ratio drugs that are highly bound to plasma proteins.

The liver is the main site of drug metabolism. It has been recognized that the metabolism of many drugs is impaired in liver diseases due to the reduction in the liver cell mass and the decrease in enzyme activity. The CYP450 enzymes in general are affected more than the conjugating enzymes in liver diseases. Also, the effect of liver diseases on different CYP450 enzymes is not uniform with some CYP enzymes affected more than the others. Administration of a single dose of a mixture of drugs that are used as probes for the different CYP enzyme activity to normal volunteers and patients with different severity of liver diseases showed that different CYP enzymes are affected by the liver diseases to different extents [14]. Phase II metabolic reactions such as glucuronidation are not affected significantly except in patients with advanced cirrhosis. It has been proposed that the sparing of glucuronidation in liver cirrhosis is due to activation of latent UDP-glucuronosyltransferase (UGT) enzymes, upregulation of the UGT activity in the viable hepatocytes, and increased extrahepatic glucuronidation in liver cirrhosis patients [15]. Obstruction of bile flow caused by stones and tumors or reduced bile formation and secretion, which can be induced by some drugs, can reduce the clearance of endogenous and exogenous substances that are eliminated mainly by biliary excretion. Also, biliary obstruction can cause hepatocellular damage with impairment of the activity of several CYP enzymes [16]. So drugs eliminated from the body mainly by metabolism may require dosage adjustment in patients with cholestasis. The potential effect of liver dysfunction on the function of the transporters involved in the hepatocellular uptake and efflux of drugs and how this may affect the elimination of drugs remains to be determined.

The progressive impairment of renal function in patients with advanced hepatic diseases, known as the hepatorenal syndrome, with no other causes of renal failure is well documented. Patients with advanced cirrhosis have been shown to have reduced renal excretion of drugs that are usually eliminated by the kidney. Evaluation of kidney function based on serum creatinine measurement or measuring the creatinine clearance usually overestimates the glomerular filtration rate (GFR) in cirrhotic patients. This is because the conversion of creatine to creatinine is reduced and the creatinine tubular secretion is increased in cirrhotic patients. So the doses of drugs that are eliminated from the body by metabolism or by renal excretion should be adjusted in patients with advanced hepatic diseases.

The change in the drug pharmacokinetics in liver diseases can lead to alteration in drug response [12]. Also, modification of the drug therapeutic effect, which is not related to the change in drug pharmacokinetics, has been reported in liver cirrhosis. The change in drug pharmacodynamics in cirrhotic patients usually results from the change in drug-receptor affinity and binding characteristics, altered receptor intrinsic activity, and other physiological changes in these patients. Reduced effect of beta-blockers and diuretics, increased effect of narcotic analgesics and sedatives, and increased adverse effects of the nonsteroidal anti-inflammatory drugs have been reported in cirrhotic patients [17,18].

24.5.2 Dose Adjustment in Hepatic Dysfunction

Dose adjustment in patients with hepatic dysfunction is not an easy task. This is because there is no single clinical test that can be used for the assessment of liver function. Also, different metabolic enzyme systems are affected to different degrees by the reduction in liver function. The Child-Pugh classification has been used in clinical practice for categorizing patients according to the severity of their liver function impairment [18]. This classification utilizes five different laboratory tests and clinical conditions to assess the severity of liver disease: serum albumin, total bilirubin, prothrombin time, ascites, and encephalopathy. Each of these parameters is classified and is given a score of 1, 2, or 3 depending on the value of the parameter as in Table 24.1. The total Child-Pugh score is calculated from the sum of the scores for all the five parameters. The severity of the liver disease is determined from the total Child-Pugh score with patients having a score of 6–7 points classified as group A (mild), score of 8–9 group B (moderate), and score of 10–15 group C (severe). The Child-Pugh score can be useful in comparing patient groups and providing guidance for dose adjustment. However, this classification lacks the sensitivity for quantitatively predicting the specific ability of the liver to metabolize individual drugs.

The general recommendation for dose adjustment based on the Child-Pugh score is that patients with score of 8–9 require 25% reduction of their initial doses of drugs that are mainly eliminated from the body by hepatic metabolism (>60% metabolized), while patients with a score of 10 or more require 50% reduction of their initial doses of drugs that are mainly eliminated from the body by hepatic metabolism. It is important to note that this is a recommendation for the starting doses of the drugs. After starting drug therapy, the therapeutic and adverse effects of the drugs should be monitored and dose adjustment should be made if necessary.

In addition to the Child-Pugh classification, dynamic liver function tests have been developed to assess the liver handling of drugs in liver dysfunction patients. This is achieved by IV administration of exogenous compounds that are mainly eliminated by the liver and then following the disappearance of the compounds from the patient's systemic circulation or the appearance of a metabolite in plasma, urine, or in the expired air as in the breath test. Examples of these chemical probes include indocyanine green, galactose, sorbitol, antipyrine, caffeine, and midazolam. The $^{14}CO_2$ breath test has been used to evaluate the rate of metabolism of drugs such as

TABLE 24.1
Child-Pugh's Classification for Patients with Liver Diseases

Parameters	Score 1	2	3
Serum albumin (g/dL)	>3.5	2.8–3.5	<2.8
Total bilirubin (mg/dL)	<2.0	2.0–3.0	>3.0
Prothrombin time (seconds over control)	<4	4–6	>6
Ascites	Absent	Mild	Moderate
Encephalopathy	None	Moderate	Severe

aminopyrine, erythromycin, and caffeine. The ^{14}C labeled drugs are administered to the patients, and the $^{14}CO_2$ collected from the expired air is determined and is used as a measure for the rate of drug metabolism. The results of the breath test have been shown to correlate well with the Child-Pugh classification. There is no approach that has been shown to be superior than the other in dose adjustment in patients with liver diseases. However, the Child-Pugh score is used more in clinical practice to guide the dose adjustment in patients with liver diseases because the information required to apply this approach is readily available.

Example

A 55-year-old female was admitted to the hospital after developing an episode of ventricular arrhythmia. The patient had history of multiple medical problems including liver cirrhosis, hypertension, and ischemic heart disease. Her laboratory values upon admission were serum creatinine 1.1 mg/dL, serum albumin 3.2 g/dL, total bilirubin 4.5 mg/dL, and prothrombin time 8 s more than control. Physical examination showed that the patient is alert without any signs of encephalopathy, and the patient has mild ascites. The physician wanted to start the patient on lidocaine and asked you to recommend an average starting dose of lidocaine.

Answer

Lidocaine is an antiarrhythmic drug that is completely metabolized. So the patient's liver condition may affect the clearance of lidocaine. It is wise to calculate the Child-Pugh score for his patient according to Table 24.1 to determine if dose reduction is necessary.

Calculation of the Child-Pugh score:

Serum albumin	3.2 g/dL	Score = 2
Bilirubin	4.5 mg/dL	Score = 3
Prothrombin time	8 s > control	Score = 3
Ascites	Mild	Score = 2
Encephalopathy	Absent	Score = 1
	Total	Child-Pugh score = 11

According to the Child-Pugh score, the starting dose of lidocaine in this patient should be 50% of the average recommended dose of lidocaine. Lidocaine dose can be adjusted after the start of therapy according to the therapeutic and the adverse effects of lidocaine.

24.5.3 ADDITIONAL CONSIDERATIONS FOR DOSE ADJUSTMENT IN LIVER DYSFUNCTION

- The Food and Drug Administration and the European Medicines Agency recommend that companies should evaluate the pharmacokinetics of drugs in patients with impaired liver function during the drug development process. These studies should be directed to determine if special dose recommendation is required in liver dysfunction patients. For performing these studies, it is recommended to use the Child-Pugh approach in patient classification and also to evaluate the liver function using external chemical probes.

- Drugs with narrow therapeutic range should be used with caution in patients with sever hepatic dysfunction. General recommendations for dose adjustment for specific drugs in patient with liver cirrhosis have been published [19].
- High extraction ratio drugs have significant increase in their bioavailability in liver dysfunction patients and their oral dose should be reduced in these patients. The plasma clearance of these drugs is usually reduced when hepatic blood flow is reduced.
- The oral and systemic clearance of low extraction ratio drugs that are highly bound to plasma protein is determined from the liver intrinsic clearance and the free fraction of the drug in plasma. The intrinsic clearance is reduced to a degree dependent on the functional status of the liver and the free fraction is usually increased in liver dysfunction patients. Pharmacokinetic evaluation should be based on the free drug concentration in plasma and dose adjustment may be necessary even if the total drug concentration is within the normal range. However, the clearance of the low extraction ratio drugs that are not bound significantly to plasma protein is affected by the reduction of the hepatic intrinsic clearance and will not be affected by the change in protein binding. Dose selection should be aimed to achieve total drug concentration within the therapeutic range.
- The elimination of drugs that are partially excreted unchanged in urine is reduced in patients with the hepatorenal syndrome. The creatinine clearance determined in these patients is usually an overestimate of the GFR. Dose adjustment is necessary for renally excreted drugs in patients with advanced liver diseases.
- The volume of distribution for drugs in patients with hepatic dysfunction is usually increased due to edema and ascites, especially for hydrophilic drugs. So higher loading doses may be required in these patients.

24.6   OBESE PATIENTS

The terms obese and overweight refer to individuals with excess body weight compared to individuals with similar height, age, and gender. Obesity is usually accompanied by increased adipose tissues that result in change in the body composition. The increased body fat has been associated with a variety of diseases including heart diseases and diabetes mellitus and other health problems.

24.6.1   Assessment of Body Composition and Body Weight

The body composition can be determined by direct methods such as underwater weight, skin fold measurements, and dual-energy x-ray absorptiometry. However, these techniques are not readily available for the clinicians, so indirect methods are used. Clinicians use demographic patients' information to evaluate their body weight

---

TABLE 24.2
Body Mass Index Values
for Classification of Obesity

BMI (kg/m²)	Class
<18.8	Underweight
18.9–24.9	Normal weight
25.0–29.9	Overweight
30.0–34.9	Class I obesity (moderate)
35.0–39.9	Class II obesity (severe)
>40	Class III obesity (morbid)

---

such as body mass index (BMI), ideal body weight (IBW), percent IBW, lean body weight (LBW), and other measures. The BMI is the preferred measure for classifying obesity by the World Health Organization. It is calculated from the total body weight and the squared height as in Equation 24.12 and depending on the value of the BMI, patients can be classified according to Table 24.2:

$$BMI = \frac{Total\ body\ weight\,(kg)}{[Height\,(m)]^2} \tag{24.12}$$

The IBW that is the ideal weight for the patient based on his or her height (calculated for male patients here) is as follows:

$$IBW\,(kg) = 49.9\,kg\,(45.4\,kg\ for\ females) + 0.89\,(height\ in\ cm - 152.4) \tag{24.13}$$

while the percent of IBW is how much the TBW represents relative to the IBW and is determined as follows:

$$Percent\ IBW = \frac{TBW}{IBW} \times 100 \tag{24.14}$$

whereas LBW, which is the weight without any adipose tissue, is calculated as follows for males:

$$LBW\,(kg) = 1.10\,TBW - 0.0128 \times BMI \times TBW \tag{24.15}$$

and for females:

$$LBW\,(kg) = 1.07\,TBW - 0.0148 \times BMI \times TBW \tag{24.16}$$

24.6.2 Alteration in Drug Pharmacokinetics in Obese Patients

Obese patients have higher total body weight, LBW, and also adipose tissue weight. However, since the excess weight in obese individuals consists mainly of fat, this can change the body composition and increases the fat component of the body weight

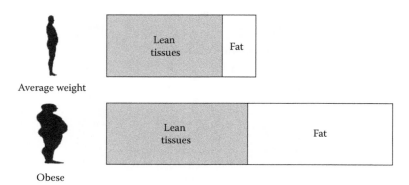

FIGURE 24.3 Diagram presenting the change in the body fat content in obese patients.

as in Figure 24.3. The drug distribution is the pharmacokinetic process that is most likely to be affected in obese patients. The Vd, which is the parameter that determines the extent of drug distribution to the tissues, is determined from the affinity of the drug to the tissues and the total body mass. In general, since the body fat content is usually increased in obese patients, the Vd/kg of relatively lipophilic drugs is usually increased in these patients [20]. The distribution of other drugs is affected to different extents.

The Vd is the parameter used for calculation of the loading dose of drugs required to rapidly achieve the desired drug concentration in the systemic circulation. If the Vd of the drug is 0.2 L/kg, the question that has to be answered is whether to calculate the total Vd of the drug based on the TBW or IBW in obese individuals. The weight descriptor that should be used to calculate the Vd depends on the distribution characteristics of the drugs. If the drug is distributed to all parts of the body including the fat component resulting from excess weight as in lipophilic drugs, the TBW should be used to calculate the total Vd, while for hydrophilic drugs that are mainly distributed in lean tissues and their distribution in fat is limited, the IBW is usually used to calculate the total Vd of the drug. Drugs with different distribution characteristics usually require different methods for calculating their Vd.

The use of different weight descriptors (TBW, IBW, LBW, etc.) to calculate the Vd of the drug has been investigated. The study concluded that there is no single weight descriptor that can predict the Vd for all drugs, and the best weight descriptor to predict the Vd of a drug is dependent on the properties of the drug of interest. The TBW was found to be the best single weight descriptor for calculating the Vd for about 40% of the studied drugs in obese patients. Weight descriptors, which account for the fat mass, such as TBW and percent IBW were preferred in moderate to highly lipophilic drugs when used in obese patients [21].

There are many examples for specific equations developed to calculate the Vd of specific drugs in obese patients, which is usually based on the distribution characteristics of the specific drug [22]. The aminoglycoside antibiotics are hydrophilic drugs that are mainly distributed in the extracellular fluid (ECF) and usually have an average Vd of about 0.26 L/kg. Since the volume of the ECF in the adipose tissues is only 40% of that in lean tissues, these drugs have lower distribution in adipose tissues. It is recommended that in obese patients (patients whose TBW is >130% of the IBW) the Vd for aminoglycosides should be calculated based on Equation 24.17. In this equation, the difference between TBW and IBW that represents the adipose tissues is multiplied by a factor of 0.4 to account for the lower extracellular fluids in adipose tissues:

$$Vd\,(L) = 0.26\,(L/kg)[IBW + 0.4(TBW - IBW)] \qquad (24.17)$$

Also, lipophilic drugs such as phenytoin usually have high affinity to fat and are distributed to adipose tissues more than their distribution to lean tissues. The Vd for phenytoin is usually calculated in obese patients using Equation 24.18. In this equation, the difference between TBW and IBW, which represents the adipose tissues, is multiplied by a factor of 1.33 to account for the higher affinity of this lipophilic drug to the adipose tissues:

$$Vd\,(L) = 0.7\,(L/kg)[IBW + 1.33(TBW - IBW)] \qquad (24.18)$$

whereas for drugs that are not distributed in adipose tissues like digoxin and theophylline, the IBW is usually used to calculate their Vd. This demonstrates that the drug characteristics are the main factor in determining the change in drug distribution in obese patients.

In addition to the effect on drug distribution, obese patients usually have higher gastrointestinal (GIT) perfusion due to the increased cardiac output, which may increase the drug absorption. Also, there is increased liver perfusion, which can increase the drug metabolism during the first-pass effect. There are no reported cases of significant alteration in drug bioavailability in case of obesity. Plasma protein binding is not significantly affected in obese patients. Obesity may have minor effect on hepatic metabolism resulting from minor increase in the activity of some enzyme systems and the change in hepatic blood flow. Since the CL_T is the pharmacokinetic parameter that relates the dosing rate and the steady-state concentration and the clearance does not change significantly in obese patients, the weight-normalized dose (mg/kg) should be calculated based on the weight descriptor that can correct for differences in absolute CL_T in obese and nonobese patients. It is important to note that the half-life for many drugs can be longer in obese patients due the larger Vd and the relatively constant CL_T. So evaluation of drug clearance in obese patients should not be based solely on the drug half-life.

24.7 PEDIATRIC PATIENTS

Pediatric patients are different from adult patients in many developmental, physiological, and psychological aspects. These differences make the drug pharmacokinetic and pharmacodynamic characteristics in children different from those in adults. So when designing dosing regimens, children should not be viewed as "miniature" adults. There are several guidelines that are used for selecting the doses for pediatric patients. This includes the age-based dosing regimen selection method that categorizes the patients according to their age to premature baby (<37 weeks gestational age), neonates

(<1 month), infants (1–24 months), children (2–12 years), and adolescence (12–16 to 18 years), and recommends the regimen for each group. However, this approach does not account for the overlap between these age groups and the variability within each group. Also, dosage regimens based on the body weight or based on weight-normalized pharmacokinetic parameters have been used; however, higher and lower dose limits have to be set to avoid overdose and undertreatment. Furthermore, doses have been calculated based on the body surface area (BSA) in pediatric patients. Besides, allometric scaling has been used to scale the drug pharmacokinetic parameters based on body weight. The scaled pharmacokinetic parameters are used to calculate the pediatric dosing regimen, which should produce plasma drug concentrations similar to the therapeutic concentrations in adults. The last two approaches can be used in children over the age of 8 years, but their utility in younger children, infants, and neonates is limited due to the numerous age-related differences in drug disposition. These dosing guidelines can be useful; however, there are developmental and physiological changes that occur in children, which can affect the pharmacokinetic behavior of drugs. These changes should be considered when selecting the dosage regimen for specific drugs in pediatric patients [23].

24.7.1 DEVELOPMENTAL CHANGES IN PEDIATRIC PATIENTS THAT AFFECT DRUG ABSORPTION

The pH of the stomach is usually neutral at birth due to the immaturity of the parietal cells. The gastric pH decreases to about pH 3 in 24 h after birth, returns to neutral after 7–10 days of birth, and then slowly declines to reach the adult value in 2 years. This can increase the absorption of acid-labile drugs such as penicillin G and erythromycin, reduce the absorption of weak acids such as phenobarbital and phenytoin, and increase in the absorption of weak bases [24]. The gastric emptying rate is usually delayed immediately after birth and reaches the adult value in 6–8 months. The GIT transit time is also prolonged immediately after birth due to the reduced intestinal motility. This can lead to slow absorption of drugs such as paracetamol and cisapride in neonates and young infants [24]. On the contrary, the short transit time in older children can cause incomplete absorption of sustained-release formulations. Other developmental differences include the immature intestinal mucosa and biliary function, increased intestinal glucuronidase activity, and reduced first-pass metabolism and transport activity. This leads to reduction in the absorption of fat-soluble vitamins in neonates and increase in the bioavailability of drugs such as midazolam and zidovudine due to the reduction in their first-pass metabolism [25]. So drugs that undergo first-pass metabolism in adults should be used with caution in children and dosage correction may be necessary in neonates and young infants because of the increased bioavailability of these drugs. Other age-related factors can also affect the drug absorption in the pediatric population. For example, frequent feeding, which is common in this population, increases the potential for drug-food interaction. Also, vomiting and diarrhea that occur frequently in this patient population can affect the absorption of drugs.

Only minor differences exist between the rectal absorption in children and in adults. For example, the rectum pH is slightly alkaline in children. Similar to adults, drugs absorbed in the upper part of the rectum are delivered to the liver where they can undergo first-pass metabolism, while drugs absorbed in the lower part of the rectum escape the first-pass metabolism. Rectal absorption of drugs such as keto-profen in children is similar to that in adults. The bioavailability of paracetamol after rectal administration has been shown to decrease with age possibly due to the increase in first-pass metabolism with age, while the lower bioavailability for trama-dol after rectal administration in children is due to the alkaline environment of the rectum in children. In general, children do not like this route of administration, so it should be used only when oral administration of drugs is not possible. Infants and children, especially breast-fed infants, usually defecate more frequently compared to adults, which may lead to incomplete absorption if defecation occurs shortly after rectal drug administration. Also, part of the administered dose can be lost when administered rectally in the form of solution. In general, there is no need for dosage alteration of drugs administered by the rectal route in children except when practical problems can alter the drug bioavailability such as diarrhea, when the drug under-goes significant first-pass metabolism (when given in the first weeks of life) and when the drugs are absorbed better in alkaline pH.

Percutaneous absorption in neonates and infants is significantly higher because this patient population has a thinner, less keratinized skin, and a well-hydrated stratum corneum. This can lead to significant increase in the absorption of drugs administered topically and may lead to toxic systemic exposure to drugs admin-istered for their local effect. Drugs that can produce significant systemic effect or toxicity should be applied on the skin with close medical supervision during the first 1 year of age, and may be avoided in the first 2 weeks of age unless it is nec-essary [26]. Absorption of drugs after intramuscular administration in neonates is unpredictable because of the variable blood flow to the muscles in the first 2–3 weeks of life, which can lead to complications. This route of administration is not accept-able by children because of the pain associated with drug injection. So intramuscular administration should be used only in emergency cases.

24.7.2 Developmental Changes in Pediatric Patients That Affect Drug Distribution

Hydrophilic drugs such as aminoglycosides and panipenem have been shown to have larger weight-normalized Vd in neonates compared to infants and adults due to the large ECF contents in neonates [27]. Also, the low protein binding in neonates due to the lower plasma protein concentration increases the unbound fraction of highly bound drugs and leads to increase in Vd especially for drugs with small Vd [27]. The drug distribution to the central nervous system (CNS) is higher in neonates due to the increased permeabil-ity of blood brain barrier (BBB), which can augment the CNS therapeutic and adverse effects of drugs. Also the volume of the CNS is relatively large in young children and reaches about 80%–90% of that in adults at 4–6 years of age. So the intrathecal dose of methotrexate is usually calculated based on age rather than body weight or BSA.

Calculation of the loading dose of drugs is usually based on Vd and the desired drug concentration. Differences in Vd between children and adults should be consid-ered when calculating the loading dose for children. The loading dose for drugs with low Vd (≤ 0.4 L/kg), which are mainly distributed in the ECF, is usually calculated in children based on the BSA according to Equation 24.19 because the BSA is correlated with the ECF of the children [23]:

$$\text{Loading dose}_{\text{infant}(\text{Vd}\leq 0.4\,\text{L/kg})} = \text{Loading dose}_{\text{adult}} \times \frac{\text{BSA}_{\text{infant}}}{\text{BSA}_{\text{adult}}} \qquad (24.19)$$

while for drugs with high Vd (≥ 0.6 L/kg), which are extensively bound to tissue proteins, the loading dose can be based on the body weight as in Equation 24.20 since the tissue binding in children is not significantly different from adults [23]:

$$\text{Loading dose}_{\text{infant}(\text{Vd}\geq 0.6\,\text{L/kg})} = \text{Loading dose}_{\text{adult}} \times \frac{\text{Body weight}_{\text{infant}}}{\text{Body weight}_{\text{adult}}} \qquad (24.20)$$

The loading dose of drugs that have Vd of 0.4–0.6 L/kg can be calculated from the average value of the doses calculated using BSA an body weight. The increase in free fraction increases the drug effect and toxicity in addition to the increase in the rate of metabolism and excretion. The increased rate of drug elimination usually leads to reduction in the total drug concentration and dose adjustment may not be necessary.

24.7.3 DEVELOPMENTAL CHANGES IN PEDIATRIC PATIENTS THAT AFFECT DRUG METABOLISM

The hepatic clearance is dependent on hepatic blood flow, enzyme activity, and transport system. At birth, both phase I and phase II metabolizing enzymes are immature, and maturation of different enzyme systems proceeds at different rates. *In vitro* studies show significant enzyme activity 2 months after birth, and maturation of most enzyme systems occurs after 1 year. Rapid drug metabolism occurs at school age and adolescence. Enzyme maturation is important in young infants for determining the appropriate dose of the drug. Once the enzyme systems are mature, hepatic blood flow, transport system, and enzyme capacity become important in determining the dose. During the first 2 months of age, most enzyme systems are not mature and the half-lives for most drugs are prolonged. So small initial doses of the drug should be used, and then the dose can be adjusted based on clinical response and blood drug concentration. At 2–6 months of age, many enzyme systems are not fully mature, but significant rate of metabolism occurs in this age group [23]. The dose in this group of patients can be based on body weight as follows:

$$\text{Dose}_{\text{infant}(2-6\,\text{months})} = \text{Dose}_{\text{adult}} \times \frac{\text{Body weight}_{\text{infant}}}{\text{Body weight}_{\text{adult}}} \qquad (24.21)$$

Once the liver enzymes are matured after the age of 6 months, the rate of metabolism is dependent on the rate of liver growth. The liver volume, liver blood flow, and biliary function are correlated well with the BSA, so doses can be calculated based on the BSA as follows:

$$\text{Dose}_{\text{infant}(\text{age}\geq 6\,\text{months})} = \text{Dose}_{\text{adult}} \times \frac{\text{BSA}_{\text{infant}}}{\text{BSA}_{\text{adult}}} \qquad (24.22)$$

In some enzyme systems that have been shown to be correlated better with the body weight such as CYP2D6 and UGT, the doses for the drugs that are predominantly eliminated by these pathways should be calculated as follows:

$$\text{Dose}_{\text{infant (age}\geq 6\,\text{months, UGT and CYP2D6)}} = \text{Dose}_{\text{adult}} \times \frac{\text{Body weight}_{\text{infant}}}{\text{Body weight}_{\text{adult}}} \qquad (24.23)$$

When considering the differences in drug metabolism in children, it is important to know the prominent metabolic pathways involved in drug metabolism. Dosing according to these guidelines should be used with caution due to the large interindividual variability.

24.7.4 DEVELOPMENTAL CHANGES IN PEDIATRIC PATIENTS THAT AFFECT RENAL DRUG EXCRETION

The GFR is usually $70\,\text{mL/min/1.73}\,\text{m}^2$ in full-term infants (gestational age ≥ 37 weeks) and much lower in preterm infants ($20\,\text{mL/min/1.73}\,\text{m}^2$). The GFR increases gradually over the first 2 years of age to reach the adult value. The tubular function is also immature during the first year of age while the reabsorption is well developed. Calculation of dose for renally eliminated drugs should be based on the maturity and function of the process mainly involved in the specific drug elimination, namely GFR, tubular secretion, or reabsorption. There is usually good correlation between the GFR and the renal excretion rate of drugs. The GFR in children is usually determined in children using the method of Schwartz, which correlated the serum creatinine and the body length and GFR as follows [28]:

$$\text{GFR}\,(\text{mL/min/1.73}\,\text{m}^2) = k \times \frac{\text{Length}\,(\text{cm})}{\text{S. Creatinine}\,(\text{mg/dL})} \qquad (24.24)$$

where k is the constant that relates the urinary creatinine excretion and body size, and this is determined by Schwartz to be 0.55 [28]. For drugs that are mainly excreted in urine (>50%), the GFR calculated in mL/min can be used to select the dose for infants at any age after 1 week of age as follows:

$$\text{Dose}_{\text{infant (age}\geq 1\,\text{week)}} = \text{Dose}_{\text{adult}} \times \frac{\text{GFR}_{\text{infant (mL/min)}}}{\text{GFR}_{\text{adult (mL/min)}}} \qquad (24.25)$$

After 2 years of age, the renal function is developed and it correlates well with the BSA, and the doses in children can be calculated as follows:

$$\text{Dose}_{\text{infant (age}\geq 2\,\text{years)}} = \text{Dose}_{\text{adult}} \times \frac{\text{BSA}_{\text{infant}}}{\text{BSA}_{\text{adult}}} \qquad (24.26)$$

24.7.5 **I**NTEGRATING THE **D**IFFERENCES IN ALL THE **P**HARMACOKINETIC
PROCESSES IN **P**EDIATRIC **P**ATIENTS

The previous discussion covers the differences in the individual pharmacokinetic processes in the pediatric population. However, the design of dosage regimen in pediatric patients requires consideration of all the possible differences between children and adults. For example, the characteristics of Vd in pediatric patients should be considered when calculating the loading dose of the drug required to achieve a certain drug concentration, while differences in metabolic and renal clearances between children and adults should be considered when calculating the dose required to achieve a certain steady-state concentration. Also, the dosage regimen should be modified when the drug absorption is expected to be different in the pediatric population. Since the variability of drug pharmacokinetics and response is very high in children and pediatric patients represent a vulnerable population, drugs should be used with great caution in these patients. All the aforementioned factors should be considered to guide the selection of the initial dosage regimen in the pediatric population. However, once drug therapy is initiated, the drug response should be monitored clinically and therapeutic drug monitoring should be applied to guide any further dose modification whenever it is necessary.

24.8   ELDERLY PATIENTS

Elderly patients usually require modification of the standard dosage regimen because the physiological and pathological changes that occur with age can alter the drug pharmacokinetics and pharmacodynamics. This is especially important in patients with poor nutrition, chronic illness, frequent hospitalization, and limited activity. Also, these patients usually receive multiple medications that increase the potential for clinically significant drug–drug interactions, which is a major problem in this patient population.

24.8.1 **P**HYSIOLOGICAL **C**HANGES IN **E**LDERLY **P**ATIENTS **T**HAT **A**FFECT
DRUG **A**BSORPTION

There is no significant difference in drug absorption in elderly with intact intestinal epithelium. However, the gastric emptying rate is slower and the GIT transit time is longer leading to slow drug absorption. Also, the gastric acid secretion is reduced with age leading to higher gastric pH, which can affect the dissolution rate of some drugs. The drug bioavailability does not change significantly except for drugs that undergo significant first-pass effect due to the change in drug metabolism and transport function in this patient population [29]. So generally dosage modification due to the change in drug absorption in elderly patients should be made based on specific drug characteristics.

24.8.2 **P**HYSIOLOGICAL **C**HANGES IN **E**LDERLY **P**ATIENTS **T**HAT **A**FFECT
DRUG **D**ISTRIBUTION

The decreased cardiac output in these patients leads to generalized reduction in tissue perfusion, which can cause slow rate of drug distribution. The body composition in elderly patients is usually different from that in adults. Older patients usually have reduced total body mass, lean body mass, and total body water contents and increased body fat contents, which can affect the Vd of drugs [29]. The drug protein binding is usually altered in elderly because of the reduced albumin plasma concentration and the reduced albumin drug affinity. On the other hand, the concentration of α_1-acid glycoprotein is usually increased in this patient population due to the underlying health conditions and disease state. In general, these changes in the body composition lead to increase in Vd for most lipophilic drugs, and no change or decrease in Vd for most hydrophilic drugs.

24.8.3 PHYSIOLOGICAL CHANGES IN ELDERLY PATIENTS THAT AFFECT DRUG METABOLISM

The hepatic blood flow is usually reduced and the liver size is usually smaller in elderly patients. This can lead to the reduction in the hepatic clearance of high extraction ratio drugs. The first-pass metabolism of these drugs is also reduced leading to higher bioavailability after oral administration [30]. So the dose of high clearance drugs should be reduced in elderly because of the reduced hepatic clearance and increased bioavailability. On the other hand, for low extraction ratio drugs the free intrinsic metabolic clearance of these drugs has been shown to decrease by 25%–60% in elderly patients. However, for drugs that are highly bound to plasma protein ($f_u > 0.9$), the reduced free intrinsic clearance is partially compensated by the increased drug-free fraction in this patient population [31]. So low extraction ratio drugs should also be used in lower doses in elderly patients due to the reduced intrinsic clearance.

24.8.4 PHYSIOLOGICAL CHANGES IN ELDERLY PATIENTS THAT AFFECT RENAL DRUG EXCRETION

The renal function is usually reduced in the elderly population due to the reduced renal blood flow. The GFR and tubular secretion are reduced in the elderly leading to reduction in renal drug elimination. The creatinine clearance can be used as a measure of the renal function in this patient population using Equations 24.1 and 24.2. The dose of renally eliminated drugs should be reduced in elderly patients taking into account the estimated renal function and the fraction of the drug dose excreted unchanged in urine.

24.8.5 INTEGRATING THE DIFFERENCES IN ALL THE PHARMACOKINETIC PROCESSES IN ELDERLY PATIENTS

Changes in drug absorption, distribution, metabolism, and excretion in elderly patients can affect the pharmacokinetic behavior of the drugs and may necessitate dose modification in elderly patients. Since this patient population is at high risk of developing toxicity, have high potential to develop drug–drug interactions, and have high variability in pharmacokinetics and response, dosing regimens for elderly patients should be selected with caution. The physiological changes in these patients that can affect the drug pharmacokinetics should be considered to guide the selection of the initial dosage regimen. Once drug therapy is started, patients should be monitored clinically and therapeutic drug monitoring should be used to guide any further dose modification.

24.9 PREGNANT WOMEN AND NURSING MOTHERS

The physiological changes that occur during pregnancy can affect the pharmacokinetic behavior of many drugs. Most of these changes start during the first trimester and become more pronounced toward the end of pregnancy. These physiological changes return to their pre-pregnancy levels at different rates after delivery [32]. Also, the formation of the placenta and the growth of the fetus can affect the distribution and clearance of drugs.

24.9.1 PHYSIOLOGICAL CHANGES THAT AFFECT DRUG ABSORPTION DURING PREGNANCY

Pregnant women usually have delayed gastric emptying rate and prolonged GIT transit time due to diminished intestinal motility which is due to the elevated progesterone levels in these women. This can result in slow rate of drug absorption without affecting the bioavailability of orally administered drugs. Also, there is reduced gastric secretion and elevation in the gastric pH that can affect the dissolution rate of some drugs [32,33]. Nausea and vomiting are common symptoms during the early course of pregnancy that can affect the absorption of drugs administered to pregnant women.

24.9.2 PHYSIOLOGICAL CHANGES THAT AFFECT DRUG DISTRIBUTION DURING PREGNANCY

The blood flow to various organs increases during pregnancy due to the decrease in peripheral resistant and the expansion in blood volume. The plasma concentration of albumin and α_1-acid glycoprotein decreases significantly during pregnancy, which leads to reduction in drug binding to plasma protein. This leads to the increase in the drug-free fraction and free drug concentration of highly bound drugs, which can amplify the drug therapeutic and adverse effects. Pregnancy is also associated with significant increase in total body weight. Most of this increase is due to the increase in water in the vascular and extracellular spaces. Large portion of this increase is due to the fetus, placenta, and amniotic fluid. This increase in the total body water usually increases the Vd of hydrophilic drugs especially those with relatively small Vd. The body fat content is also increased during pregnancy, which can increase the Vd for lipophilic drugs also. This increase in Vd during pregnancy may necessitate the use of larger loading doses of drugs in pregnant women to achieve a certain drug concentration.

24.9.3 PHYSIOLOGICAL CHANGES THAT AFFECT DRUG METABOLISM AND EXCRETION DURING PREGNANCY

The metabolizing enzyme activity is usually altered during pregnancy because estrogens and progesterone induce some CYP enzyme systems and inhibit others [34]. Both phase I and phase II enzymes are affected during pregnancy. The metabolic clearance of some drugs, especially high extraction ratio drugs, is increased due to the increased liver blood flow. Also, the hepatic clearance of low extraction ratio drugs, which are highly bound to plasma protein, is increased because of the increase in the free fraction of these drugs during pregnancy. High extraction ratio drugs administered orally usually have higher bioavailability during pregnancy. This is because the increased liver blood flow results in slight reduction in the extraction ratio of high extraction ratio drugs, which increases the bioavailability of these drugs. The contribution of fetal drug metabolism to the overall maternal metabolism is minimal, so it does not have major effect on the maternal drug and metabolite blood concentrations.

The renal blood flow increases significantly during pregnancy reaching about 160%–180% of the normal flow rate during the third trimester. This causes significant increase in the renal excretion of many drugs such as ampicillin, cephradine, cefazolin, lithium, atenolol, digoxin, and many other renally eliminated drugs. The doses of these drugs used in pregnant women should be increased to maintain therapeutic drug concentration [35]. For drugs that are eliminated by metabolism and renal excretion, the calculation of dose should be based on the effect of pregnancy on the metabolic and renal clearance and the contribution of each of these clearances to the drug total body clearance.

24.9.4 Drug Pharmacokinetics in Nursing Women

Drugs used by nursing women can be excreted in milk to different extents. The amount of drug excreted in milk is usually small compared to the total amount of the drug in the mother's body and should not affect the drug pharmacokinetic behavior in the mother. However, the small drug amount excreted in milk can represent a significant dose of the drug and may produce pharmacological and adverse effects especially in premature infants. The extent of drug excretion in breast milk and the drug effect in infants are usually affected by many factors that are related to the drug properties, maternal pharmacology, and infant-related factors.

24.9.4.1 Factors Related to the Drug Properties

Drug properties are important in determining the extent of drug excretion in milk. Human milk is slightly more acidic than plasma and has pH of approximately 7.1. So basic drugs excreted in milk will be more ionized and trapped because ionized drug molecules cannot diffuse back to the plasma. In general, the milk to plasma ratio for basic drugs (e.g., erythromycin) is >1, while that of acidic drugs (e.g., penicillin) is <1. Also, since the excretion of drugs in milk occurs mainly by passive diffusion, lipophilic drugs are excreted in milk more than hydrophilic drugs. Furthermore, drugs with very large molecular weight such as heparin (MW is 15,000) are too large to cross a lipid barrier, and hence are not excreted in milk. Besides, drugs that are not highly bound to plasma protein are excreted in milk more than those that are highly bound to plasma protein because only free drug molecules can be excreted in milk.

24.9.4.2 Factors Related to Maternal Pharmacology

Since drug excretion from plasma to milk occurs by passive diffusion along a concentration gradient, high maternal plasma drug concentration usually produces high milk drug concentration. The drug dose, route of administration, frequency of administration, and time of feeding relative to maternal dosing are important factors in determining the amount of drug that will be available for excretion into milk.

24.9.4.3 Factors Related to the Infant

The total amount of drug ingested by the infant is dependent on the volume of milk consumed and the average plasma drug concentration in the mother [36]. The drug received by the infants in most cases does not accumulate to concentrations that can produce adverse effects. However, neonates, especially premature infants, are at high risk of developing serious toxicities from drug exposure via the ingested milk because of their immature function of their eliminating organs. So breast-fed infants whose mothers are taking medications should be monitored for any signs of pharmacological and adverse effects of these drugs.

PRACTICE PROBLEMS

24.1 A patient admitted to the hospital because of acute myocardial infarction was started on oral antiarrhythmic medication. He was given 600 mg every 12 h from an oral formulation that is known to be rapidly absorbed but only 80% bioavailable. At steady state, the maximum and minimum plasma concentrations were 30 and 10.5 µg/mL, respectively.
   a. Calculate mathematically the half-life and the volume of distribution of this drug in this patient.
   b. The patient suddenly developed acute renal failure and the kidney function dropped to 30% of its normal value. If the renal clearance of this drug is 75% of the total body clearance, recommend an appropriate dose for this patient after developing the renal failure.
   c. Calculate the maximum and minimum plasma concentration achieved at steady state from the regimen you recommended in part (b).

24.2 A 65-year-old man was taking his antihypertensive medication as 500 mg every 12 h. He was taking his medication in the form of an oral tablet that is rapidly and completely absorbed. After administration of a single oral 500 mg dose, 375 mg is excreted unchanged in urine and the drug half-life is 8 h. The average plasma concentration of this antihypertensive drug in this patient while taking 500 mg every 12 h was 20 mg/L.
   a. Calculate the volume of distribution of this drug in this patient.
   b. This patient developed acute renal failure and his creatinine clearance decreased from the normal value of 120–30 mL/min. Calculate the new total body clearance for this drug in this patient after developing the renal failure assuming that the deterioration in the kidney function does not affect the drug distribution characteristics.
   c. Recommend a maintenance dose for this patient after developing the renal failure if the usual dose in patients with normal kidney function is 500 mg every 12 h.
   d. Calculate the maximum and minimum plasma concentrations achieved at steady state from the regimen you recommended in part (c).

24.3 A patient was admitted to the hospital because of severe pneumonia. An IV loading dose of an antibiotic followed by IV maintenance doses of 300 mg q12 h were prescribed. The creatinine clearance was 120 mL/min, which is considered normal for this patient. After 7 days of therapy (300 mg q12 h), the maximum and minimum plasma concentrations were 38 and 12.5 mg/L, respectively.

    a. Calculate mathematically the half-life and the volume of distribution of this drug in this patient.

    b. At steady state (while receiving 300 mg q12 h), 180 mg of the drug is excreted unchanged in urine during one dosing interval. What is the renal clearance of this drug?

    c. After 15 days of antibiotic therapy, the kidney function of this patient deteriorated and his creatinine clearance was found to be 40 mL/min. What is the new half-life of the drug after this change in the patient's kidney function?

    d. What will be the steady-state maximum and minimum plasma concentrations if this patient continues taking 300 mg q12 h IV despite the change in his kidney function?

24.4 After IV administration of procainamide (an antiarrhythmic drug), 60% of the administered dose is excreted unchanged in urine. The rest of the dose is metabolized in the liver. The average volume of distribution of procainamide is 2 L/kg and the half-life is 3 h in patients with normal kidney function.

    a. Calculate the renal clearance of procainamide in patients with normal kidney function.

    b. Calculate the half-life of procainamide in a patient with creatinine clearance of 30 mL/min (normal creatinine clearance is 120 mL/min).

    c. Calculate the daily oral maintenance dose required in a patient with creatinine clearance of 30 mL/min (normal creatinine clearance is 120 mL/min). (The average daily oral maintenance dose in patients with normal kidney function is 3 g/day.)

    d. If a patient with creatinine clearance of 30 mL/min (normal creatinine clearance is 120 mL/min) receives 750 mg every 6 h, calculate the maximum and minimum plasma concentrations at steady state in this patient.

24.5 A new antihypertensive drug is rapidly but incompletely absorbed.

    • When 800 mg is given intravenously to normal volunteers:
        600 mg can be recovered in the urine unchanged from time zero to infinity.
        The AUC obtained from time zero to infinity is 400 mg h/L.
        The elimination half-life is 8 h.

    • When 400 mg is given orally:
        The AUC from time zero to infinity is 125 mg h/L.

    a. If a patient with normal kidney function is receiving 800 mg every 12 h orally, what will be the average plasma concentration at steady state ?

    b. Calculate the maximum and the minimum plasma concentrations achieved at steady state for the regimen in part (a) (800 mg every 12 h orally) if the drug is rapidly absorbed after oral administration.

    c. If the average maintenance dose for patients with normal kidney function is 800 mg IV every 12 h, what will be the maintenance dose for a patient whose creatinine clearance is only 10% of normal.

    d. What will be the maximum and the minimum plasma concentrations at steady state for the IV regimen you recommended in part (c) for the patient with 10% of the normal kidney function assuming that the change in kidney function does not affect the volume of distribution.

REFERENCES

1. European Medicines Agency. Note for guidance: Pharmacokinetic studies in man [no. 3CC3A; online]. http://www.emea.europa.eu/pdfs/human/ewp/3cc3aen.pdf, last accessed June 15, 2011.
2. European Medicines Agency Committee for Proprietary Medicinal Products. Note for guidance [no. CPMP/ICH/379/95; online]. http://www.emea.europa.eu/pdfs/human/ich/028995en.pdf, last accessed June 15, 2011.
3. Center for Drug Evaluation and Research, U.S. Food and Drug Administration, Guidance for industry (1999): Population pharmacokinetics.
4. Vanholder R, DeSmet R, Glorleux G, and Arglles A (2003) Review in uremic toxins: Classification, concentration, and interindividual variability. *Kidney Int* 63:1934–1943.
5. Sun H, Frassetto L, and Benet LZ (2006) Effect of renal failure on drug transport and metabolism. *Pharmacol Ther* 109:1–11.
6. Koup JR, Jusko WJ, and Elwood CM (1979) Digoxin pharmacokinetics: Role of renal failure in dosage regimen design. *Clin Pharmacol Ther* 18:9–21.
7. Jusko WJ, Szefler SJ, and Goldfarb AL (1974) Pharmacokinetic design of digoxin dosage regimen in relation to renal function. *J Clin Pharmacol* 14:525–535.
8. DiPiro JT, Spruill WJ, and Wade WE (2005) *Concepts in Clinical Pharmacokinetics*, 4th edn., American Society of Hospital Pharmacist, Inc., Bethesda, MD.
9. Giusti DL and Hayton WL (1973) Dosage regimen adjustments in renal impairment. *Drug Intell Clin Pharm* 7:382–387.
10. Graziani G, Bordone G, Bellato V, Finazzi S, Angelini C, and Badalamenti S (2006) Role of the kidney in plasma cytokine removal in sepsis syndrome: A pilot study. *J Nephrol* 19:176–182.
11. Pea F, Viale P, Pavan F, and Furlanut M (2007) Pharmacokinetic considerations for antimicrobial therapy in patients receiving renal replacement therapy. *Clin Pharmacokinet* 46:997–1038.
12. MacKichan JJ (2006) Influence of protein binding and use of unbound (free) drug concentration, in Burton ME, Shaw LM, Schentang JJ, and Evans WE (Eds.) *Applied Pharmacokinetics and Pharmacodynamics—Principles of Therapeutic Drug Monitoring*, Lippincott Williams & Wilkins, Philadelphia, PA.
13. Blaschke TF (1977) Protein binding and kinetics of drugs in liver diseases. *Clin Pharmacokinet* 2:32–44.
14. Frye RF, Zgheib NK, Matzke GR, Chaves-Gnecco D, Rabinovitz M, Shaikh OS, and Branch RA (2006) Liver disease selectivity modulates cytochrome P450-mediated metabolism. *Clin Pharmacol Ther* 80:235–245.
15. Hoyumpa AM and Schenker S (1991) Is glucuronidation truly preserved in patients with liver disease? *Hepatology* 13:786–795.
16. George J, Murray M, Byth K, and Farrell GC (1995) Differential alterations of cytochrome P450 proteins in livers from patients with severe chronic liver disease. *Hepatology* 21:120–128.

17. Davis M (2007) Cholestasis and endogenous opioids—Liver disease and endogenous opioid pharmacokinetics. *Clin Pharmacokinet* 46:825–850.
18. Rossat J, Maillard M, Nussberger J, Brunner HR, and Burnier M (1999) Renal effects of selective cyclooxygenase-2 inhibition in normotensive salt-depleted subjects. *Clin Pharmacol Ther* 66:76–84.
19. Hebert MF (1998) Guide to drug dosage in hepatic disease, in Holford N (Ed.) *Drug Data Handbook*, 3rd edn., Adis International, Auckland, New Zealand.
20. Blouin RA and Warren GW (1999) Pharmacokinetic considerations in obesity. *J Pharm Sci* 88:1–7.
21. Green B and Duffull SB (2004) What is the best size descriptor to use in pharmacokinetic studies in the obese? *Br J Clin Pharmacol* 58:119–133.
22. Bauer LA (2008) *Applied Clinical Pharmacokinetics*, 2nd edn., McGraw-Hill Companies, Inc. New York.
23. Bartelink IH, Rademaker CMA, Schobben AF, and van den Anker JN (2006) Guidelines on pediatric dosing on the basis of developmental physiology and pharmacokinetic consideration. *Clin Pharmacokinet* 46:1077–1097.
24. Strolin Benedetti M and Baltes EL (2003) Drug metabolism and disposition in children. *Fundam Clin Pharmacol* 17:281–299.
25. Capparelli EV, Mirochnick M, Dankner WM, Blanchard S, Mofenson L, McSherry GD, Gay H, Ciupak G, Smith B, and Connor JD (2003) Pharmacokinetics and tolerance of zidovudine in preterm infants. *J Pediatr* 142:47–52.
26. Ginsberg G, Hattis D, Miller R, and Sonawane B (2004) Pediatric pharmacokinetic data: Implications for environmental risk assessment for children. *Pediatrics* 113:973–983.
27. Kimura T, Sunakawa K, Matsuura N, Kubo H, Shimada S, and Yogo K (2004) Population pharmacokinetics of arbekacin, vancomycin, and panipenem in neonates. *Antimicrob Agents Chemother* 48:1159–1167.
28. Schwartz GJ, Haycock GB, Edelmann CM Jr., and Spitzer A (1976) A simple estimate of glomerular filtration derived from body length and plasma creatinine. *Pediatrics* 58:259–263.
29. Schwartz JB (2007) The current state of knowledge on age, sex, and their interactions on clinical pharmacology. *Clin Pharmacol Ther* 82:87–96.
30. El Desoky E (2007) Pharmacokinetic-pharmacodynamic crisis in elderly. *Am J Ther* 14:488–498.
31. Butler JM and Begg EJ (2008) Free drug metabolic clearance in elderly people. *Clin Pharmacokinet* 47:297–321.
32. Frederiksen MC (2001) Physiologic changes in pregnancy and their effect on drug disposition. *Semin Perinatol* 25:120–123.
33. Simpson KH, Stakes F, and Miller M (1988) Pregnancy delays paracetamol absorption and gastric emptying in patients undergoing surgery. *Br J Anaesth* 60:24–27.
34. Loebstein R and Koren G (2002) Clinical relevance of therapeutic drug monitoring during pregnancy. *Ther Drug Monit* 24:15–22.
35. Anger GJ and Piquette-Miller M (2008) Pharmacokinetic studies in pregnant women. *Clin Pharmacol Ther* 83:184–187.
36. Anderson GD (2007) Pregnancy-induced changes in pharmacokinetics: A mechanistic-based approach. *Clin Pharmacokinet* 46:989–1008.

25 Pharmacokinetic Drug–Drug Interactions

OBJECTIVES

After completing this chapter you should be able to

- Discuss the different basis for classifying drug–drug interactions
- Describe the different mechanisms of drug–drug interactions
- Describe the mechanisms by which a drug can affect the absorption of another drug
- State the pharmacokinetic processes that are affected by the change in drug protein binding and how these changes affect the overall pharmacokinetic behavior of the drug
- Give examples of commonly used enzyme inhibitors and enzyme inducers
- Evaluate the effect of administration of enzyme inhibitors and enzyme inducers on the pharmacokinetic behavior of drugs after IV and oral administration
- Describe the effect of induction and inhibition of drug transporters on the drug absorption, distribution, and elimination of drugs
- Give examples of clinically significant drug interactions that affect the absorption, distribution, metabolism, excretion, and transport of drugs
- Describe the general in vitro and in vivo approaches used to study the potential for drug–drug interactions during drug development

25.1 INTRODUCTION

The term drug interaction means the interaction of the drug with other factors that can lead to modification of the drug response. These factors can be another drug, food, beverage, nutrient, herb, disease, alcohol, or tobacco. So drug–drug interaction (DDI) can be defined as the change in the therapeutic and/or adverse effects of a drug by prior or concurrent administration of a second drug. It is also possible that the effect of both drugs is modified when used together. This definition can be expanded to include the situations when administration of two drugs that do not affect each other can diminish or amplify the therapeutic and/or adverse effects of the two drugs. For example, when two drugs that have opposite effect on blood glucose concentration, two antihypertensive drugs, or two nephrotoxic drugs, are administered concurrently.

Large variation exists in the reported incidence of DDI in the literature. This is because the incidence of DDI depends on the studied population, the clinical site of the study, and the criteria used to identify a DDI. The increase in the number of drugs used by the patients increases the potential for DDI. So hospitalized patients usually have higher incidence of DDI compared to ambulatory patients, with critically ill patients having the highest potential for experiencing DDI because of the large number of drugs they usually get. Also, the severity of DDI outcome is different and can range from causing major life-threatening effects, to moderate effect that requires further treatment, to minor effect that does not require any other treatment. The certainty that the DDI will happen also varied from theoretical, unlikely, possible, suspected, probable, to reputable. So the different criteria used to identify DDI in the different studies can contribute to the variability in the reported incidence. Even with the lowest estimated incidence of DDI and due to the large number of prescriptions written every day, DDI represent a major concern because these interactions can affect large number of patients [1].

Studying the potential for the interaction of new drug molecules with other drugs is very important and it is usually required by regulatory authorities as a part of the new drug application. This is important because studying the mechanism of DDI and identifying the outcome of DDI is important to determine the best approach for handling DDI. Handling DDI involves avoiding the use of the interacting drugs together when the interaction can cause a life-threatening effect or permanent harm to the patient. Other less severe DDI can be handled by modifying the dosing regimen for one or both interacting drugs or the use of noninteracting drug alternative from the same or different drug class. In clinical practice, this information can be helpful for clinicians when prescribing medications for the patients, while for new drug molecules this information is usually useful for recommendation of dosing and labeling.

25.2 CLASSIFICATION OF DRUG–DRUG INTERACTIONS

The classification of DDI can be based on the mechanism of interaction or the outcome of the interaction as discussed later. DDI can also be classified based on severity and documentation.

25.2.1 MECHANISM OF DRUG–DRUG INTERACTIONS

DDI can be classified according to their mechanism of interaction which can result from pharmacokinetic, pharmacodynamic, and pharmaceutical alterations. Pharmacokinetic DDI are drug interactions that occur due to change in the absorption, distribution, metabolism, or excretion of one or both of the interacting drugs. So these interactions cause change in the concentration time profile in the body and at the site of action for one or both interacting drugs causing modification of the observed effect. This chapter focuses on the pharmacokinetic DDI. On the contrary, pharmacodynamic DDI are interactions that result in modification of therapeutic and/or toxic effects of one or both drugs without affecting the pharmacokinetics of the drugs. This can occur due to competition between interacting drugs for the same receptors, alteration of the drug receptors rendering them more or less sensitive to the drug effect, or effect on different body systems that produce similar or opposite effects. Occasionally, DDI results from pharmacokinetic and pharmacodynamic changes. Pharmaceutical DDI are those interactions that occur during manufacturing, storage, dispensing, or administration due to physical or chemical incompatibilities.

25.2.2 DESIRABLE VERSUS UNDESIRABLE DRUG–DRUG INTERACTIONS

The term DDI is usually viewed as interactions between drugs that lead to unfavorable consequences. Although this is true for some DDI, there are other DDI that can produce beneficial effects to the patients. There are drug combinations that are used together to produce drug interaction that can improve the therapeutic effect of one of the drugs. The classical example is the use of probenecid in combination with penicillin G to inhibit penicillin G renal tubular secretion, which slows penicillin G rate of elimination and prolongs its effect. Other beneficial combinations include the use of carbidopa with L-dopa in Parkinson's disease to inhibit the peripheral decarboxylation of L-dopa and increase its central nervous system (CNS) availability. Also, clavulanic acid salts are used with amoxicillin to inhibit the β-lactamase enzyme and increase the susceptibility of the β-lactamase secreting bacteria to amoxicillin. Furthermore, the use of cilastatin with imipenem inhibits the renal dehydropeptidase enzyme responsible for imipenem metabolism in the kidney and increases its urinary tract concentration.

25.3 PHARMACOKINETIC DRUG–DRUG INTERACTIONS

The pharmacokinetic DDI affects the concentration of at least one of the interacting drugs in the body leading to modification of the drug response. These DDI occur due to alteration of the absorption, distribution, metabolism, or elimination of one or both of the interacting drugs.

25.3.1 PHARMACOKINETIC DRUG–DRUG INTERACTIONS THAT AFFECT DRUG ABSORPTION

Pharmacokinetic DDI can affect the rate and/or extent of drug absorption. Interactions that affect the rate of drug absorption are usually important after single drug administration, while interactions that affect the extent of drug absorption can have significant effect after a single dose and during multiple drug administration. The rate of drug absorption can result from the change in the rate of drug dissolution in the gastrointestinal tract (GIT) and modification of the gastric emptying rate or GIT motility. The drug dissolution rate after oral administration can be altered if the gastric pH is changed by drugs, food, or beverages. Antacids and proton pump inhibitors usually raise the gastric pH, which slows the dissolution rate of basic drugs leading to slower rate of absorption. Administration of drugs such as propantheline delays the gastric emptying and metoclopramide increases the gastric emptying rate, which can affect the rate of drug absorption. Opiates and drugs with anticholinergic activity such as tricyclic antidepressants, phenothiazines, and antihistaminics usually decrease the GIT motility and prolong the GIT transit time. Although the outcome of these effects is variable, the delay in gastric emptying rate usually leads to delayed absorption and the longer GIT transit time increases the extent of absorption especially for drugs with limited solubility.

Interactions that affect the extent of drug absorption can have more clinically significant effect because these interactions can decrease the steady-state drug concentration leading to reduction in the therapeutic effect of the drug. The decrease in the extent of drug absorption can happen as a result of the decrease in the drug dissolution due to modification of the gastric pH. For example, H_2-histamine blockers can reduce the dissolution and bioavailability of ketoconazole. Adsorption and complexation can also reduce the bioavailability of drugs due to the formation of nonabsorbable complex. For example, cholestyramine can reduce the bioavailability of digoxin, warfarin, and levothyroxine. Also, antacids can reduce the bioavailability of ofloxacin. Drug bioavailability can also be affected due to changes in the first-pass metabolism, which is discussed under interactions that affect drug metabolism. DDI that results from altered drug dissolution due to changes in gastric pH or due to complexation can be avoided in most cases by allowing enough time between administration of the different drugs.

25.3.2 Pharmacokinetic Drug–Drug Interactions That Affect Drug Distribution

DDI that can alter drug distribution usually results from changes in the plasma or tissue protein binding. This is because the Vd of drugs is dependent on the drug binding in plasma and tissues as discussed in Chapter 3 and as described by Equation 25.1:

$$Vd = V_p + V_t \left(\frac{f_{uP}}{f_{uT}} \right) \tag{25.1}$$

where
    Vd is the volume of distribution
    V_p is the volume of the plasma
    V_t is the volume of the tissues
    f_{uP} is the free fraction of the drug in plasma
    f_{uT} is the free fraction of the drug in tissues

This relationship indicates that the decrease in the plasma protein binding without change in the drug tissue binding causes increase in Vd, while the decrease in tissue binding without a change in the plasma protein binding causes decrease in Vd.

DDI leading to alteration in protein binding results from concurrent administration of two drugs that compete for the same protein binding sites. The drug with the higher affinity to the plasma proteins can displace the other drug from its binding sites resulting in higher free fraction and higher free concentration of the displaced drug. DDI that involves displacement from binding to plasma proteins usually occur between drugs that are highly bound to plasma protein ($f_u < 0.1$) and when the majority of the protein binding sites are occupied. Since the unbound drug is the species that can cross the biological membranes and can reach the site of action, the free drug concentration is highly correlated with the drug's therapeutic and adverse effects. Changes in free drug concentration should cause modification of the drug response and toxicity.

To evaluate the clinical significance of DDI involving changes in the drug plasma protein binding, the effect of the change in free drug concentration on drug elimination has to be considered. The effect of the change in free drug concentration on drug elimination is different for high extraction ratio and low extraction ratio drugs. For low extraction ratio drugs, the increase in the free fraction and free drug concentration is usually accompanied by an increase in drug clearance. The higher drug clearance leads to a reduction in the average total plasma drug concentration during multiple drug administration. These drugs have limited first-pass metabolism that is not significantly affected by the increase in the drug-free fraction. This means that the change in protein binding does not significantly affect the bioavailability of low extraction ratio drug. So the outcome of this interaction is a decrease in the total drug concentration, and an increase in the free fraction of the drug, so the free drug concentration is not affected significantly. This indicates that DDI that involves changes in the protein binding of low extraction ratio drugs usually does not have clinical significance.

The change in the plasma protein binding of high extraction ratio drugs does not affect the clearance or the steady-state concentration during multiple IV administration of these drugs. So the increase in the drug-free fraction will cause an increase in the free drug concentration. However, after oral administration the increase in the free fraction of the drug can decrease the bioavailability of high extraction ratio drugs due to the increased first-pass metabolism leading to lower average total drug concentration at steady state. The outcome of this DDI is the decrease in the total drug concentration due to the reduction in bioavailability and the increase in the free fraction of the drug, which leads to insignificant change in free drug concentration. So DDI that involve changes in the plasma protein binding should be interpreted carefully because most of these interactions do not have clinical significance and do not require any regimen modification [2].

25.3.3 Pharmacokinetic Drug–Drug Interactions That Affect Drug Metabolism

Drugs can affect the metabolism of other drugs by inhibition or induction of the drug metabolizing enzyme systems. Inhibition of drug metabolism leads to reduction of the drug metabolic clearance, and hence the drug CL_T. This causes increase in the drug steady-state concentration if the metabolic clearance has a significant contribution to the drug total clearance. Inhibition of drug metabolism can be competitive or noncompetitive. In competitive inhibition, the drug and the inhibitor compete for the same enzyme system and the inhibitor prevents the drug from reaching the catalytic site of the enzyme and reduces its metabolism. The inhibitor concentration usually determines the degree of inhibition in competitive inhibition with higher inhibitor concentration causing more inhibition [3,4]. Noncompetitive inhibition occurs when the drug and the inhibitor bind to different domains of the enzyme, but inhibitor binding to the enzyme alters the binding of the drug to the catalytic site of the enzyme. The onset of metabolic inhibition is usually immediate and inhibition occurs once the inhibitor concentration is accumulated to the concentration required to cause significant metabolic inhibition. Metabolic inhibition is usually reversible and the drug metabolic rate returns to the normal rate once the inhibitor is cleared from the body. Some enzyme inhibitors such as clarithromycin, erythromycin, and verapamil form irreversible complex with the metabolizing enzymes. The effect of these inhibitors may last for 2–3 weeks since it will continue until new enzymes are synthesized [3].

Enzyme inducers increase the drug metabolic rate by stimulating the liver to synthesize new enzymes. This can lead to increase in the hepatic drug clearance and reduce the steady-state drug concentration especially for low extraction ratio drugs. The effect of an enzyme inducer occurs gradually until the full induction state and the highest hepatic clearance is achieved in 2–3 weeks. The effect of enzyme inducers usually decreases gradually after termination of the inducer to reach the baseline (uninduced) state in 2–3 weeks [5,6]. Enzyme inhibition and enzyme induction can also affect the first-pass metabolism leading to alteration in the drug bioavailability. High extraction ratio drugs undergo extensive first-pass metabolism that leads to their low bioavailability after oral administration. Even small change in the first-pass metabolism of these drugs, due to metabolic enzyme inhibition or induction, can lead to significant change in the fraction of dose that escapes the first-pass metabolism and cause significant change in bioavailability. Enzyme induction decreases the oral bioavailability, while enzyme inhibition increases the bioavailability of the drugs that undergo significant first-pass metabolism. These interactions are most significant in drugs with extensive first-pass metabolism that have bioavailability less than 10% such as lovostatin, saquinavir, simvastatin, quetiapine, and buspirone and also in drugs with bioavailability between 10% and 30% such as atorvastatin, indinavir, verapamil, felodipine, sirolimus, tacrolimus, and zeleplon [6].

Predicting DDI that can alter the drug metabolism is possible if the drug metabolic pathways are identified. The U.S. Food and Drug Administration (FDA) requires that all new drugs undergo in vitro metabolic studies with different CYP 450 isoforms and other enzyme systems to determine the specific metabolic pathways for all new drugs. Once the metabolic pathways and the metabolizing enzyme systems that catalyze each pathway are identified for a specific drug, it is possible to predict the potential DDI that can alter the metabolism of this particular drug. The literature and the online resources include plenty of information about the different enzyme systems involved in drug metabolism and tables of known substrates, inhibitors, and inducers for each of these enzyme systems [7–9]. When the metabolic pathways for a drug are known, the tables of inhibitors and inducers can be used to predict all the potential metabolic DDI with this drug.

Examples of the common enzyme inhibitors include cimetidine, erythromycin, fluoxetine, ketoconazole, fluconazole, verapamil, ciprofloxacin, enoxacin, metronidazole, allopurinol, disulfiram, sulphinpyrazone, and many other drugs. Some of these drugs can inhibit more than one enzyme system and some drugs are more potent inhibitor than others. When any of these common enzyme inhibitors are prescribed, it is important to check if the other drugs used by the patient are eliminated mainly by metabolism and if metabolic inhibition can occur. Examples of clinically significant DDI that involves inhibition of drug metabolism include the inhibition of anticoagulant metabolism by metronidazole leading to enhanced anticoagulant effect and possible bleeding, inhibition of corticosteroid metabolism by erythromycin, inhibition of terfenadine metabolism by clarithromycin, inhibition of simvastatin metabolism by ciprofloxacin, inhibition of haloperidol metabolism by fluoxetine, and inhibition of theophylline metabolism by enoxacin. When such an interaction is detected, it is necessary to try to find an alternative drug that is not an enzyme inhibitor. When an alternative drug is not available and when the use of the two interacting drugs is not contraindicated, reduction of the dose and close monitoring of the patient is necessary.

Examples of common potent enzyme inducers include barbiturates, carbamazepine, aminoglutithimide, phenazone, rifampicin, phenytoin, primidone, tobacco, and many other drugs. Prescriptions that include any of these drugs should be checked to examine if DDI due to enzyme induction can occur. Examples of clinically significant DDI that involves enzyme induction include the use of oral anticoagulants, contraceptives, and corticosteroids with any of the enzyme inducers mentioned previously that can reduce the therapeutic effects of these drugs. Also, tobacco smoke induces the metabolism of haloperidol, rifampicin induces the metabolism of phenytoin, and barbiturates induce the metabolism of theophylline. When DDI that involves enzyme induction is detected, it is necessary to try to find an alternative drug that is not an enzyme inducer if possible. Drug induction interaction can be managed by increasing the dose of the affected drug gradually with close monitoring of the patient until the desired therapeutic effect is achieved. This higher dose of the affected drug should be reduced again when the enzyme inducer is stopped.

25.3.4 Pharmacokinetic Drug–Drug Interactions That Affect Drug Transporting Proteins

Transport proteins are specialized efflux or influx pumps that can transport endogenous and exogenous substances across biological membranes. These transport proteins are involved in the absorption, distribution, and elimination of a wide variety of drugs. Drug transport across the intestinal membrane, brain uptake across the blood brain barrier (BBB), renal tubular secretion, hepatocyte uptake, and placental distribution involves different transport proteins. The transport proteins can be inhibited and induced causing alteration of the pharmacokinetic behavior of the substrates for these transport proteins leading to drug interactions. Among the most studied transport protein is the p-glycoprotein (P-gp) transporter that is present in almost all organs in the body including the epithelial cells of the small and large intestine, the proximal renal tubules, the biliary canalicular membrane of hepatocytes, the ductules of the pancreas, the surface cells of the medulla and cortex of the adrenal glands, and the endothelial cells of the BBB. So the P-gp decreases the drug absorption in the GIT, increases drug excretion in urine and bile, and reduces drug entry to the brain [10].

Substrates for P-gp include many anticancer drugs, antibiotics, antivirals, calcium channel blockers, immunosuppressive agents, and many other drugs. Drugs that are substrates for P-gp can compete with each other for this transporter and drugs that have high affinity to P-gp can inhibit the transport of other drugs. Examples of drugs that have been shown to inhibit the P-gp include clarithromycin, cyclosporine, diltiazem, verapamil, tacrolimus, quinidine, dipyridamole, felodipine, nicardipine, propranolol, nifedipine, ritonavir, telmisartan, tamoxifen, and other drugs [10,11]. Interaction between these P-gp inhibitors with drugs that are substrates for P-gp leads to alteration of the pharmacokinetics of these drugs. The outcome of this interaction depends on the drug pharmacokinetic characteristics and may include one or more changes such as the increase in intestinal absorption, reduction in renal and biliary secretion, and increase in brain distribution. The P-gp transport protein can also be induced by drugs such as clotrimazole, nifedipine, phenytoin, rifampicin, dexamethasone, and phenobarbital. These inducers increase the expression of this transport protein and amplify its activity, leading to a change in the pharmacokinetics of P-gp substrates [10,11]. The outcome of the DDI that results from induction of the P-gp again depends on the drug pharmacokinetic characteristics, and may include one or more changes such as the reduction of the intestinal absorption, increase in the renal and biliary secretion, and reduction in the brain distribution. An interesting observation is the overlap of the substrates, inhibitors, and inducers of P-gp transport protein and CYP3A4 metabolizing enzymes in the small and large intestine. The function of P-gp is the efflux of substrates to the intestinal lumen, which decreases the drug bioavailability. CYP3A4 contributes to the first-pass metabolism, which also decreases the drug bioavailability. Inhibition and induction of P-gp and CYP3A4 also have similar effect on the drug bioavailability, which makes it difficult to separate the effect of these two systems on the drug bioavailability when interpreting the results of in vivo studies investigating such DDI.

25.3.5 PHARMACOKINETIC DRUG–DRUG INTERACTIONS THAT AFFECT DRUG EXCRETION

Clinically significant DDI that involves the urinary excretion process usually affect drugs or pharmacologically active metabolites that are mainly eliminated by the urinary route. Drugs are excreted in urine by glomerular filtration, tubular reabsorption, and active tubular secretion. The glomerular filtration of a drug depends on the free plasma drug concentration and the GFR. Drugs that can alter the GFR usually have minor and clinically insignificant effect on the glomerular filtration rate of drugs, while tubular reabsorption usually occurs by passive diffusion, which is dependent on the drug lipid solubility. Ionization of drugs in the lumen of the renal tubules usually affects the drug reabsopriton. Acidic drugs are ionized in alkaline urinary pH and are excreted faster due to the limited tubular reabsorption of the ionized drug, while basic drugs are excreted faster in acidic urinary pH because of the limited reabsorption of the ionized drugs. For example, the urinary elimination of the basic drugs such as quinidine and amphetamine is enhanced by urine acidification with ammonium chloride, while urinary alkalinization with sodium bicarbonate usually increases the rate of excretion of salicylates. Modification of the urinary pH is one of the approaches used to enhance the elimination of weakly acidic and basic drugs in case of toxicity [1].

Drug elimination by active tubular secretion can be altered when more than one drug compete for the same active transport system. Compounds with higher affinity for the transport system can competitively inhibit the active secretion of other drugs. Probenecid is known to inhibit the renal excretion of penicillins, cephalosporins, dapsone, rifampin, and thiazide diuretics by inhibition of their active tubular secretion. This leads to increase in their serum concentrations, which potentiates their therapeutic effect and possibly increases their toxic effects. Also, aspirin can inhibit methotrexate active tubular secretion, which necessitates reduction in methotrexate dose when these two drugs are used together.

DDI can also affect the pharmacokinetics of drugs undergoing biliary excretion. Drugs excreted in bile as conjugates can be hydrolyzed by the bacterial flora in the small intestine where the drug can be reabsorbed leading to enterohepatic recycling and prolongation of the drug effect. Some antibiotics can reduce the activity of the bacterial flora in the small intestine reducing this enterohepatic recycling.

25.4 EVALUATION OF PHARMACOKINETIC DRUG–DRUG INTERACTIONS

The outcome of DDI depends on the specific circumstances of the interactions. This includes factors related to the mechanism of the interaction, and the interacting drug characteristics and effects. These factors have to be considered when evaluating the clinical significance of DDI [1].

25.4.1 TIME COURSE OF THE INTERACTION

Some DDI occur rapidly after administration of the interacting drugs, while others may take days or even weeks to develop. Understanding the mechanism of DDI usually helps in determining the time course for the appearance and the disappearance of the effect of the interaction. For example, inhibition of drug metabolism occurs rapidly once the inhibitor concentration in the body reaches the level that can cause significant inhibition of the metabolizing enzymes. However, enzyme induction may take weeks before the patient reaches the full induction state. Similarly, the effect of the enzyme inhibitor disappears rapidly once the patient stops taking the inhibitor, while the effect of enzyme inducers will continue until the patient returns to the uninduced state, which may take weeks after stopping the administration of the enzyme inducer.

25.4.2 EXTRAPOLATION FROM A DRUG TO ANOTHER

Some drug classes are relatively homogeneous and all members of the class probably interact with other drugs in essentially the same way. However, for most therapeutic classes the pharmacokinetic and pharmacodynamic characteristics of the different drugs within the class are different, which results in different interaction pattern for the different drugs of the same therapeutic class. This can be useful when selecting noninteracting drug alternatives to avoid DDI. For example, cimetidine inhibits the metabolism of many other drugs, while other H_2 antagonists such as ranitidine and famotidine are unlikely to do so.

498   Basic Pharmacokinetics

25.4.3   THERAPEUTIC INDEX OF THE DRUG

The dose of the drugs with narrow therapeutic index is selected with the aid of specific monitoring parameter that can be used to adjust the dose based on these parameters, such as in case of oral anticoagulants where the dose is adjusted based on the value of the prothrombin time. In this case, DDI may result in alteration of the anticoagulant steady-state concentration and modification of the anticoagulant activity, which may necessitate readjustment of the oral anticoagulant dose. While in other instances drugs may be administered in large doses for a short period of time to treat some acute conditions. For example, corticosteroids can be administered in large doses over a short period of time to treat acute conditions such as acute severe asthma or severe lupus cases. In this case, DDI that can alter the corticosteroid drug concentrations are less likely to have clinical significance.

25.4.4   SEQUENCE OF ADMINISTRATION OF THE INTERACTING DRUGS

The order in which the interacting drugs are given can have an important effect on the possibility for developing serious consequences due to the DDI. In general, when a drug is added to the drug therapy of a patient who is taking an enzyme inducer, for example, the dose of the drug is increased and decreased until the desired therapeutic effect is achieved. The dose selected this way is the optimum dose of the drug for the patient in the full induction state. The problem can arise if the enzyme inducer is stopped while still using the drug, because the patient will gradually return to the uninduced state, which can lead to increase in the drug steady-state concentration and possible toxicity if the dose is not reduced, while if a patient who is stabilized on the dose that produces the desired therapeutic effect starts taking an enzyme inducer, modification of the drug dose is usually necessary to maintain the desired therapeutic effect. For example, if a patient who is taking an enzyme inducer was started on oral anticoagulants, the dose of oral anticoagulants is adjusted until the desired prothrombin time is achieved. Dose modification of the oral anticoagulants will be necessary if the enzyme inducer is stopped while the patient continues to take the oral anticoagulant. On the contrary, if the patient who is taking an oral anticoagulant that maintains the desired prothrombin time was started on an enzyme inducer, the dose of the oral anticoagulant will have to be modified to maintain the desired prothrombin time.

25.4.5   INFLUENCE OF DRUG DOSE

The outcome of DDI varies depending on the dose of the drugs involved with larger doses producing more significant interactions in most cases. The clinical significance of some DDI is also dependent on the dose. For example, salicylates administered in dose below 2 g/day are eliminated mainly by metabolism with small fraction of dose eliminated unchanged in urine. At this dose, urinary alkalinization is not likely to affect the renal elimination of salicylate to a great extent. However, when salicylate doses are above 5 g/day, the metabolic pathways are saturated and a large fraction of dose is excreted unchanged in the urine. In this case, urinary alkalinization can significantly enhance the elimination rate of salicylate by increasing its renal excretion.

25.5 DRUG–DRUG INTERACTION STUDIES IN DRUG DEVELOPMENT

Evaluation of the drug interaction potential for new molecular entity is an important component of the drug development process. The FDA has published several guidance documents for evaluating the drug interaction potential for new drugs during the development process [12–14]. Evaluation of drug interactions includes in vitro studies to explore the potential for metabolic and transporters drug interactions with the new drug. The significant interactions uncovered from the in vitro studies are investigated further for their clinical significance by in vivo studies in humans. The results of these in vivo and in vitro studies in addition to other information from population pharmacokinetic assessment are used to develop the dosing guidelines and provide the information included in the label of the new drug.

25.5.1 IN VITRO STUDIES

The in vitro studies usually include investigation of the new drug potential for interaction with CYP metabolizing enzymes, other metabolic enzymes, and transporters [15]. The interaction with the CYP enzymes includes the inhibitory and the induction effects of the new drug on different CYP metabolizing enzymes. The CYP inhibition studies usually utilize different in vitro systems including human liver microsomes, expressed enzymes, hepatocytes, and liver slices. Liver tissues used in the in vitro studies have to be obtained from more than one individual because of the inter-subject variability in drug metabolism and genetic polymorphism. Investigation of the ability of the new drug to inhibit CYP enzymes involves studying the enzyme kinetics of a specific probe substrate for the specific CYP enzyme system using different substrate concentrations above and below the K_m. Then the enzyme kinetics of the same substrate is studied in the presence of different concentrations of the new drug that is investigated for its inhibitory effect to the CYP enzymes. The relationship between the enzymatic reaction rate and substrate concentration can be described by the Michaelis-Menten equation as in Equation 25.2, and in the presence of an inhibitor the reaction rate is described by Equation 25.3:

$$\text{Rate} = \frac{V_{max}S}{K_m + S} \tag{25.2}$$

$$\text{Rate} = \frac{V_{max}S}{K_m(1+(I/K_i)) + S} \tag{25.3}$$

where
V_{max} is the maximum rate of the enzymatic reaction
K_m is the Michaelis-Menten constant
S is the substrate concentration
I is the inhibitor concentration
K_i is the in vitro inhibition constant

These parameters can be estimated from the results of the in vitro study. The ratio I/K_i is calculated using the highest expected inhibitor (new drug) concentration while using the highest recommended dose. If the ratio is <0.1, this means that the new drug is not likely to have any inhibitory effect on the CYP enzyme used in the experiment and no further in vivo studies are required, while if the ratio I/K_i is >0.1, this means that there is a potential for inhibition of the CYP enzyme used in the experiment by the new drug and further investigation of the inhibitory effect of the new drug by in vivo studies may be necessary. These experiments are repeated for all other CYP enzymes [15–17].

In vitro studies can also be performed to evaluate the potential enzyme induction effect of the new drug molecule. The in vitro system used in the evaluation depends on the stage of drugs development and the purpose of the study. Usually, freshly pre-pared hepatocyte system is incubated with the new drug at concentration relevant to the expected clinical drug concentration for 2–5 days. Positive controls are prepared using known inducers for the specific CYP enzyme being studied. After induction, the enzyme activity is studied using a specific probe substrate for the CYP enzyme. If the in vitro studies demonstrate that the increase of enzyme activity after incuba-tion with the new drug is less than 40% of the positive control, no further in vivo studies are required, while if the enzyme activity is more than 40% of the positive control, in vivo studies should be performed to examine if induction can happen in clinical doses and if the extent of induction can cause significant DDI [16]. Similar experiments are performed to test the new drug as an inhibitor or inducer for other non-CYP metabolizing enzymes.

Additional in vitro experiments can also be performed to screen for P-gp sub-strates, inducers or inhibitors utilizing techniques such as Caco-2 cells or other tech-niques. Experiments performed to test if the new drug molecule is a P-gp substrate usually utilize digoxin as a positive control, while testing for P-gp inhibition utilizes digoxin and vinblastine as probe substrates. When the in vitro experiments provide evidence of P-gp inhibition by the new drug molecule, further in vivo experiments can be performed to see if clinically significant interaction can occur. Similar in vitro experiments can be performed to test if the new drug is a substrate, inducer, or inhibitor for other transporters [17].

25.5.2 In Vivo Studies

In vivo studies are designed to confirm or refute the information obtained in the in vitro studies. For example, when the in vitro studies indicate that the new investi-gational drug is metabolized by a specific CYP enzyme system, in vivo drug inter-action study is performed to determine if selective inducer and inhibitor for that specific CYP can change the clearance of this new drug. Also, if the new drug is a potential inhibitor or inducer for a specific CYP enzyme, interaction studies are performed to determine the effect of the drug on the clearance of the most selective substrate for that specific CYP enzyme. In these studies, the most selective substrate and the most potent inducer or inhibitor should be used. If the studies performed under these harsh conditions fail to detect significant interaction, no further drug interaction studies are required. However, if DDI is detected in these in vivo studies, further studies with other substrates, inhibitors, and inducers are performed. Also, the information generated in population pharmacokinetic studies can be used to confirm the presence or absence of DDI. The following points should be considered when designing in vivo DDI studies [15,17]:

- These studies are performed in healthy volunteers when the study end-point is to evaluate the pharmacokinetic changes resulting from the DDI. However, patients should be used when the studies involve pharmacodynamic measurements.
- Both genders should be included in the studies except when the drug under investigation is intended for use in only one gender.
- The number of subjects included in these studies depends on the results of the in vitro studies and the intra- and interindividual variability. If the results of the in vitro studies indicate that the interaction is likely to occur, small number of subjects is needed to detect the interaction in the in vivo studies, while if the results of the in vitro studies indicate that the interaction is unlikely, large number of subjects should be used in the in vivo studies to reach the right conclusion.
- The largest dose and the shortest dosing intervals recommended for use in patients are usually used in these in vivo interaction studies. Smaller doses should be used in these studies if the drug interactions may cause significant increase in drug concentration that can lead to increased risk of toxicity.
- DDI studies are usually performed after administration of a single dose of the drug as long as the drug does not accumulate significantly during repeated administration and does not follow time-dependent pharmacokinetics. Multiple-dose studies are recommended when pharmacodynamic measurements are obtained during the study. Also, when both the drug and its metabolite have inhibitory effect, multiple-dose studies are performed to allow the accumulation of metabolite to detect the full inhibitory effect. When the induction effect is investigated, multiple doses of the enzyme inducer should be administered.
- The randomized crossover study design is usually used in these studies. However, fixed sequence crossover studies or parallel study design can be used when some of the drugs used in the study have long half-life or long-lasting effect.
- In these studies, the substrate concentration is usually monitored to characterize the pharmacokinetic behavior of substrate under different study conditions. However, substrates and inhibitor concentrations can be measured to determine if the pharmacokinetic behaviors of the two interacting drugs are affected.
- The pharmacokinetic parameters obtained in these studies are evaluated to determine if there is significant DDI. The 90% confidence interval of the geometric mean ratio of the pharmacokinetic parameters for the substrate such as AUC and C_{max} estimated in the presence and absence of the interacting drug is used in the evaluation. When the calculated 90% confidence interval is within the 80%–125% range (no effect boundaries), this means that the change in the systemic exposure is considered not clinically meaningful. This means that the DDI is not clinically significant. When the drug exposure-response relationship for the efficacy and toxicity measures is established, other no effect boundaries may be used.

25.5.3 LABELING CONSIDERATIONS

The information obtained from the in vitro and in vivo drug interaction studies has to be carefully analyzed to determine the new drug potential for interaction with other drugs. This information has to be included in the drug label [18]. Information about the metabolic pathways, metabolites, and pharmacokinetic interactions is usually included in the appropriate section of the new drug label. When the interaction study results suggest that the new drug should not be used, should be used in modified doses, or should be used with caution in patients receiving some other specific drugs, this information should be included in the appropriate section of the label. Additional information based on studies performed in other drugs that have similar metabolic interaction characteristics to the new drug being developed can be included in the label with an indication that similar interactions may occur.

REFERENCES

1. Baxter K (Ed.) (2010) *Stockley's Drug Interactions: A Source Book of Interactions, Their Mechanisms, Clinical Importance and Management*, 9th edn., Pharmaceutical Press, Chicago, IL.
2. Rowland M and Tozer TN (2010) *Clinical Pharmacokinetics and Pharmacodynamics: Concepts and Applications*, 4th edn., Lippincott Williams & Wilkins, Philadelphia, PA.
3. Thummel KE and Wilkinson GR (1998) In vitro and in vivo drug interactions involving human CYP3A. *Annu Rev Pharmacol Toxicol* 38:389–430.
4. DuBuske LM (2005) The role of p-glycoprotein and organic anion–transporting polypeptides in drug interactions. *Drug Saf* 28:789–801.
5. Shapiro LE and Shear NH (2002) Drug interactions: Proteins pumps, and P-450s. *J Am Acad Dermatol* 47:467–484.
6. Dresser GK and Bailley DG (2002) A basic conceptual and practical overview of interactions with highly prescribed drugs. *Can J Clin Pharmacol* 9:191–198.
7. Mann HJ (2006) Drug-associated disease: Cytochrome P450 interactions. *Crit Care Clin* 22:329–345.
8. Sweeney BP and Bromilow J (2006) Liver enzyme induction and inhibition: Implication of anaesthesia. *Anesthesia* 61:159–177.
9. Micromedex® 1.0 Healthcare Series, Clinical Decision Support, Drug Interactions, Thomson Reuters, Greenwood Village, CO. http://www.thomsonhc.com (last accessed June 15, 2011).
10. Endres CJ, Hsiao P, Chung FS, and Unadkat JD (2006) The role of transporters in drug interactions. *Eur J Pharm Sci* 27:501–517.
11. Balimane PV, Han Y-H, and Chong S (2006) Current industrial practices of assessing permeability and p-glycoprotein interaction. *AAPS J* 8:Article 1, E1–E13.
12. Center for Drug Evaluation and Research, U.S. Food and Drug Administration, Guidance for industry (1997): Drug metabolism/drug interactions in the drug development process: Studies in vitro.
13. Center for Drug Evaluation and Research, U.S. Food and Drug Administration, Guidance for industry (1999): In vivo drug metabolism/drug interaction studies: Study design, data analysis and recommendation for dosing and labeling.
14. Center for Drug Evaluation and Research, U.S. Food and Drug Administration, Guidance for industry (2006): Drug interaction studies: Study design, data analysis and implications for dosing and labeling.

15. Huang S-M, Temple R, Throckmorton DC, and Lesko LJ (2007) Drug interaction studies: Study design, data analysis and implications for dosing and labeling. *Clin Pharmacol Ther* 81:298–304.
16. Huang S-M and Lesko LJ (2004) Drug-drug, drug-dietary supplement and drug-citrus fruit and other food interactions. What have we learned? *J Clin Pharmacol* 44:559–569.
17. Huang S-M (2004) Drug-drug interactions, in Krishna R (Ed.) *Applications of Pharmacokinetic Principles in Drug Development* Kluwer Academic, New York.
18. U.S. Food and Drug Administration Advisory Committee for Pharmaceutical Sciences and Clinical Pharmacology Subcommittee meeting. Issues and challenges in the evolution and labeling of drug interaction potentials of NME, Rockville, MD. April 23, 2003, http://www.fda.gov/ohrms/dockets/ac/03/slides/3947S2_02_Huang_files/frame.htm, Last accessed June 15, 2011.

26 Pharmacogenetics
The Genetic Basis of Pharmacokinetic and Pharmacodynamic Variability

OBJECTIVES

After completing this chapter you should be able to

- Define the common terms used in the field of pharmacogenetics
- Describe the basic gene structure and the consequences of gene variation
- List a few examples of clinically significant genetic polymorphism involving CYP450 and non-CYP450 metabolizing enzymes
- Give examples of genetic polymorphism involving drug pharmacodynamics
- Evaluate the clinical significance of genetic polymorphism that involves drug pharmacokinetics and pharmacodynamics
- Discuss the benefits of pharmacogenetic testing for optimization of drug therapy

26.1 INTRODUCTION

The genetic variation in drug response has been recognized since the 1950s when some patients experienced prolonged neuromuscular blockade after receiving the muscle relaxant suxamethonium chloride in preparation for surgical procedures. These patients were found to have a less efficient genetic variant of the butylcholinesterase enzyme (atypical pseudocholinesterase) responsible for the hydrolysis of suxamethonium chloride. The reduced cholinesterase activity resulted in prolongation of the half-life of this muscle relaxant and slowed the recovery from surgical paralysis. Also, the genetic variation in the *N*-acetyltransferase enzyme divides patients to slow acetylators and rapid acetylators, who metabolize drugs through the acetylation pathway at two distinct rates. When these two patient populations receive the same dose of drugs that are metabolized through the acetylation pathway such as the antituberculosis drug isoniazid and the antiarrhythmic drug procainamide, higher steady-state drug concentration is achieved in the slow acetylator population.

These clinical observations resulted in the development of the field of pharmacogenetics, which deals with the genetic variations that give rise to differences in drug pharmacokinetics and/or pharmacodynamics. The interest in the relationship between genetic variation and patient response to drug therapy led to the development of the field of pharmacogenomics, which is the broader application of the genomic technology in understanding the disease characteristics and in drug discovery. The knowledge gained from the human genome project allowed the perception of why in some diseases different patients with different genetic characteristics respond differently to the same treatment. In some diseases, the patient's specific genetic characteristics can be used to predict the patient's response to a particular medication and the probability of developing adverse effects. Understanding the patient's genetic makeup is the key for the development of personalized medications with greater efficacy and safety. The current clinical applications of pharmacogenetics are limited and are mainly directed to screening patients for variation in some of the cytochrome P450 (CYP450) genes and selecting the drug dose based on the results of these tests. Few pharmacogenetic tests are currently used to screen patients before the start of therapy when the drug therapeutic and toxic effects are influenced by the patient's genotype. However, the continuous progress in this field should provide the primary care providers with the tools that can help in clinical decision making for the selection of the drug and dose, and prediction of response based on the genetic makeup of the patient.

26.2   GENE STRUCTURE AND GENE VARIATIONS

The gene is a linear sequence of nucleotides joined together by the phosphodiester bond and represents the unit of heredity in a living organism. It is defined as "a locatable region of genomic sequence, corresponding to a unit of inheritance which is associated with regulatory regions, transcribed regions, and or other functional sequence regions" [1]. Variations in the gene structure that occur in more than 1% of the population are referred to as genetic polymorphism. Genetic polymorphism occurs in different forms including complete gene deletion, gene duplication, or genetic translocation to form a new gene hybrid. The most common genetic polymorphism is the single nucleotide polymorphisms (SNPs) in which only one nucleotide at a specific position in the sequence is deleted, inserted, or changed. Each change in the nucleotide sequence introduces a variant form of the gene that is designated as an allele of the original gene. So the gene has the original specific sequence of nucleotides, and the alleles are the variants of this gene. Thus, the alleles of the original gene are responsible for determination of the specific characteristics of an individual such as the color of the eye, the color of hair, or the blood group etc. The human genome has over 1.5 million SNPs locations where differences in the nucleotides exist, forming different alleles in different individuals.

Understanding the nature of polymorphism can help in interpreting the genotype-phenotype relationship. The genotype is the inherited instructions the individual carries within his or her genetic code, while the phenotype is the observable characteristics or traits of an individual. These observable characteristics can be morphological, developmental, biochemical, physiological, or behavioral.

Phenotypes result from the expression of the genes and the influence of environmental factors and interaction between the two. The type of genetic polymorphism can be classified based on the effect on protein expression or phenotype. Deletion of a gene results in loss of function and absence of the gene product such as in CYP2D6 alleles associated with loss of gene products, which leads to the common phenotype of metabolic deficiency, while gene duplication results in increased function and higher formation rate of gene products such as in CYP2D6 alleles associated with excessive gene product, which leads to the common phenotype of ultrarapid metabolism. Additionally, gene translocation usually results in the formation of nonfunctioning gene and absence of gene products.

The mode of inheritance is dependent on whether it is transmitted by a gene at a single locus (monogenic) or by genes at multiple loci (polygenic) on the chromosome. When the genetic change occurs at a single locus and leads to the absence of a protein product, all the resulting alleles will form the same phenotype. The activity of CYP2D6 is inherited as a monogenetic trait. The different CYP2D6 alleles are usually associated with the absence or excessive formation of the gene product. In this case, the genetic polymorphism in the rate of CYP2D6 metabolism is observed in the general population as three distinct clusters: poor, extensive, and ultrarapid metabolizers, that is, polymodal frequency distribution [2]. On the contrary, the different CYP2C9 alleles have different amino acid substitutions that encode for allozymes (variant forms of an enzyme) with unequal catalytic activities, which is not uniform for the different substrates. In this case, the genetic polymorphism in the rate of CYP2C9 metabolism is detected in the general population as variation in the metabolic rate around a mean value, that is, unimodal frequency distribution [3]. Polygenic or multifactorial inheritance is a phenotypic characteristic or trait attributed to two or more genes or the interaction with environment. For example, the therapeutic effect of warfarin has been linked to numerous genes, with the strongest association with CYP2C9, which affects the rate of warfarin metabolism, and the vitamin K reductase, which is the therapeutic target for warfarin. So warfarin response is considered a polygenic trait and the variation in warfarin dose required to achieve adequate anticoagulant effect is observed in the general population as unimodal frequency distribution [4]. A haplotype is when a combination of alleles at different locations in the gene is transmitted together. For many proteins, the association between gene structure and phenotype may be poor in reference to a single polymorphism, whereas the association is stronger when a number of specific polymorphisms within a defined haplotype are included in analysis.

A standardized format for the nomenclature of the different alleles has been developed to help in communicating and cataloguing the specific attributes of specific genetic polymorphism. The allele name consists of the gene name followed by an asterisk and a numerical value [5]. The numerical value will take 1 for the most common allele that encodes the active protein, and the other alleles will take numbers in the chronological order of their identification. For example, the alleles for the gene that encode the CYP2D6 enzymes can have the following names: CYP2D6*1, CYP2D6*2, CYP2D6*3, CYP2D6*4, and so on. The name includes the supergene family [CYP], family [2], subfamily [D], and the specific gene [6] followed by * and the number that denotes the different alleles.

Because of the diploid nature of the human genome, each cell has two copies of the same gene one inherited from the male and the other from the female. Individuals having two copies of the same allele on the corresponding positions on paired chromosomes are said to have homozygous genotype while any combination of two different alleles yields a heterozygous genotype. For example, if the gene CYP2C9 has three different alleles: CYP2C9*1, CYP2C9*2, and CYP2C9*3, there will be six possible genotypes: CYP2C9*1/*1, CYP2C9*2/*2, CYP2C9*3/*3, CYP2C9*1/*2, CYP2C9*1/*3, and CYP2C9*2/*3. The first three genotypes are considered homozygous because they have similar alleles and the last three genotypes are considered heterozygous because they have different alleles. The allele is considered dominant if it is expressed in observable trait and influences the phenotype of the individual and recessive if it does not. Both dominant and recessive alleles of drug metabolizing enzymes have been described. The phenotype is usually influenced by the number of alleles that encode the active protein. A good example to demonstrate the relationship between the number of alleles encoding the active metabolizing enzyme and the metabolic phenotype has been described for CYP2D6. Homozygous individuals with two inactive alleles usually have absence or very little metabolizing enzymes and have the least metabolic activity (poor metabolizers). Heterozygous individuals with one active CYP2D6 allele have metabolizing enzymes and metabolic activity less than those with two active alleles (extensive metabolizers), whereas homozygous individuals with two active alleles usually have duplication of the CYP2D6 on the same chromosome, excessive formation of the metabolizing enzymes, and the highest metabolic activity (ultrarapid metabolizers) [6].

26.3   GENETIC POLYMORPHISM IN PHARMACOKINETICS

The majority of the clinically significant inherited variability in pharmacokinetics is related to variation in drug metabolism. However, genetic variations in drug transporters have been identified and changes in the pharmacokinetics behavior of substrates for these transporters have been characterized. Most of the genetic polymorphisms in drug metabolism have been identified by observation of a group of patients experiencing adverse effects or therapeutic failure while receiving the usual doses of the drug. Further investigations usually reveal the genetic basis of these variations in drug response.

26.3.1   CYTOCHROME P450 ENZYMES

The genetic variation in CYP2D6 is a well-characterized genetic polymorphism in the CYP450 enzymes. It was discovered when some of the patients taking the antihypertensive drug debrisoquine (currently not used clinically), which is specifically metabolized by CYP2D6, experienced severe hypotension that was accompanied by higher plasma debrisoquine concentrations. This increased drug effect was explained by inherited deficiency in debrisoquine metabolizing enzymes as determined by further investigations. Approximately 20% of the prescribed drugs are metabolized in the CYP2D6. Genetic polymorphism in the CYP2D6 gene have been discovered in most of the world populations leading to large variation in the enzyme metabolizing activity ranging from complete deficiency, intermediate activity, extensive activity to ultrarapid activity [7]. The prevalence of poor metabolizers is around 6%–10% in Caucasians, slightly higher in African American, and around 2% in Asians. The ultrarapid metabolizers represent about 7% of the Caucasian population, while in the Middle East and north Africa the percentage of ultrarapid metabolizers is much higher and can reach up to 35%.

CYP2D6 deficiency can lead to amplification of the pharmacological effect of the drug if CYP2D6 represents the major route of its elimination such as in case of fluoxetine and tricyclic antidepressants. The drug effect can be reduced significantly if CYP2D6 is involved in the activation of the drug. For example, CYP2D6 deficiency can lead to the lack of the analgesic effect of codeine because the metabolism of codeine to morphine is catalyzed by CYP2D6 [8]. Gene duplication of CYP2D6 can lead to inheritance of ultrarapid metabolite phenotype that has been associated with reduced effect of some antidepressant and antipsychotic drugs due to their fast rate of metabolism [7]. Because of the good correlation between the in vitro genotype and the patient phenotype with regard to CYP2D6 activity, genotyping has been recommended before using CYP2D6 substrates with low safety margins to protect poor metabolizers from developing adverse effects. This is specifically important in patients with personal or family history of adverse effects or reduced activity of drugs metabolized by CYP2D6.

CYP2C9 is the main enzyme system for the metabolism of a number of drugs with narrow therapeutic range including warfarin, phenytoin, losartan, glipizide, and a number of nonsteroidal anti-inflammatory drugs (NSAIDs). Many CYP2C9 alleles have been identified with three allele variants that can encode allozymes with significantly different catalytic activities for the metabolism of S-warfarin. The allele expressing the wild-type protein is designated as CYP2C9*1/*1, while the CYP2C9*2/*2 allele encodes allozymes with about 30%–40% of the metabolic activity of the wild type for S-warfarin metabolism, and the CYP2C9*3/*3 allele encodes allozymes with almost no activity for S-warfarin metabolism. Modest reduction in the metabolism of S-warfarin has been observed in the heterozygous genotypes, for example, CYP2C9*1/*2, CYP2C9*1/*3, and CYP2C9*2/*3. So one would expect that patients carrying one or more of the alleles associated with the reduced metabolic activity should have higher S-warfarin concentration for a given warfarin dose. These patients usually require lower doses of warfarin to produce therapeutic anticoagulant effect compared with the patients who do not have these variant alleles [9]. Also, the incidence of gastrointestinal (GIT) bleeding in patients receiving NSAIDs and the incidence of hypoglycemia in patients treated with glimepiride or glibendamide were significantly higher in patients with the CYP2C9 genotypes associated with the lower metabolic activity. Epidemiological studies demonstrated that individuals heterozygous for the inactive CYP2C9 allele with intermediate metabolic activity are about 35%–40% among Caucasians and 3.5% in Japanese, while subjects who are homozygous for the two inactive CYP2C9 alleles with presumed poor metabolizers phenotype are 4% among Caucasian and 0.2% among Japanese [10].

CYP2C19 is associated with the metabolism of the S-enantiomer of the antiepileptic drug mephenytoin and other drugs such as diazepam, citalopram, propranolol, omeprazole, and proguanil. Similar to the CYP2D6 isoenzyme, specific gene variations in the gene encoding CYP2C19 lead to the poor metabolizer phenotype with respect to the number of therapeutic agents metabolized by these enzymes. However, the ultrarapid phenotype has not been detected for this enzyme isoform. The frequency of poor metabolizers is about 2%–5% in Caucasian and African American, 10%–23% in the Asian population, and about 70% in the south pacific populations. A dose reduction is recommended for drugs that are completely or partially metabolized by CYP2C19 such as the tricyclic antidepressants and citalopram, fluoxetine, and sertraline in poor metabolizers because higher plasma concentrations of these drugs have been reported in these patients. Higher frequency of adverse effects have been reported in poor metabolizers while receiving narrow therapeutic index drugs metabolized by the CYP2C19 such as phenytoin, warfarin, mephobarbital, and hexobarbital. Studies have shown that the proton pump inhibitors metabolized by CYP2C19 such as omeprazole, rabeprazole, and lansoprazole are more effective in the management of peptic ulcer in patients with one or more of the CYP2C19 alleles associated with the poor metabolizer phenotype. Also, the antimalarial prodrugs proguanil and chlorproguanil, which have to be activated by the CYP2C19, are not effective in patients carrying defective CYP2C19 allele because of their inability to activate the prodrug [11].

CYP3A4 is the predominant metabolizing enzyme present in the adult liver and small intestine. Large variation in the CYP3A4 activity is observed between individuals because of the large variability in the isoenzyme expression and the overlap in substrate specificity. A variety of alleles has been identified for the CYP3A4 gene; however, most of these alleles occur at low frequencies and do not alter the phenotype to any appreciable extent. Despite the genetic influence on the activity of CYP3A enzymes, it does not significantly contribute to the variability in the metabolic clearance of these enzymes. The CYP3A5 is expressed in only 50% of the African Americans and about 20% of Caucasians. Individuals who have both CYP3A4 and CYP3A5 usually have higher metabolic rate for the drugs that are metabolized by both enzyme isoforms [11].

26.3.2 THIOPURINE METHYLTRANSFERASE

The genetic polymorphism of the thiopurine methyltransferase (TPMT) is well documented. The enzyme TPMT catalyzes the S-methylation of the thiopurine drugs such as azathioprine, mercaptopurine, and thioguanine, which are used in patients with leukemia, rheumatoid diseases, inflammatory bowel disease, and organ transplantation. The thiopurine drugs are inactive prodrugs that require activation to thioguanine nucleotide to produce their cytotoxic effect. In the hematopoietic tissues, TPMT is the main metabolizing enzyme of these drugs. The activity of TPMT in the red blood cells is variable and polymorphic with around 90% of patients have high activity, 10% have intermediate activity, and 0.3% have very low or undetectable enzyme activity. This makes the patients with low TPMT activity at high risk of developing life-threatening hematological toxicity while taking these thiopurine drugs. Determination of the functional TPMT status before the start of azathioprine, or mercaptopurine therapy, can be very useful in selecting the dose of these drugs to avoid the severe hematological toxicity of these drugs in the patients with low TPMT activity [12]. TPMT-deficient patients who are at high risk of developing toxicity while taking thiopurine drugs may require dose reduction to 20%–50% of the standard dose [11].

26.3.3 N-ACETYLTRANSFERASE

Acetylation is the main metabolic pathway for the elimination of drugs such as isoniazid, hydralazine, amrinone, and phenelzine. The bimodal distribution of the rate of isoniazid acetylation in different individuals has been one of the first observed genetic controls of drug metabolism. Isoniazid is metabolized by the enzyme N-acetyltransferase2 (NAT2), which has many variants. Genetically controlled differences in acetylation activity have been observed with individuals carrying the slow acetylation allele and exhibit the "slow acetylator" phenotype, and those with the heterozygous alleles exhibit the "rapid acetylator" phenotype. Large ethnic differences exist in the distribution of the acetylation status. The percentage of slow acetylators in Caucasians and African Americans is between 50% and 60%, while the percentage is about 20% in Chinese, and 10%–15% in Japanese and Eskimos. The genetic polymorphism in the acetylation pathway has to be considered when using drugs that are eliminated mainly via this pathway. Smaller doses of isoniazid should be administered in slow acetylators to avoid the development of peripheral neuropathy, which usually results from the elevated isoniazid concentrations achieved if they receive the standard doses. Also, rapid acetylators are more susceptible to isoniazid hepatotoxicity, which may result from the faster rate of formation of the metabolite implicated in isoniazid-induced hepatotoxicity [13].

   Also, slow acetylators are more susceptible to the development of systemic lupus erythematosus-like syndrome while using the antihypertensive drug hydralazine. This adverse effect is probably associated with the elevated plasma hydralazine concentration in this patient population. The topoisomerase II inhibitor amonafide is metabolized through the acetylation pathway to N-acetyl-amonafide, which is an active metabolite that contributes to the toxicity of this anticancer drug. Large interindividual variability exists in the pharmacokinetics of amonafide with higher incidence of myelosuppression reported in rapid acetylators compared to slow acetylator. This adverse effect has been attributed to the larger amount of the active metabolites formed in this patient population. It was recommended to use the acetylation status as the basis for amonafide dose selection with slow acetylators receiving higher doses compared to the rapid acetylator [14]. Amonafide is no longer in clinical use because of the large inter-patient variability in pharmacokinetics and toxicity; however, it represents a good example of the significant contribution of the genetic polymorphism to the pharmacokinetics and pharmacodynamics variability of drugs.

26.3.4 UDP-GLUCURONOSYLTRANSFERASE

Glucuronidation is the major metabolic pathway for numerous drugs and endogenous compounds. Genetic polymorphism has been reported in the different UDP-glucuronosyltransferase (UGT) families, which can contribute to the large interindividual variability in the rate of the glucuronidation process. Unconjugated hyperbilirubinemia as in Gilbert's and Crigler-Najjar syndromes has been associated with UGT1A1 polymorphism and occurs in individuals carrying the enzyme variant that produces slow glucuronidation [15]. Another example for the UGT1A1 polymorphism involves the disposition of the anticancer drug irinotecan, which is a prodrug metabolized to the active metabolite SN-38. The active metabolite SN-38 is eliminated by metabolism through the glucuronidation pathway. Irinotecan can cause severe and sometimes fetal toxicities including myelosuppression and diarrhea. It was suggested that patients with the UGT1A1 allele associated with the low glucuronidation activity are more susceptible to these toxicities [16]. The association between the UGT1A1 polymorphism and irinotecan toxicity is included in the label of irinotecan; however, there is no clear recommendation for the need of pharmacogenetic screening for UGT1A1 before initiation of irinotecan therapy.

26.3.5 DRUG TRANSPORTERS

Drug transporters such as the ATP binding cassette (ABC) transporters and the solute carrier (SLC) transporters play a significant role in drug absorption, distribution, metabolism, and excretion. The key ABC transporters involved in drug disposition are ABCB1 (P-gp, MDR1), the ABCC (MRP 1–9), and the ABCG2 (breast cancer resistant protein). ABCB1 plays significant role in drug disposition; however, the role of polymorphism in its function is not clear. There have been more than 100 genetic variants for the ABCB1 gene identified. Some of these variants have been associated with increased susceptibility to renal cell carcinoma, Parkinson's disease, inflammatory bowel disease, refractory epilepsy, and response to HIV therapy. A number of clinical studies have shown a link between ABCB1 polymorphisms and the pharmacokinetics of drugs such as the lower exposure to amlodipine associated with a specific haplotype of ABCB1 [17]. Also, ABCC2 polymorphism has been correlated with a twofold increase in methotrexate concentration specially after administration of high methotrexate dose, resulting in an increased need for the folate rescue in these patients [18]. Higher concentrations of pravastatin during multiple administration, and lower frequency of diarrhea in patients taking irinotecan, have been associated with ABCC2 polymorphisms. Also, ABCG2 polymorphism have been linked to alteration in the pharmacokinetics of several drugs such as achieving higher plasma concentrations of diflomotecan, lower plasma concentrations of rosuvastatin, and alteration of irinotecan conversion to its active metabolite, SN-38. However, the clinical significance of these observations is yet to be determined and should be studied further in larger number of patients [11].

The SLC transporters that are engaged in drug disposition include the organic cation transporter (OCT), organic anion transporter (OAT), nucleoside transporter, and the polypeptide transporters (OATPs). Polymorphisms in SLCO1B1, which is one of the members of the polypeptide transporters, have been linked to variation in pravastatin and fexofenadine pharmacokinetics, and increased exposure to repaglinide and nateglinide during multiple administration [11,19]. The genetic polymorphism in different transporters is well established, and the association between these polymorphisms and variation in the drug pharmacokinetic behavior is well documented as mentioned before.

However, the majority of the reported transporter polymorphism does not have the clinical significance necessary to suggest the importance of determining the transporter genetic status before using drugs that are substrates for these transporters.

26.4 GENETIC POLYMORPHISM IN PHARMACODYNAMICS

Most drugs produce their therapeutic effects by interaction with a specific target that can be an enzyme or a receptor. Genetic polymorphism that can alter the interaction between the drug and its specific target can increase or decrease the activity of the drug. This can explain why some patients respond better than other patients to a specific treatment. There are few documented examples that link polymorphism to the pharmacodynamic of the drug, for example, the β_1-adrenergic receptor gene polymorphism and the β-blocker response. Studies have demonstrated that in hypertensive patients some specific haplotypes respond better to β-blockers and had greater reduction in blood pressure compared to patients with other haplotypes. These observations can explain the better blood pressure response to β-blockers of Caucasians compared to African Americans. This is because the frequency of the allele associated with the higher β_1-receptor activity is higher in Caucasians than in African Americans [20].

Another well-documented effect of genetic polymorphism on the drug pharmacodynamics is the vitamin K epoxide reductase complex subunit 1 (VKORC1) gene polymorphism and warfarin response. This gene encodes vitamin K reductase that is inhibited by warfarin. This inhibition interferes with carboxylation of vitamin K-dependent coagulating factors and proteins C and S. Two haplotypes have been linked to the daily warfarin dose required to maintain adequate anticoagulation effect. The different haplotypes produce different amounts of VKORC1, which is the target site for warfarin. The haplotype associated with the lower VKORC1 amount require lower doses of warfarin compared to the other haplotype. The higher frequency of the haplotype associated with lower VKORC1 amounts in the Asian population can explain the lower warfarin dosage requirement in these patients [21]. Also, polymorphism near the human interferon gene has been used to predict the response of hepatitis C to interferon treatment. Genotype 1 hepatitis C patients carrying certain genetic variant alleles achieve sustained virological response after treatment with Pegylated-interferon-alpha-2a or Pegylated-interferon-alpha-2b. Additional examples include the mutation in the angiotensin-converting-enzyme (ACE) gene, which has been proposed as a possible reason for the variation in response to ACE inhibitors. Furthermore, β_2-adrenergic receptor mutations have been linked to the reduction of the bronchodilator effect of albuterol.

26.5 IMPLEMENTATION OF PHARMACOGENETIC TESTING IN CLINICAL PRACTICE

The development in the field of pharmacogenetics demonstrating the association between the genetic polymorphism and the pharmacokinetic and pharmacodynamic characteristics of drugs has been slowly adopted in clinical practice. This knowledge can help clinicians in identifying responders from nonresponders, optimizing drug dose, and avoiding adverse effects based on the patient's specific genetic characteristics.

The pharmacogenetic biomarkers that are strongly associated with pharmacokinetic and pharmacodynamic characteristics of drugs can be utilized in guiding the clinical use of these drugs. Information about these pharmacogenetic biomarkers is usually included in the drug label, and if these pharmacogenetics tests are required, recommended, or may be performed when using the drugs. The U.S. Food and Drug Administration (FDA) provides an updated list of all FDA-approved drugs with pharmacogenomic information in their labels [22].

For example, cetuximab is a recombinant monoclonal antibody that binds specifically to the human epidermal growth factor receptor (EGFR) and used in the treatment of some types of cancer. The use of this drug should be restricted to tumors that express EGFR, which is the target for this drug. Also, treatment with the antiretrovirus drug maraviroc is restricted to patients with confirmed infection with CCR5-tropic HIV-1, because this drug is effective only against this type of infection. Furthermore, the antileukemic drug dasatinib is only effective against Philadelphia chromosome-positive acute lymphoblastic leukemia (Ph+ ALL). Moreover, the anticancer drug trastuzumab is effective against human epidermal growth factor receptor 2-overexpressing cancers, so it should only be used in tumors that are tested positive for this receptor.

In some drugs, the pharmacogenetic biomarker tests are recommended to optimize drug therapy and avoid adverse effects. For example, testing for the allele associated with the increased incidence of carbamazepine-induced Stevens-Johnson syndrome (HLA-B*1502) is recommended in the Asian population when they start taking carbamazepine. Also, it is recommended to test patients taking irinotecan for the UGT allele associated with the lower metabolic rate of its active metabolite SN-38, and has been implicated for the serious adverse effects observed after irinotecan therapy. Other recommended pharmacogenetic tests include testing for CYP2C9 and VKORC1 variants during warfarin therapy, testing for TPMT variants during azathioprine, mercaptopurine, and thioguanine therapy, and testing for glucose-6-phosphate dehydrogenase deficiency during rasburicase use.

26.6 FUTURE DIRECTIONS

Pharmacogenetic discoveries provide important information that can be utilized in making clinical decisions involving drug selection and doses to improve patient care. However, additional work is needed to improve the utility of this information in clinical practice. Clinical trials are needed to demonstrate that the use of the pharmacogenetic testing can improve the clinical outcome. Determination of the cost-effectiveness of pharmacogenetic testing can greatly promote the utilization of these tests in clinical practice. Regulatory authorities and professional organizations should develop more guidelines for utilizing pharmacogenetic testing in different clinical conditions. All healthcare professionals have to be adequately educated about the interpretation of pharmacogenetic test results and utilization of these results in clinical decision making. Collaboration between the healthcare professionals is necessary to implement a practice model to order, perform, interpret, and utilize pharmacogenetic testing. Utilization of the pharmacogenetic discoveries in clinical decisions can help in promoting safe and effective drug use and predicting the patient response to drug therapy.

REFERENCES

1. Pearson H (2006) Genetics: What is a gene? *Nature* 441:398–401.
2. Linder MW, Evans WE, and McLeod HL (2006) Application of pharmacogenetic principles to clinical pharmacology, in Burton ME, Shaw LM, Schentag JJ, and Evans WE (Eds.) *Applied Pharmacokinetics and Pharmacodynamics: Principles of Therapeutic Drug Monitoring*, Lippincott Williams & Wilkins, Philadelphia, PA.
3. Lee CR, Goldstein JA, and Pieper JA (2002) Cytochrome P450 2C9 polymorphism: A comprehensive review of the in-vitro and human data. *Pharmacogenetics* 12:251–263.
4. Krynetskiy E and McDonnell P (2007) Building individualized medicine: Prevention of adverse reaction to warfarin therapy. *J Pharmacol Exp Ther* 322:427–434.
5. Ingelman-Sundberg M, Daly AK, and Nebert DW Human cytochrome p450 (CYP) allele nomenclature committee. http://www.cypalleles.ki.se/, last accessed June 15, 2011.
6. Agundez JAG, Ledesma MC, Ladero JM, and Benitez J (1995) Prevalence of CYP2D6 gene duplication and its repercussion on the oxidative phenotype in a white population. *Clin Pharmacol Ther* 57:265–269.
7. Meyer UA (1994) Pharmacogenetics: The slow, the rapid, and the ultrarapid. *Proc Natl Acad Sci USA* 91:1983–1984.
8. Sindrup SH and Brosen K (1995) Pharmacogenetics of codeine hypoalgesia. *Pharmacogenetics* 5:335–346.
9. Higashi MK, Veenstra DL, Kondo LM, Wittkowsky AK, Srinouanprachanh SL, Farin FM, and Rettie AE (2002) Association between CYP2C9 genetic variants and anticoagulation-related outcomes during warfarin therapy. *JAMA* 287:1690–1698.
10. Nasu K, Kubota T, and Ishizaki T (1997) Genetic analysis of CYP2C9 polymorphism in a Japanese population. *Pharmacogenetics* 7:405–409.
11. Williams JA, Anderson T, Anderson T, Blanchard R, Behm MO, Cohen N, Edeki T, et al. (2008) PhRMA white paper on ADME pharmacogenomics. *J Clin Pharmacol* 48:849–889.
12. Evans WE, Hon YY, Bomgaars L, Coutre S, Holdsworth M, Janco R, Kalwinsky D, et al. (2001) Preponderance of thiopurine S methyltransferase deficiency and heterozygosity among patients intolerant to mercaptopurine or azathioprine. *J Clin Oncol* 19:2293–2301.
13. Bonicke R and Reif W (1953) Enzymatic inactivation of isonicotinic acid hydrizide in human and animal organism. *Naunyn Schmiedebergs Arch Exp Pathol Pharmakol* 220:321–323.
14. Innocenti F, Iyer L, and Ratain MJ (2001) Pharmacogenetics of anticancer agents: Lessons from amonafide and irinotecan. *Drug Metab Dispos* 29:596–600.
15. Kadakol A, Ghosh SS, Sappal BS, Sharma G, Chowdhury JR, and Chowdhury NR (2000) Genetic lesions of bilirubin uridine-diphosphoglucuronate glucuronosyltransferase (UGT1A1) causing Crigler-Najjar and Gilbert syndromes: Correlation of genotype to phenotype. *Hum Mutat* 16:297–306.
16. Paoluzzi L, Singh AS, Price DK, Danesi R, Mathijssen RH, Verweij J, Figg WD, and Sparreboom A (2004) Influence of genetic variants in UGT1A1 and UGT1A9 on the in vivo glucuronidation of SN-38. *J Clin Pharmacol* 44:854–860.
17. Leschziner GD, Andrew T, Pirmohamed M, and Johnson MR (2007) ABCB1 genotype and PGP expression, function and therapeutic drug response: A critical review and recommendations for future research. *Pharmacogenomics J* 7:154–179.
18. Rau T, Erney B, Gores R, Eschenhagen T, Beck J, and Langer T (2006) High-dose methotrexate in pediatric acute lymphoblastic leukemia: Impact of ABCC2 polymorphisms on plasma concentrations. *Clin Pharmacol Ther* 80:468–476.
19. Chung JY, Cho JY, Yu KS, Kim JR, Oh DS, Jung HR, Lim KS, Moon KH, Shin SG, and Jang IJ (2005) Effect of OATP1B1 (SLCO1B1) variant alleles on the pharmacokinetics of pitavastatin in healthy volunteers. *Clin Pharmacol Ther* 78:342–350.

20. Shin J and Johnson JA (2007) Pharmacogenetics of beta-blockers. *Pharmacotherapy* 27:874–887.
21. Rieder MJ, Reiner AP, Gage BF, Nickerson DA, Eby CS, McLeod HL, Blough DK, Thummel KE, Veenstra DL, and Rettie AE (2005) Effect of VKORC1 haplotypes on transcriptional regulation and warfarin dose. *N Engl J Med* 352:2285–2293.
22. U.S. FDA-approved drugs with pharmacogenomic information in their labels. http://www.fda.gov/Drugs/ScienceResearch/ResearchAreas/Pharmacogenetics/ucm083378.htm, last accessed June 15, 2011.

27 Applications of Computers in Pharmacokinetics

OBJECTIVES

After completing this chapter, you should be able to

- Discuss the different purposes for using computers in the field of pharmacokinetics
- Differentiate between the educational, research, and clinical applications of computers in the field of pharmacokinetics
- List specific commonly used examples of teaching, simulation, data analysis, and dose calculation computer programs that are used in pharmacokinetics

27.1 INTRODUCTION

Computers have been used extensively in the field of pharmacokinetics as instructional tool, in addition to simulations, data analysis, and dosage calculation. Pharmacokinetic classes are ideal for computer-based instruction because the different pharmacokinetic parameters that govern the drug concentration–time profile in the body can be related together by mathematical expressions. This makes graphical presentation of the drug concentration–time profile very useful for presenting the interplay between the different pharmacokinetic parameters. Computer-based pharmacokinetic simulations can be used for educational as well as research purposes. Pharmacokinetic simulations can be used to visualize how the change in any of the pharmacokinetic parameters can affect the drug concentration–time profile in the body, which can be useful for understanding the basic pharmacokinetic concepts. For research, simulations of the gastrointestinal tract (GIT) factors that can affect drug absorption have been used to predict the absorption of compounds with different properties. Besides, simulation of the drug concentration–time profiles in different body organs based on in vitro tissue distribution information have been used for developing physiologically based pharmacokinetic models (PBPK). Furthermore, simulation of the expected drug pharmacokinetic and pharmacodynamic behavior under different drug administration conditions is used for guiding the design of clinical studies.

In pharmacokinetic studies, the drug concentrations determined at different time points after drug administration are fitted to the mathematical expression that describes the drug concentration–time profile to estimate the pharmacokinetic parameters. When the experiments involve measuring the drug response in addition to the drug concentration, the data are used to estimate the pharmacokinetic and pharmacodynamic parameters from the mathematical expressions that describe the pharmacokinetic–pharmacodynamic (PK/PD) model. Pharmacokinetic data analysis is usually performed using statistical programs that are designed specifically to estimate the different pharmacokinetic and pharmacodynamic parameters from the available data. Population pharmacokinetic data analysis programs can utilize sparse pharmacokinetic information obtained from a large number of patients to estimate the drug pharmacokinetic parameters and to identify measurable factors that can cause changes in the drug pharmacokinetic behavior. Practitioners also use specialized computer programs to calculate the patient dosage requirement and recommend the appropriate dosing regimen based on the patient's specific characteristics and the measured blood drug concentration.

27.2   COMMONLY USED PHARMACOKINETIC COMPUTER PROGRAMS

The following is a list of the commonly used pharmacokinetic computer programs arranged in alphabetical order with a brief description of each program. The information included in the program description does not represent a critical review of the program, since this information was supplied by the program developer or obtained from the available information on the program website.

27.2.1   acslX

The acslX program provides an environment for modeling, simulation, and analysis of complex nonlinear systems and processes. Widely used for PBPK and PK/PD modeling, acslX supports both textual and graphical languages for specifying complex biological models, and a MATLAB®-like scripting language for specification of parameter estimation, sensitivity analysis, Monte-Carlo, or Markov Chain Monte Carlo analyses. Data integration capabilities with Microsoft Excel and Access are provided, and a PBPK/PK/PD toolkit is also available that includes linear and nonlinear PBPK models of various organs, exposure models for inhalation, oral and dermal exposures, and a variety of pharmacodynamic dose response models.

Web site: http://www.acslx.com
Platform: Windows

27.2.2   ADAPT II

ADAPT II is a computational modeling platform developed for pharmacokinetic and pharmacodynamic applications. The program allows individual pharmacokinetic parameter estimation using weighted least squares, maximum likelihood, generalized least squares, maximum a posterior Bayesian estimation, and includes capabilities for single and multi-subject simulations. It also performs parametric population PK/PD modeling. ADAPT II is distributed by the Biomedical Simulations Resource

(BMSR) in the Department of Biomedical Engineering at the University of Southern California at no charge, under the terms of a release agreement. S-ADAPT is a version of ADAPT II that contains an augmented interface as well as additional simulation and optimization abilities.

Web site: http://bmsr.usc.edu/Software/ADAPT/SADAPTsoftware.html
Platform: Windows, and requires Intel Visual Fortran 9.1-11.1 or Compaq 6.6

27.2.3 BOOMER AND MULTIFORTE

Boomer and MultiForte are general purpose modeling and simulation programs. They allow the estimation of parameter values by nonlinear weighted least squares regression and the simulation of complex systems of differential equations. Parameter estimation can be performed by normal or Bayesian methods. Five techniques for approaching the minimum sums of weighted residuals (WSS) are included. These are the Gauss-Newton, Damped Gauss-Newton, Marquardt, Simplex, and the grid search methods. A comprehensive list of weighting schemes is also included. The model to be analyzed can be entered as a system of integrated equations or as a system of differential equations. Simulations with random error in parameters or data are also possible. A batch run can be repeated many times to assist in Monte Carlo type studies.

Web site: http://boomer.org/
Platform: Windows and Mac

27.2.4 CALCUSYN

CalcuSyn V 2.0 is the definitive analyzer of combined drug effects able to automatically quantify phenomena such as synergism and inhibition. Mixed drug treatment is becoming common in the treatment of cancer, AIDS, etc., and CalcuSyn is the widely used software for establishing efficacy in this field. It performs multiple drug dose-effect calculations using the median effect methods.

Web site: www.biosoft.com
Platform: Windows and Online

27.2.5 CYBER PATIENT

Cyber Patient is a multimedia pharmacokinetic simulation program that can be used for the development and presentation of problem-solving case studies. This simulation program is appropriate for use in pharmacy or medical schools to assist the instructor in the development of pharmacokinetic drug models. The Cyber Patient simulation is based on a numerical method for one- and two-compartment oral and IV models. In addition to the simulation of pharmacokinetics, Cyber Patient contains help system that is a "hypertext" introduction to basic pharmacokinetics.

Website: www.labsoft.com
Platform: Windows

27.2.6   DATAKINETICS

Datakinetics allows the user to quickly analyze and select the appropriate dosing regimen for a number of drugs including aminoglycosides, digoxin, phenytoin, theophylline, and vancomycin based on the patient's characteristics and drug concentrations. This program is designed to be used by healthcare professionals who have knowledge of pharmacokinetic dosing and desire a tool for optimizing dosage regimens.

Web site: www.datakin.com
Platform: Windows, Palm OS and Pocket PC

27.2.7   e-PHARMACOKINETICS

This is a teaching and simulation program that consists of three parts: the basic pharmacokinetic concepts, the pharmacokinetic simulations, and the PK/PD simulations. The basic pharmacokinetic concepts section is a self-instructional, computer-based, interactive pharmacokinetic tutorial consisting of 22 different modules that deal with the basic pharmacokinetic concepts. The pharmacokinetic simulations section of the program allows the user to simulate the plasma concentration–time profiles for 37 different pharmacokinetic models on the linear and semilog scales, while the PK/PD simulations section of the program allows the user to simulate the plasma concentration–time profiles and the drug effect-time profile for 20 different PK/PD models. The companion CD of the current volume includes all the three parts.

Web site: www.e-pharmacokinetics.com
Platform: Windows and Online

27.2.8   GASTROPLUS

GastroPlus is an advanced software program that simulates the absorption, pharmacokinetics, and pharmacodynamics for drugs in human and preclinical species. The underlying model is the Advanced Compartmental Absorption and Transit (ACAT) model. Simulations Plus, the developer of GastroPlus, has evolved the ACAT model to a high state of refinement, providing accurate, flexible, and powerful simulation program. Its smoothly integrated platform combines a user-friendly interface with sophisticated science to help the user in making better project decisions. It includes modules for additional functions such as the module for predicting drug–drug interaction, modules for predicting drug absorption after ocular or pulmonary administration, and modules for whole-body physiological models for human (fasted and fed), beagle dog (fasted and fed), rat (fasted and fed), mouse (fasted and fed), and monkey.

Simulations Plus also has additional related software such as Dose Disintegration and Dissolution Plus (DDDPlus), which simulates the in vitro dissolution of active pharmaceutical ingredients and formulation excipients under various experimental conditions. Also, ADME Predictor is a program that uses the chemical structure of a compound to predict over 120 properties including pKa(s), logP/logD, solubilities, permeabilities, toxicities, metabolic rates for CYP hydroxylation, CYP inhibitor classification, UGT metabolism classification, and likely sites of metabolic attack for

CYP oxidation. Besides, MedChem Designer is a new tool that combines innovative molecule drawing features with a few fast and accurate ADMET property predictions from the ADME Predictor.

Web site: http://www.simulations-plus.com/
Platform: Windows

27.2.9 KINETICA

Kinetica provides standardized PK/PD analysis for drug development. It facilitates data analysis and reporting in a structural, yet flexible and easy-to-automate, environment. The program includes 60 different validated templates, including noncompartmental, pharmacokinetic, pharmacodynamic, and PK/PD fitting for standard compartmental and population analyses, absorption, convolution, deconvolution, renal, protein binding, enzyme kinetics, transdermal, in vivo and in vitro correlation, and in vitro dissolution. It also includes a subset of Microsoft Visual Basic Applications to build custom workflow, analysis settings, data import, data handling and reporting.

Web site: http://www.thermoscientific.com
Platform: Windows

27.2.10 MODERN BIOPHARMACEUTICS

Modern Biopharmaceutics is a computer-based training software that provides a complete information base for both university biopharmaceutics courses and continuing-education minicourses for active professionals. The program teaches both basic principles and important applications. It includes information for predicting fraction absorbed, absorption analysis using the Wagner–Nelson method, dissolution models and data fitting, pharmacokinetic simulation models, section on biopharmaceutics classification system and absorption prediction, and section on basic pharmaceutics concepts. Video presentations of the key concepts in dissolution and absorption are included in modern biopharmaceutics. This educational program is available in English and Spanish.

Web site: www.tsrlinc.com
Platform: Windows and Mac

27.2.11 MONOLIX

MONOLIX 3.2 is free software dedicated to the analysis of nonlinear mixed effects models. The objectives of using this software include parameter estimation by computing the maximum likelihood estimator of the parameters, without any approximation of the model and calculating standard errors for the maximum likelihood estimator. The software can also be used for model selection by comparing several models using some information criteria (AIC, BIC), testing hypotheses using the Likelihood Ratio Test, and testing parameters using the Wald Test. The software also provides goodness of fit plots and data simulation.

Web site: www.monolix.org
Platform: Windows

27.2.12 MwPharm

MwPharm 4.0 is a clinical pharmacokinetic program used primarily to calculate the proper dosing regimen for patients from population pharmacokinetic parameters and individual patient parameters. The dosage regimen is determined by modeling of plasma drug concentration versus time based on pharmacokinetic parameters from an extensive drug database and individual patient physiological parameters. The program can simulate and optimize the parameter values by curve fitting to the measured data, which enables to refine the dosage regimen. The program includes a database of drugs (over 180) together with their kinetic parameters. Data for existing drugs can be modified and new drugs can be added to the database.

Web site: http://www.mediware.cz/aktuality.php?lang=eng
Platform: Windows

27.2.13 NCOMP

NCOMP performs noncompartmental analysis of pharmacokinetic data obtained from IV bolus, continuous infusion, and oral modes of administration. Integration of AUC and AUMC is done by either Lagrange polynomials or the hybrid method of Purves, which uses parabola-through-the-origin and log trapezoidal algorithms. Written for Microsoft Windows, NCOMP is designed to be used in conjunction with a spreadsheet program for graphical display and handling of data. NCOMP interactively aids the user in determining how best to extrapolate the areas to time infinity and in estimating the time zero concentration for IV bolus data.

Contact: astatine@freeshell.org
Platform: Windows

27.2.14 NLMEM Macro

NLMEM is a SAS macro implementing nonlinear mixed effects models, including models expressed in terms of an ordinary differential equation. In particular, it allows analyzing data from population PK/PD studies.

Contact: Andrzej Galecki <agalecki@umich.edu>
Platform: Windows and Mac

27.2.15 NONMEM

NONMEM is a population PK/PD analysis that was developed originally in the 1970s by Stuart Beal and Lewis Sheiner of the University of California San Francisco. It is a nonlinear mixed effects modeling tool used in population PK/PD analysis. The current versions of NONMEM allow PK/PD modelers to use the software with a user-friendly interface. It also provides a comprehensive tool kit in an easier-to-use package to facilitate population-based data analyses and improves the rate of success of analyzing complex PK/PD models. NONMEM 7 is programmed in Fortran 90/95 code and can be used with Windows, Linux, or Solaris operating systems incorporating a Fortran 90/95-compliant compiler

Web site: http://www.iconplc.com/
Platform: Windows, Linux, or Solaris operating system

27.2.16   PCCAL

Three pharmacokinetic-related educational packages were developed by the Pharmacy Consortium for Computer Aided Learning (PCCAL), which is based in the School of Pharmacy and Pharmacology at the University of Bath, England, and are available from CoAcs. The Biopharmaceutics package is designed to introduce the student to biopharmaceutics, then continues by looking at the application of biopharmaceutics to oral drug delivery and regulatory standards for oral drug delivery. The Pharmacokinetic Simulations package is designed to teach the basic principles of pharmacokinetics through computer simulations. The easy-to-use simulations cover IV and oral drug administration, IV infusions, single and multiple drug administration, linear and nonlinear drug elimination, and one- and two-compartment pharmacokinetic models. The Introductory Pharmacokinetics Workshop package provides an introduction to methods and principles involved in the calculation of pharmacokinetic parameters such as clearance, half-life, elimination rate constant, volume of distribution, absorption rate constant, and area under the curve.

Web site: http://www.coacs.com
Platform: Windows and Online

27.2.17   PDx-Pop

PDx-Pop provides an easy to use graphical user interface to expedite the iterative process of population pharmacokinetic modeling and analysis. Working in concert with NONMEM, for population pharmacokinetic and PK/PD modeling, MS Excel and R or S-PLUS Analytic Software, PDx-Pop delivers optimal flexibility, increased efficiency, and added functionality.

Web site: http://www.iconplc.com/
Platform: Windows, Linux and Mac OS X

27.2.18   PK Solutions

PK Solutions is an automated Excel-based program for both research and education. The program performs single- and multiple-dose pharmacokinetic data analysis of concentration–time data from biological samples following IV or extravascular routes of administration. It provides tables of the published pharmacokinetic parameters for 75 of the most widely used drugs. PK Solutions calculates results using noncompartmental (area) and compartmental (exponential disposition terms) methods without presuming any specific compartmental model. Multiple dose and steady state parameters are automatically projected from single dose results.

Web site: http://www.SummitPK.com
Platform: Windows and Mac

27.2.19   PK-SIM

PK-Sim is a unique software tool for summary and evaluation of preclinical and clinical experimental results on absorption, distribution, metabolism, and excretion by means of whole-body PBPK modeling and simulation. It allows for straightforward construction of highly specific PBPK models by incorporation of in vitro and in vivo experimental data. The resulting pharmacokinetic model allows to extrapolate to various scenarios to support the preparation of study design of succeeding preclinical and clinical experiments. The programs come with several modules that can be used depending on the nature of the data analysis such as the species, absorption, distribution, metabolism, excretion, PK/PD, population pharmacokinetics, and clearance scaling modules.

Web site: http://pksim.com/
Platform: Windows

27.2.20   PKSOLVER

PKSolver 2.0 is a menu-driven add-on program for Microsoft Excel written in Visual Basic for Applications, for solving basic problems in pharmacokinetic and pharmacodynamic data analysis. It provides a range of modules including noncompartmental analysis, compartmental analysis, and pharmacodynamic modeling. Two special built-in modules, multiple absorption sites, and enterohepatic circulation are included for fitting the double-peak concentration–time profile based on the classical one-compartment model. In addition, twenty frequently used pharmacokinetic functions were encoded as a macro and can be directly accessed in an Excel spreadsheet. It is a fast and easy-to-use tool with a user-friendly interface.

Web site: http://dx.doi.org/10.1016/j.cmpb.2010.01.007
Platform: Windows

27.2.21   RxKINETICS

RxKinetics is the vendor for three different pharmacokinetic programs. APK that provides pharmacokinetic dosing calculation of the most commonly used drugs that follow the one-compartment model. It involves a simplified serum level entry and fast patient and drug model data access. APK allows users to design dosage regimens for patients from infants to geriatrics. Antibiotic Kinetics is similar to APK but oriented toward antibiotics. Kinetics for Windows is designed for the practicing pharmacist. This program provides the pharmacists with an easy to use pharmacokinetic dosing tool for adult patients.

Web site: http://www.rxkinetics.com/index.php
Platform: Windows, PalmOS, Windows Mobile

27.2.22   SCIENTIST FOR WINDOWS

Scientist for Windows 3.0 is a general mathematical modeling and data analysis application specifically designed to fit model equations to experimental data. It can fit almost any mathematical model from the simplest linear functions to complex systems of differential equations, nonlinear algebraic equations or models expressed as Laplace transforms. Scientist for Windows has libraries of mathematical models for chemical kinetics, diffusion and pharmacokinetics. PKAnalyst for Windows is another program designed to simulate and perform parameter estimation for pharmacokinetic models. With over two dozen built-in models, it can calculate micro rate constants for compartmental models, analyze saturable kinetics, handle bolus and zero/first-order input for finite and infinite time periods, and produce concentration-effect Sigmoid-E_{max} diagrams.

Web site: www.micromath.com
Platform: Windows and Online

27.2.23 SIMCYP

The Simcyp population-based simulator streamlines drug development through the modeling and simulation of pharmacokinetics and pharmacodynamics in virtual populations. The Simulator is used for the prediction of drug–drug interactions and pharmacokinetic outcomes in clinical populations. It contains numerous databases containing human physiological, genetic, and epidemiological information. By integrating this information with the in vitro or clinical data, the Simulator allows the prediction of the drug PK/PD behavior in "real-world" populations and provides information for key management decisions relating to clinical trial design, clinical trial avoidance, and drug–drug interaction information, which is important in the drug development process.

Web site: www.simcyp.com
Platform: Windows and Mac

27.2.24 STELLA

STELLA is a simulation program with an icon-based graphical interface for model building. It offers a practical way to dynamically simulate, visualize, and communicate how complex systems and ideas really work. STELLA models provide endless opportunities to explore different situations by asking "what if," and watching what happens. Many educators and researchers are using STELLA to study everything from economics to physics, literature to calculus, chemistry, and of course can be used in pharmacokinetic simulations. Pharmacokinetic simulations can run over a certain time and summary of the simulation results can be tabulated and graphed.

Web site: www.iseesystems.com
Platform: Windows and Mac

27.2.25 T.D.M.S.2000

T.D.M.S.2000 is a clinical pharmacokinetic program that estimates individual patient's population pharmacokinetic parameters and refines them when serum drug concentrations become available. Both Bayesian and least-squares curve fitting can be used to fit serum concentrations. Population estimates are based on height, weight, serum creatinine, drug interactions, and disease states that affect pharmacokinetics.

Population estimates are available for vancomycin (two compartment), phenytoin (Michaelis-Menten), plus aminoglycosides and several other one-compartment drugs. A one-compartment general model is available for use with user-supplied parameters. A database for storage of previous patient data and a report function for generating printed reports suitable for medical records are included.

Web site: http://tdms2000.com/
Platform: Windows

27.2.26 TRIAL SIMULATOR

The Pharsight Trial Simulator is a powerful and easy-to-use simulation program for defining and testing interactive drug models, exploring and communicating study design attributes, and performing statistical and sensitivity analysis through graphical and statistical summaries. The Trial Simulator models encapsulate existing scientific knowledge, to help the entire clinical development team communicate and test ideas, and plan relevant, effective trials for every phase of clinical testing. Pharsight Trial Simulator can anticipate risks and preview the range of expected results before performing the costly trials and exposing human subjects to experimental therapies.

Web site: http://www.pharsight.com/main.php
Platform: Windows

27.2.27 USC PACK PHARMACOKINETIC PROGRAMS

1. *Program for population pharmacokinetic modeling*: This program uses the nonparametric EM (NPEM) algorithm to compute the location and probability mass of the overall joint probability density function (PDF) and can run on PCs. It is suitable for researchers and community hospitals to make population models for patients under their care and to couple this with the USC*PACK PC clinical software for Bayesian individualization of drug dosage regimens.
2. *The USC*PACK clinical programs*: This program and the new MM-USC*PACK programs for maximally precise multiple model (MM), are used to design of dosage regimens. There are population models available for clinical use to guide and adjust therapy with gentamicin, tobramycin, netilmicin, and amikacin. There are also models for digoxin, digoxin with quinidine, quinidine, and digitoxin. The software permits development of dosage regimens to achieve target goals in the peripheral compartment as well as to achieve target serum concentration goals.
3. *Programs for infectious diseases*: The USC*PACK clinical EFFECTS program takes literature data of the growth of organisms and their kill by various drugs, puts it together with data of a particular patient's MIC, and computes the time course of bacterial growth and kill in the central compartment, and the peripheral compartment. These analyses are an important adjunct to planning drug dosage regimens to ensure an adequate margin of safety.

4. *Programs for cardiology*: The USC*PACK clinical digoxin program computes dosage regimens of digoxin, digitoxin, and lidocaine to achieve specifically chosen therapeutic goals. These may be stated as desired trough serum concentrations or better yet as desired peak concentrations in the peripheral compartment.

Web site: http://www.lapk.org/software.php
Platform: Windows

27.2.28 WINNONLIN

WinNonlin is a pharmacokinetic, pharmacodynamic, and noncompartmental data analysis program. In addition to its extensive library of built-in pharmacokinetic, pharmacodynamic, and PK/PD models, WinNonlin supports custom, user-defined models to address any kind of data. WinNonlin provides a complete solution with data management, statistical, modeling, and visualization tools. It has worksheet interface that facilitates data handling and transformations. Its descriptive statistics and linear mixed effects modeling engines provide flexible pre- and post-modeling analyses. It also includes bioequivalence wizard that supports U.S. Food and Drug Administration standards for average, individual and population bioequivalence assessment. Additional tools enable exploration of your drug's properties through nonparametric superposition, semicompartmental modeling, deconvolution, and nonparametric analysis of crossover studies. The IVIVC Toolkit for WinNonlin expands the capabilities of WinNonlin, enabling the use of WinNonlin for in vivo in vitro correlations (IVIVC). This Toolkit brings enhanced deconvolution methods, numerical convolution, new plotting capability, and the "IVIVC Wizard" to pharmacokineticists and formulators. This allows the use of WinNonlin to speed formulation development and improve chances of success in bioequivalence studies.

Web site: http://www.pharsight.com/main.php
Platform: Windows

27.2.29 WINNONMIX

The Pharsight WinNonMix is designed to meet the need for population PK/PD analysis, particularly important in later phases of clinical trials. It is a program for nonlinear mixed-effects modeling, to estimate the parameters in nonlinear PK/PD models, to approximate the distribution of those parameters in a population, and estimate fixed and random effects in the model from the observed data. WinNonMix provides these features in an interactive and easy-to-use Windows application, with a user interface similar to that of WinNonlin to select PK/PD models from a predefined library or create user-defined compiled models. The library of predefined models includes numerous pharmacokinetic, pharmacodynamic, and PK/PD models. WinNonMix can estimate population parameter means as well as the between-individual variability in those parameters.

Web site: http://www.pharsight.com/main.php
Platform: Windows

28 The Companion CD

OBJECTIVES

After going through the CD contents you should be able to

- Define the different pharmacokinetic parameters
- Identify the pharmacokinetic parameters that affect the plasma drug concentration–time profile after different routes of administration
- Describe the interplay of different pharmacokinetic parameters
- Analyze the effect of changing the pharmacokinetic parameters on the plasma drug concentration–time profile after single and multiple drug administration by different routes
- Design and recommend the dosing regimens required to achieve specific plasma drug concentration–time profiles
- Evaluate the appropriateness of certain dosing regimens for patients
- Describe the different pharmacokinetic–pharmacodynamic models that relate the drug concentration–time profile to the drug effect-time profile for directly and indirectly acting drugs
- Predict and explain the effect of changing the pharmacokinetic or pharmacodynamic parameters on the drug concentration-effect relationship for drugs administered by different routes

28.1 INTRODUCTION

The pharmacokinetic teaching and simulation program included in the companion CD consists of a collection of modules developed with the objective of utilization of computer capabilities to illustrate the different pharmacokinetic concepts. The pharmacokinetic concepts are ideal for computer-based presentations and simulations because the drug concentration–time profile in the body can be described by mathematical expressions that include the drug pharmacokinetic parameters that control the rate of drug absorption, distribution, and elimination. This makes graphical presentations very useful in visualizing the effect of each pharmacokinetic parameter on the drug concentration–time profile and the overall drug disposition. The pharmacokinetic program is interactive and relies mainly on graphical presentations and simulations to illustrate the pharmacokinetic concepts.

28.2 PHARMACOKINETIC PROGRAM

The pharmacokinetic program included in the CD is developed as a stand-alone Windows® application of the commercially available Authorware® software (Adobe Inc.). This Windows application can also run on the Mac computers with the aid of conversion software such as crossover. The program starts once the CD is inserted in the computer drive; the user can then navigate through the different program components. It consists of three main parts: the basic pharmacokinetic concepts, the pharmacokinetic simulations, and the pharmacokinetic–pharmacodynamic simulations.

28.2.1 BASIC PHARMACOKINETIC CONCEPTS

This is a self-instructional, computer-based, interactive pharmacokinetic tutorial. The tutorial consists of 22 different modules that deal with most of the basic pharmacokinetic concepts covered in this book. The topics covered in this basic pharmacokinetic section of the program are listed in Table 28.1. Each module consists of three parts: the concept presentation, the simulation exercise, and the self-assessment questions.

TABLE 28.1
Topics Covered in the Basic Pharmacokinetic Concepts Part of the Companion CD

Introduction to Pharmacokinetics

IV administration
    Elimination rate constant
    Volume of distribution
    Half-life
    Total body clearance
    Area under the curve
    IV drug administration
Oral administration
    Bioavailability and bioequivalence
    Absorption rate constant
    Oral drug administration
Steady-state concept
    Constant rate IV infusion
    Multiple drug administration
Drug elimination
    Renal excretion of drugs
    Metabolite kinetics (I)
    Metabolite kinetics (II)
Drug elimination during disease state
Multiple compartment pharmacokinetics
    Two-compartment pharmacokinetic model (I)
    Two-compartment pharmacokinetic model (II)
Nonlinear pharmacokinetics
Intermittent IV infusions
Physiological approach to the clearance concept
Kinetics of the pharmacological effects
Therapeutic drug monitoring

The concept presentation part includes an introduction to the pharmacokinetic concept. This part relies mainly on graphs and simulations with a small amount of text to illustrate the concept. The simulation exercise allows changing the values of one or more of the pharmacokinetic parameters and then simulates the plasma concentration–time profile. These simulations can help the users visualize how the change in each pharmacokinetic parameter affects the overall drug disposition in the body. The self-assessment questions consist of a set of multiple-choice questions related to the presented concept. Immediate feedback is given to the user after answering each question and the general performance is evaluated at the end of the question set. The educational value of these tutorials has been formally assessed and showed great benefits to the users [1,2]. The portfolio describing these modules was selected as one of the winning portfolios in the American Association of Colleges of Pharmacy (AACP) Council of Faculty Innovation in Teaching Competition.

28.2.2 PHARMACOKINETIC SIMULATIONS

This part of the program allows the user to simulate the plasma concentration–time profiles for 37 different pharmacokinetic models on the linear and semilog scales. The simulations allow the user to change the value of one or more of the drug pharmacokinetic parameters and then simulate the plasma drug concentration–time profile. These simulations cover

- Drug administration by IV bolus, oral, constant rate IV infusion, and intermittent IV infusion
- Single and multiple drug administration
- One- and two-compartment pharmacokinetic models
- Linear and nonlinear drug elimination

28.2.3 PHARMACOKINETIC/PHARMACODYNAMIC SIMULATIONS

This part of the program allows the user to simulate the plasma concentration–time profiles and the drug effect-time profile for 20 different pharmacokinetic/pharmacodynamic models after single and multiple drug administration. These simulations allow the user to change the value of one or more of the drug pharmacokinetic or the pharmacodynamic parameters and then simulate the plasma concentration–time and the drug effect-time profiles. These simulations cover

- The direct link pharmacodynamic models
- The indirect link pharmacodynamic models (effect compartment models)
- The indirect response models

28.3 SUGGESTIONS FOR USING THE COMPANION CD

The companion CD included with this book can be used to reinforce the concepts presented in the textbook. The basic pharmacokinetic concepts are presented in the computer program as interactive graphs and simulations that can clearly illustrate the concepts, while the detailed theoretical background and mathematical derivations for the different pharmacokinetic concepts are covered in the textual materials of the textbook. Hence, the computer-based information complements the printed information to help the reader with better understanding and comprehension of the pharmacokinetic concepts. So users may go through the computer-based presentation of the pharmacokinetic concepts to obtain the general idea of the concepts and then the detailed information can be obtained from the textual materials.

The pharmacokinetic simulation part of the program can be used to visualize how the change in each of the pharmacokinetic parameters affects the drug concentration–time profile after different routes of administration for drugs that follow different models covered in the simulations. The idea is to simulate the drug concentration–time profile using a set of pharmacokinetic parameters. Then, the value of one of the pharmacokinetic parameters is changed while keeping the values of all the other pharmacokinetic parameters unchanged. The user should try to predict the change in the drug concentration–time profile due to the change in the pharmacokinetic parameter value, and then run the simulation to evaluate the agreement between the predictions and the simulated drug concentration–time profile. The same principle can be applied for the pharmacokinetic–pharmacodynamic simulations, which allows examining the change in any one of the pharmacokinetic or pharmacodynamic parameters on the drug concentration–time and the drug effect-time profiles.

REFERENCES

1. Hedaya MA (1998) Development and evaluation of an interactive internet-based pharmacokinetic teaching module. *Am J Pharm Ed* 62:12–16.
2. Hedaya MA and Collins P (1999) Pharmacokinetic teaching utilizing the world wide web: A flashlight™ assessment. *Am J Pharm Ed* 63:415–421.

Solutions for the Practice Problems

Chapter 2

2.1 a. $7^2 = 49$
    b. $12^2 = 144$
    c. -1
    d. $3 - 1 = 2$
    e. 2
    f. $3 \times 2 = 6$

2.2 a. 100 mg
    b. 60 h

2.3 a. Slope = 3 mg/h, y-intercept = 280 mg/L
    b. Concentration = 280 mg/L − 3 (mg/L h) t

Chapter 3

3.4 a. 30 L
    b. 600 mg IV
    c. 66.6 mg/L

3.5 a. 40 L
    b. 480 mg

Chapter 4

4.1 a. Quinidine
    b. Theophylline

4.2 a. Renal clearance = $Q \times E = 1.5 \times 0.2 = 0.3$ L/min
    b. Hepatic clearance = $1.2 \times 0.3 = 0.36$ L/min
    c. $CL_T = 0.3 + 0.36 = 0.66$ L/min

4.3 The $CL_T = k\,Vd$ = before renal disease = 6.93 L/h and after renal disease = 3.47 L/h. The renal disease decreased the efficiency of the kidney for eliminating the drug. This is reflected in the lower total body clearance and smaller elimination rate constant

Chapter 5

5.1 a. Drug A because the half-life is dose independent
    b. $k = 0.1155$ h^{-1}

    c. Drug A: Increasing the dose increases the initial rate of drug elimination, while the elimination rate constant and half-life remain constant (dose independent)

        Drug B: Increasing the dose does not affect the elimination rate and the elimination rate constant, while the half-life increases

5.2 a. A plot of the amount versus time is a straight line on the Cartesian scale, so the elimination follows zero-order kinetics

    b. The elimination rate constant = 11 mg/h

    c. The half-life immediately after drug administration = 18.2 h

    d. If the dose is 600 mg, the elimination rate constant will be 11 mg/h

    e. The amount of drug remaining 20 h after administration of 400 mg = 180 mg

    f. No drug will be remaining 40 h after administration of 400 mg

5.3 a. A plot of the amount versus time is a straight line on the semilog scale, so the elimination follows first-order kinetics

    b. The elimination rate constant, $k = 0.4617 \, h^{-1}$

    c. The dose is equal to the y-intercept = 500 mg

    d. The equation: $A = 500 \, mg \, e^{-0.4617t}$

    e. The amount of the drug after 10 h = 4.94 mg

    f. Half-life = 1.5 h

5.4 a. Half-life = 3 h, $k = 0.231 \, h^{-1}$, Vd = 30 L, and $CL_T = 6.93 \, L/h$

    b. AUC = 144.1 mg h/L

    c. If the dose is only 500 mg, Cp_0 will be 16.65 mg/L, and the AUC will be 72.05 mg h/L. Half-life, k, Vd, and CL_T will not change

    d. Dose = 1500 mg

5.5 a. Half-life = 0.9 h, $k = 0.77 \, h^{-1}$, Vd = 50 L, $CL_T = 38.5 \, L/h$, AUC = 5.195 mg h/L

    b. The concentration will be 0.5 mg/L after 2.7 h

    c. If the dose is only 400 mg, Cp_0 will be 8 mg/L, and the AUC will be 10.39 mg h/L. Half-life, k, Vd, and CL_T will not change

    d. The plasma concentration after 10 h = 0.0018 mg/L

5.6 Calculate the plasma concentrations at different time points by substituting different values for time in the equation. Then plot the concentrations on semilog graph paper

5.7 a. Half-life = 3 h, $k = 0.2303 \, h^{-1}$, Vd = 400 L, $CL_T = 92.12 \, L/h$, AUC = 4.342 mg h/L

    b. The slope will be the same and the y-intercept will be 2.5 mg/L

    c. The concentration will be 0.25 mg/L after 6 h

    d. Dose = 1600 mg

5.8 a. Half-life = 5 h, $k = 0.1382 \, h^{-1}$, Vd = 0.5 L/kg, $CL_T = 0.0691 \, L/h$, AUC = 72.46 mg h/L

    b. The slope will be the same and the y-intercept will be 40 mg/L

    c. The concentration will be 1 mg/L after 16.69 h

    d. The initial concentration should be 5.238 mg/L, so the dose = 2.62 mg/kg

5.9 a. Ampicillin, largest k

    b. Ampicillin, smallest Vd

    c. Propranolol, highest clearance (k × Vd)

    d. Propranolol, largest Vd

    e. Ampicillin, fastest rate of elimination

5.10 a. Before renal disease: half-life = 2 h, k = $0.3465\,h^{-1}$, Vd = 20 L, CL_T = 6.93 L/h, AUC = 86.6 mg h/L

         After renal disease: half-life = 4 h, k = $0.1733\,h^{-1}$, Vd = 20 L, CL_T = 3.47 L/h, AUC = 173 mg h/L

    b. The renal disease decreased the efficiency of the kidney for eliminating the drug. This is reflected in the lower total body clearance, smaller elimination rate constant, and longer half-life

5.11 a. Half-life = 7 h, k = $0.099\,h^{-1}$, Vd = 40 L, CL_T = 3.96 L/h, AUC = 202 mg h/L

    b. The plasma concentration after 14 h = 5 mg/L

    c. The slope should be the same −0.043

    d. The initial plasma concentration = 10 mg/L

5.12 a. Half-life = 3 h

    b. The MEC is dose independent = 2 mg/L

    c. Duration = 9 h

    d. Dose = 60 mg

    e. The concentration will always be lower than the MEC, so no effect is observed

Chapter 9

9.1 a. k = $0.13\,h^{-1}$ Half-life = 5.33 h

    b. t_{max} = 6 h

    c. C_{max} = 2.7 mg/L

9.2 a. t_{max}: Drug A = 2.0 h   Drug B = 2.0 h

    b. C_{max}: Drug A = 33.44 mg/L   Drug B = 16.72 mg/L

9.3 a. t_{max} = 2.746 h

    b. C_{max} = 50.66 mg/L

    c. t_{max} will be the same, C_{max} = 10.1 mg/L

9.4 a. Cp after 6 h = 10 mg/L

    b. Half-life = 6 h

    c. k_a = $0.624\,h^{-1}$

    d. Vd = 29.2 L

    e. t_{max} = 3.32 h

    f. C_{max} = 11.69 mg/L

    g. Slope = $-0.05\,h^{-1}$

9.5 a. Half-life = 4.5 h

    b. Vd = 59.6 L

    c. CL_T = 9.18 L/h

    d. t_{max} = 2.28 h C_{max} = 5.9 mg/L

    e. AUC = 54.5 mg h/L

9.6 a. k_a = $0.693\,h^{-1}$

    b. Equation: Cp = 154 ng/mL $(e^{-0.332t} - e^{-0.693t})$

    c. t_{max} = 2.04 h C_{max} = 40.7 ng/mL

9.7 a. A plot of the fraction remaining to be absorbed versus time is linear on semilog graph paper indicating first-order absorption

   b. $k_a = 0.354\,h^{-1}$

9.8 a. $k_a = 1.0\,h^{-1}$

   b. Half-life $= 3\,h$ $Vd = 50\,L$

Chapter 10

10.1 $F = 0.638$

10.2 a. $F_{capsule} = 0.4$

   b. $F_{IM} = 0.9$

   c. $F_{suspension}/F_{capsule} = 1.25$

   d. IV > IM > suspension > capsule

10.3 a. Formulation A, because it has shorter t_{max}

   b. $F_A/F_B = 0.75$ This means that the absolute bioavailability of formulation A is only 75% of the absolute bioavailability of formulation B

10.4 a. Half-life $= 2.31\,h$ $Vd = 20\,L$

   b. The syrup has the fastest absorption rate

   c. Absolute bioavailability: syrup $= 0.742$ capsules $= 0.558$ tablets $= 0.466$

   d. $F_{capsule}/F_{syrup} = 0.75$

   e. $F_{tablet}/F_{capsule} = 0.835$

10.5 a. Half-life $= 4\,h$

   b. AUC $= 64.6\,mg\,h/L$

   c. $F_{tablet} = 0.54$

   d. $CL_T = 4.17\,L/h$ $Vd = 24\,L$

10.6 a. Half-life $= 9\,h$ $Vd = 20\,L$

   b. Bioavailability $= 0.36$

10.7 a. Bioavailability $= 0.809$

   b. AUC $= 43.3\,mg\,h/L$

Chapter 12

12.1 Loading dose $= 450\,mg$ Infusion rate $= 52\,mg/h$

12.2 a. At steady state, rate of elimination = rate of administration $= 70\,mg/h$

   b. $Cp_{ss} = 10.1\,mg/L$

   c. $k = 0.231\,h^{-1}$

   d. Cp_{ss} is not affected by loading dose $= 10.1\,mg/L$

   e. Approximately $15\,h$

   f. $Cp_{ss} = 20.2\,mg/L$

12.3 a. Half-life $= 7\,h$ $Vd = 40.4\,L$

   b. Loading dose $= 485\,mg$ Infusion rate $= 48\,mg/h$

12.4 a. Half-life $= 5\,h$

   b. $Vd = 45.2\,L$

   c. $Cp_{ss} = 16\,mg/L$

   d. $Cp_{ss} = 32\,mg/L$

12.5 a. $Cp_{ss} = 16\,mg/L$

   b. Elimination rate $= 100\,mg/h$

   c. Half-life $= 5\,h$

    d. $Cp_{ss} = 16\,mg/L$
    e. $Cp_{ss} = 32\,mg/L$
12.6 a.   Elimination rate = 60 mg/h
    b.   Half-life = 7 h
    c.   Vd = 30.3 L
    d.   Loading dose = 455 mg   Infusion rate = 45 mg/h
12.7 a.   Elimination rate = 20 mg/h
    b. $Cp_{ss} = 4.95\,mg/L$
    c. $k = 0.1155\,h^{-1}$
    d. $Cp_{ss} = 4.95\,mg/L$
    e.   Approximately 30 h
    f. $Cp_{ss} = 9.9\,mg/L$

Chapter 13

13.1 a. $Cp_{min\ ss} = 18.16\,mg/L$ $Cp_{max\ ss} = 8.16\,mg/L$
    b. $Cp_{average} = 12.8\,mg/L$
    c.   Dose = 400 mg every 8 h
13.2 a.   Half-life = 13.3 h
    b.   Vd = 20 L
    c. $Cp_{average} = 20\,mg/L$
13.3 a. $Cp_{average} = 16.67\,mg/L$
    b. $Cp_{average} = 16.67\,mg/L$
    c.   Dose = 240 mg every 12 h
13.4 a. $Cp_{average} = 9\,mg/L$
    b.   Dose = 444.4 mg
    c.   Dose = 333.3 mg
    d. $Cp_{min\ ss} = 27.8\,mg/L$ $Cp_{max\ ss} = 13.9\,mg/L$
13.5 a. $Cp_{average} = 20\,mg/L$
    b. $Cp_{average} = 40\,mg/L$
    c. $CL_T = 2.5\,L/h$
    d.   Dose = 750 mg every 8 h
    e. $Cp_{average} = 25\,mg/L$
13.6 a. $Cp_{min\ ss} = 16.58\,mg/L$ $Cp_{max\ ss} = 6.58\,mg/L$
    b. $Cp_{average} = 10.8\,mg/L$
    c. $Cp_{min\ ss} = 33.16\,mg/L$ $Cp_{max\ ss} = 13.16\,mg/L$
13.7 a.   Half-life = 6 h
    b.   Vd = 15 L
    c. $Cp_{average} = 21.6\,mg/L$
    d.   Approximately 30 h
    e.   At steady state rate of elimination = rate of administration = 450 mg
13.8 a.   Half-life = 9.43 h   Vd = 40 L
    b.   Dose = 1268 mg
13.9 a.   Loading dose = 600 mg
    b.   Dosing interval = $11.5\,h \cong 12\,h$
    c.   Dose = $308\,mg \cong 300\,mg$

      d. $Cp_{average} = 13.9\,mg/L$
      e. Dosing regimen = 400 mg every 12 h
13.10 a. Dosing interval = 11.5 h $\cong$ 12 h
      b. Dose = 613.4 mg $\cong$ 600 mg
      c. $Cp_{average} = 14.3\,mg/L$

Chapter 14

14.1   a. Amount = 720 mg
      b. Renal excretion rate = 30 mg/h = 0.5 mg/min
      c. CrCL = 50 mL/min
      d. CL_R = CrCL = 50 mL/min
14.2   a. Renal excretion rate = 140.7 μg/h
      b. Renal excretion rate = 25 μg/h
      c. CL_R = 50 mL/h
      d. Slope = $-k/2.303 = 0.3\,h^{-1}$
14.3   a. Bioavailability = 0.875
14.4   a. Half-life = 1.61 days
      b. CL_R = 140 L/day CL_T = 215 L/day
      c. Fraction = 0.65
      d. Amount = 1.165 mg
      e. $k_m = 0.15\,day^{-1}$
14.5   a. Half-life = 3 h
      b. CL_R = 7 L/h
      c. Fraction = 0.6
      d. $k_m = 0.091\,h^{-1}$

Chapter 15

15.1   a. Metabolite I: Formation rate limited
         Metabolite II and Metabolite III: Elimination rate limited
15.2   a. CL_T = 4.33 L/h   AUC = 23 μmol h/L
      b. CL_R = 0.866 L/h
      c. Fraction = 0.3
      d. CL_T = 3.0 L/h
      e. CL_R = 3.0 L/h
      f. Formation clearance metabolite 1 = 1.3 L/h
         Formation clearance metabolite 2 = 2.165 L/h
      g. AUC of drug = 69 μmol h/L
         AUC of metabolite 1 = 30 μmol h/L
      h. Amount of metabolite 1 = 100 μmol, amount of metabolite 2 = 0 μmol
      i. Ratio = 0.433
      j. No, because we do not have information about the elimination rate constants of the parent drug and the metabolite

15.3 a.   Fraction metabolized = 0.924
$CL_{T(m)} = 10.87 L/h$
$Vd_{(m)} = 35.7 L$
Metabolite formation clearance = 7.65 L/h, formation rate constant = $0.1159 h^{-1}$
   b. $Cp_{ss(m)} = 21 \mu mol/L$
   c.   Ratio = 0.82
15.4 a. $CL_{T(m)} = 8 L/h$ $Vd_{(m)} = 20 L$
   b.   Fraction = 0.546
   c.   Metabolite formation clearance = 2.87 L/h, formation rate constant = $0.109 h^{-1}$
   d.   Amount = 800 mg
   e. $Cp_{ss} = 12.7 mg/L$ $Cp_{ss(m)} = 4.55 mg/L$
15.5 a. $CL_R = 4.16 L/h$
   b. $CL_m = 9.70 L/h$
   c.   Formation clearance = 9.702 L/h
   d. $CL_{T(m)} = 7 L/h$, $CL_{m(m)} = 0 L/h$, and $CL_{R(m)} = 7 L/h$
   e. $k_{(m)} = 0.233 h^{-1}$, $k_{(m)} < k$ (i.e., elimination rate limited)
   f.   AUC = 8.66 μmol h/L $AUC_{(m)} = 12$ μmol h/L
   g.   Ratio = 1.39

Chapter 16
16.1 a. $V_{max} = 590 mg/day$ $K_m = 9.8 mg/L$
   b.   Concentration = 30 mg/L   half-life = 1 day
   c.   Cpss = 10.1 mg/L
   d.   Dose = 396 mg/day
16.2 a. $V_{max} = 630 mg/day$ $K_m = 7.2 mg/L$
   b.   Dose = 425 mg/day
   c.   Half-life = 0.986 day
   d.   Elimination rate when $Cp = K_m$ is equal to $\frac{1}{2}V_{max} = 315 mg/day$
16.3 a. $V_{max} = 640 mg/day$ $K_m = 5.6 mg/L$
   b.   Dose = 466 mg/day
   c.   Half-life = 1.01 day $CL_T = 31.1 L/day$
   d. $Cp_{ss} = 13.3 mg/L$
16.4 a. $V_{max} = 790 mg/day$ $K_m = 5.6 mg/L$
   b.   Enzyme induction will increase V_{max} without affecting K_m
New $V_{max} = 830 mg/day$ $K_m = 5.6 mg/L$
   c.   Dose = 648 mg/day
16.5 a. $V_{max} = 340 mg/day$ $K_m = 8.8 mg/L$
   b. $Cp_{ss} = 17.2 mg/L$
   c.   Half-life = 1.1 day $CL_T = 13.0 L/day$

Chapter 17

17.1 The drug concentration will be different in different tissues depending on the affinity of the drug to each tissue

17.2 During the alpha-phase the decline in drug concentration is due to the distribution and elimination processes, while during the beta-phase the decline in drug concentration is due to the elimination process only

17.3 a. After 0.5 h: $Cp = 10.1$ mg/L
    After 3 h: $Cp = 4.32$ mg/L
    After 12 h: $Cp = 1.60$ mg/L

   b. Cp (mg/L) $= 36e^{-2.8t} + 12e^{-0.11t}$

17.4 a. $t_{1/2\alpha} = 0.0775$ h $t_{1/2\beta} = 3.65$ h
    $V_c = 14.26$ L $AUC = 3.885$ mg h/L
    $CL_T = 19.3$ L/h $k_{10} = 1.353$ h^{-1}
    $k_{21} = 1.255$ h^{-1} $k_{12} = 6.52$ h^{-1}
    $Vd_{ss} = 88.3$ L $Vd_\beta = 101.6$ L

   b. Cp (8 h) $= 0.14$ mg/L   Amount remaining $= 14.2$ mg

17.5 a. $A = 53.0$ mg/L $B = 17$ mg/L
    $\alpha = 1.34$ h^{-1} $\beta = 0.13$ h^{-1}
    $t_{1/2\alpha} = 0.52$ h $t_{1/2\beta} = 5.3$ h
    $V_c = 7.14$ L $AUC = 170.0$ mg h/L
    $CL_T = 2.94$ L/h $k_{10} = 0.412$ h^{-1}
    $k_{21} = 0.423$ h^{-1} $k_{12} = 0.635$ h^{-1}
    $Vd_{ss} = 17.8$ L $Vd_\beta = 22.6$ L

   b. Cp (12 h) $= 3.57$ mg/L

   c. $Cp_0 = 210$ mg/L

   d. A, B, and AUC

   e. $A = 159$ mg/L $B = 51$ mg/L $AUC = 510$ mg h/L

   f. Infusion rate $= 29.4$ mg/h

17.6 a. $A = 1.356$ mg/L $B = 0.431$ mg/L
    $\alpha = 0.124$ min^{-1} $\beta = 0.0072$ min^{-1}
    $t_{1/2\alpha} = 5.59$ min $t_{1/2\beta} = = 96.0$ min
    $V_c = 28.0$ L $AUC = 70.8$ mg min/L
    $CL_T = 0.706$ L/min $k_{10} = 0.0252$ min^{-1}
    $k_{21} = 0.0354$ min^{-1} $k_{12} = 0.0706$ min^{-1}
    $Vd_{ss} = 83.8$ L $Vd_\beta = 98.0$ L

   b. The equation describes the best curve that describes the best profile

   c. Amount $= 7.94$ mg

   d. The concentration when 5 mg is remaining $= 0.051$ mg/L

Chapter 18

18.1 a. Regimen: 75 mg every 8 h administered as IV infusion of 1 h duration

   b. $Cp_{max\ ss} = 6.02$ mg/L $Cp_{min\ ss} = 0.998$ mg/L

18.2 a. Half-life $= 2.22$ h

   b. $Vd = 15$ L

   c. Regimen: 130 mg every 8 h administered as IV infusion of 1 h duration

   d. $Cp_{max\ ss} = 8.1$ mg/L $Cp_{min\ ss} = 0.9$ mg/L

18.3 a. Half-life = 3.0 h

   b. Vd = 15 L

   c. Regimen: 140 mg every 8 h administered as IV infusion of 1 h duration

   d. $Cp_{max\ ss}$ = 9.89 mg/L $Cp_{min\ ss}$ = 1.96 mg/L

18.4 a. CrCL = 26.7 mL/min

   b. 22%

   c. Estimated half-life = 11.36 h

   d. Half-life = 8.5 h   Vd = 14 L

   e. Cp_{max} = 5.15 mg/L

   f. $Cp_{max\ ss}$ = 8.25 mg/L $Cp_{min\ ss}$ = 3.37 mg/L

   g. Concentration increases due to drug accumulation

   h. Regimen: 90 mg every 24 h administered as IV infusion of 1 h duration

18.5 a. Half-life = 3 h   Vd = 5.09 L

   b. Regimen: 90 mg every 12 h administered as IV infusion of 1 h duration

   c. $Cp_{max\ ss}$ = 8.9 mg/L $Cp_{min\ ss}$ = 0.625 mg/L

   d. Approximately the half-life will be 6 h

18.6 a. Estimated half-life = 9.2 h

   b. Four samples should be obtained:
       Before drug administration, then 1, 4, and 10 h after drug administration

   c. Half-life = 9 h   Vd = 8.57 L

   d. Regimen: 65 mg every 24 h administered as IV infusion of 0.5 h duration

   e. $Cp_{max\ ss}$ = 8.67 mg/L $Cp_{min\ ss}$ = 1.48 mg/L

Chapter 20

20.1 a. MRT = 5.97 h

   b. CL_T = 4.14 L/h

   c. Vdss = 24.7 L

20.2 a. F for A = 0.6, B = 0.4, C = 0.7
       The extent of absorption: C > A > B

   b. MRT for IV = 6.5 h, A = 8.5 h, B = 7 h, and C = 9 h
       The rate of absorption: B > A > C

20.3 a. MRT_{IV} = 6.59 h

   b. $MRT_{capsule}$ = 9.9 h MRT_{tablet} = 9.1 h

   c. $MAT_{capsule}$ = 3.31 h MAT_{tablet} = 2.51 h

   d. CL_T = 7.41 L/h   Vdss = 48.9 L

Chapter 21

21.1 Small variability in the extraction ratio for high extraction ratio drugs results in significance variability in the drug bioavailability

21.2 Enzyme induction significantly affects the hepatic clearance of low extraction ratio drugs and has little effect on the hepatic clearance for high extraction ratio drugs

21.3 a. CL_H = 38.96 mL/min

   b. CL_H = 38.5 mL/min

   c. CL_H = 85.0 mL/min

21.4 a. $CL_H = 1.33 \, L/min$
     b. $CL_H = 0.923 \, L/min$
     c.   Extraction ratio: Before CHF = 0.89   After CHF = 0.92
     d.   Bioavailability: Before CHF = 0.11   After CHF = 0.08

21.5 Note: The arrows represent the significant change in the CL_T, half-life, or bioavailability, while small or minor changes are considered no change
     a.   Effect of enzyme induction

Drug	CL_T	Half-Life	Bioavailability
A	↑	↓	↔
B	↔	↔	↔
C	↔	↔	↓
D	↑	↓	↔
E	↔	↔	↔
F	↑	↓	↔
G	↑	↓	↔
H	↔	↔	↓

     b. Effect of enzyme inhibition

Drug	CL_T	Half-Life	Bioavailability
A	↓	↑	↔
B	↔	↔	↔
C	↔	↔	↑
D	↓	↑	↔
E	↔	↔	↔
F	↓	↑	↔
G	↓	↑	↔
H	↔	↔	↑

     c. Effect of displacement from the plasma protein binding sites

Drug	CL_T	Half-Life	Bioavailability
A	↑	↓	↔
B	↔	↔	↔
C	↔	↔	↔
D	↑	↓	↔
E	↔	↔	↔
F	↔	↔	↔
G	↔	↔	↔
H	↔	↔	↔

d. Effect of the decrease in hepatic blood flow

Drug	CL_T	Half-Life	Bioavailability
A	↔	↔	↔
B	↔	↔	↔
C	↓	↑	↓
D	↔	↔	↔
E	↔	↔	↔
F	↔	↔	↔
G	↔	↔	↔
H	↓	↑	↓

Chapter 24

24.1 a. Half-life 7.9 h   Vd = 24.6 L
   b. Dose = 285 mg every 12 h
   c. Half-life in failure = 16.6 h
   $Cp_{max\ ss} = 23.5\ mg/L$ $Cp_{min\ ss} = 14.2\ mg/L$
   The maximum and the minimum concentration change due to the reduction in dose, but the average concentrations resulting from the full dose and the reduced dose before and after developing the renal failure are similar

24.2 a. Vd = 24 L
   b. $CL_T = 0.91\ L/h$
   c. Dose = 219 mg every 12 h
   d. $Cp_{max\ ss} = 57.0\ mg/L$ $Cp_{min\ ss} = 36.2\ mg/L$

24.3 a. Half-life = 7.5 h   Vd = 11.76 L
   b. $CL_R = 0.65\ L/h$
   c. Half-life in failure = 12.5 h
   d. $Cp_{max\ ss} = 52.8\ mg/L$ $Cp_{min\ ss} = 27.3\ mg/L$

24.4 a. $CL_R = 0.277\ L/h/kg$
   b. Half-life = 5.45
   c. Dose = 1.65 g every day
   d. $Cp_{max\ ss} = 10.0\ mg/L$ $Cp_{min\ ss} = 4.67\ mg/L$

24.5 a. $Cp_{average} = 20.9\ mg/L$
   b. $Cp_{max\ ss} = 33.6\ mg/L$ $Cp_{min\ ss} = 11.89\ mg/L$
   c. The IV dose = 260 mg every 12 h
   d. $Cp_{max\ ss} = 39.4\ mg/L$ $Cp_{min\ ss} = 28.1\ mg/L$

Index

A

AACP, *see* American Association of Colleges of Pharmacy

Abbreviated new drug application (ANDA), 175–177

ABC transporters, *see* ATP binding cassette transporters

Absolute bioavailability, 159

Absorption phase, 129–130

Absorption rate constant (k_a), 127, 145
- clinical importance, 145
- determination, 132
  - residuals, method of, 132–138
  - Wagner–Nelson method, 138–144
- and elimination rate constant (k), 136–138
- extent of drug absorption, 171

ACAT, *see* Advanced Compartmental Absorption and Transit

ACE inhibitors, *see* Angiotensin converting enzyme inhibitors

Acid-labile drugs, 2, 102

acslX program, 518

Active drug ingredient, in vivo BA study for, 163

Acute pharmacodynamic effect, for BE demonstration, 180

ADAPT II program, 518–519

ADME Predictor, 520–521

Advanced Compartmental Absorption and Transit (ACAT), 520

Albumin, 26

Alkaline drugs, 25

Alpha-1-acid glycoprotein, 26

American Association of Colleges of Pharmacy (AACP), 530

Aminoglycoside
- estimation based on patient information
  - half-life, 350–351
  - volume of distribution, 351
- estimation from blood concentrations
  - first dose, 351–353
  - before steady state, 353
  - during steady-state, 353–355
- extended-interval dosing regimen, 349
- pharmacokinetic characteristics, 348
- plasma concentration, guidelines, 348

Aminopyrine, 32

Ampicillin, 164

Analysis of variance (ANOVA), 185–186

Analytical method validation, in BE study, 183
- accuracy, 183–184
- calibration curve, 184
- extraction efficiency/recovery, 184
- precision, 184
- selectivity, 183
- stability, 184–185

ANDA, *see* Abbreviated new drug application

Angiotensin converting enzyme (ACE) inhibitors, 157

Area under drug concentration–time curve (AUC), 65–66, 165–169

ATP binding cassette (ABC) transporters, 155, 512

Atropine, 102

AUC, *see* Area under drug concentration–time curve

Authorware® software, 529

B

BBB, *see* Blood brain barrier

BC, *see* Bioavailability

BCRP, *see* Breast cancer resistance protein

BCS, *see* Biopharmaceutics classification system

BDDCS, *see* Biopharmaceutics drug disposition classification system

BE, *see* Bioequivalence

Beal, Stuart, 522

Best line, graphical determination, 19–20

Beta-blockers, 403

Biliary drug excretion, 234

Bioavailability (BC)
- clinical importance, 164
- extent of drug absorption, 170
- regulatory requirement for, 157–158

Bioequivalence (BE), 175
- approaches, 179
  - acute pharmacodynamic effect, 180
  - clinical studies, 180
  - in vitro dissolution testing, 180
- bioequivalent products, 176
- definition, 152
- determination, 187
  - drug metabolites measurement, 189–190
  - drugs with long half-lives, 188
  - drug urinary excretion data, 188–189
  - enantiomers *vs.* racemates, 192
  - endogenous substances, 191
  - first point C_{max}, 192–193
  - fixed dose combination, 189